DISEASES OF THE KIDNEY AND URINARY TRACT

Dr. Shipra Chandra

ALLIED HEALTH PRESS

Diseases of the Kidney and Urinary Tract

Author: **Dr. Shipra Chandra**

Allied Health Press
4164 Lakeshore Road
Burlington ON L7L 1A4
Canada
www.alliedhealthpress.com
Email: orders@arclereducation.com

ISBN: 978-1-77956-800-7

General Disclaimer:

This book is a summation of information from different sources and encompasses a wide range of medical conditions, the latest therapy methods, principals and techniques that are used in current practice, at the time of publication. This book offers general information with educational purposes, it is not to be applied or relied on for any diagnostic or treatment purposes. Please do not use the data/matter as a substitute for professional diagnosis and treatment. Please consult your healthcare provider or a licensed physician before making any healthcare queries or treatment choices. The medical information and research findings presented in this book are for educational purposes only and should not be used for the treatment of specific individual patients, as individual cases may vary. The author(s), editors(s) and publisher cannot be held accountable and make no guarantees that the information provided in this book will apply to each and individual patient. This book is meant to serve as a basic guideline and other relevant literature sources should be used for more specific information. This text can be a vital resource for students, trainees, and practitioners, covering essential topics. This book encompasses a wide range of medical conditions and the latest therapy options used in current practice. Through the utilization of many different medical studies this book provides the basics of different medical conditions, which can be used as a basic guide from where medical students, trainees and practitioners can extract necessary information. Further, some of the books have graphic images to explain anatomy for medical/educational purposes only. Hence, the book is intended for students or teachers/staff or individuals with a mature outlook looking to learn or enhance their knowledge.

Allied Health Press publishes wide variety of books and eBooks. For more information about Allied Health Press and its products, visit our website at www.alliedhealthpress.com

ABOUT THE AUTHOR

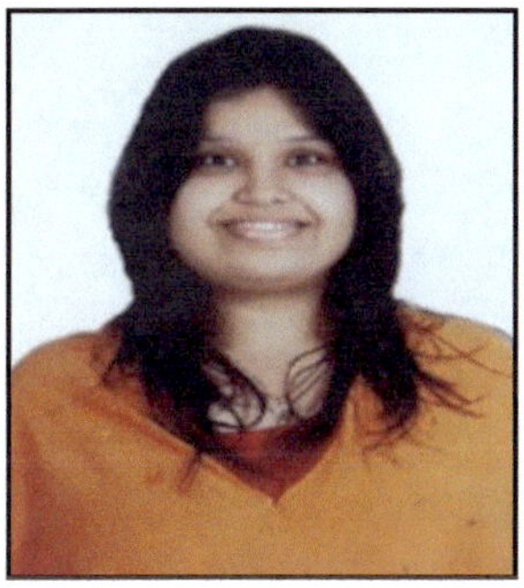

Dr. Shipra Chandra born in Delhi in 1983, completed school from a government school in Delhi in 2001 with First division. Being a science student , took admission in Chemistry Honors at Kirori Mal College, Delhi University. But the wonders of Human Body always fascinated me and I continued preparing for Pre Medical Test (PMT) despite being in a reputed college and course.

By the Grace of God and blessings of my family I secured 5th rank in CPMT 2002 along-with being waitlisted at DPMT and securing rank in AIEEE exam. Joined MBBS on 14/11/2002 at the most prestigious King George Medical College, Lucknow, U.P. Completed MBBS in First division in 2008 and joined AIIMS, New Delhi Department of Emergency Medicine for work experience in 2009 but continued the preparation for Post Graduation Entrance Test and cracked the UP-PGME in 2010 and was allotted MD Physiology from King George Medical University.

After completing the MD in 2013, I again cleared AIIMS, New Delhi entrance test for Senior Residency. Learned a lot during my 3 year tenure from 2013 to 2016 at AIIMS. Following which I joined Fortis Hospital Shalimar Bagh and continued search for a Government Job. Gave the interview at U.P. Public Service Commission in 2017, cracked it and joined as Assistant Professor at Sarojini Naidu Medical College, Agra in 2017. I have 7 research publications , one book chapter and guided 3 MD students during my tenure . Promoted to the post of Associate Professor in 2022 and currently working in the same capacity.

Brief Table of Contents

Detailed Table of Contents

CHAPTER 5

Polycystic Kidney Disease and Congenital Disorders 141

CHAPTER 6

Hypertensive and Diabetic Nephropathy 175

CHAPTER 7

Renal Involvement in Systemic Diseases 211

CHAPTER 8

Acute Kidney Injury (AKI) 249

CHAPTER 9

Chronic Kidney Disease (CKD) 283

CHAPTER 10

Urinary Tract Infections (UTIs) 321

CHAPTER 11

Obstructive Uropathy and Urolithiasis (Kidney Stones) 355

CHAPTER 14

Renal Replacement Therapy (RRT) and Dialysis 463

CHAPTER 15

Kidney Transplantation and Immunosuppressive Therapy 497

Index 533

LIST OF FIGURES

PREFACE

The urinary tract and human kidney perform vital functions essential to homeostasis, fluid and electrolyte balance, endocrine regulation, and waste elimination. Although they are structurally small, these organs support a substantial physiological burden, cooperating with other systems to maintain equilibrium within fluctuating internal conditions. Their role is not limited to filtration only but includes the generation of erythropoietin, control of blood pressure through the renin-angiotensin mechanism, and maintenance of acid-base balance. When those processes are disrupted by illness or injury, their impact is not just on the kidneys but on the whole body—systemic dysfunctions that can quickly escalate if not caught and treated in a timely fashion.

Over the past decades, the clinical burden of renal and urinary tract disease has risen steadily. Increased rates of population aging, hypertension and diabetes prevalence, universal use of nephrotoxic medications, and shifting patterns of infections have all contributed to the increasing frequency of kidney disease. At the same time, better diagnosis and treatment have improved the accuracy with which these disorders are diagnosed and treated. Health workers of all types—general practitioners, nephrologists, urologists, or critical care specialists—must handle a growing volume of knowledge in order to correctly interpret symptoms, select appropriate investigations, and offer personalized treatment plans. Knowledge of normal physiology and the broad range of pathologies affecting the kidney and urinary system is essential for making informed decisions.

Diseases of the Kidney and Urinary Tract is envisioned as a significant clinical reference text that integrates vital concepts in renal anatomy, physiology, diagnostic methodology, and pathological disease. Envisioned to serve both as an academic text and a working reference, the book traces the progression from normal to disease expression, and from diagnosis to therapeutic intervention. It summarizes physiological mechanisms, clinical findings, laboratory correlations, and therapeutic management into a reasonable and user-friendly pattern. The material is not limited to primary renal disease but also addresses renal complications in systemic disorders and has dedicated chapters on modern modalities of treatment, such as dialysis and transplantation. The scheme allows for a gradual progression, enabling readers to establish a solid foundation before tackling more complex or overlapping disease presentations.

Chapter 1 provides the functional and structural profile of the kidneys and urinary tract, including gross and microstructure, blood supply, filtration mechanism, and the nephron's role in maintaining systemic equilibrium. Such fundamental information is essential for appreciating disease processes in relation to disrupting normal function. Chapter 2 addresses the clinical diagnostics—renal function tests, such as serum creatinine, eGFR, urinalysis, imaging modalities, and newer biomarkers used in the detection of early renal impairment.

Chapter 3 covers glomerular diseases, which include glomerulonephritis, detailing immune and non-immune mechanisms, histopathological classification, and therapeutic considerations. Chapter 4 covers the interstitium and the tubules, detailing conditions such as acute and chronic interstitial nephritis and their etiologies, such as infection, drugs, and autoimmune diseases. Chapter 5 covers inherited and congenital disease entities such as autosomal dominant polycystic kidney disease, nephronophthisis, and congenital structural abnormalities.

Chapter 6 describes hypertensive and diabetic nephropathy, the two most common causes of chronic renal failure worldwide. The chapter provides an overview of the pathophysiological impact of these systemic diseases on the kidney and techniques for early intervention. Chapter 7 describes how systemic diseases, such as lupus, amyloidosis, and vasculitides, impact the kidney, typically in an indirect manner, yet with significant clinical implications.

Chapter 8 covers acute kidney injury, with a focus on etiologies of ischemia, toxins, infection, and sepsis. It includes classification schemas like RIFLE and KDIGO, and guides readers through diagnostic work-up and management principles. Chapter 9 covers a comprehensive review of chronic kidney disease, including staging, progression, complications, and care burden. Patient monitoring, meal planning, and disease management slowing are especially highlighted.

Chapter 10 discusses urinary tract infections, ranging from uncomplicated cystitis to complicated pyelonephritis, covering risk factors, microbial pathogens, resistance patterns, and treatment recommendations. Chapter 11 deals with obstructive uropathies and kidney stones, such as mechanical obstruction, its presentation, imaging diagnosis, and interventional techniques.

Chapter 12 presents data on renal and urothelial cancers, including renal cell carcinoma and transitional cell carcinoma. It consolidates diagnostic imaging, histological presentations, staging, and treatment from nephron-sparing surgery to systemic chemotherapy. Chapter 13 covers fluid, electrolyte, and acid-base disorders commonly encountered in kidney conditions such as hyperkalemia, metabolic acidosis, and hyponatremia, with helpful clinical guidelines.

Chapter 14 is devoted to renal replacement treatments, including hemodialysis, peritoneal dialysis, and continuous renal replacement therapy (CRRT). It covers indications, modalities, complications, and patient care considerations. Chapter 15 is kidney transplantation and outlines donor selection, fundamental transplant surgery, immunosuppressive therapy, and post-transplant complications like graft rejection and infection risk.

Medical students will appreciate the book as a well-organized and straightforward summary of renal pathophysiology. Nephrology, internal medicine, and urology residents, as well as fellows, may consult it for clinical decision-making and for exam preparation. Practicing clinicians, nurses, and allied health professionals caring for patients with nephrology conditions will appreciate the step-by-step discussion of diagnosis and treatment. It is also of use to scientists and educators in its integration of clinical and scientific information for pedagogical purposes. Integrating mandatory facts into physiological, diagnostic, and therapeutic contexts, this work is a valuable resource for anyone seeking to optimize patient outcomes in individuals with kidney and urinary tract disease.

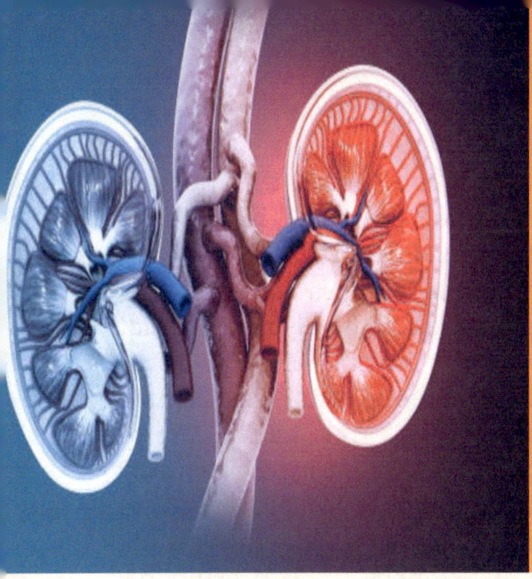

Chapter 1

ANATOMY AND PHYSIOLOGY OF THE KIDNEY AND URINARY TRACT

Contents

Introduction

The anatomy and physiology of the urinary system and the kidney are fundamental parts of human anatomy, which have crucial roles in maintaining homeostasis. The kidneys play a significant role in regulating blood pressure and volume, maintaining electrolyte balance, and removing waste products from the blood. These processes are facilitated by elaborate structures, such as nephrons, which filter blood, reabsorb essential materials, and secrete waste materials as urine. Additionally, the urinary system, consisting of the ureters, bladder, and urethra, facilitates the storage and expulsion of urine from the organism. It is essential to know the details of these systems to appreciate their function in health as well as to identify the potential diseases and disorders, which tend to arise due to malfunctioning of these structures. The rise in incidence of renal diseases, particularly conditions reflects such conditions as urolithiasis, underscoring the importance of this information. As evidenced by research, around 12,000 hospital admissions each year are due to kidney stones alone, a health concern of significant proportions (Al-Modhefer et al., 2016). Kidney stones also have the potential to cause severe complications like urinary obstruction, infection, and, if left untreated, irreversible damage to the kidneys. Adequate diagnosis and management rely heavily on knowledge of both renal anatomy and physiology. Recent technological advances in imaging techniques, such as ultrasound, have progressively enhanced our capacity to diagnose and monitor kidney pathologies, such that medical physicians can treat conditions more effectively, especially in obstructive urolithiasis cases, a highly pertinent condition in populations with specific diet and environmental factors (Al-Lugami et al., 2017). Moreover, the implications of renal physiology extend beyond direct health care to impact the broader societal context, including healthcare access and preventive care. By learning about the structure and function of the kidneys and urinary tract, we not only improve clinical skills but we are also made more aware of risk factors and lifestyles that may affect renal health. Educational interventions aimed at spreading knowledge about the kidneys could presumably reduce the incidence of associated diseases. With a greater focus on public health interventions, an understanding of the associated biological processes will become increasingly significant in shaping the best interventions and policies to restrict the cost of kidney and urinary tract diseases. Ultimately, a thorough understanding of these anatomical and physiological concepts is essential for both the advancement of medical science and improved patient care (Figure 1.1).

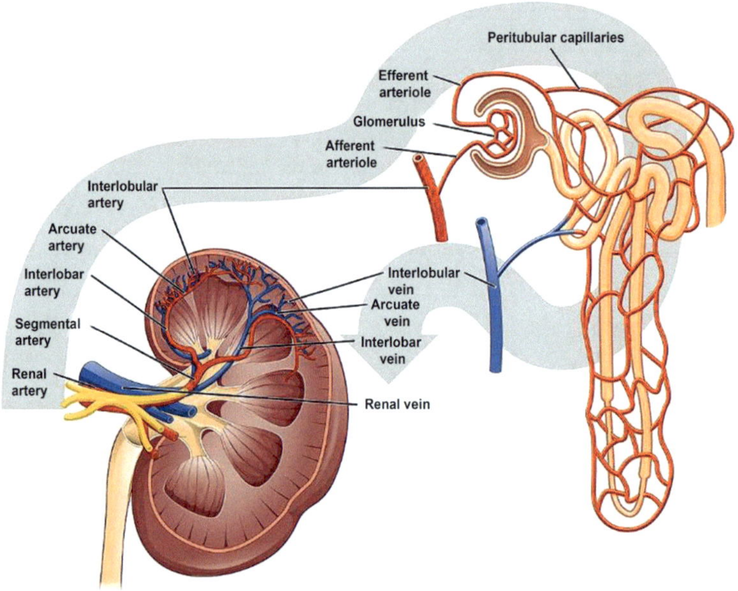

Figure 1.1. Anatomy and physiology of the kidney.

Source: https://wtcs.pressbooks.pub/app/uploads/sites/47/2024/02/2612_Blood_Flow_in_the_Kidneys.jpg.

Overview of the Kidney and Urinary Tract

The two retroperitoneal, bean-shaped organs, the kidneys, play a critical role in maintaining homeostasis in the body. The primary functions include filtering blood, regulating fluid and electrolyte balance, and removing waste materials in the form of urine. Comprising numerous nephrons, the functional organs of the kidneys, the kidneys facilitate the intricate processes of filtration, reabsorption, and secretion. The kidneys effectively filter metabolic waste, excess ions, and toxins through the glomerulus and renal tubules, ensuring the stability of blood composition, which is vital to their overall health. Additionally, the kidneys regulate blood pressure through the renin-angiotensin-aldosterone system, highlighting their multifunctional role in ensuring not only waste removal but also systemic physiological stability (Beebe et al., 2019). The urinary organs, which include the kidneys, ureters, bladder, and urethra, play a central role in the production and ejection of urine. Urine is transported from the kidneys via the ureters to the bladder, where it is stored until it is expelled. The process of storage allows strategic regulation of urination for convenience and management of the body's excretory needs. The bladder, being a muscular organ, enlarges and contracts in size to store varying amounts of urine and employs mechanisms, such as the detrusor muscle, to facilitate urination. The urethra, a channel for urination, has a varying structure and length in both sexes and includes specialized sphincters that regulate urination. The physiological activities and the anatomical arrangement of these structures work in tandem to ensure efficient waste elimination, and any derangement will lead to complications, including urinary tract infection (UTI), attesting to the urinary system's central role (Musa et al., 2025). Apart from their physiological roles, the kidneys and the urinary tract play a significant role in broader health contexts, particularly when it comes to UTIs. UTIs are prevalent and can affect individuals of all age groups, and can be linked to tragic results if not treated. The symptoms typically manifest as dysuria, frequency, and suprapubic discomfort. It is essential to understand the risk factors associated with UTIs, including anatomical factors and personal hygiene practices. Early diagnosis and prompt treatment are crucial, as complications can progress rapidly. Systematic management of UTIs encompasses not only drug therapy but also education in preventive practices. Therefore, the kidneys and urinary tracts' anatomical and physiological intricacies have direct bearing on not only normal bodily functions but on consequential health consequences as well, further necessitating study and public education about urinary health (Musa et al., 2025) (Figure 1.2).

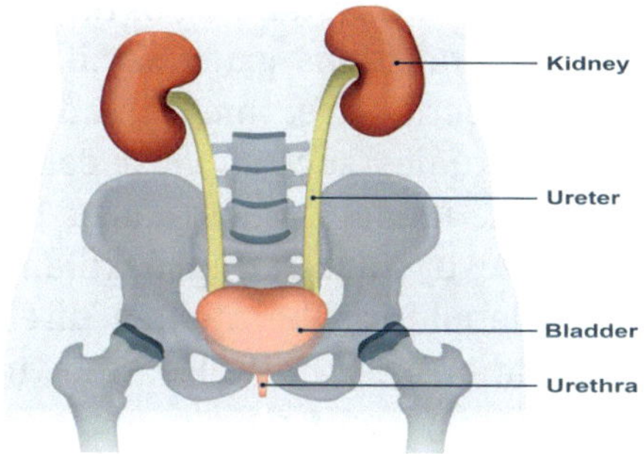

Figure 1.2. Overview of the kidney and urinary tract.

Source: https://media.healthdirect.org.au/images/inline/original/urinary-system-295b22.png.

Importance of Studying Anatomy and Physiology

It is essential that medical students, as well as physicians, have knowledge about the physiology and anatomy of the urinary tract and the kidney, because it allows them to understand how the body maintains homeostasis, especially in terms of fluid balance, waste excretion, and electrolyte balance. By studying the intricate architecture of the kidneys, with nephrons serving as functional units, students can appreciate how the kidneys clean blood, reabsorb essential substances, and eliminate waste. Such a fundamental appreciation is necessary, not only for those who opt for healthcare-related careers, but also for the general populace, in order to make informed decisions regarding healthy lifestyles. Additionally, knowledge of the physiological processes underlying kidney function can enlighten us on the pathogenesis of certain diseases and disorders, thereby highlighting the necessity for anatomy and physiology training in developing health awareness. The increasing prevalence of renal ailments, such as kidney stones, further underscores the need to learn anatomy and physiology. With an estimated 12,000 hospitalizations per year because of this disease, an exact understanding of the involved structures and functions gains significance in coming to effective treatment plans. Going through case studies, such as those concerning calcium oxalate kidney stones, makes learning more effective by illustrating firsthand how anatomical details can be applied directly to real-life situations. For instance, knowing the etiology of kidney stone development and the pathology that goes with it is equally essential to diagnosis and treatment. Incorporating this information in the learning experience offers a well-rounded understanding of how the disorders arise, how they compromise kidney function, and what interventions can be used to address the condition, making anatomy and physiology studied in a clinical context essential. Besides that, the study of the anatomy and physiology of the kidney and urinary system has the twofold advantage: it benefits upcoming medical professionals in the identification and management of disease, and also assists in medical research. As new techniques are being researched to manage kidney problems, familiarity with the foundational anatomical and physiological principles allows for innovation in therapy. For example, a careful review of kidney stone treatment reveals various approaches, including pain control, medical therapies, and dietary interventions, all based on the physiological principles of renal function. By providing individuals with knowledge of anatomy and physiology, we not only equip healthcare workers with the capability to manage conditions better but also enable them to contribute to research and public health programs aimed at preventing disease (Valparaiso University, 1911; Al-Modhefer et al., 2016).

1.1. Anatomy of the Kidney

The human kidney possesses an elaborate anatomy that matches its multifunctional role in homeostasis. One kidney is roughly the size of a fist, situated retroperitoneally on either side of the spinal column. The renal cortex, an outer layer, harbors the renal corpuscles as well as the proximal and distal convoluted tubules, which play a key role in the formation of urine. Beneath the cortex lies the renal medulla, distinguished by cone-shaped structures known as renal pyramids. These pyramids drain urine to the renal pelvis, which then transfers it to the ureters for transport to the bladder. The elaborate nephron pattern, the functional unit of the kidneys, provides a vast surface area for filtration and reabsorption processes, enabling the compensation of body fluid balance, electrolyte balance, and waste disposal from the blood, thereby determining the body's overall homeostasis, as per available anatomical texts (N/A, 1997). Additionally, the renal vascular anatomy also contributes to the efficient functioning of the kidneys. The blood supply is regulated mainly by the renal artery that bifurcates from the abdominal aorta and is relayed through a system of smaller arteries that gradually taper. The afferent arterioles supply the blood to the glomeruli, where it is filtered. The efferent arterioles subsequently create a peritubular capillary network that surrounds the nephron, facilitating the exchange of substances. Filtered blood is returned to the inferior vena cava by renal veins. Knowledge about the vascular organization is essential, as any alterations in the blood supply will have a direct impact on renal function and can lead to profound physiological consequences. Research on the renal vasculature offers more insight into disease states such as hypertension and renal insufficiency, indicating that renal hemodynamics must be regulated for overall well-being (Al-Lugami et al., 2017).

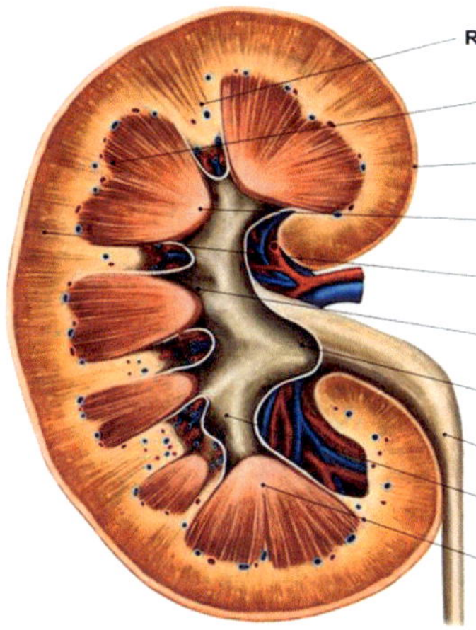

Figure 1.3. Anatomy of the kidney.

Source: https://www.kenhub.com/thumbor/6h_vqbnkREKCXdDQX7uHtc3jI6U=/fit-in/800x1600/filters:watermark(/images/logo_url.png,-10,-10,0):background_color(FFFFFF):format(jpeg)/images/library/10923/renal-cortex_englishMA.jpg.

Beyond their physical form, the kidneys are also crucial in regulating fluid and electrolyte balance through an intricate interplay of hormonal interactions. Nephrons respond to hormones such as aldosterone and antidiuretic hormone (ADH), which control reabsorption of sodium and water, respectively. Aldosterone causes the retention of sodium in exchange for potassium and hydrogen ions, thereby balancing the fluid in the body. ADH increases the permeability of the collecting ducts to water, consequently facilitating the production of concentrated urine. All this helps prevent dehydration and maintain blood pressure in the event of changes in body condition. It is essential to understand these hormonal impacts in the understanding of various renal pathologies because disruption of these signals typically results in diseases such as diabetes insipidus or hyperaldosteronism, which demonstrates that the kidneys are significant in endocrine and systemic homeostasis (N/A, 1997) (Figure 1.3).

1.1.1. Structure and Location of the Kidneys

The kidneys, such vital organs of the human system, are located in the posterior cavity of the abdomen, specifically in the retroperitoneal space. Being so located, they are shielded by the lower ribs yet continue to perform well in purifying the blood. The single kidney measures approximately the size of a fist and weighs between 10 and 12 centimeters in length, with a bean-like shape. This structure of the body is necessary for its multitudinous functions, including regulation of electrolyte balance, acid-base homeostasis, and excretion of waste products. The kidneys also possess a rich vascular supply, with blood being supplied through the renal arteries, which branch out directly from the abdominal aorta. Their relative position within the body not only enables optimum filtering efficiency but also provides access to various physiological systems necessary for maintaining homeostasis. At the internal level, kidneys possess a highly organized anatomy comprising renal cortex, renal medulla, and renal pelvis. The outer cortex appears granular in structure, with nephrons as the structural and functional components of urine secretion. Within the renal medulla, anatomy includes the renal pyramids, which are covered by collecting ducts that drain to the renal pelvis. The renal pelvis serves as a funnel to channel the urine from the nephrons, gathered together, into the ureters. Such an intricate structure provides for effective filtration and reabsorption. Therefore, any alteration within this tightly regulated system can produce significant physiological dysfunctions, thereby illustrating the vital role the kidneys play in ensuring overall body health. The interaction of these organs illustrates just how fundamental the kidneys are in managing both fluid balance and waste elimination. The function of the kidneys is not merely excretion; they are essential to systemic health and are impacted by multiple disease states. Among such issues is the development of kidney stones, a condition that has increased in prevalence across most populations.

Kidney stones form in the renal pelvis due to various factors, including metabolic disorders and dietary habits. Kidney stones may lead to interference with the free flow of urine, hence complications requiring surgery. It is imperative, therefore, to be aware of the anatomical sites and structures in the kidneys so that conditions can be diagnosed and managed effectively. Based on Al-Modhefer et al. (2016), the complexity of kidney structure organization heavily influences pathological processes, which is why there is a need for further research and improved management methods for renal illnesses. Practitioners can gain a better understanding of renal health and its implications for overall well-being by understanding the complex relationship between structure and function.

1.1.2. Internal Anatomy: Cortex, Medulla, and Pelvis

The intrarenal anatomy of the kidney is generally divided into three central regions: cortex, medulla, and pelvis, with each serving different but complementary functions in renal physiology. The outer cortex is the outermost layer of the kidney, containing numerous renal corpuscles and convoluted tubules. It is within this layer that blood filtration occurs. Podocytes and mesangial cells play a vital role in maintaining the function of glomeruli's integrity, whereas densely packed nephron structure plays a crucial role in efficient reabsorption and secretion. The cortex needs to be healthy because damage here will predispose it to reduced kidney function and potential chronic disease, which again makes it necessary to study its anatomy and physiology in relation to kidney disease and disorders. Internally, the renal medulla consists of a series of pyramidal structures known as renal pyramids through which urine becomes concentrated.

The primary structures of the medulla include the loops of Henle and collecting ducts, which are essential for controlling water and electrolyte balance. As the filtrate passes through these complexes, water is reabsorbed, forming concentrated urine, a process that relies mainly on the osmotic gradient established by the medulla. Medullary abnormalities, such as those found in certain congenital diseases that result in hydronephrosis, can disrupt this balance, having deleterious effects on renal function as a whole. The complexity of the medullary structure is thus critical in providing homeostasis in the body, further supporting the study of this renal segment to a large extent. Finally, the renal pelvis is a funnel-shaped structure that collects urine from the renal calyces and directs it toward the ureter. It plays a critical role in the drainage of urine, which is crucial in preventing conditions like hydronephrosis. Observations in some genetic mouse models, such as Crim1 hypomorphic mice, reveal that pelvicalyceal developmental abnormalities may lead to significant renal anomalies, including obstructive nephropathy and contractile dysfunction of the pelvic smooth muscle (Abraham et al., 2012). Furthermore, understanding the anatomical interaction between the pelvis and the surrounding structures may help design targeted therapy for urinary tract disorders (Beebe et al., 2019). This interconnectedness illustrates how the integrity of the pelvis directly influences kidney function and health (Figure 1.4).

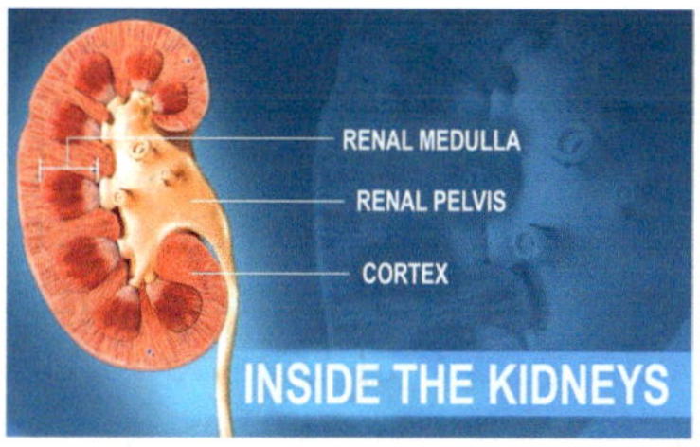

Figure 1.4. Internal anatomy: cortex, medulla, and pelvis of the kidney.

Source: https://www.visiblebody.com/hubfs/4C_Inside_the_Kidneys.jpg.

1.1.3. Blood Supply and Nephron Structure

The subtle interaction between blood supply and nephron architecture is at the heart of the kidneys' function in filtering and regulating the body's internal environment. The individual nephron, the functional unit of the kidney, comprises a renal corpuscle and renal tubule, its architecture specially suited to effective filtration and reabsorption. The blood comes into the nephron through the afferent arteriole to the glomerulus, where the majority of plasma is filtered into Bowmans capsule. This initial process of filtration is crucial in removing excess solutes and waste, while retaining vital components of blood. The unique nephron design, for example, its position in relation to various blood vessels, enables optimal exchange and the kidney's ability to adapt to changes in blood composition and pressure, thereby maintaining the body in a homeostatic state.

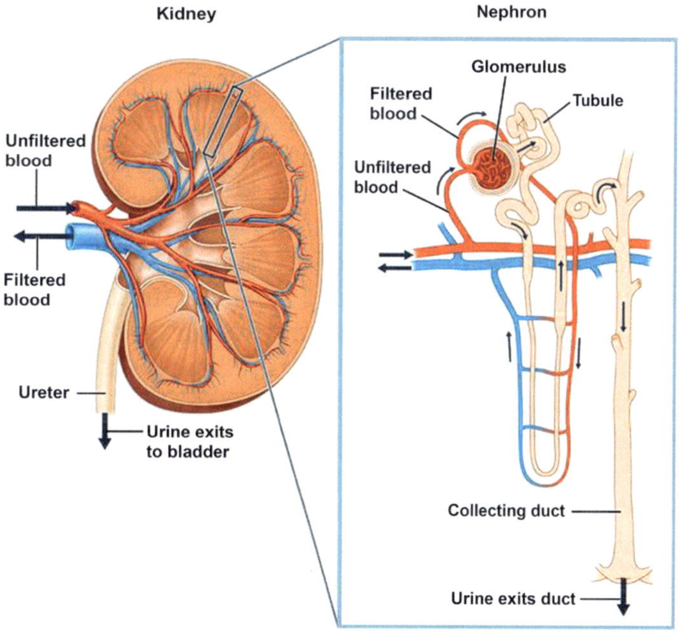

Figure 1.5. Blood supply and nephron structure of the kidney.

Source: https://www.niddk.nih.gov/media-assets/11236/B2-Image03-Kidney+Nephron-FINAL_thumbnail.jpg.

During the course of blood flowing through the nephron, the renal tubule segments listed below have different functions that are integral to their vascular supply. The major reabsorption of water, ions, and nutrients such as glucose and amino acids is effected by the proximal convoluted tubule. The dense microvilli here serve to maximize reabsorptive surface area, and thus the requirement for optimal blood flow to supply substrates of demand for active transport mechanisms becomes evident. In contrast, the thick ascending limb of the loop of Henle utilizes a sodium-potassium-chloride cotransporter to actively reabsorb ions, which is particularly relevant to hypertension states. Mechanisms for sodium reabsorption in this segment of the nephron confirm its key role in regulating blood pressure and fluid balance, indicating the interdependence of nephron perfusion and structure in maintaining physiological homeostasis (Dominiczak et al., 2017). Renal function specificity is also made possible by the unusual pattern of vessels around the nephron. Peritubular capillaries, which are derived from the efferent arterioles, accompany the renal tubules and have direct roles in substance exchange between the blood and tubular fluid. This thin network of capillaries is not only involved in the reabsorption of essential nutrients and water but also in the secretion of waste products into the renal tubule. This dual role thus underscores the importance of an adequate blood supply in maintaining nephron function. Furthermore, the architecture of medullary vasa recta is significant in creating a hyperosmotic environment to obtain the kidney concentration of urine. Therefore, knowledge of the relationship between nephron architecture and blood supply is crucial to understanding the physiology of the kidney and its implications for broader health concerns (Beebe et al., 2019) (Figure 1.5).

1.2. Function of the Kidneys

The kidneys play a central role in maintaining homeostasis in the human body, primarily through their filtration and excretory functions. Retroperitoneally placed, the bean-shaped organs filter blood to remove metabolic waste products, thereby preventing the accumulation of toxins that can disrupt cellular function. Filtration occurs at the nephron, the functional unit of the kidney, where glomerular filtration initiates the creation of urine. The kidneys also regulate fluid and electrolyte balance, which is crucial for maintaining blood pressure and ensuring the effective functioning of other organ systems. Through the regulation of ion excretion, such as sodium and potassium, the kidneys maintain acid-base balance and overall body homeostasis, highlighting the vital role of the kidneys in physiological stability and health. In addition to filtration, the kidneys play a significant role in endocrine function by secreting hormones that are essential for the body's functions. For instance, erythropoietin, which is produced under conditions of hypoxia, stimulates the formation of red blood cells in the bone marrow and consequently regulates oxygen delivery around the body. The kidneys also play a crucial role in converting vitamin D into its active metabolite, calcitriol, which is necessary for calcium absorption and maintaining bone health. These endocrine activities demonstrate that the kidneys are not solely excretory organs, but are actively involved in other physiological processes that influence metabolism and overall health, thereby bridging the gap between the endocrine and excretory systems. These dependency functions prove the intricate nature of renal physiology and the significance of the kidneys. Optimal renal function requires a symphony of interaction between multiple organ systems, highlighting the role of the kidneys within the broader context of human physiology. Such intersystem cooperation is essential, as deficiency in renal activity can have severe systemic implications, such as fluid overload or metabolic disturbance. Routine radiologic examinations can provide useful information regarding renal anatomy and physiology, enabling clinicians to be mindful of the accurate pathologies that affect kidney function, as suggested by the interdisciplinary correlation among pediatricians, urologists, and radiologists (Grossman et al., 1973). Thus, a clear understanding of kidney function is critical not only for diagnosing kidney disease but also for informed clinical decision-making that affects patient treatment. The kidneys serve as a fulcrum for various bodily functions, demonstrating their crucial role in bodily welfare and physiological equilibrium (Figure 1.6).

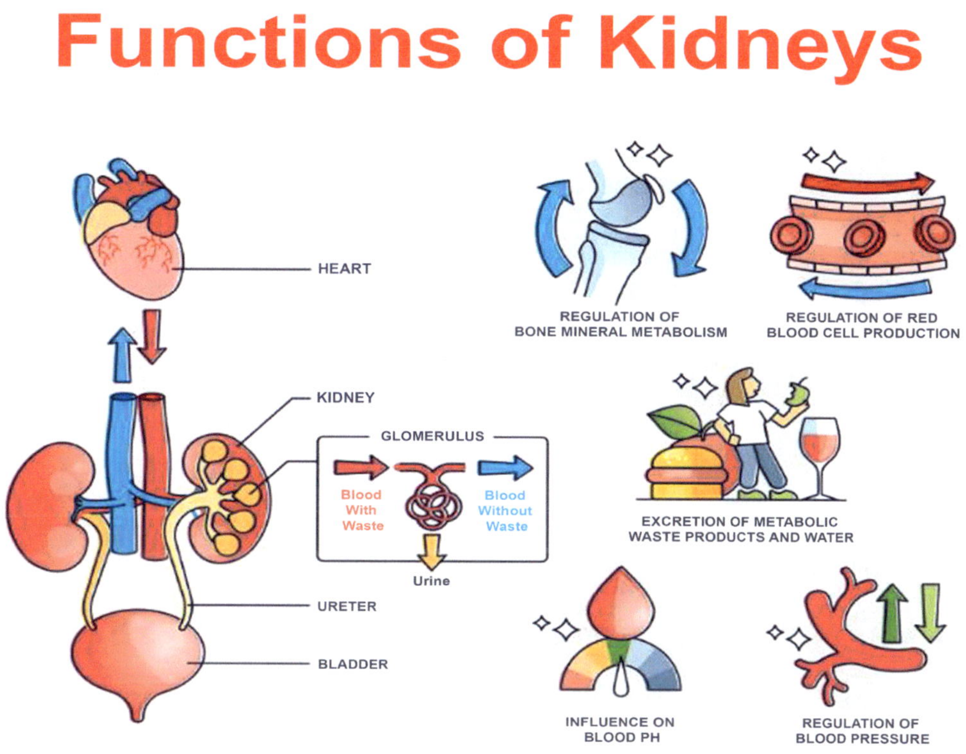

Figure 1.6. Function of the kidneys.

Source: https://assets.lybrate.com/imgs/tic/enadp/function-of-kidney.jpg.

1.2.1. Filtration of Blood and Formation of Urine

The filtration of blood in the kidneys is a critical process by which waste products are eliminated while essential substances are conserved for homeostasis. This happens in nephrons, the functional and structural units of the kidney, where the blood flows through the glomerulus. The glomerular capillaries act as a filter barrier, allowing water, ions, and small molecules to pass through, while holding back larger proteins and blood cells. This sieving results in glomerular filtrate, which is then further processed as it flows along the renal tubules. The kidneys filter approximately 180 liters of blood daily, emphasizing their crucial role in maintaining fluid and electrolyte balance. By maintaining reasonable control of blood composition, the kidneys are essential to the overall metabolic health, showing their integral role in the anatomy and physiology of the urinary system. Once the preliminary filtration in the glomerulus has occurred, the glomerular filtrate passes through the renal tubules, where essential functions such as reabsorption and secretion take place. Most of the nutrients, including glucose, amino acids, and bicarbonate, are reabsorbed by the proximal convoluted tubule into the blood, while it secretes waste products, such as hydrogen ions and certain drugs. As the filtrate enters the loop of Henle, further reabsorption of salts and water occurs, serving an essential function in urine concentration. The collecting duct and distal convoluted tubule give more opportunity for electrolyte regulation and acid-base balance alteration by the kidneys. This intricate processing transforms the filtrate into urine, demonstrating the kidneys' dynamic response to the body's physiological needs. Understanding the mechanisms helps generate valuable information regarding kidney function and its position within the urinary system. The coexistence of filtration, reabsorption, and secretion results in the formation of urine, the primary route of waste excretion. Urine formation is not merely the removal of excess, but a highly controlled process that maintains the stability of the internal environment. Interruptions to such processes can lead to various pathological conditions, such as acute kidney injury or chronic kidney disease, which significantly impact health. For instance, kidney stones, as described in Al-Modhefer et al. (2016), can inhibit proper urine flow and result in severe complications. Similarly, urinary tract infections, highlighted in Musa et al. (2025), can arise when the urinary system becomes compromised, interfering with filtration and urine secretion. Therefore, a thorough understanding of how blood filtration is converted into urine production is essential for comprehending the broader implications of kidney function on health and disease management (Figure 1.7).

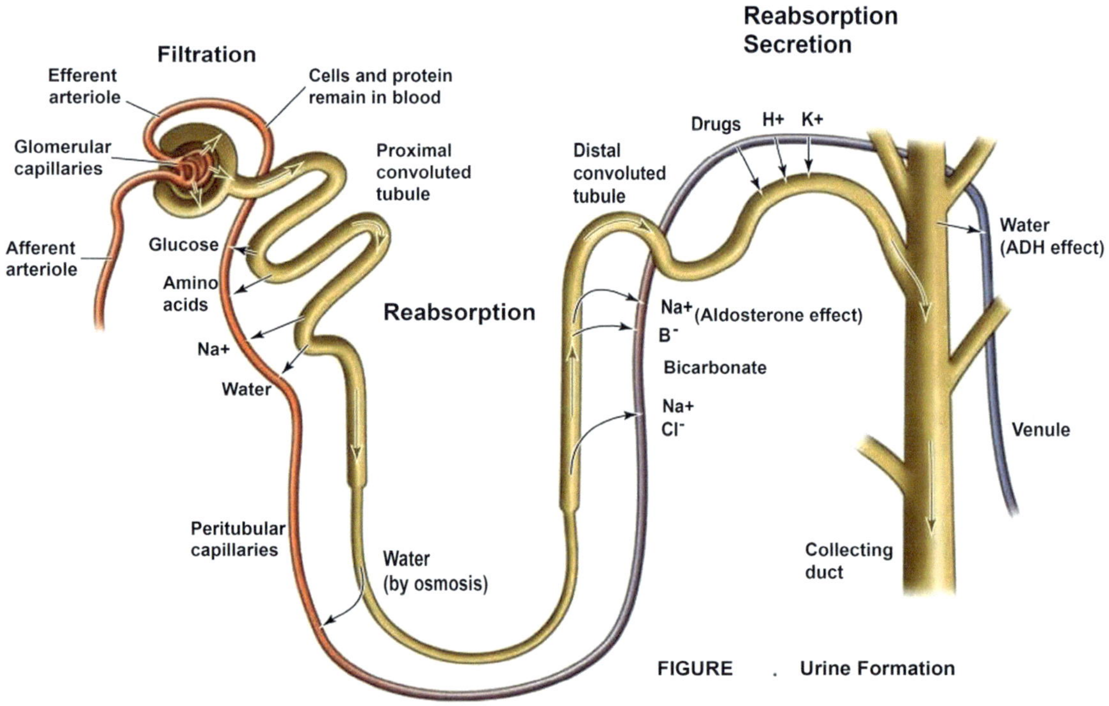

Figure 1.7. Filtration of blood and formation of urine.

Source: https://img.brainkart.com/article/article-Urine-Formation-1G9.jpg.

1.2.2. Regulation of Electrolytes and Acid-Base Balance

The kidneys also play an important role in electrolyte management and acid-base balance, which is essential for homeostasis maintenance. The kidneys accomplish this by facilitating minute interactions between filtration, reabsorption, and secretion in the various segments of the nephrons. Sodium (Na^+) is one of the most essential electrolytes controlled by the kidneys; it is reabsorbed primarily in the proximal tubule as well as the thick ascending limb of the loop of Henle. This regulation is essential because excessive amounts of sodium can induce hypertension, which threatens overall cardiovascular health. The kidneys also regulate the excretion of potassium (K+) and calcium (Ca2+) in response to dietary intake and hormonal influences. The ability of the kidneys to finely adjust these electrolytes reinforces its critical role in physiological homeostasis, thereby preventing derangement that can lead to severe disease. Acid-base balance is another critical renal physiology function that interacts with electrolyte control. The kidneys control the body's pH by secreting hydrogen ions (H^+) and reabsorbing bicarbonate (HCO_3^-). The intricate process enables the blood pH to remain within a narrow range of 7.35 to 7.45. In normal homeostasis, bicarbonate reabsorption is located in the proximal tubule, while H^+ secretion is closely linked with processes of Na^+ reabsorption. Metabolic acidosis and alkalosis are clinical conditions that highlight the kidneys' function in maintaining acid-base balance. The awareness of these renal functions highlights the body's ability to adapt to dietary and environmental changes, and demonstrates the kidneys' contribution to overall metabolic homeostasis. Moreover, the intricate interaction between electrolyte homeostasis and hypertension illustrates the clinical relevance of renal function. The pathophysiology of hypertension is mediated by high dietary salt, partly through its action on the reabsorption of sodium in renal organs, specifically the thick ascending limb of the loop of Henle (TAL; Dominiczak et al., 2017). Research indicates that alterations in Na+ homeostasis in this nephron segment have significant implications for blood pressure regulation. As hypertension contributes to approximately 9.4 million deaths annually, renal mechanisms controlling electrolytes are essential in the formulation of therapeutic options. Aiming to understand the renal mechanisms regulating electrolyte homeostasis may not only provide an enhanced understanding of hypertension but also pave the way for new, targeted treatments in the management of this widespread public health condition (Dominiczak et al., 2017). Through careful examination of these interactions, the regulation of electrolytes and acid-base balance, a cornerstone of renal physiology, is unveiled.

1.2.3. Role in Blood Pressure Regulation

Kidneys play a significant role in blood pressure homeostasis by multiple physiological mechanisms, the majority of which are sodium (Na^+) and volume-related. The nephron, or the renal functional unit, is key to this process because it participates in the filtration and reabsorption of water and electrolytes. One of the primary mechanisms for controlling blood pressure is the distal nephron segments, particularly the thick ascending limb of the loop of Henle (TAL). In this segment, sodium reabsorption is enhanced under various conditions, leading to increased blood volume and, consequently, higher blood pressure. This mechanism indicates the importance of renal Na^+ handling and its direct correlation with hypertension, whereby disruption of Na^+ reabsorption can aggravate blood pressure issues, as quoted in current controversy about salt sensitivity and its role in health outcomes (Dominiczak et al., 2017). It is also important to determine the cellular and molecular characteristics of the kidney for the purpose of understanding its role in blood pressure regulation. Advances in transcriptomics have, in recent times, enabled one to demarcate exclusive cell populations through the nephron. The techniques determine cell-type-specific expression patterns of genes associated with hypertension and other renal pathophysiologies. The expression profiles of certain proximal tubule populations, for instance, are characteristic of conditions related to hypertension and provide crucial information regarding potentially targeted treatments. Furthermore, new technologies such as single-nucleus RNA sequencing have highlighted the kidneys' complex cellular organization and the role of various cell types in the development of systemic hypertension, thereby opening up therapeutic avenues targeting individual cellular mechanisms implicated in high blood pressure conditions (Chen et al., 2019). Finally, the kidneys regulate systemic vascular resistance through the renin-angiotensin-aldosterone system (RAAS), which is a key component involved in blood pressure regulation. Renin, an enzyme secreted by the juxtaglomerular cells of the kidney, initiates a cascade that leads to the production of angiotensin II. This potent vasoconstrictor increases blood pressure by constricting blood vessels and stimulating the release of aldosterone, which in turn increases sodium and water reabsorption. The equilibrium between renal function and the RAAS system illustrates how the kidneys regulate blood pressure, not just through direct control of sodium, but also through systemic vascular effects. Consequently, dysregulation of this system can lead to chronic hypertension, underscoring the crucial role of the kidneys in the intricate dynamics of blood pressure regulation. Clarification of such overlapping mechanisms is crucial to developing effective interventions against hypertension and its implications (Figure 1.8).

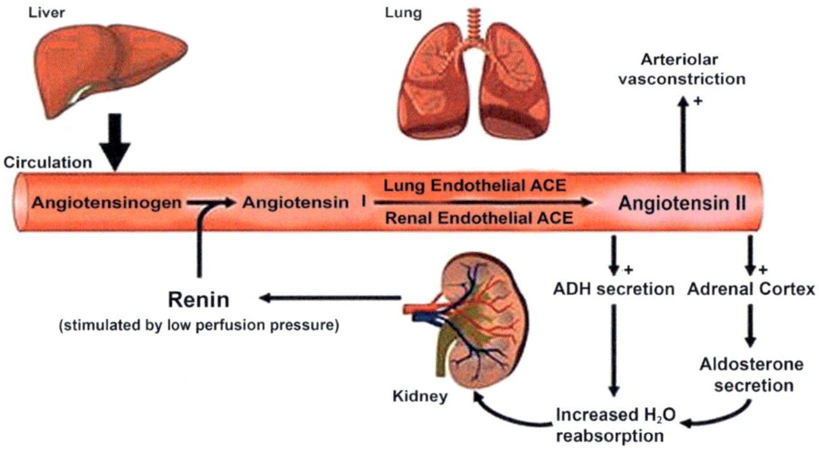

Figure 1.8. Kidneys role in blood pressure regulation.

Source: https://www.cusabio.com/statics/images/BPR-img1.jpg.

1.3. Anatomy of the Urinary Tract

The urinary system is a vital component of the human body, primarily responsible for removing waste and regulating electrolytes, as well as maintaining fluid balance. The system comprises various major organs, including the kidneys, ureters, bladder, and urethra. Each of them plays a vital role in maintaining homeostasis. The kidneys, which many would consider the body's primary filtration system, are responsible for removing waste from the blood, regulating blood pressure, and secreting essential hormones. The organization of kidneys, through their filtration units called nephrons, enables filtration, reabsorption, and excretion to occur in a sophisticated manner, ultimately leading to the production of urine, which is transported via the ureters to the bladder to be held. This anatomy serves as the basis for understanding the complex physiology of the urinary system and the cooperation between various organs and their activities. As the bladder fills with urine, its muscular layers can distend, signaling the central nervous system to void. The bladder's anatomy is in three layers: mucosa, detrusor muscle, and adventitia, which all work harmoniously together to perform its role effectively. Micturition, or urination, is facilitated through the coordinated contraction of the detrusor muscle, while the internal and external urethral sphincters relax, allowing urine to exit the body. Such a process demonstrates the interaction between the urinary tract and the nervous system, thereby highlighting the need for precise anatomical coordination. Moreover, knowledge regarding interactions of the urinary tract's anatomical components enhances knowledge of normal urinary tract disorders. Conditions such as kidney stones and urinary tract infections have anatomical origins, which illuminate preventive strategies and therapeutic options, demonstrating the value of a richly detailed model of anatomy in practice. Beyond mere anatomy, the form of the urinary tracts communicates an essential set of implications for its physiology. The Foundational Model of Anatomy (FMA) formalizes these correspondences in an integrated framework for exploring the spatial truth of the urinary system. By expressing the relationships among anatomy and organ position that are involved in urine production and removal, the FMA is able to more clearly disclose our knowledge of normal function and disease in the system. It is a valuable resource for researchers and clinicians working to explain the complexity of anatomical and functional defects. This ontology not only supports spatial thinking in anatomical situations but also offers avenues for contributions to anatomical information science, hence improving both teaching and research on the urinary system and its critical roles in the human body (Valparaiso University, 1911; Kumar et al., 2005) (Figure 1.9).

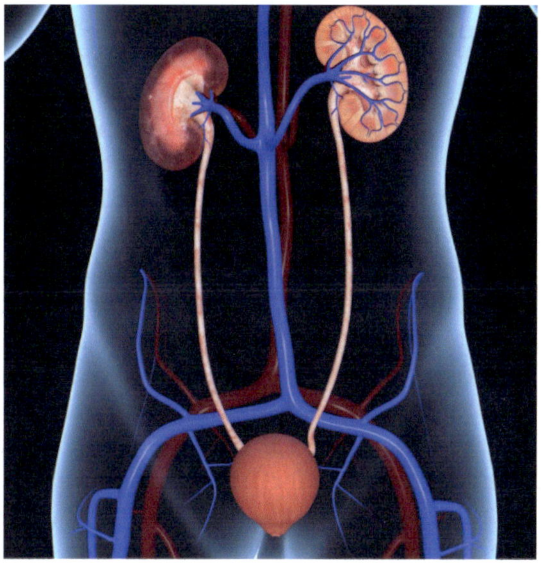

Figure 1.9. Anatomy of the urinary tract.

Source: https://external-content.duckduckgo.com/iu/?u=https%3A%2F%2Fres.cloudinary.com%2Fgrohealth%2Fimage%2Fupload%2Ff_auto%2Cfl_lossy%2Cq_auto%2Fv1583507687%2FDCUK%2FContent%2FHuman-Kidney-Urinary-System-Suprarenal-Gland-Healthcare-And-Medicine-Medicine_Medium.jpg&f=1&nofb=1&ipt=8b28634940f2bdcced4ae58830280573fcb92e67c2683739a3d379c6ac1a7df1.

1.3.1. Structure of the Ureters

The ureters, an essential component of the urinary system, are muscular tubes that facilitate the flow of urine from the kidneys to the bladder. The shape of each ureter is approximately 25 to 30 centimeters long and is formed of three layers: the mucosa, muscularis, and adventitia. The innermost layer, or mucosa, consists of transitional epithelium, which allows it to expand while urine flows through. Surrounding the mucosa is the muscularis layer, composed of smooth muscle in the guise of an inner longitudinal layer and an outer circular layer, harmonizing peristaltic movements for urine propulsion. Such a structural basis is essential, as it not only facilitates the effective transport of urine but also prevents reflux, allowing the urine to move unidirectionally toward the bladder, thereby maintaining the efficiency and integrity of urinary function. Additionally, the anatomical positioning of the ureters is significant for both functional and clinical purposes. The tubes originate in the renal pelvis of the kidneys, flowing downward into the retroperitoneal space, crossing over at the pelvic brim before entering the bladder. The ureter course is mapped out by adjacent structures, i.e., blood vessels and the psoas major muscle. This anatomical relationship is not only critical for the passage of urine but also highlights the significance of the ureters in pathology, such as kidney stones. The prevalence of kidney stones has been shown to exponentially escalate hospitalizations, further establishing the importance of being aware of the structure and functioning of the ureter, particularly when examining the impact of ureteral obstruction by calculi (Al-Modhefer et al., 2016). In the domain of imaging and diagnostic tests, advanced methods such as multi-slice computed tomography (MSCT) have more precisely characterized ureteral anatomy and pathology. MSCT urography provides the imaging ability of visualizing urinary tract anatomy so that normal and abnormal states, such as ureteral obstructions caused by stones, can be properly identified. This imaging technique highlights the fine anatomy of the ureters and is particularly notable for its ability to produce clear anatomical images without the use of contrast media, thereby improving safety and accessibility in diagnostic procedures (Izzudin et al., 2021). Conversely, an understanding of the ureter anatomy, in conjunction with contemporary imaging modalities, highlights the intrinsic value of the ureters within the broader context of kidney and urinary tract anatomy and physiology (Figure 1.10).

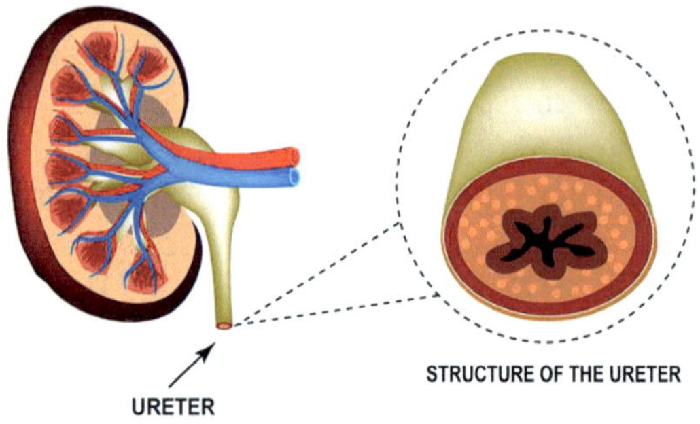

Figure 1.10. Structure of the ureters.

Source: https://www.southvalleyurology.net/wp-content/uploads/2025/04/UTUC-upper-tract-tumors-2-AdobeStock_140174285.jpg.

1.3.2. Anatomy of the Bladder

The bladder, a muscular sac located in the pelvis, has an essential role in storing and expelling urine, which the kidneys produce. The anatomy of the bladder reveals its unique composition, which consists of four major layers: the mucosa, submucosa, muscularis, and adventitia. The innermost layer, the mucosa, is lined with transitional epithelium that is flexible enough to allow for expansion and recoil as the bladder fills and drains. Beneath this lies the submucosa, which consists of connective tissue and blood vessels that provide nourishment and support. The muscular layer, composed of smooth muscle, is essential for the bladder's ability to contract and accommodate urination. Finally, there is adventitia, a protective tissue that attaches the bladder to surrounding tissues, thus keeping it anchored in the pelvic cavity. The storage capacity of the bladder is remarkable, typically containing 300 to 500 milliliters before voiding is required. There are stretch receptors in the bladder wall that send a message to the brain, indicating fullness, which initiates a series of reflex actions leading to urination. This intricate relationship highlights the coordination between the bladder and the nervous system and also underlines the contribution of anatomical as well as physiological factors in the act of urination.

During micturition, there is a synchronized contraction of the detrusor muscle, while the internal urethral sphincter relaxes to allow urine to flow out to the urethra. This intricate mechanism highlights the role of the bladder not only in storage but also in effectively regulating urine ejection, which is crucial for maintaining bodily homeostasis. Awareness about bladder anatomy also sheds light on other medical conditions that can undermine urinary health.

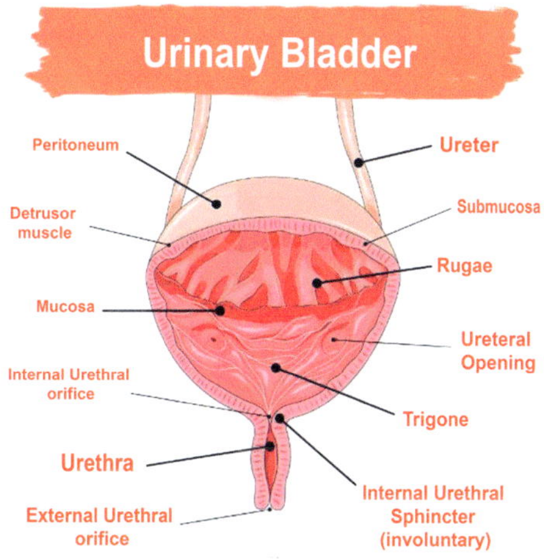

Figure 1.11. The urinary bladder anatomy.

Source: https://cdn.medizzy.com/SKZgm6kqzyDBW560v4UnzPgDciw=/img/posts/65a1e752-4e68-46cd-a1e7-524e6816cdb0.

For instance, urinary tract infections (UTIs) can occur in the bladder, leading to inflammation and discomfort. Clinical management of such illnesses typically entails a multi-faceted approach comprising symptom recognition and treatment plans tailored to individual patients. For instance, one recent case report reported a 45-year-old woman with acute cystitis, exemplifying the importance of prompt medical intervention in preventing bladder infection complications. Hence, bladder anatomy is a critical factor not only in normal function but also in disease, which underscores the significance of broad knowledge in both anatomical and physiological fields for proper health management (Beebe et al., 2019; Musa et al., 2025) (Figure 1.11).

1.3.3. Urethra: Structure and Function

The urethra, being a vital structure of the urinary tract, is really the tube through which urine is excreted from the body. Structurally, the urethra in men and women differs widely, with the male urethra measuring approximately 20 centimeters long and serving a double role as an area of both the urinary and reproductive tracts for males. On the other hand, the urethra of females is approximately 4 centimeters in length and is all dedicated to urinary function. This difference in anatomy not only affects urinary flow but also increases susceptibility to certain diseases, such as urinary tract infections, which are more prevalent among females due to the shorter length of the urethra. Thus, the urethra's anatomy is closely related to its function as an excretory channel and urinary tract well-being. Functionally, the urethra facilitates the controlled emission of urine, which is achieved through both neurologic and anatomical mechanisms. The external urethral sphincter provides voluntary control at the termination of the urethra, thus allowing patients to control urination voluntarily. This sphincter, in conjunction with the internal urethral sphincter at the bladder neck, is a working unit required for urinary continence. Besides, pelvic innervation increases the sensitivity of the urethras so that contractions can occur at the appropriate moment to urinate. When urine travels through the urethra, several mechanisms, including peristalsis, are observed, most notably in the male urethra, where the path also includes ejaculation, demonstrating the urethra's multifunctional role in the male body. Despite its comparatively minor yet often underappreciated significance, the urethra plays a crucial role in maintaining bodily homeostasis, underscoring its structural and functional relevance within the context of kidney and urinary tract physiology. It not only serves as a conduit for the discharge of urine but also helps regulate fluid and electrolyte content by managing the discharge of urine. Moreover, studies show that an understanding of the urethra's anatomy and function can enhance diagnostic strategies in urology in assessing disorders of obstruction or incontinence of the urine (Grossman et al., 1973). Educational resources, as produced for anatomy and physiology courses, are critical because they outline the anatomical consequences and physiological processes at play, giving students and doctors alike insightful comprehension of urological well-being (Beebe et al., 2019).

1.4. Physiology of Urine Formation

The process of urine formation is a complex physiological phenomenon and is primarily conducted inside the nephrons, the functional units of the kidney. It is a three-step process and involves filtration, reabsorption, and secretion. By means of filtration, the plasma of blood is filtered by the glomerulus, which is a network of capillaries found within the renal corpuscle. These various solutes, including water, ions, and small molecules, pass from the blood into the Bowman's capsule and are converted into a fluid known as filtrate.

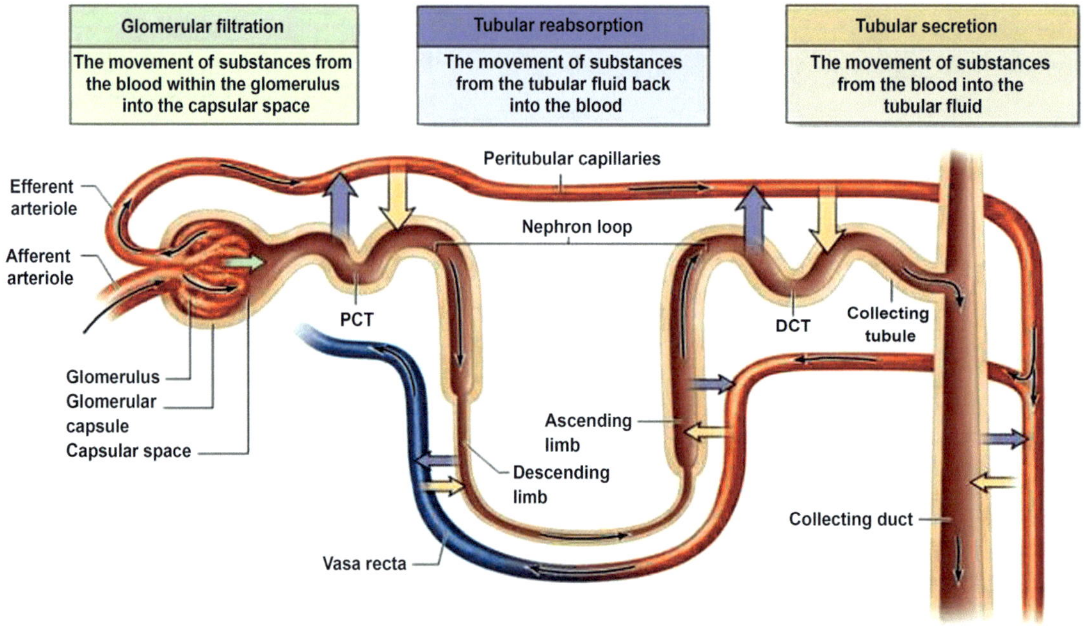

Figure 1.12. Physiology of urine formation.

Source: https://nurseslabs.com/wp-content/uploads/2017/04/Urine-Formation-Urinary-System-Anatomy-and-Physiology.png.

Through the movement of this filtrate inside the nephron, particularly the proximal tubule, essential elements such as glucose, amino acids, and specific ions are reabsorbed back into the bloodstream actively to enable the body to conserve nutrients, while , such as waste products and excess factors, flow towards excretion. The reabsorption, the second mechanism of urine production, plays a critical role in facilitating homeostasis within the body. In the segments of all nephrons, especially the loop of Henle and the collecting ducts, selective permeability is crucial for reabsorbing water and essential ions, allowing for the regulation of fluid balance. The countercurrent multiplier mechanism of the loop of Henle enables urine to become concentrated, allowing the body to retain water in conditions of low hydration. The hormone aldosterone also regulates sodium reabsorption and potassium secretion, exerting a significant effect on blood pressure and fluid status.

The complexity of such interactions highlights the crucial role of the kidneys in filtering blood, as well as regulating essential fluid and electrolyte levels necessary for overall physiological function. The third and final step in urine formation is secretion, which, in addition to reabsorption, helps eliminate excess unwanted substances from the blood into the tubular fluid. Here, ions, creatinine, and a few medications are filtered into the nephron, which fine-tunes the composition of urine before it is excreted. Such a subtle balance plays a crucial role in regulatory processes, particularly in acid-base balance regulation and waste expulsion. A major clinical problem arises when disruptions occur within this system, as illustrated by the increased prevalence of kidney stones, where calcium oxalate crystals can deposit due to changes in urine composition. Understanding the physiology of urine development is important not only for appreciating normal kidney function but also for designing effective management plans for disorders such as this one, which lead to a maximum of 12,000 hospitalizations annually due to complications of kidney stones (Al-Modhefer et al., 2016) (Figure 1.12).

1.4.1. Glomerular Filtration Process

Glomerular filtration is a critical initial step in kidney function that initiates the urine formation process and enables body fluid homeostasis. It occurs in the glomeruli, a cluster of capillaries covered by Bowman's capsule, where blood plasma is removed. The three-layer filtration barrier consists of the fenestrated endothelium, the basement membrane, and the podocytes. Each layer plays a crucial role in selectively allowing substances such as water, ions, and small molecules to cross while excluding large proteins and blood cells. As a result of this selective permeability, the kidneys can efficiently regulate plasma composition in the blood, ensuring fluid balance and electrolyte homeostasis. Additionally, it serves another protective function, as a malfunction at this level can lead to diseases such as end-stage renal disease (ESRD), a severe health issue for patients (Astuti et al., 2017). Regulation of glomerular filtration is necessary to maintain renal and body homeostasis. The filtration rate is regulated by multiple factors, including blood pressure, blood flow, and the structure of the nephrons. Glomerular filtration rate (GFR) is a crucial parameter that determines the kidneys' filtering capacity. A decreased GFR may be indicative of compromised kidney function and requires a clinical examination. Second, hormonal regulation via the renin-angiotensin-aldosterone system is also pertinent in regulating renal blood flow and filtration pressure. This compensatory response is responsible for stabilizing the GFR under various physiological states. With such forces in operation, an understanding of how glomerular filtration operates concerning cardiovascular health is essential, since differences are behind diseases such as hypertension and chronic kidney disease (CKD) (Daminet et al., 2017). The clinical utility of the glomerular filtration process extends beyond basic renal function to encompass diagnostics and disease management. Technologies such as contrast-enhanced ultrasound have emerged to quantify renal perfusion and highlight alterations within this filtration capacity, particularly in patients with chronic kidney disease. Such technologies indicate a shift towards non-invasive methods that can provide information about kidney status without requiring invasive access. By quantifying perfusion dynamics, healthcare practitioners can detect alterations that may arise before overt dysfunction develops, allowing for earlier intervention and more appropriately tailored therapy. Hence, glomerular filtration is not only a vital physiological process but also an essential component of renal diagnostics, enabling healthcare workers to monitor kidney function and act upon possible complications before their development (Daminet et al., 2017) (Figure 1.13).

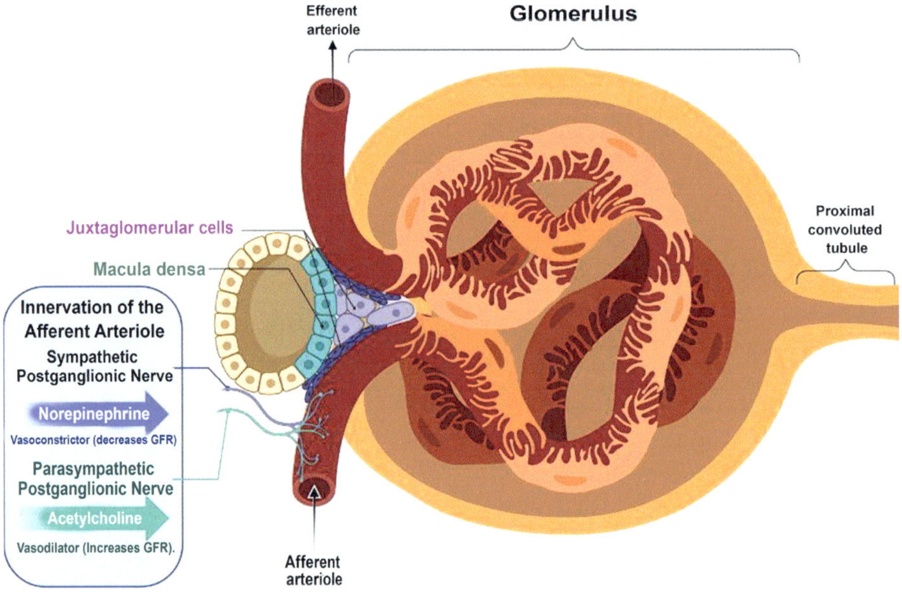

Figure 1.13. Glomerular filtration.

Source: https://uen.pressbooks.pub/app/uploads/sites/462/2024/06/U19-019-Neural-Regulation-of-GFR-v2.png.

1.4.2. Tubular Reabsorption and Secretion

The kidneys play a crucial role in homeostasis regulation through tubular reabsorption and secretion, which are natural mechanisms of urine formation. Tubular reabsorption involves the transport of water and solutes from the tubular fluid to the blood, with most occurring in the proximal convoluted tubule. Reabsorption is a selective process that enables the kidneys to recover vital substances such as glucose, bicarbonate, and ions. Notably, the thick ascending limb of the loop of Henle is particularly significant for sodium reabsorption, osmolarity control, and blood pressure regulation, as excessive dietary salt intake can lead to salt-sensitive hypertension. The concerted activity in other nephron segments explains the complexity of renal physiology, allowing for responsiveness to changing physiological conditions and dietary intakes (Dominiczak et al., 2017). Secretion, in conjunction with reabsorption, is a crucial process by which the kidneys eliminate waste products and maintain electrolyte balance. It is particularly active in the collecting ducts and distal convoluted tubule, where ions such as potassium, hydrogen ions, and certain drugs are actively secreted into the tubular fluid. These secretory functions are regulated by several factors, including hormonal control from the endocrine system.

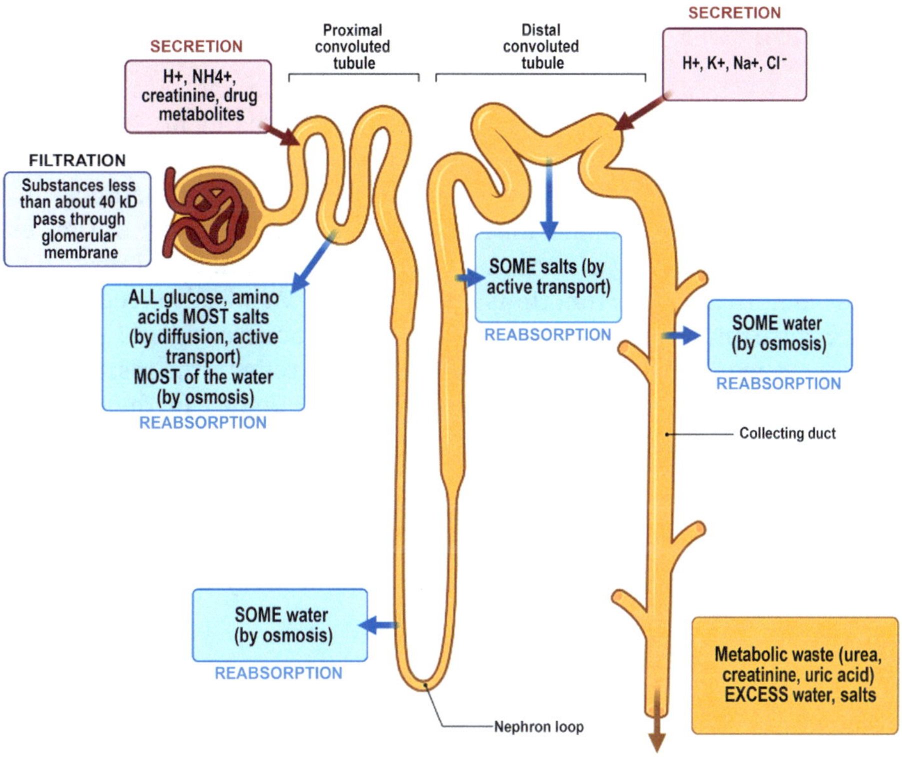

Figure 1.14. Tubular reabsorption and secretion.

Source: https://uen.pressbooks.pub/app/uploads/sites/462/2024/06/U19-011-Reabsorption-in-the-Nephron-v3.png.

For example, aldosterone activates sodium reabsorption and potassium secretion, illustrating the interconnection between renal physiology and systemic homeostasis. This mutual relationship of reabsorption and secretion enables the kidneys to control body processes to a great extent and influence the overall physiological equilibrium (Speck et al., 2020). The simultaneous occurrence of tubular secretion and reabsorption not only emphasizes the kidneys' pivotal role in electrolyte and fluid regulation but also their sophisticated anatomical design. The nephron, the functional unit of the kidney, possesses a remarkable design that aids these intricate processes. The vascular architecture of the nephron, specifically the peritubular capillaries, is designed for the effective transport of materials between the blood and the tubules. In addition, the countercurrent mechanism created in the medulla provides for the output of a concentrated urine and maintains essential ions. This efficiency testifies to the evolution of kidneys as an adaptation that links disparate physiological systems to achieve an internal balance irrespective of external variations. This degree of sophistication in design testifies to a precision that implies orchestration for a purpose in the renal system (Speck et al., 2020) (Figure 1.14).

1.4.3. Concentration and Dilution of Urine

The kidneys play a pivotal role in the processes of urine concentration and dilution, which are essential for maintaining fluid and electrolyte balance within the body. The functional unit of the kidney, the nephron, employs various mechanisms to accomplish these functions through filtration, reabsorption, and secretion. Urine concentration is primarily achieved in the loop of Henle, where the counter-current multiplication system creates a hyperosmotic medullary interstitium. This osmotic gradient enables the kidneys to reabsorb water from the collecting ducts in response to antidiuretic hormone (ADH) stimulation. In high ADH levels, water is reabsorbed, and concentrated urine is produced; in low ADH, water is excreted, and dilute urine is produced. This sophisticated regulation of response shows the capacity of kidneys to adjust to the body's hydration status dynamically. In addition to hormonal influences, the renal tubules' structure and permeability have great impact on urine concentration and dilution. Aquaporin 3 plays explicitly a significant role in water transport within the bladder urothelial cells and is fundamental in maintaining fluid balance (Manso et al., 2025). Moreover, reabsorptive mechanisms in the proximal convoluted tubule and Loop of Henle are controlled by active transport and osmotic gradients, thereby influencing the end-product composition of urine. Alterations in these mechanisms can have far-reaching effects on hydration status, and clinical illnesses such as diabetes insipidus or renal insufficiency can disrupt the concentrating mechanisms for urine. Kidneys also need to respond to various physiological and pathological insults, regulating water and solute excretion in appropriate amounts while ensuring homeostasis. Understanding the mechanisms of urine concentration and dilution is essential, particularly the clinical correlates such as urinary tract infection (UTI) and management. UTI cases within long-term care facilities are significantly high, and bacterial concentrations can influence renal function and osmotic balance in bladder volume (Kirdis et al., 2011). Additionally, the role of hydration status in UTI development highlights the importance of maintaining adequate urine concentration as a preventive measure against urinary pathogens. The development of advanced diagnostic methods and antibacterial agents, such as silver-coated catheters, reflects the research directions in this field that support further urinary tract health. Hence, a complete understanding of kidney physiology not only enables one to recognize parameters that influence urine concentration but also enhances the methodologies towards treating urinary disorders properly.

1.5. Regulation of Kidney Function

The regulation of kidney function is a crucial aspect of homeostasis that maintains the body's balance in terms of fluid, electrolyte, and acid-base balance. The kidneys regulate this intricate control through several mechanisms, including glomerular filtration, tubular reabsorption, and secretion. Glomerular filtration is the process by which blood plasma is filtered through the walls of glomerular capillaries, allowing water, ions, and small molecules to pass into the renal tubule while excluding larger constituents, such as proteins. This action forms the initial filtrate, which is then modified as it flows along the nephron. The key regulation of these actions is required in order to accommodate the body's evolving demands, underlining the kidneys' key role in establishing overall physiological balance. Tubular reabsorption is a vital component of renal function, facilitating the recovery of essential materials from the filtrate into the bloodstream.

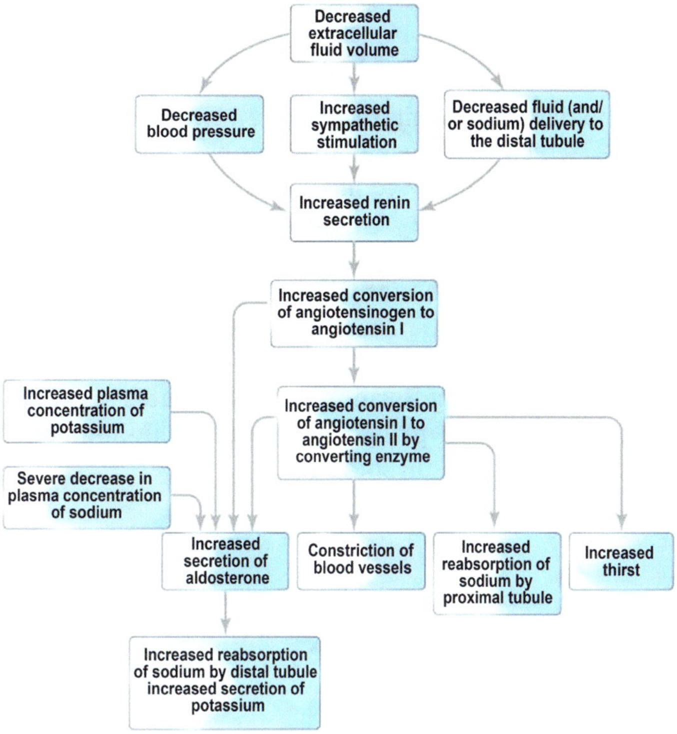

Figure 1.15. Regulation of kidney function.

Source: https://img.brainkart.com/imagebk34/wluN4vk.jpg.

As the filtrate is transported through the proximal convoluted tubule and into the loop of Henle, specific transport mechanisms reclaim certain nutrients, including glucose, amino acids, and other ions. There is significant hormonal regulation throughout this process, with ADH and aldosterone of particular significance. ADH stimulates water reabsorption to concentrate urine and conserve body fluids, while aldosterone regulates the balance of sodium and potassium with direct implications on blood pressure and volume. An understanding of these hormonal influences helps portray how the kidneys dynamically respond to physiological conditions, such as fluid balance and intake, ultimately providing a rich understanding of their regulatory ability in maintaining homeostasis. The dynamic interplay between these regulatory pathways and the intrinsic cellular identities of kidney cells also further explains the significance of kidney function. Recent developments in genomic technologies, such as single-nucleus RNA sequencing, have revealed thirty unique molecular profiles between different cell populations in the human kidney. These profiles enhance our understanding of the ways in which specific cellular and molecular identities play distinct roles in kidney function and disease, particularly in disease conditions such as chronic kidney disease and hypertension (Chen et al., 2019). Furthermore, new evidence underscores the point that targeted therapies based on molecular information may advance clinical interventions and treatment processes for renal diseases. Additionally, research into hydration needs, particularly in novel environments such as space, underscores the kidneys' versatility and their underlying function in maintaining water balance (Roth et al., 2025). This compound view highlights the kidneys' essential contributions to the overall physiology of urinary tracts (Figure 1.15).

1.5.1. Hormonal Control: ADH and Aldosterone

The regulation of body fluid homeostasis primarily relies on two key hormones: antidiuretic hormone (ADH) and aldosterone. ADH, which is released from the posterior pituitary gland, plays a crucial role in osmotic balance regulation through the modification of water reabsorption by the kidneys. During conditions of reduced fluid volume or heightened plasma osmolality, the body increases ADH levels, resulting in the insertion of aquaporin channels in the kidneys' collecting ducts. This mechanism aids in reabsorbing water back into the blood, thereby reducing the volume of urine and concentrating it. ADH therefore plays a crucial role in renal water management, enabling the body to maintain hydration in response to varying physiological demands. Aldosterone, on the other hand, is an adrenal cortex-secreting hormone that regulates sodium and potassium balance in the kidneys. Its release is stimulated primarily by the renin-angiotensin-aldosterone system (RAAS) due to decreased blood pressure or sodium.

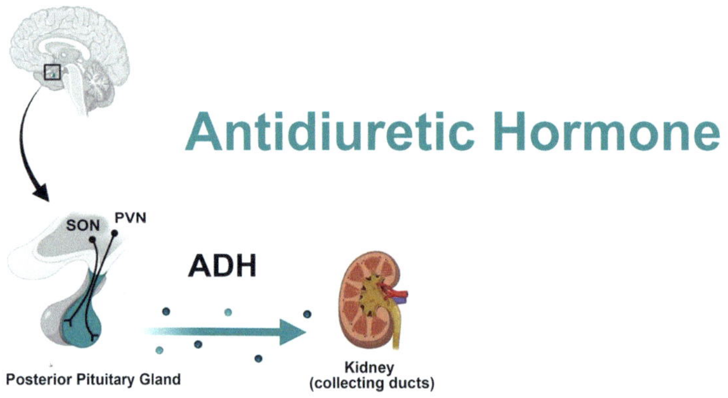

Figure 1.16. Antidiuretic hormone (ADH) control.

Source: https://microbenotes.com/wp-content/uploads/2024/04/Antidiuretic-Hormone-ADH.jpeg.

Aldosterone acts on the distal convoluted tubule and collecting ducts to promote sodium retention and potassium excretion. By promoting increased sodium retention, aldosterone indirectly affects water retention through osmosis, also helping to regulate blood volume and pressure. Moreover, the interaction between aldosterone and ADH suggests a more complex mechanism whereby the kidneys fine-tune electrolyte and fluid balance, a key to overall physiological homeostasis. The significance of learning about ADH and aldosterone goes beyond rudimentary physiology; it has critical implications for many diseases. Hormonal dysregulation has also been linked with disorders like diabetes insipidus, in which inappropriate urinary frequency and thirst are seen with inadequate ADH, and hyperaldosteronism, which can result in hypertension and hypokalemia due to sodium over-retention. Recent space physiology research has illustrated the impact of microgravity on hormonal homeostasis, where fluid shifts induce deranged ADH and aldosterone responses, affecting renal function and electrolyte control (Doty et al., 1994). As researchers further explore these hormonal pathways, they clarify our understanding of kidney function and open avenues for site-directed intervention in the clinic, highlighting the significance of such hormones in modern medical science (Shokr et al., 2016) (Figure 1.16).

1.5.2. Neural Regulation and Feedback Mechanisms

Neural control of renal function is mainly mediated by sympathetic and parasympathetic mechanisms that modulate renal activity under different physiological states. The sympathetic nervous system plays a vital role in the control of glomerular filtration rate (GFR) and renin release, mechanisms which are essential during stress or hypotensive conditions. By stimulating the juxtaglomerular cells to release renin, the sympathetic messages thereby form angiotensin II, a key hormone that constricts the renal arteries and induces sodium reabsorption. Moreover, sympathetic nerve modulation encompasses transport mechanisms in the kidney, specifically in the renal tubules, including the collecting tubules, whose handling of water and sodium is neurally controlled, demonstrating an interaction between neural processes and renal excretory mechanisms (Burnstock et al., 2016). The feedback mechanism within the kidney plays an important role in homeostasis in the sense that it maintains body fluids and electrolytes under equilibrium, even during fluctuations in external conditions. An example worthy of note is the myogenic response, whereby afferent arterioles constrict as blood pressure and flow increase, thereby maintaining a constant GFR. This autonomic response is complemented by hormonal feedback mechanisms, such as the renin-angiotensin-aldosterone system (RAAS), which helps stabilize blood pressure and volume by regulating sodium and water reabsorption. Additionally, the interaction of neural signals with such feedback mechanisms optimizes their effectiveness; sympathetic stimulation not only modulates renal blood flow but also interacts with local mediators to modify responses of the kidney to the varying physiological needs, thus emphasizing the intrinsic role of neuronal input in renal regulation (Leiz et al., 2023). The relationship between neural control and feedback processes within the kidney is crucial for adaptation to diverse physiological conditions, particularly in the context of hypertension and diabetes pathologies. Maladaptive mechanisms, typically evoked by chronic sympathetic overdrive, can predispose to renal damage and dysfunction. In conditions like hypertension, excessive stimulation of the sympathetic nerves has been reported to elevate renal vascular resistance and alter renal tubular function, leading to dysregulation of sodium handling and fluid balance. Renal sympathetic nerve modulation has also been shown in experiments to induce the progression of renal disease by affecting the expression of genes responsible for tubule form and function. This highlights the importance of understanding the mechanisms of neural and feedback interactions in building therapies aimed at minimizing renal complications (Burnstock et al., 2016) (Figure 1.17).

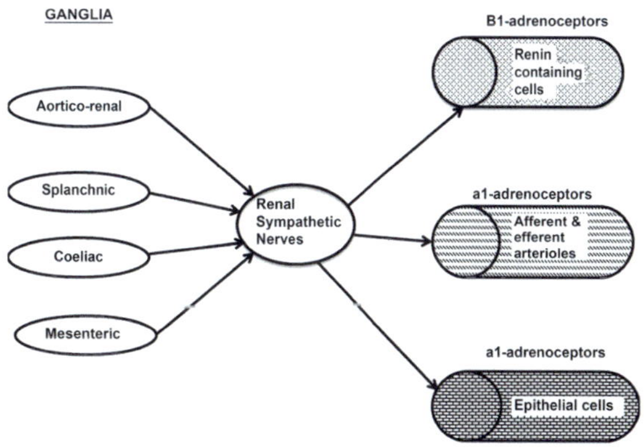

Figure 1.17. The neural regulation of the kidney in hypertension and renal failure.

Source: https://physoc.onlinelibrary.wiley.com/cms/asset/cc2e2246-c9dc-4330-8a38-55b78cb2296b/eph1321-fig-0001-m.jpg.

1.5.3. Impact of Hydration Status on Kidney Function

Hydration level is a key to maintaining the normal function of the kidneys, as the kidneys are responsible for fluid regulation and the excretion of waste. In a well-hydrated state, the kidneys efficiently filter the blood and remove excess electrolytes and metabolic end-products through the urine. Dehydration, conversely, significantly disrupts this process, resulting in a high solute concentration in the renal tubules. This condition not only potentially compromises the kidneys' ability to clear toxins effectively, but can also lead to the formation of kidney stones and other nephrological conditions.

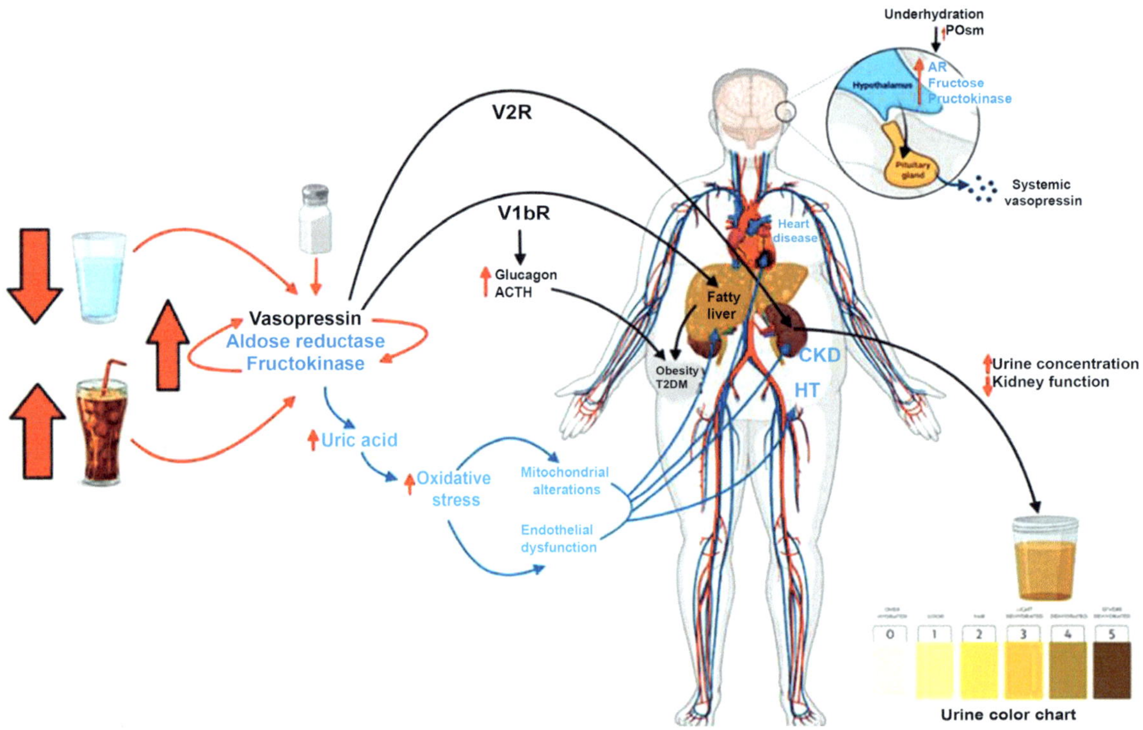

Figure 1.18. Impact of hydration status on kidney function.

Source: https://pub.mdpi-res.com/nutrients/nutrients-14-02070/article_deploy/html/images/nutrients-14-02070-g001.png?1652777790.

Physiological mechanisms by which fluid status affects renal function underscore the need for ongoing surveillance of fluid intake, particularly in vulnerable populations, such as the elderly, who may have unique risks from inadequate hydration. While hydration is essential to preserving kidney function, quantification of hydration status is not without difficulty. Several methods for evaluation of body fluid compartments exist, but the majority are in fact very impractical in a clinical setting, and the absence of a gold-standard compels further confusion. As discussed in prior literature, therapeutic practice gaps may be created by the difficulty in measuring hydration status effectively. For instance, older people often develop decreased thirst perception, and this puts them at risk for dehydration and subsequent renal dysfunction. In this case, clinicians must exert extra efforts to apply existing evaluation techniques, weighing their strengths and weaknesses, to institute timely interventions that are advantageous for kidney function in their patients (Bak et al., 2017). The consensus on adequate fluid intake is particularly pertinent to higher age groups, as recommendations are based on physiological differences. From a review of the literature, it is evident that intake in individuals aged 65 years and above is inconsistent, with mean consumption ranging from 311 to 2390 mL/day. These changes pose a challenge to come up with overall guidelines on hydration for maintaining kidneys. Organizational guidelines, such as those provided by the European Society for Clinical Nutrition and Metabolism (ESPEN), suggest that the daily fluid intake should be approximately 1.6 L for women and 2.0 L for men, including fluid consumption through food and beverages (Botigué et al., 2020). By doing so, they can minimize the risks of kidney failure due to dehydration and ultimately ensure renal well-being, thereby improving the health of older adults (Figure 1.18).

1.6. Common Kidney and Urinary Tract Disorders

Anatomy and physiology of the urinary tract and kidney are crucial in the pathogenesis and treatment of prevalent diseases, such as urinary tract infections (UTIs) and renal calculi. UTIs are most commonly caused by bacterial infections and cause colossal morbidity if not treated and diagnosed promptly. This infection affects millions annually and is characterized by frequent urination, dysuria, and lower abdominal pain. Understanding the mechanisms of the kidneys' filtering and collection, and the ureters' role in conveying urine, is vital in knowing how infection can flourish. The prevalence of UTIs highlights the importance of urine hygiene and hydration intake in maintaining the anatomical and physiological integrity of the urinary tract (Roth et al., 2025). Kidney stones are also a common disorder related to the structural and functional features of the kidney. The pathophysiology of stone formation is multifactorial, involving urine supersaturation, crystallization, and agglutination of substances such as calcium oxalate or uric acid. Risk factors for the development of stones include dehydration, dietary habits, and metabolic disturbances, reflecting the correlation between physiology and anatomy. The obstructive actions of kidney stones can potentially result in pain and complications, such as infection and renal injury, further underscoring the crucial relationship between the renal structures and their physiological roles. Therefore, it is essential to have a comprehensive understanding of kidney anatomy for effective prevention and intervention procedures in addressing kidney stone formation (Astuti et al., 2017). Chronic kidney disease (CKD) and end-stage renal disease (ESRD) are severe health conditions that result from the long-term impairment of renal function, and are often the culmination of numerous underlying diseases. Hypertension, diabetes mellitus, and recurring urinary tract infections are common conditions that can gradually decline kidney function over time. In CKD patients, it is essential to monitor renal function regularly and manage comorbidities to retard the progression to ESRD, which requires dialysis or transplant. The consequences of these conditions extend beyond the physical realm to impact the patient's quality of life and psychological well-being. Consequently, healthcare providers must address these complex interrelations by adopting a multifaceted approach to treatment and prevention that considers both the anatomical structures and their physiological roles in maintaining kidney health (Astuti et al., 2017).

1.6.1. Kidney Stones: Causes and Treatment

Kidney stone development, or nephrolithiasis, is a multifactorial process regulated by many variables, including nutritional intake, metabolic derangements, and hydration status. Calcium stones, the most prevalent type, typically develop due to an excess of calcium in the urine, often exacerbated by inadequate fluid intake or dietary imbalance. Other types of stones, such as uric acid stones, may develop in patients who are dehydrated or have a high protein intake. Also playing a role are intrinsic conditions, such as metabolic disturbances or gastrointestinal disease, which influence the chemical makeup of urine and facilitate stone development. It is essential to acknowledge these etiological factors for effective prevention and management, as they reflect the intricate interplay between kidney physiology and overall health, as detailed in recent studies (Ismail et al., 2001). After the development of kidney stones, their removal or dissolution is necessary, especially for the alleviation of symptoms such as severe pain and urinary obstruction. Treatment varies depending on the size, type, and location of the stones in the urinary tract. Small stones can pass through without requiring treatment, with measures focused on controlling pain and managing fluid intake to facilitate their passage. Medical attention becomes necessary for larger stones or for stones that lead to complications. Techniques such as extracorporeal shock wave lithotripsy (ESWL) break up stones into small fragments that can be easily eliminated. Surgical procedures like ureteroscopy or percutaneous nephrolithotomy are reserved for more complex cases. Selecting an appropriate treatment modality highlights the importance of having comprehensive knowledge about kidney and urinary tract anatomy and physiology, as every treatment impacts these structures and systems differently (Ismail et al., 2001). Preventive and follow-up management are necessary to reduce the risk of recurrence, particularly in individuals with a propensity to develop nephrolithiasis. Crucial actions include dietary modification, increased hydration, and, as appropriate, pharmacologic management aimed at modifying urine composition. Physicians typically order patients to improve their urinary output in order to dilute the stone-forming materials. They may prescribe dietary changes that can limit oxalate and sodium intake, thereby reducing calcium and uric acid excretion in the urine. Furthermore, new guidelines emphasize the coordination between nephrologists and urologists in the treatment of idiopathic calcium nephrolithiasis, citing the importance of a multidisciplinary approach in searching for underlying systemic etiologies (Bartoletti et al., 2016). Through awareness of these preventive and treatment measures, patients can significantly improve their outcomes and quality of life in kidney stone disease (Figure 1.19).

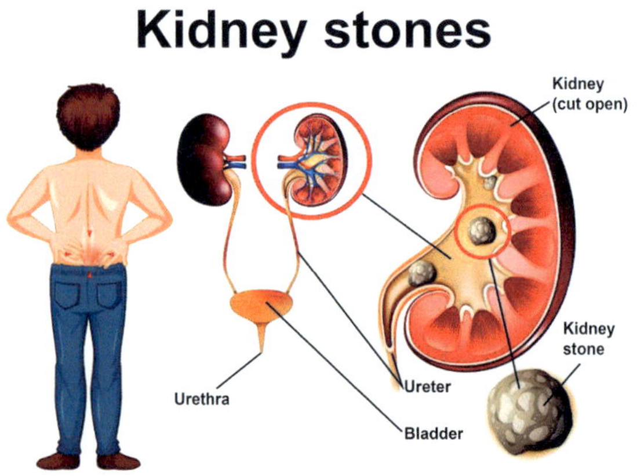

Figure 1.19. Understanding kidney stones.

Source: https://handehospital.org/wp-content/uploads/2024/04/Kidney-Stones-scaled.jpg.

1.6.2. Urinary Tract Infections: Symptoms and Prevention

The frequency and onset of urinary tract infections (UTIs) indicate a significant public health problem, particularly in women. UTI symptoms are frequently presented as dysuria, urgency, frequency of micturition, and lower abdominal pain. These are manifestations of the body's response to inflammation caused by bacterial invasion, typically with organisms such as *Escherichia coli*. The anatomical structure of the urinary tract, e.g., the urethra, bladder, and kidneys, plays a decisive role in susceptibility and symptom occurrence in UTIs. In women, a shorter urethra is a predisposing factor for bacteria to ascend up to the bladder. Recognizing these symptoms is significant as, if not treated, UTIs have the potential to create more severe complications like pyelonephritis or kidney involvement, which may necessitate more intense medical intervention, thus showing the significance of awareness and early intervention.

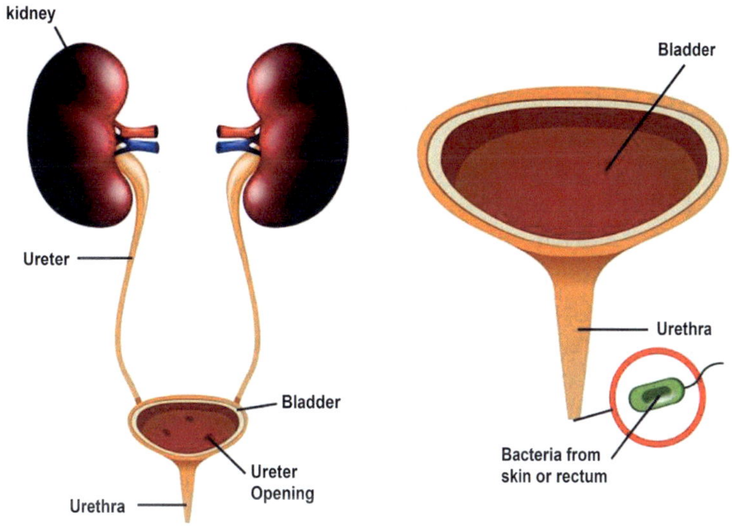

Figure 1.20. Urinary tract infections (UTIs).

Source: https://www.omegahospitals.com/blog/storage/2024/10/17843052-935x765.jpg.

UTI prevention is crucial in preventing the occurrence and improving the overall quality of life in affected individuals. Personal hygiene plays a crucial role in prevention, particularly in women, as poor hygiene practices may lead to bacterial colonization. Recommended are urinating immediately after intercourse, wiping from front to back, and maintaining adequate fluid intake to thicken urine so that it can effectively flush out bacteria. In addition, the interaction between diabetes and UTIs can be significant enough to influence prevention behaviors, most notably among women with diabetes, who are at higher risk due to a variety of factors including impaired immune function and hyperglycemia. A. d. v. s study showed that pre-interventional awareness among diabetic women was relatively low towards the etiological factors in UTIs, reflecting an essential educational need for improving preventive strategies in risk groups (Sayied et al., 2021). Treatment of urinary tract infection typically involves both symptomatic relief and antimicrobial therapy. Clinicians will normally give antibiotics to eliminate offending pathogens, but recurrence may necessitate a more conservative approach, such as prophylactic antibiotics or other modalities like cranberry extract, which is somewhat effective in the prevention of recurrence. Additionally, an understanding of the anatomy and physiology of the urinary tract can inform therapy as well as individual preventive strategies. Current trends indicate a rising incidence of UTIs, likely due to lifestyle changes and growing antibiotic resistance, necessitating ongoing research and adjustments to management practices. Constant education on the signs and symptoms of UTIs and prevention can be of significant benefit in controlling their burden, particularly among vulnerable populations (Al-Modhefer et al., 2016) (Figure 1.20).

1.6.3. Chronic Kidney Disease: Stages and Management

Chronic kidney disease (CKD) is characterized by progressive loss of kidney function, which is classified into five stages based on the estimated glomerular filtration rate (eGFR). Stage 1 is minimal damage with an eGFR of 90 mL/min or more, and stages progress towards end-stage renal disease (ESRD) with an eGFR less than 15 mL/min. There are different clinical manifestations and complications in every stage; early stages have minimal symptomatology, so it is hard to recognize. As the disease advances, patients can have low urine output, electrolyte disturbances, and high blood pressure. Additionally, CKD patients are at higher risk of cardiovascular morbidity and other systemic complications, underlining the need for early identification and appropriate management in a bid to arrest progression and enhance patient outcomes. CKD management is complex and involves modulating intrinsic risk factors, arresting disease progression, and controlling complications. Essential strategies include optimizing blood pressure control, improving glycemic control in diabetic patients, and implementing renal-protective dietary modifications. Renal function monitoring and electrolyte levels are also crucial to adjust therapeutic interventions. Pharmacologic intervention can be facilitated by the administration of angiotensin-converting enzyme (ACE) inhibitors or angiotensin receptor blockers (ARBs), which have shown efficacy in reducing proteinuria and maintaining renal function in patients with CKD. For patients heading toward ESRD, renal replacement therapy counseling involving hemodialysis or kidney transplantation is critical to maximize survival and life quality when kidney function is no longer sustainable. New developments in diagnostic technology, such as contrast-enhanced ultrasound (CEUS), have been termed potential breakthroughs in the evaluation of CKD. CEUS enables the real-time assessment of renal perfusion, potentially facilitating the early detection of kidney impairment. Examination has shown that this imaging method can exhibit significant changes in renal hemodynamic dynamics, a valuable factor to identify the course of the disease (Daminet et al., 2017). Furthermore, identifying the causes of ESRD—such as hypertension, diabetes, and urinary tract infections—is useful for formulating individualized treatment schedules for patients. By resolving these issues in a timely manner, healthcare professionals can more effectively prevent the progression of CKD and enhance clinical management, thereby improving the overall patient prognosis and quality of life (Astuti et al., 2017).

SUMMARY

In outlining the kidneys' and urinary tract's pivotal role within human physiology, it is evident that these organs have more than simply a waste elimination function. Instead, they are fundamentally involved in maintaining homeostasis, regulating fluid balance, and controlling electrolyte levels. The subtlety of renal anatomy—ranging from the intricate organization of nephron units to the elegant vascular supply—allows for the dynamic filtration mechanisms that condition blood composition. Furthermore, alterations in renal pathophysiology, as demonstrated in cases of kidney stones, underscore the importance of comprehending these structures in an integrated manner. The incidence of kidney stones, resulting in approximately 12,000 hospital admissions per year, argues for an understanding of anatomical and physiological concepts and their clinical relevance (Al-Modhefer et al., 2016). Also, innovative renal imaging technologies are a progressive development in nephrology research that facilitates the body's improved comprehension of kidney functions and diseases. Through the identification of imaging biomarkers required, researchers can study not only prevailing conditions but also potential conditions that are caused by the failure of the kidneys to keep pace with metabolic demands. The addition of new imaging technology enhances diagnostic capabilities, enabling early intervention and improved outcomes. These advances, as discussed in meetings such as the "Advances in Renal Imaging" symposium, facilitate interdisciplinary dialogue to advance our current understanding of renal abnormalities (Symposium IIR, 2016). Multidisciplinary collaboration is necessary to condense management approaches and create effective treatment strategies for urinary tract disease. Lastly, the intricate functions of the kidneys and the urinary tract are required by the body's equilibrium. Familiarity with their intricate anatomy and physiology is a point of reference in managing urinary tract disorders. The nature of renal disease, such as stones, demands a keen eye towards both preventive and therapeutic avenues. With the advancement of research, incorporating a sense of respect for anatomy, pathology, and therapeutic modalities will not only enhance clinical practice but also foster a deeper appreciation for the complex nature of renal health. Ultimately, ongoing education and development of imaging and treatment technologies will enable an environment in which improved patient care is more feasible, and future research and therapeutic strategies will be realized.

In kidney and urinary tract anatomy and physiology, it is essential to emphasize the intricate functions that these organs play in regulating homeostasis and overall body function. The kidneys play a crucial role in filtering blood, removing waste, and maintaining electrolyte balance, among other functions. Their intricate structure, with the inclusion of nephron units, facilitates various processes such as glomerular filtration, tubular reabsorption, and secretion. The overloading of these processes not only impacts fluid balance but also is critical to the regulation of blood pressure via mechanisms such as the renin-angiotensin-aldosterone system. An understanding of these interactions is necessary during the assessment of renal function and its effect on overall health. Furthermore, altered renal physiology can have significant clinical implications, particularly within the setting of spinal cord injury (SCI). Studies indicate that SCI can lead to polyuria, characterized by an overproduction of urine, due to changes in neural tracts responsible for regulating kidney function. SCI at various levels has been experimentally examined for its effect on the secretion of hormones such as arginine vasopressin (AVP) and atrial natriuretic peptide (ANP), which are crucial in regulating urine volume and electrolyte balance (Gumbel et al., 2021). This shift explains how neurologic impairments manifest in conjunction with renal dysfunction, and further research into targeted therapies may prove helpful in enhancing the quality of life for these individuals. Furthermore, building an in-depth knowledge of renal anatomy and physiology is crucial to clinical practice and education. Educational tools such as hands-on lab manuals provide helpful information on urinary system function and anatomy, in addition to examinations like urinalysis and physiologic experiments (Beebe et al., 2019). Utilizing these educational tools enables students and professionals to gain a deeper understanding of how the kidney system functions in relation to overall systemic health issues. By combining anatomical data with physiological processes, students can gain a deeper understanding of the intricacies of renal health and the potential impact of various clinical disorders on the urinary system, making them better prepared for real-life situations in healthcare environments.

CLOSER LOOK

ANTIDIURETIC HORMONE (ADH)

ADH, or vasopressin, is a peptide hormone involved in the crucial regulation of body fluid balance, blood pressure, and renal function. ADH is synthesized in the hypothalamus and released from the posterior pituitary gland. It is essential for homeostasis because it helps maintain body water balance. When the body is dehydrated, has increased blood osmolality, or is hypotensive, osmoreceptors in the hypothalamus and baroreceptors in the vascular compartment stimulate the release of ADH into the bloodstream. Secreted, ADH exerts its action in the kidneys, specifically in the collecting ducts and distal tubules, where it binds to V2 receptors on the cells. This binding initiates the insertion of aquaporin-2 water channels into cellular membranes, enabling the more efficient reabsorption of water from the filtrate back into the blood. The volume of urine output is reduced, and blood pressure and volume are increased, restoring the body's balance of fluids.

ADH discharge is under strict control and can be influenced by various factors. Plasma osmolality and decreased blood volume are the primary physiological stimuli, although stress, trauma, pain, and certain drugs can also stimulate its release. Alcohol suppresses ADH release, resulting in urine output during and following ingestion of alcohol and leading to dehydration. The importance of ADH is most starkly evident in clinical states where its equilibrium is disturbed. A case in point is Diabetes Insipidus (DI), which is central (due to the insufficiency of ADH secretion) or nephrogenic (where the kidneys are resistant to ADH). Both result in polyuria, polydipsia, and risk of dehydration. Another condition, the Syndrome of Inappropriate Antidiuretic Hormone Secretion (SIADH), is associated with hypersecretion of ADH in the setting of normal or reduced plasma osmolality, causing water retention, dilutional hyponatremia (low sodium levels), and concentrated urine. Head trauma, infections, tumors, or drugs can elicit SIADH.

Clinically, ADH has significant diagnostic and therapeutic implications—serum and urine osmolality and ADH measurement aid in distinguishing fluid balance disorders. Therapeutically, synthetic ADH analogs such as desmopressin are used in the treatment of central diabetes insipidus and conditions like nocturnal enuresis (bedwetting). Knowledge of ADH's role is also significant in critical care and nephrology, particularly among patients with fluid imbalances, shock, or head injuries. Its vasoconstrictor actions also make it significant in the management of certain types of hypotension. Overall, antidiuretic hormone is a crucial molecule that enables the body to regulate water homeostasis and vascular tone. A dysfunction in its regulation or action has significant clinical implications, underscoring its role in physiology and medicine. It is imperative to know ADH's mechanism, provoking factors, and concomitant disorders to make a diagnosis and management in various healthcare settings effectively.

References

1. Wilkinson, L., Kurniawan, N. D., Phua, Y. L., Nguyen, M. J., Li, J., Galloway, G. J., Hashitani, H., Lang, R. J., & Little, M. H. (2012). Association between congenital defects in papillary outgrowth and functional obstruction in Crim1 mutant mice. *The Journal of Pathology*, *227*(4), 499–510. https://doi.org/10.1002/path.4036AlLugami, A., Sickinger, M., von Pückler, K., Wehrend, A., et al. (2017). Sonography of the distal urethra in lambs. https://core.ac.uk/download/84118352.pdf (accessed on 25th June 2025).
2. Al-Modhefer, A. K., Cunningham, P., Noble, H., Walsh, D., et al. (2016). Kidney stones: Pathophysiology, diagnosis and management. https://core.ac.uk/download/74406360.pdf (accessed on 25th June 2025).
3. Astuti, A. Y., & Mohammad, A. M. (2017). Gender-based health disorders in end-stage renal disease patients in the hospital Elmarj City of Libya. https://media.neliti.com/media/publications/164690-EN-gender-based-health-disorders-in-end-sta.pdf (accessed on 25th June 2025).
4. Bak, A., Greene, C., & Tsiami, A. (2017). Methods of assessment of hydration status and their usefulness in detecting dehydration in the elderly. https://core.ac.uk/download/84342531.pdf (accessed on 25th June 2025).
5. Bartoletti, R., Buchholz, N., Buchholz, N. N. P., Bushinsky, D., et al. (2016). Metabolic diagnosis and medical prevention of calcium nephrolithiasis and its systemic manifestations: A consensus statement. https://core.ac.uk/download/72001809.pdf (accessed on 25th June 2025).
6. Beebe, L., Hesse, D., & Massey, A. (2019). *UGA Anatomy and Physiology 2 Lab Manual* (3rd ed.). https://core.ac.uk/download/217306575.pdf (accessed on 25th June 2025).
7. Botigué, T., Lavedán, A., Masot, O., Miranda Iglesias, A., et al. (2020). Fluid intake recommendation considering the physiological adaptations of adults over 65 years: A critical review. https://core.ac.uk/download/361357072.pdf (accessed on 25th June 2025).
8. Burnstock, G., & Loesch, A. (2016). Sympathetic innervation of the kidney in health and disease: Emphasis on the role of purinergic cotransmission. https://core.ac.uk/download/79521483.pdf (accessed on 25th June 2025).
9. Chen, S., Gao, D., Gaut, J., Hoshi, M., et al. (2019). A single-nucleus RNA-sequencing pipeline to decipher the molecular anatomy and pathophysiology of human kidneys. https://core.ac.uk/download/223009535.pdf (accessed on 25th June 2025).
10. Daminet, S., Duchateau, L., Paepe, D., Saunders, J., et al. (2017). Contrast-enhanced ultrasound examination for the assessment of renal perfusion in cats with chronic kidney disease. https://core.ac.uk/download/158348152.pdf (accessed on 25th June 2025).
11. Dominiczak, A., Ferreri, N. R., & Graham, L. A. (2017). The role of renal transporters and novel regulatory interactions in the TAL that control blood pressure. https://core.ac.uk/download/82893296.pdf (accessed on 25th June 2025).
12. Doty, S. E. (1994). Water and electrolyte regulation during space flight and exercise. https://core.ac.uk/download/38900928.pdf (accessed on 25th June 2025).
13. El Sayied, H., Hemida, S., Mohamed, H., Ragheb, M., et al. (2021). Effect of Web Causation Epidemiological Model on preventive behaviors of diabetic females with genitourinary tract infection. https://core.ac.uk/download/524771923.pdf (accessed on 25th June 2025).

14. Grossman, H. (1973). *Pediatric Uro-Radiology*. https://core.ac.uk/download/51294704.pdf (accessed on 25th June 2025).
15. Gumbel, J. H. (2021). Investigations of potential mechanisms underlying spinal cord injury-induced polyuria. https://core.ac.uk/download/519866981.pdf (accessed on 25th June 2025).
16. Ismail, H. S. (2001). Comparative study between ultrasound and KUB and IVU in renal colic patients in Kelantan. https://core.ac.uk/download/132566828.pdf (accessed on 25th June 2025).
17. IUPUI Imaging Research Symposium. (2016). *2016 Advances in Renal Imaging Symposium*. https://core.ac.uk/download/55533168.pdf (accessed on 25th June 2025).
18. Izzudin, M. (2021). *Analysis of Window Width Variation on Image Anatomical Information MSCT Stenography*. https://core.ac.uk/download/478598064.pdf (accessed on 25th June 2025).
19. Kirdis, H. (2011). Development of novel methods for microbiological evaluation of urology products. https://core.ac.uk/download/622419122.pdf (accessed on 25th June 2025).
20. Kumar, A., Mejino, J. L. V., Rosse, C., Schultz, J., et al. (2005). Anatomical information science. https://core.ac.uk/download/pdf/9412314.pdf (accessed on 25th June 2025).
21. Leiz, J. (2023). Molecular functions of the transcriptional regulator AP-2 alpha (TFAP2A) in the renal collecting duct. https://core.ac.uk/download/574719590.pdf (accessed on 25th June 2025).
22. Manso, M. (2025). Fluid reabsorption across pig urinary bladder. https://core.ac.uk/download/328760428.pdf (accessed on 25th June 2025).
23. Musa, S., & Rrustemi, Q. (2025). Urinary tract infections classification and nursing management. https://core.ac.uk/download/656543434.pdf (accessed on 25th June 2025).
24. N/A. (1997). Change of relative size of renal cortex and medulla related to age. https://core.ac.uk/download/48532388.pdf (accessed on 25th June 2025).
25. Patwardhan, K. (2008). Concepts of human physiology in Ayurveda. https://core.ac.uk/download/pdf/87482.pdf (accessed on 25th June 2025).
26. Roth, E. M. (2025). *Water*. https://core.ac.uk/download/pdf/85242878.pdf (accessed on 25th June 2025).
27. Shokr, E. (2016). *Introduction to Human Physiology for Medical Students*. https://core.ac.uk/download/322470167.pdf (accessed on 25th June 2025).
28. Speck, P. L. (2020). The kidney: A designed system for plasma homeostasis. https://core.ac.uk/download/351114222.pdf (accessed on 25th June 2025).
29. Valparaiso University. (1911). *Old School Catalog 1911–12, Chicago College of Medicine and Surgery*. https://core.ac.uk/download/216810581.pdf (accessed on 25th June 2025).

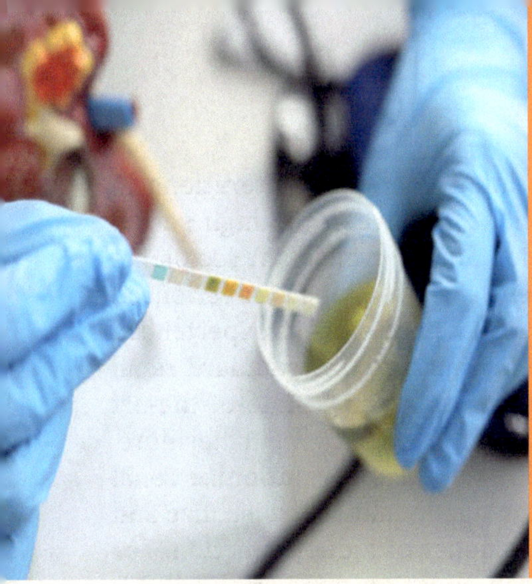

Chapter 2

RENAL FUNCTION TESTS AND DIAGNOSTIC TOOLS

Contents

Introduction

The measurement of renal function is of paramount value in the clinical and research settings and serves as a cornerstone to the diagnosis and treatment of many conditions involving the kidneys. Tests of renal function provide essential information about the kidneys, organs whose basic function is the removal of waste products, the control of electrolytes, and the general homeostasis. With the growing incidence of chronic kidney disease (CKD) globally, awareness and use of appropriate diagnostic tools become more essential. Advances in technology have enhanced the accuracy of testing procedures, paving the way for more sensitive identification of renal dysfunctions. Application of new biomarkers and imaging techniques into routine clinical practice is not only aimed at improving the precision of diagnostics but also to facilitate early intervention measures that play a significant role in patient outcomes. Of the array of tests available for diagnosis, biomarker measurement, such as lipocalin-2 or neutrophil gelatinase-associated lipocalin (NGAL), has been of specific interest. Current evidence suggests that NGAL is a sensitive early marker of acute kidney injury, detecting alterations in kidney function more effectively than traditional tests. The association between the high serum and urine levels of NGAL in deceased donors and later graft function among transplant recipients demonstrates its possible clinical application. Median donor NGAL levels whose kidneys experienced delayed graft function were statistically significantly greater than those whose kidneys experienced early function, demonstrating the relevance of incorporating these biomarkers into standard renal function assays (Minoo et al., 2024). This vision of heading toward embracing state-of-the-art diagnostic practice is a sign of growing interest in precision medicine in nephrology. Furthermore, the advent of advanced imaging technologies and machine learning will also revolutionize renal diagnostics. These technologies can even complement traditional imaging modalities to visualize and characterize the renal anatomy better and make real-time measurements of kidney function. For instance, magnetic resonance imaging (MRI) combined with positron emission tomography (PET) enables the assessment of renal perfusion and metabolic function, providing information about underlying pathology that standard imaging modalities may miss. Additionally, pairing artificial intelligence (AI) with next-generation sequencing technologies can accelerate diagnosis and usher in more personalized treatment regimens. Through the ongoing creation and integration of these advanced diagnostic technologies, healthcare workers can continue to close gaps in the early treatment and diagnosis of renal impairment, thereby promoting better outcomes for patients in terms of renal well-being (Massironi et al., 2024) (Figure 2.1).

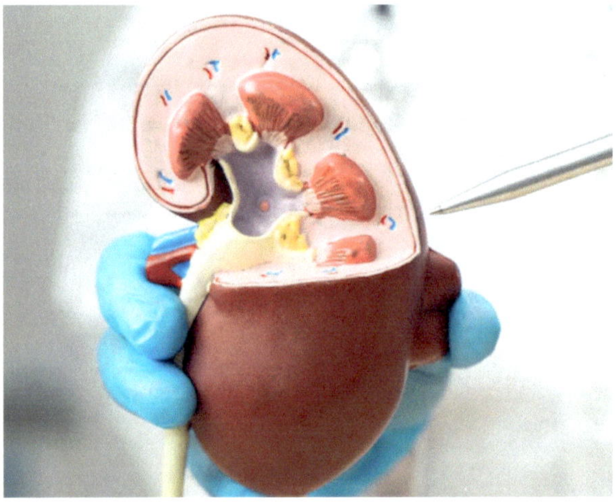

Figure 2.1. Renal function tests for kidney health.

Source: https://hrdiagnostic.in/blog/wp-content/uploads/2024/09/Renal-Function-Tests.jpg.

Definition of Renal Function Tests

Renal function tests are critical diagnostic tests utilized to assess the functionality and health of the kidneys. Renal function tests primarily measure renal functionality in eliminating waste products and assessing the body's general electrolyte status. Serum creatinine, blood urea nitrogen (BUN), and creatinine clearance are the most significant indicators of renal function. An increase in serum creatinine is an indicator of a reduction in glomerular filtration rate (GFR), which means that kidney function is impaired. The tests can diagnose acute kidney injury, chronic kidney disease (CKD), and other renal derangements. Furthermore, knowledge of renal function is essential for managing comorbid conditions such as hypertension and diabetes, as the kidneys play a crucial role in regulating fluid balance, blood pressure, and the metabolism of substances essential for maintaining homeostasis. The value of renal function tests extends beyond the delivery of basic diagnostics; they are also used to convey public health knowledge about CKD incidence and associated risks. CKD has been recognized as a high-priority global health challenge, affecting millions of individuals worldwide. According to research, an estimated 697.5 million CKD cases were reported in 2017, with a global prevalence of approximately 9.1% (Bikbov et al., 2020). This highlights the importance of early detection and follow-up through renal function tests, which can allow for prompt interventions and improve patient outcomes. The tests also enable medical professionals to monitor disease progression and assess sensitivity to treatment, particularly for groups at a higher risk of kidney complications. By integrating renal function tests into regular health screenings, clinicians can significantly help reduce the broader impact of kidney disease on healthcare systems overall. In addition to standard laboratory work, novel diagnostic measures are being explored to enhance the accuracy of renal assessment. More recent technologies, such as imaging and biomarker assays, provide additional data that is beneficial for optimizing diagnoses and directing the treatment plan. For instance, imaging systems can visualize kidney morphology and blood flow, while novel biomarkers may be better predictors of disease behavior or drug responsiveness. Medical professionals must keepstay up-to-date with these developments, as the ESC/EAS Guidelines affirm, recommending the integration of new medical knowledge into clinical practice to ensure the highest quality patient care (François et al., 2019). Therefore, while traditional renal function tests remain the cornerstone of kidney evaluation, the advancement in diagnostic methods emphasizes the importance of adopting a holistic strategy to manage renal well-being effectively.

Importance of Renal Health

Renal function is most important due to its crucial contribution to overall body function. The kidneys are essential regulators of homeostasis, controlling fluid balance, electrolytes, and acid-base balance. They filter waste products out of the blood and excrete them in the urine. With compromised renal function, an accumulation of wastes can lead to severe resultant health effects, from cardiovascular disease to increased mortality. In 2017, approximately 1.2 million people died from chronic kidney disease (CKD), presenting the need for early diagnosis and control measures to promote renal health. Additionally, being aware of the preventability and treatability of CKD is crucial in curbing its incidence globally, particularly in the low and middle-socio-demographic index (SDI) nations, where the disease burden is most disproportionately high (Bikbov et al., 2020). Thus, an active approach to renal health will prevent a significant amount of morbidity and improve the quality of life in various populations. Apart from impacting individual health, the importance of renal health also has significant public health implications. The kidneys not only function as a filter system but are also involved in blood pressure regulation and hormone secretion, such as erythropoietin, which stimulates red blood cell production. Declined kidney function will disrupt these vital processes, resulting in hypertension and anemia, with compounded health risks. The Global Burden of Diseases study demonstrates the intricate association between CKD and elevated cardiovascular disease mortality, an association that identifies the need for comprehensive CKD management (Bikbov et al., 2020). Regular renal function tests play a crucial role in identifying populations at risk and delivering early intervention. By putting renal well-being in the center of health policy, stakeholders can address the structural determinants of CKD occurrence and improve population-level health. Diagnostic testing and renal function tests are essential in monitoring kidney health and preventing further complications. These include serum creatinine tests, urine testing, and imaging tests, which provide vital information on renal status. These tests are of special importance as they not only contribute to the diagnosis of CKD but also to information regarding its etiology, course, and potential impact on other conditions. Current guidelines place strong emphasis on integrating these diagnostic tests into routine healthcare practice to enhance patient care and enable earlier intervention. As the medical community becomes more proactive in applying advances in renal diagnosis, education, and awareness of the necessity to protect the health of the kidneys continues to be crucial. By fostering a culture of preventive care through regular checks and assessments, medical professionals can reduce the burden of kidney disease and its complications, ultimately leading to improved public health management (Figure 2.2).

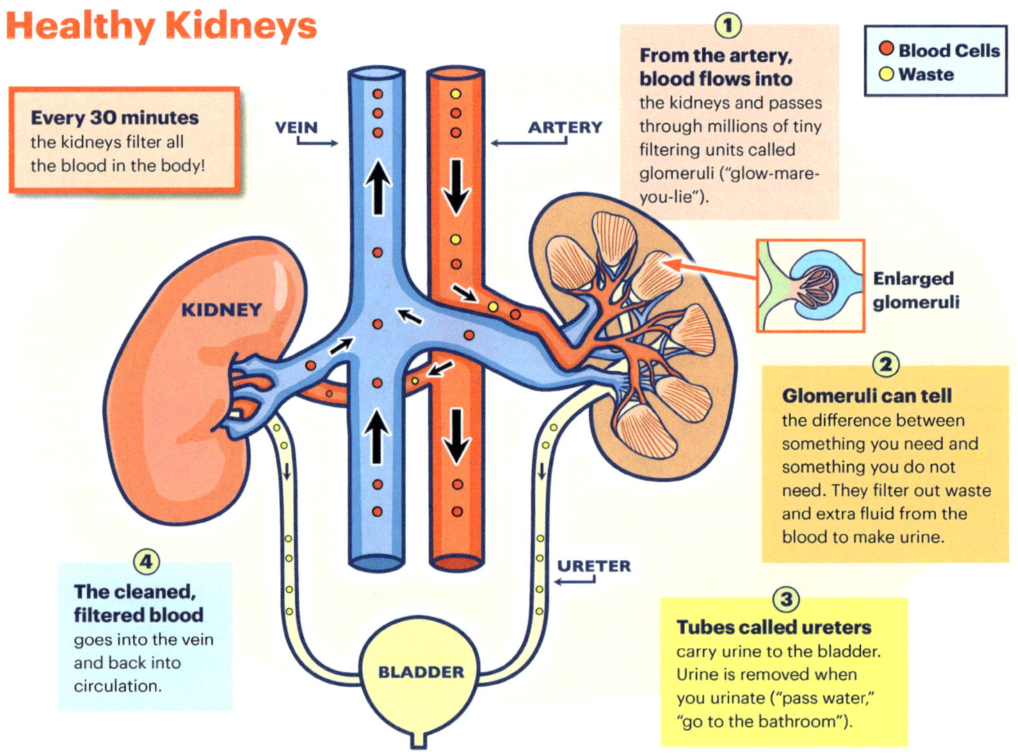

Figure 2.2. Healthy kidneys.

Source: https://www.kidney.org/sites/default/files/2024-10/11-10-0101_GBH_LearnAboutKidneys_4-5%20%281%29.png.

Overview of Diagnostic Tools Available

A range of investigative tools is essential for evaluating renal function as much as for diagnosing kidney-related conditions. Renal function tests (RFTs) are the primary means of checking kidney function. Serum creatinine levels and calculated estimates of glomerular filtration rate (eGFR) are crucial laboratory investigations included in RFTs. Serum creatinine, a byproduct of muscle metabolism, is a measure of a person's intrinsic renal function. An elevated serum creatinine level generally indicates impaired kidney function, as the kidneys are less able to clear this waste product from the body. Furthermore, eGFR offers a more integrated view by considering the impact of age, gender, and body surface area, thereby enabling clinicians to make more precise diagnoses and stage chronic kidney disease (CKD). These tools enable clinicians to make real-time clinical choices and track disease progression longitudinally. In addition to laboratory investigations, imaging modalities are equally crucial in the diagnostic evaluation of renal function. Ultrasonography is a non-invasive imaging technique used routinely for visualizing kidney morphology and assessing abnormalities, such as renal size or parenchymal changes. It has been demonstrated that renal parenchymal thickness, measured by ultrasound, is a significant predictor of the progression of CKD. Compared between CKD patients and healthy controls, the differences in parenchymal thickness were striking, with the measurements of CKD patients being significantly lower. This finding demonstrates the utility of ultrasonography not only for diagnosis but also for monitoring kidney function, thereby solidifying its value as an essential diagnostic aid in addition to RFTs. With the innovations in imaging devices, these enhance the clinician's capacity for gaining insights into renal condition unique to the patient. Additionally, new diagnostic modalities like biomarker analysis and novel imaging modalities are extending renal evaluation broadly. The biomarkers cystatin C and urine markers have shown promise for distinguishing between kidney diseases, with added levels of specificity in diagnosis. Similarly, new imaging techniques, such as magnetic resonance imaging (MRI) and computed tomography (CT), provide enhanced resolution and visualization of kidney architecture and perfusion. However, while new methodology holds excellent potential for future progress, its application may be limited by accessibility, cost, and need for expertise. Therefore, integrating these technologies with traditional RFTs and ultrasonography provides a comprehensive picture of renal function, enabling enhanced patient management and results. These tools, together, form a strong foundation for effective clinical evaluation and treatment of renal well-being, and illustrate the necessity of multidimensional diagnosis in contemporary medicine.

2.1. Anatomy and Physiology of the Kidneys

The kidneys, which are vitally essential organs in the body, are responsible for the upkeep of homeostasis by virtue of their complex form and function. These kidney organs, located in the retroperitoneal space, consist of distinct parts: the renal cortex, renal medulla, and renal pelvis. The nephron is the functional unit of the kidney that performs the tasks of filtering blood, regulating electrolytes, and eliminating waste products. There are approximately one million nephrons in each kidney, which is made up of a glomerulus and a renal tubule. The glomerulus is a filtration membrane in that water, ions, and some solutes pass through it, but it retains larger molecules like proteins. The renal tubules, including the proximal and distal convoluted tubules and loop of Henle, play a crucial role in reabsorption and secretion to enable the body to retain essential nutrients and remain in fluid equilibrium. Renal function tests (RFTs) are highly crucial in determining kidney function and identifying disease. These examinations evaluate renal function to clear waste products from the blood, primarily by measuring the serum creatinine level and estimating the glomerular filtration rate (eGFR).

The eGFR is a crucial parameter that reflects the kidneys' efficiency; a considerable decline typically indicates impaired renal function. Additionally, imaging modalities of the kidneys, such as ultrasonography, allow for assessment of kidney size and parenchymal thickness, which is crucial in the case of disease conditions such as CKD and congenital structural abnormalities. In recent years, research has shown that renal parenchymal thickness, measured by ultrasound, can be a useful predictor of CKD progression, adding to the value of imaging and complementing conventional RFTs (Ahmad et al., 2025).

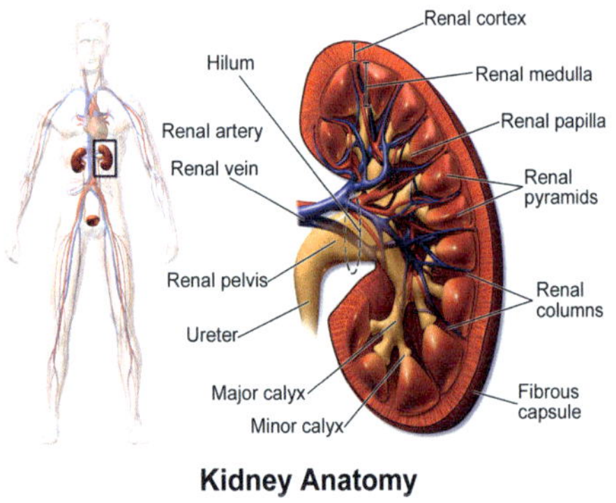

Figure 2.3. Anatomy of the kidneys.

Source: https://upload.wikimedia.org/wikipedia/commons/d/d6/Blausen_0592_KidneyAnatomy_01.png.

Additionally, enhanced diagnostic technology increases the potential to differentiate between various forms of anemia, which can be associated with renal function. For instance, serum hepcidin is an essential marker that distinguishes iron deficiency anemia (IDA) from anemia of chronic disease (ACD), which is more common in the elderly population. In view of the challenge presented by bone marrow tests, which are invasive, hepcidin offers a less burdensome alternative for clinical assessment. This refers to the importance of applying a combination of serum hepcidin and standard iron profiles in their diagnosis to guarantee an accurate diagnosis for anemia, thus providing a broader range of patient care. Eventually, the incorporation of these innovative biomarkers with conventional renal function tests can lead to more accurate diagnoses in patients with renal-related disorders (Manna et al., 2025) (Figure 2.3).

2.1.1. Structure of the Kidneys

The structure of the kidneys is central to their function, serving as the body's principal organ for purifying blood and regulating various physiological processes. Located retroperitoneally along the sides of the vertebral column, each kidney is individually bean-shaped. Internally, the kidney is divided into the cortex and the medulla. The renal cortex, the outer layer, houses the glomeruli and renal tubules that are responsible for blood filtration. Adjacent to this is the renal medulla, consisting of renal pyramids that contribute to urine production. Distinguishing between these areas is crucial when evaluating renal function tests to assess the efficacy of nephron function and overall kidney health (Ahmad et al., 2025). Abnormal findings in the renal structure, including parenchymal thinning, can represent chronic kidney disease and aid in the structural assessment during diagnosis. Ultrasonography is a powerful non-invasive imaging modality for identifying kidney structure and function. In producing accurate definitions of renal anatomy, ultrasound enables physicians to visualize abnormalities such as cysts, tumors, and alterations in the renal parenchyma. For instance, studies have found that significant decreases in renal parenchymal thickness are common in patients with chronic kidney disease and thus structures are related to renal function tests like serum creatinine and estimated glomerular filtration rate (Ahmad et al., 2025). Additionally, the ability to quantify changes in kidney size and shape can assist in identifying congenital defects or obstructions that impact renal function. Therefore, regular ultrasonographic examination plays a crucial role in the diagnosis and treatment of renal disease in its initial stages. In addition to imaging techniques, urine cytology has also proven to be an essential method for evaluating the kidneys' structure and function. Urine analysis enables the evaluation of cellular changes indicative of kidney pathology, such as kidney stones or cancer. For example, it has been demonstrated through research that patients with kidney stones exhibit significant nuclear atypical changes in urinary sediments that may be related to renal dysfunction as assessed through eGFR. The specificity of the eGFR in detecting such abnormalities also identifies the relationship between structural evaluation and measurement of renal function. Thus, a total understanding of kidney anatomy is essential not only for accurate diagnosis but also for the design of targeted treatment plans, thereby bridging the gap between structural assessment and kidney health management.

2.1.2. Functions of the Renal System

The renal system performs vital functions required to establish homeostasis within the body. The primary function of the kidneys is to filter blood and produce urine, essentially removing waste products, excess substances, and toxins. Filtration plays a crucial role in electrolyte balance, acid-base homeostasis, and fluid volume.

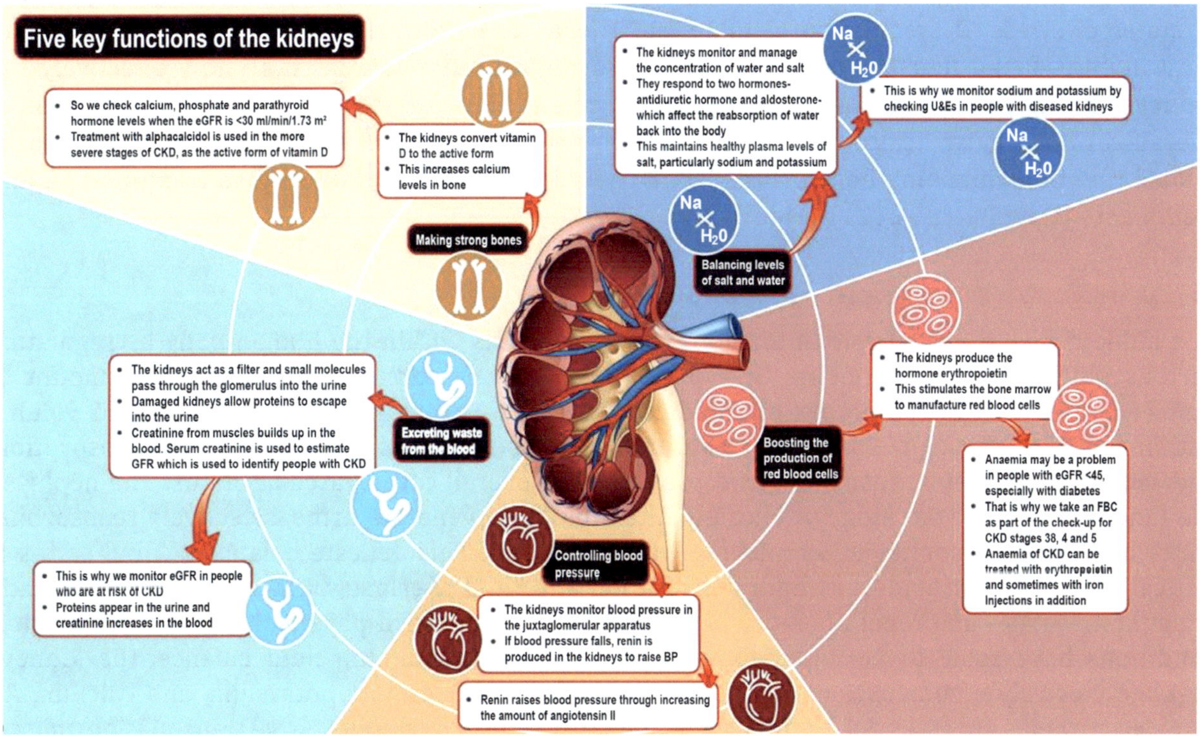

Figure 2.4. Key kidney functions.

Source: https://www.issuesandanswers.org/wp-content/uploads/2020/02/828fffe53a98f0c1514968a7bec47b66-scaled.jpg.

For example, the kidneys filter out urea and creatinine, waste products of protein metabolism that need to be eliminated to prevent toxic accumulation. Furthermore, the renal system regulates the concentration of various ions, including sodium and potassium, thereby helping to control blood pressure and overall cardiovascular function. The role of the kidney in regulating the composition of blood is directly associated with various tests of renal function, as they check how practical and functional the kidneys are in eliminating waste (David et al., 2021). In addition to waste elimination, the renal system also plays a role in hormone secretion. Erythropoietin is a hormone secreted by the kidneys to stimulate red blood cell production when the blood lacks sufficient oxygenation. This function plays a crucial role in maintaining the body's adequate oxygen-carrying capacity. The renal process also metabolizes vitamin D into calcitriol, which is essential for calcium absorption and bone health. Kidney hormone regulation impacts not only organ function but also overall body health, showing the symbiotic interaction between kidney function and bodily demand. Hormonal activity can be measured as crucial in diagnosing certain conditions such as anemia or metabolic bone disease, thus, making integral renal function tests a necessity (Bikbov et al., 2020). Moreover, the kidney system is also responsible for regulating blood pressure through the renin-angiotensin-aldosterone system (RAAS). When blood pressure decreases, the kidneys release renin, an enzyme that triggers a cascade of events leading to vasoconstriction and fluid retention. This system not only raises blood pressure but also raises kidney perfusion to maintain filtration processes even in states of stress. Dysregulation of this system leads to serious diseases like hypertension and heart failure. Renal function tests, therefore, provide information regarding how effectively the kidneys are managing fluid and electrolyte balance and illustrate their key role in the process of overall cardiovascular health and disease. The intricate roles of the renal system underscore its crucial role in maintaining homeostasis, which necessitates specialized diagnostic equipment and treatments (David et al., 2021) (Figure 2.4).

2.1.3. Role of Kidneys in Homeostasis

The kidneys play a crucial role in maintaining homeostasis within the human body by regulating various physiological parameters. One of their primary functions is regulating the amount of fluid, which is crucial for proper physiological function. The kidneys regulate the fluid volume within the body through a set of intricate mechanisms that encompass filtration, reabsorption, and secretion, thereby influencing blood pressure and overall cardiovascular status. The nephron, the functional unit of the kidney, delicately filters blood to generate urine, selectively reabsorbing water and essential solutes and removing waste products. This delicate balance of fluid status is critical; dysregulation underlies both dehydration and fluid overload, both of which significantly affect homeostasis and renal function, as renal responses to varied physiological and pathological conditions have come to be understood. In addition to maintaining fluid balance, the kidneys regulate electrolyte homeostasis by controlling the levels of sodium, potassium, and calcium. All these electrolytes are essential for numerous cellular functions, including nerve transmission, muscle contraction, and enzyme activity. The kidneys achieve this balance, in large part, by depending on hormones such as aldosterone and antidiuretic hormone (ADH), which modulate sodium and water reabsorption according to the body's needs. Electrolyte imbalance can lead to severe health issues, including muscular dysfunction and cardiac arrest. Therefore, assessment of renal function through diagnostic tests, such as serum electrolytes and glomerular filtration rate (GFR) tests, is crucial for understanding a patient's homeostatic potential and guiding follow-up interventions, particularly in patients with signs of renal dysfunction. Kidney function also impacts acid-base balance. The kidneys help to maintain the body's pH in a minimal range, which is essential for metabolic functions. By excreting hydrogen ions and reabsorbing bicarbonate in the urine, the kidneys assist in buffering dietary, metabolic, or pathophysiologic acid-base changes. These conditions, like chronic kidney disease (CKD), can alter these regulatory mechanisms, leading to metabolic acidosis and other accompanying disturbances. Monitoring and tracking of these changes through renal function tests are crucial in advancing timely and efficient medical intervention. Highly advanced diagnosis tools, including genetic testing as supported by research focusing on TMEM216 gene mutations, illustrate the importance of intensive assessment techniques considering both renal function and homeostatic control, thereby enhancing patient therapy and outcomes in renal pathology, as shown in recent research (Manna et al., 2025; Sun et al., 2025) (Figure 2.5).

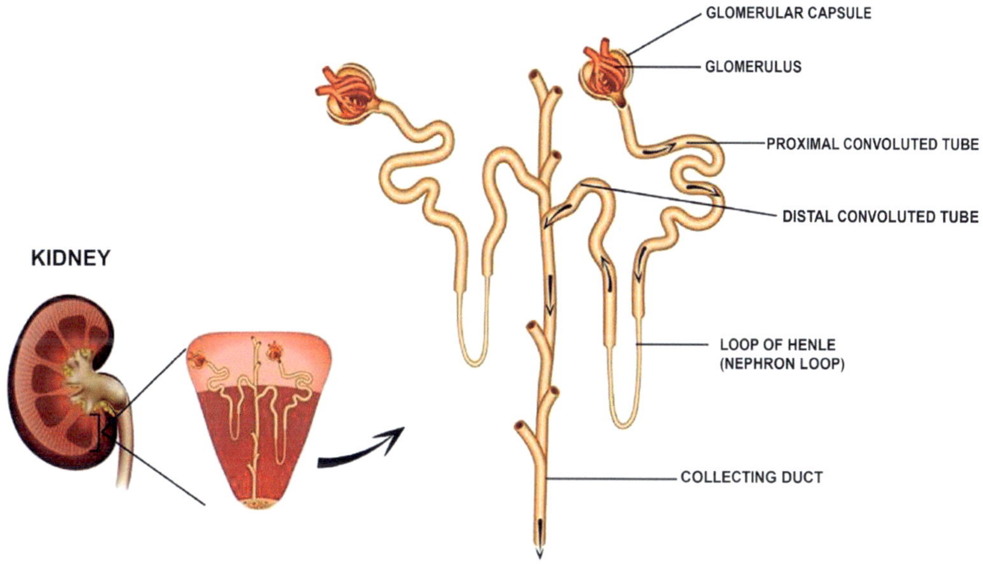

Figure 2.5. Role of the kidneys in homeostasis.

Source: https://external-content.duckduckgo.com/iu/?u=https%3A%2F%2Fwww.ase.org.uk%2Fsites%2Fdefault%2Ffiles%2Fabpi_homeostasis_kidney_small.jpg&f=1&nofb=1&ipt=1e7e06abe844aa417091abf183af93bc188a97304b1e5c5de539ec258dfd7bd4.

2.2. Common Renal Function Tests

Kidney function tests are essential diagnostic procedures utilized for evaluating the kidneys' efficacy in waste product filtration, fluid balance regulation, and maintenance of various levels of electrolytes in the body. Amongst the most common tests are serum creatinine, blood urea nitrogen (BUN), and glomerular filtration rate (GFR) measurements. Serum creatinine is a byproduct of muscle metabolism, and its concentration in blood provides a reliable estimate of kidney function. An elevated serum creatinine typically indicates deranged nephron function and merits investigation and treatment. BUN, however, is used to assess kidney filtration function but can also be influenced by non-renal conditions, such as nutrition and circulatory volume. Hence, the employment of these tests in conjunction delivers comprehensive information about renal function and health. Aside from regular tests, urinary testing is also crucial in evaluating kidney function. Determination of abnormalities, such as proteinuria or hematuria, which can be evidence of existing kidney disease, can be made through urine testing. For instance, albuminuria can be utilized as an indicator of diabetic kidney disease early on, alerting clinicians to the potential for future complications. Additionally, a 24-hour urine collection can provide information regarding the kidneys' capacity for excreting certain substances and assess electrolyte balance. This test, contributes to a comprehensive assessment of renal health, along with spot urine samples. A combination of urinary analysis with serum testing increases diagnostic sensitivity so that clinicians can better customize treatment plans. New technologies and new diagnostic methods continue to advance in renal function testing. As the healthcare landscape continues to evolve, promising methods such as liquid biopsies and advanced biomarkers are being increasingly recognized as having the potential to aid in diagnosis. These emerging tools can detect subtle changes in renal function and have significant potential as an adjunct to routine tests. For instance, progress in identifying epigenetic modifications could lead to the discovery of diagnostic biomarkers that enable the detection of kidney disease at an earlier stage, ultimately achieving improved outcomes for patients. The discovery of such advancements highlights the urgency for identifying kidney disease at an early stage, along with effective interventions to manage kidney diseases. The integration of novel methodologies and conventional tests promotes a comprehensive approach to renal health assessment, thereby ensuring best-in-class care for patients with kidney disease (Liu et al., 2025; Dybiec et al., 2024) (Figure 2.6).

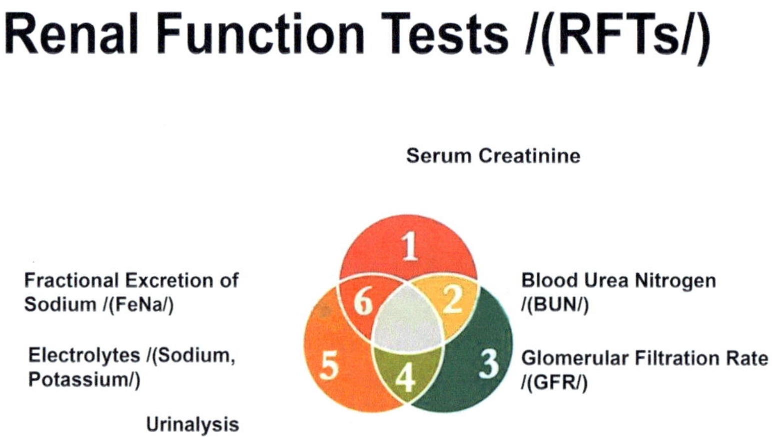

Figure 2.6. Common renal function tests.

Source: https://fastercapital.co/i/Clinical-Laboratory-Value-Understanding-Common-Clinical-Laboratory-Values--A-Comprehensive-Guide--Renal-Function-Tests---RFTs--.webp.

2.2.1. Serum Creatinine Test

Serum creatinine is a vital laboratory test used in assessing renal function, particularly in determining the presence of chronic kidney disease (CKD). Creatinine is a waste product of muscle metabolism that is usually excreted by the kidneys. Elevated serum creatinine levels can indicate impaired kidney function, prompting further diagnostic testing. This is a relatively straightforward test, which involves a blood test to assess the level of creatinine, providing a reflection of the glomerular filtration rate (GFR). Serum creatinine should be carefully interpreted, as age, sex, and muscle mass can alter baseline levels. Therefore, the serum creatinine test is a screening used in initial assessments that can lead to more specific tests or examinations, thus facilitating early interventions in individuals at risk of kidney disease. In CKD, the serum creatinine test is critical for the estimation of incidence and prevalence rates globally, as demonstrated in recent research. Studies have evidenced that, as of 2017, approximately 697.5 million individuals worldwide were afflicted with varying stages of CKD, illustrating the increasing disease burden. Furthermore, the numbers indicate that mortality due to CKD has increased immensely in the past decades, highlighting an urgent need for earlier identification through the utilization of practical diagnostic tools such as the serum creatinine test (Bikbov et al., 2020). This upsurge in CKD incidence has serious consequences for the public health system, and it demands a focus on increasing renal function screening to facilitate early detection and treatment of the disease, preceded by severe morbidity and mortality. The serum creatinine test, so practical as it is, cannot be judged in isolation. It should be considered as one of a wide range of renal function tests and diagnostic procedures that further the overall evaluation of kidney health. Additional tests, such as urine examination and imaging studies, can provide additional data regarding renal status. Agency standards emphasize the value of a multi-faceted treatment and diagnosis approach to CKD (Williams et al., 2018). By integrating the serum creatinine test with other diagnostic technologies, clinicians can better detect renal dysfunction and administer interventions that target the underlying causes of kidney disease, resulting in improved patient outcomes and reduced treatment of renal-related diseases (Figure 2.7).

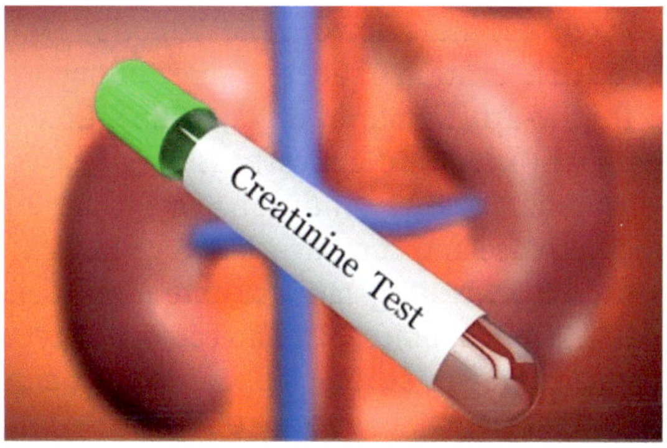

Figure 2.7. Serum creatinine test.

Source: https://images.apollo247.in/pd-cms/cms/2025-05/AdobeStock_293261041%20(1).jpg?tr=q-80,f-webp,w-400,dpr-2.5,c-at_max%201000w.

2.2.2. Blood Urea Nitrogen (BUN) Test

The BUN is an essential diagnostic tool for renal function evaluation, a reflection of the ability of the body to excrete waste through the kidneys. Urea is a by-product of protein metabolism, and concentration in the blood may be utilized as a reflection of the effectiveness of kidney function in excreting it from the blood. Normal BUN levels typically range from 7 to 20 mg/dL; a value outside this range may indicate various pathophysiological conditions. Elevated BUN is generally indicative of renal dysfunction or impairment, although it may be caused by causes other than renal, e.g., gastrointestinal hemorrhage, excessive high-protein intake, and dehydration. Isolated estimation of BUN will therefore often be inadequate to provide true and accurate impression of renal function, and thus clinicians employ the estimation along with other investigations, e.g., serum creatinine and urine analysis. When considering the clinical usefulness of BUN levels, attention must be given to their shortcomings and potential interference with other measures of renal function. For instance, as research indicates, BUN levels are influenced by factors unrelated to kidney function, such as age, gender, and muscle mass, making the test value challenging to interpret. Moreover, accuracy in BUN is often enhanced when measured in conjunction with serum creatinine, which is a more direct indicator of renal function. In a review, it was noted that certain clinical conditions, such as dehydration or acute kidney injury, exhibit changes in BUN that warrant further examination and follow-up (Kumaran et al., 2025). Consequently, while the BUN test is essential, it should be part of an integral diagnostic strategy that utilizes several parameters to provide an integrative assessment of renal condition. The value of BUN testing is also in evaluating the progression of kidney disease and complications. For individuals with chronic diseases leading to renal impairment, repeated BUN testing can facilitate monitoring of treatment efficacy and enable timely adjustment of patient management. In one retrospective study, increased BUN was found to be associated with poor outcomes in several populations, including patients with life-threatening infections, such as COVID-19 (Ziamajidi et al., 2024). This underscores the applicability of the test beyond routine renal assessment because BUN levels may reflect systemic disease and inflammation. As technology advances in medicine and the pathophysiologic basis for renal disease is better understood, the BUN test will undoubtedly remain a mainstay in renal function testing and patient care in a variety of clinical arenas (Figure 2.8).

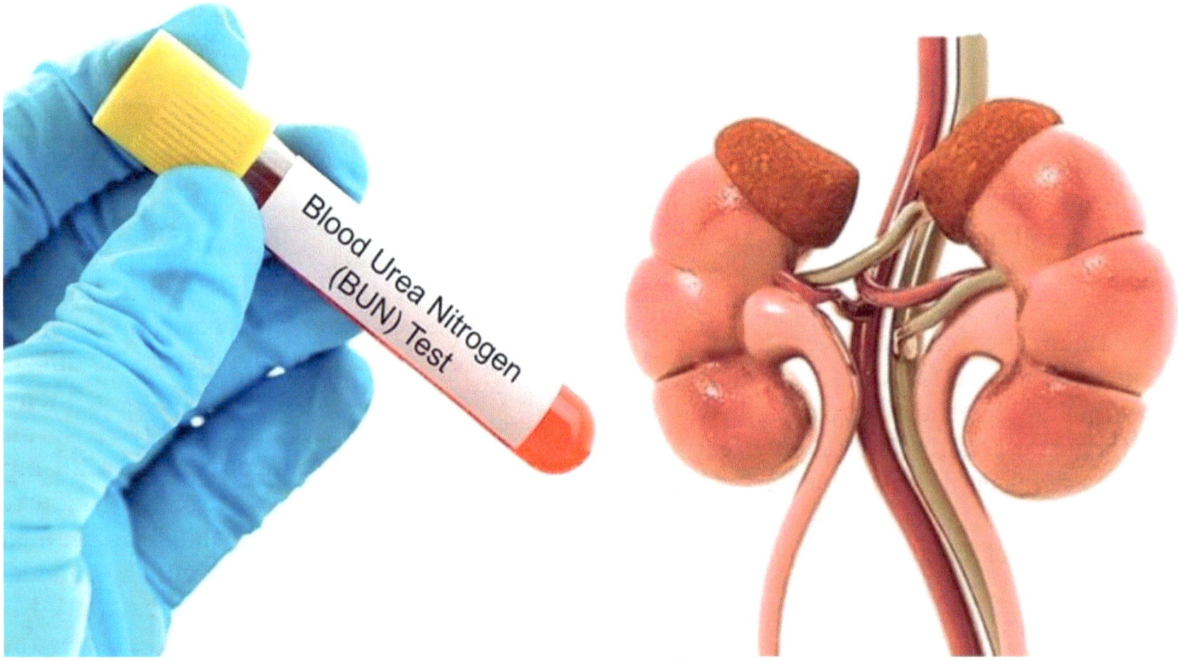

Figure 2.8. Blood urea nitrogen (BUN) test.

Source: https://requestatest.com/includes/uploads/blog/BUN.jpg.

2.2.3. Glomerular Filtration Rate (GFR) Estimation

GFR estimation is a critical component of renal function assessment and a principal marker for kidney health. Estimation of GFR is used to diagnose CKD, predict its stage, and guide appropriate management. In the past, GFR was measured directly by inulin clearance, an invasive procedure that has progressively been supplanted by estimates from serum creatinine concentrations due to ease of performance and cost-effectiveness. The development of equations such as the Cockcroft-Gault and, more recently, the Chronic Kidney Disease Epidemiology Collaboration (CKD-EPI) equation allows clinicians to approximate GFR from available serum creatinine, allowing timely interventions that are capable of preventing CKD progression and complications as outlined in the 2024 revised KDIGO guidelines (Levin et al., 2024). Cystatin C is a helpful alternative to creatinine in estimating GFR, particularly in populations where creatinine results can be affected by variables such as muscle mass or diet. The protein, which is secreted at a relatively constant rate by all nucleated cells, yields a more stable assessment of renal function, particularly in patients with compromised muscle metabolism or in the elderly. Additionally, it has been recommended that combining creatinine and cystatin C measurements could enhance the precision of GFR estimation, aligning with current clinical practice guidelines and emphasizing the importance of precise and accurate kidney function tests in patient management (Levin et al., 2024). The integration of these markers in routine assessment reflects the dynamic nature of renal diagnostics and supports improved outcomes for CKD patients. Moreover, accurate estimation of GFR not only plays a critical role in the diagnosis and staging of CKD but also in therapeutic management and allocation of resources in health systems. New evidence shows an increasing prevalence of CKD worldwide with related morbidity and mortality due to decreased renal function. Burden to the health system calls for robust diagnostic tools in effective detection of at-risk populations. The application of eGFR formulas facilitates the early identification of CKD, enabling preventive measures and timely referral to nephrology. Further, ongoing research on novel diagnostic markers and newer technologies endeavors to further refine GFR estimation to increase accuracy and reducing variability, thereby facilitating optimal patient management in the spectrum of CKD (Figure 2.9).

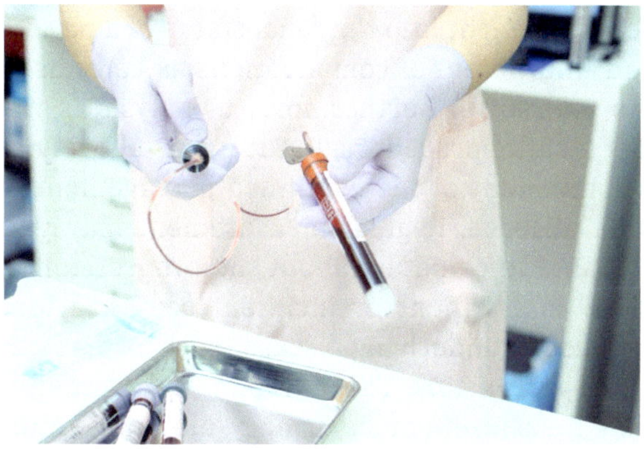

Figure 2.9. Estimated glomerular filtration rate (eGFR) test.

Source: https://www.verywellhealth.com/thmb/1PnIoq7cxjYWj1PoFZLo_p0PSLU=/1500x0/filters:no_upscale():max_bytes(150000):strip_icc()/instruments-collect-patient-s-blood-935307896-84ddb23d2ea040a8a01c43176cf7d58b.jpg.

2.3. Urinalysis as a Diagnostic Tool

Urinalysis is a fundamental diagnostic tool in the discipline of nephrology, playing a significant role in evaluating renal function. It is a non-invasive examination in which urine features, such as color, clarity, concentration, and pH, are examined, as well as the presence of biochemical substances. Among the most significant findings that are tested are proteins, glucose, and creatinine, which, when found at abnormal levels, can indicate the presence of kidney disease or impairment. Remarkably, the 2024 KDIGO Clinical Practice Guideline emphasizes the application of urinalysis, along with serum creatinine-based estimated glomerular filtration rate (eGFR) estimation, to increase precision in the detection of chronic kidney disease (CKD) (Levin et al., 2024). By using urinalysis in combination with other exams, health care professionals can gain general insight into the renal status of a patient and find potential complications as early as in the course of. Furthermore, urinalysis is not just a static procedure, but it works actively as a component of the continued management of renal disease. Regular measurement may give valuable information about the progression of renal impairment or incipient complications because of underlying diseases such as diabetes or hypertension. The guideline recommends that measurement of urinary albumin—most often by albumin-to-creatinine ratio (ACR)—is crucial for risk stratification and prediction of unfavorable health outcomes in individuals with known CKD (Bryan et al., 2021). This ongoing surveillance facilitates the effective adjustment and adaptation of therapeutic methods according to changing health trends in the patient. Consequently, urinalysis becomes not only a diagnostic tool but also a marker of disease progression and therapy efficacy, thereby illustrating its valuable contribution to overall management of renal health. In addition, it has enhanced the role of urinalysis in the clinical setting by incorporating cutting-edge technologies, including point-of-care testing (POCT). POCT enables quick analysis and instant feedback, which is able to improve decision-making processes in acute care situations, hence making patient management efforts more streamlined. This ability is most crucial in facilities where laboratory access is limited, so that vital information can be made available for timely interventions. KDIGO guidelines advocate for the standardization of urinalysis protocols to ensure comparability and accuracy in diverse clinical environments, thereby optimizing patient outcomes (Levin et al., 2024; Bryan et al., 2021). In summary, with growing awareness and advancements in urinalysis technology, it remains a valuable tool in the diagnostic armamentarium for assessing renal function and guiding efficient patient care (Figure 2.10).

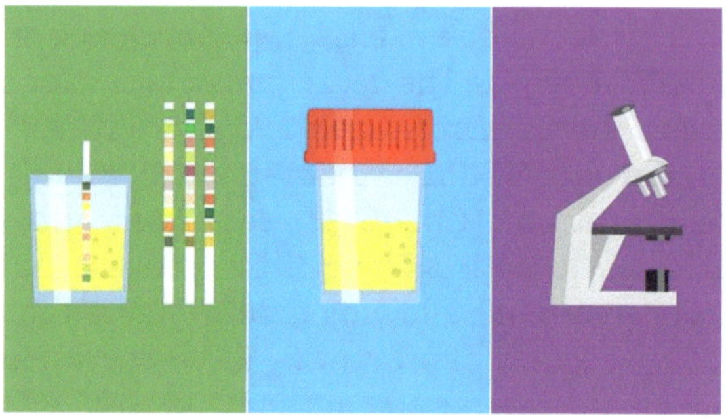

Figure 2.10. Urinalysis as a diagnostic tool.

Source: https://images.everydayhealth.com/images/urinary-conditions/urine/what-is-urinalysis-and-how-is-it-done-722x406.jpg?sfvrsn=425c2827_1.

2.3.1. Components of Urinalysis

Urinalysis is a valuable component of renal function evaluation and overall health status, providing a view into pathological processes. Physical, chemical, and microscopic urine analysis is usually part of the evaluation. Physical characteristics such as color, clarity, and specific gravity are assessed to yield information about hydration status and potential urinary tract disease. For instance, dark urine typically means dehydration, while turbid urine can signal infection. The chemical analysis measures pH, protein, glucose, and blood parameters, providing vital information about the metabolic condition and kidney function. Elevated protein levels might be a sign of renal injury, which could warrant further investigation of conditions like diabetes or hypertension. Therefore, the meticulous procurement and interpretation of urinalysis results are essential elements of the diagnosis and evaluation of renal function. Microscopic examination of urine is crucial for identifying cellular and crystalline elements that may indicate underlying pathology. This examination includes the presence of red blood cells, white blood cells, casts, and crystals, which collectively render a composite impression of renal pathology. The amount of red blood cells, for example, may indicate glomerular injury or damage to the urinary tract, while elevated white blood cell counts tend to suggest infections or urinary tract inflammation. Additionally, urine casts, which are composed of proteins secreted by injured renal tubules, may indicate certain forms of kidney disease. Identification of these factors is both science and detail-oriented as slight variations in outcome contribute significantly to clinical decision-making. Thus, microscopic analysis needs to be employed to correlate the results of urinalysis with clinical manifestations and direct subsequent diagnostic procedures. The auxiliary use of ultrasound and renal function tests also enhances renal function assessment beyond routine urinalysis. For instance, ultrasonography is a non-invasive technique used to investigate anatomical structures and measure kidney size, parenchymal thickness, and the presence or absence of obstructions. It has been determined through research that there are significant differences in renal parenchymal thickness among healthy individuals and individuals with CKD, which can be assessed by ultrasound parameters (Ahmad et al., 2025). Additionally, renal function tests such as serum creatinine and the estimated glomerular filtration rate (eGFR) are used to complement urine analysis and provide a more comprehensive picture of renal function. For pediatric patients with ureteropelvic junction obstruction (UPJO), urinary findings correlated with sonographic renal pelvic diameter (RPD) can also establish renal function status (Mahasin et al., 2025). Together, these strategies highlight the interdependent nature of urinalysis and other renal evaluation methods in developing effective diagnostic strategy.

2.3.2. Interpretation of Urinalysis Results

Urinalysis interpretation is one of the leading roles in the assessment of renal function and diagnosis of renal abnormalities. Urinalysis is composed of several elements, including physical, chemical, and microscopic evaluation, that offer essential information regarding kidney health. A physical examination involves observing urine color, clarity, and specific gravity, which can indicate hydration status or kidney insufficiency. The chemical profile determines the levels of such compounds as protein, glucose, and ketones, and essential deviations from normal tend to reflect underlying disease conditions like nephrotic syndrome or diabetes mellitus. Notably, the correlation between abnormal urinalysis and renal impairment has been well addressed in clinical practice guidelines, emphasizing the importance of critical interpretation to optimize effective management of the patient, particularly in chronic kidney disease, as outlined in KDIGO guidelines (Levin et al., 2024). Microscopic evaluation of urine also adds to the diagnostic information by identifying cellular elements, casts, and crystals that may represent renal or systemic diseases. For instance, the presence of red blood cells may indicate glomerular damage or bleeding from the urinary tract, while the presence of white blood cells suggests infection or inflammation. Crystals and casts generated in the renal tubules also provide diagnostic specificity, enabling clinicians to differentiate between acute and chronic processes. With an awareness of the significance of these findings and how they align with existing clinical guidelines, clinical professionals can tailor diagnostic and therapeutic strategies accordingly. Most significantly, the interpretation of urinalysis results should consider the patient's clinical context and history to avoid misdiagnosis due to passing aberrancies or non-pathological states that mimic pathology, as emphasized by the KDIGO 2024 Clinical Practice Guideline and its commitment to inclusive evaluation protocols (Levin et al., 2024). Furthermore, the integration of point-of-care testing (POCT) for urinalysis has transformed clinical practices, thanks to the timely nature of the results that enable instant decision-making. This innovation is crucial in the effective management of acute conditions, such as urinary tract infections or worsening chronic kidney disease. POCT equipment provides real-time feedback on urine quality, allowing clinicians to respond immediately, which is invaluable in time-critical circumstances. To ascertain accuracy and timely reliability, however, uniform procedures in collecting and processing specimens must be utilized. The KDIGO 2024 guidelines suggest robust practices in POCT implementation for the purpose of making valid interpretations to inform patient care and outcomes. As technology improves and nephrology continues evolving, ongoing education regarding the interpretation of urinalysis remains critical for healthcare providers as they navigate the nuances of renal diagnostics and patient management (Figure 2.11).

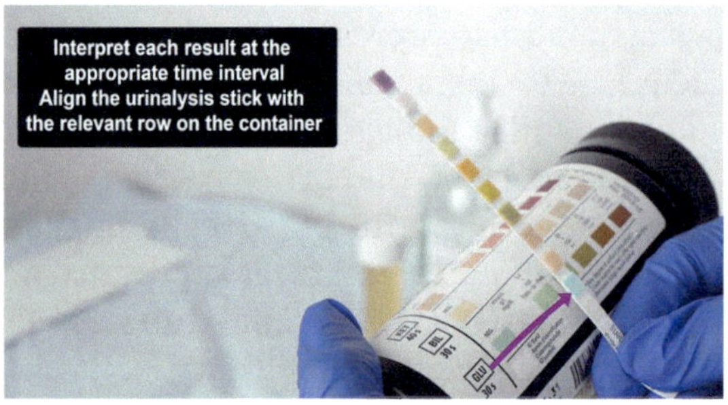

Figure 2.11. Interpretation of urinalysis results.

Source: https://geekymedics.com/wp-content/uploads/2023/09/interpret_results_urinalysistwo.jpg.

2.3.3. Clinical Significance of Urinalysis Findings

Urinalysis is one of the most important tests used in renal function evaluation and determining if renal disease exists. Urine analysis can provide very significant information about the kidneys' ability to filter and metabolize. Routine urinalysis would include specific gravity, pH, and the absence or presence of some compounds such as glucose or protein within particular limits. Abnormalities of these norms can be reflective of underlying renal pathology and may require additional diagnostic workup. As a case in point, hematuria or urine protein content that is above normal tends to precede glomerular damage or systemic diseases like hypertension or diabetes mellitus and, if untreated, can ultimately lead to CKD. Thus, urinalysis not just aids in diagnosing renal pathologies but also plays an integral part in monitoring long-term health follow-up in patients with predisposing conditions (Steven et al., 2017). There is more to the clinical value of urinalysis results than mere diagnosis; they play a crucial role in prescribing treatment and assessing disease progression. For example, urinalysis facilitates the monitoring of proteinuria levels, a significant parameter for evaluating patients with conditions such as diabetic nephropathy. Through ongoing evaluation, healthcare providers can quantify the efficacy of therapeutic interventions designed to prevent renal damage. Additionally, urinalysis results can also prompt referrals to nephrology so that patients receive ideal care in accordance with their individual renal needs. However, characteristics such as the presence of casts or crystals can help in proposing an underlying pathology for renal impairment and hence facilitate immediate, effective management. Last but not least, the inclusion of urinalysis in the evaluation of renal function remains central to optimizing patient care and improving long-term prognosis (Lurbe et al., 2016). Furthermore, urinalysis findings can serve as an indicator of overall health, suggesting comorbidities that require intervention. Changes in urinalysis parameters can be indicative of multiple conditions, including infections, metabolic abnormalities, and hematologic disorders. For example, the presence of leucocytes or nitrites in the urine can be indicative of a UTI, which necessitates early management to prevent further renal issues. Likewise, an increase in glucose can be indicative of poorly controlled diabetes, which needs utmost caution for renal health. Thus, urinalysis provides a good amount of information that impacts decisions regarding management and patient education. The ability to explore the discoveries of urinalysis regarding renal as well as systemic health underlines the necessity of incorporating such information in daily clinical practice and finally leads to improved patient outcomes as well as improving renal health dynamics (Steven et al., 2017).

2.4. Imaging Techniques in Renal Assessment

Imaging modalities are becoming increasingly central to the assessment of renal function and disease, thereby raising diagnostic accuracy above that of conventional blood tests. Among them is MRI, which becomes a valuable tool due to its ability to produce high-definition and detailed images of renal anatomy. Notably, phase-contrast magnetic resonance imaging (PC-MRI) offers the unique ability to measure renal blood flow non-invasively. Evidence suggests that PC-MRI can accurately measure blood flow volumes in both native and transplanted kidneys by assessing flow dynamics within the renal arteries. PC-MRI has been included in quality improvement studies, establishing normal ranges of renal blood flow and hence improving screening for diseases such as transplant renal artery stenosis (TRAS). In this way, PC-MRI presents a promising pathway for developing renal imaging protocols, which can potentially lead to enhanced patient management and outcomes (Martin et al., 2024). Single-photon emission computed tomography (SPECT) is also an essential imaging modality in renal assessment, particularly in measuring glomerular filtration rates (GFR). While traditional SPECT scans reveal some aspect of renal function, their planar imaging limitations inherently lead to inaccuracies. Recent advances have been aimed at increasing this modality's precision with advances in tracers, such as the application of 68Ga-Ethylenediaminetetraacetic acid (68Ga-EDTA). Dynamic positron emission tomography (PET) scanning provides a more accurate evaluation of renal function by accurately measuring tracer elimination processes under dynamic conditions. Empirical data from studies involving 68Ga-EDTA substantiate its capability to discriminate between varying levels of renal compromise, even before changes in normal serum parameters.

Thus, this discovery places 68Ga-EDTA dynamic PET on the verge of becoming a revolutionary renal imaging tool with extensive implications for clinical practice (Ding et al., 2023). Moreover, ultrasonography remains a reference point in renal imaging, primarily due to its accessibility and extensive application in clinical practice. This technique excels in visualizing kidney anatomy and identifying structural abnormalities, such as cysts, masses, or hydronephrosis. With Doppler ultrasound, clinicians can assess renal blood flow patterns, something essential in the assessment of disease like renal artery stenosis. Invasive diagnostic methods are not required because ultrasonography is portable, inexpensive, and non-invasive. While operator dependency and interobserver variability are the technique's drawbacks, the development of ultrasound technology, like three-dimensional imaging and contrast-enhanced ultrasound, continues to push its diagnostic capabilities. Hence, the combination of ultrasonography with other imaging tests can yield a comprehensive approach to renal evaluation, comprising both structural and functional analysis, which enables patient diagnosis and management (Figure 2.12).

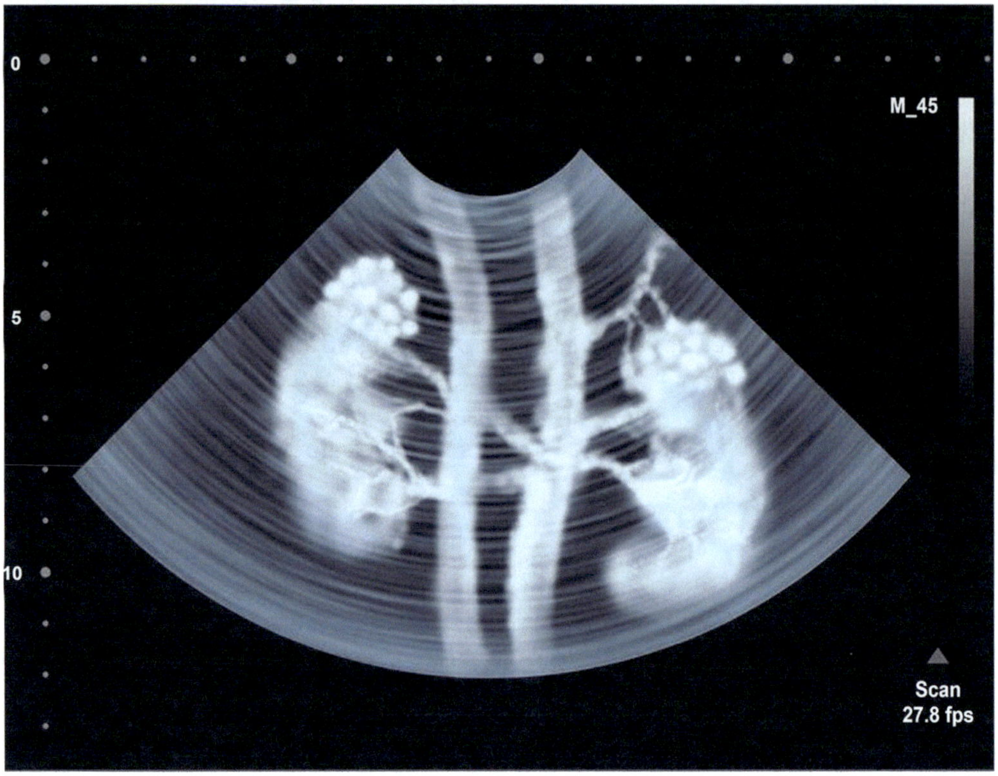

Figure 2.12. Imaging techniques in renal assessment.

Source: https://media.post.rvohealth.io/wp-content/uploads/2020/08/renal-scan_thumb.jpg.

2.4.1. Ultrasound of the Kidneys

Ultrasound imaging has emerged as a vital imaging modality for assessing kidney function and health, particularly due to its affordability and non-invasive nature. This imaging modality provides critical information regarding renal anatomy and pathology, making it highly valuable in the assessment of chronic kidney disease (CKD) and other kidney diseases. According to research, renal parenchymal thickness, assessed using ultrasound, is a key marker of kidney function. For instance, studies have established that CKD patients exhibit significantly thinner renal parenchymal thickness compared to normal subjects, correlated with elevated serum creatinine and decreased estimated glomerular filtration rates (eGFR) (Ahmad et al., 2025). The ability of ultrasound to visualize structural changes in the kidneys facilitates the early detection of diseases that can lead to detrimental consequences for kidney function. In addition to its application in detecting structural disorders, ultrasound also provides additional information on renal function through indices such as the renal artery resistance index (RI). RI measurement can be helpful in acute kidney injury (AKI), where the resistance index has been found to identify at-risk patients effectively. Among a comparative study of AKI and non-AKI patients, significant variation in renal function parameters like RI was observed, and increasing values of RI were observed to indicate a higher risk for sepsis-related

AKI (Wang et al., 2024). This finding highlights the versatility of ultrasound as a multi-parameter imaging technique that combines anatomical and functional assessments. This dual capability enhances clinicians' diagnostic proficiency and improves the establishment of appropriate treatment planning in patients with renal impairment. Furthermore, the incorporation of ultrasound with other tests of renal function strengthens the diagnostic scenario for kidney disease. While everyday laboratory tests such as serum creatinine and 24-hour urine output provide critical information, the gathering of these findings, coupled with ultrasound findings, can give a more comprehensive understanding of a patient's kidney condition. For example, by comparing renal parenchymal thickness with serological tests such as serum creatinine and cystatin C, medical professionals are more capable of identifying the progression of CKD. With an increase in kidney disease cases being reported from various regions worldwide, the use of ultrasound and supportive diagnostic equipment is a promising method for enhancing patient outcomes through early treatment and customized management of kidney function (Figure 2.13).

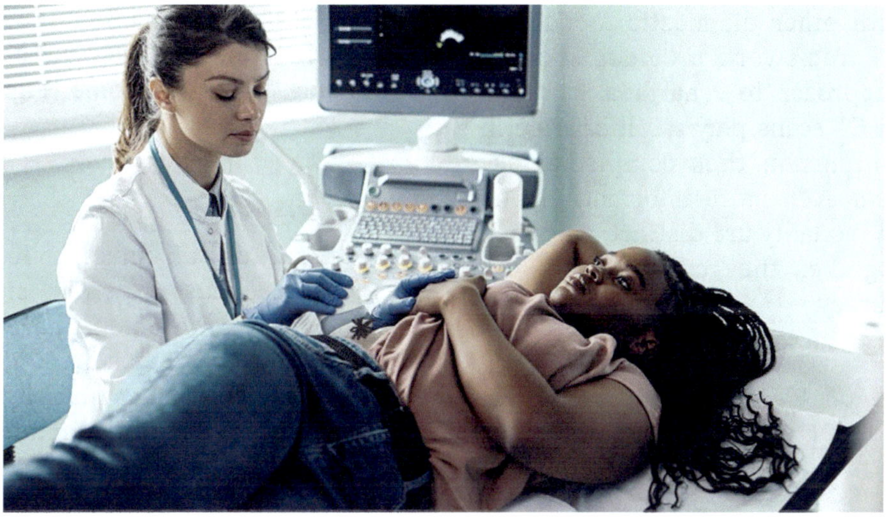

Figure 2.13. Kidney ultrasound scans.

Source: https://i0.wp.com/post.medicalnewstoday.com/wp-content/uploads/sites/3/2023/07/kidney_ultrasound_GettyImages1495030757_Header-1024x575.jpg?w=1155&h=1528.

2.4.2. CT Scans and MRIs

In renal diagnosis, imaging modalities such as CT scans and MRIs are valuable tools for a comprehensive understanding of kidney anatomy and function. Although primarily used for imaging anatomical structures, these modalities are also greatly useful in identifying underlying pathology that compromises renal function. For example, CT scans are particularly useful in identifying renal masses, stones, and vascular malformations. Their respective ability to detect high-resolution cross-sectional images allows clinicians to estimate lesion size and location with precision, a factor highly relevant to developing an adequately targeted treatment protocol. Finally, advances in CT technology, such as multiphasic methods, enhance renal perfusion contrast, allowing diagnoses that include alterations in blood flow to reflect associated pathophysiological mechanisms. MRI is increasingly being recognized for renal diagnostic needs, particularly in patients who are predisposed to be radiation sensitive or who have impaired renal function. MRIs, unlike CT scans, do not expose patients to ionizing radiation and hence are a safer choice for serial imaging. This aspect is particularly relevant to monitoring chronic renal disease or assessing complications of interventions. Furthermore, MRI can produce excellent soft tissue contrast, better differentiating between complex renal cysts and potential malignancies. The inclusion of functional MRI techniques with renal imaging in recent years enables the evaluation of renal perfusion and oxygenation, providing a comprehensive assessment of renal function that can inform management decisions. Integration with other diagnostic modalities within an MRI framework provides support for a unified approach to renal health. While both MRIs and CT scans play a critical role in assessing renal function, their complementary use makes them even more informative. The data from each modality are distinct, yet when interpreted together, they contribute to the diagnostic accuracy.

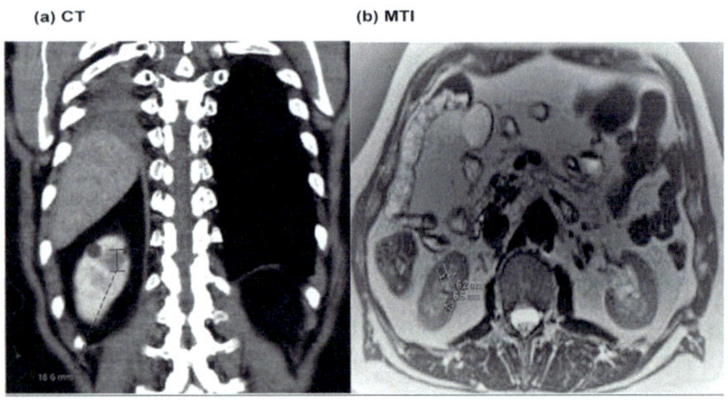

Figure 2.14. CT scan and MRI showing right renal lesions. (a): CT scan showing a 1.3 cm hypodense mass in the upper pole of the right kidney; and (b): MRI show two similar hypodense lesions in the lower pole of the right kidney.

Source: https://www.researchgate.net/publication/333473820/figure/fig1/AS:822830497280003@1573189486167/CT-Scan-and-MRI-showing-right-renal-lesions-a-CT-Scan-showing-a-13cm-hypodense-mass.ppm.

For instance, a CT scan is able to reveal structural abnormalities, while an MRI can assess renal perfusion and function, too. Such a comprehensive approach is particularly beneficial in complex cases where renal pathology may coexist with systemic disease. Furthermore, ongoing research and guidelines, such as the 2022 ACC/AHA and ESC/ERS guidelines, continue to emphasize the importance of multidimensional imaging methods in providing comprehensive patient management (Eric et al., 2022; Humbert et al., 2022). Finally, the complementarity of these diagnostic instruments facilitates the effective identification and management of renal disease, optimizing patient outcome (Figure 2.14).

2.4.3. Role of Imaging in Diagnosing Renal Diseases

The utilization of imaging for diagnosing renal disease has grown in significance as technological advancements have expanded the range of diagnostics beyond traditional methods. Imaging devices, such as ultrasound, computed tomography (CT), and magnetic resonance imaging (MRI), provide critical information about renal anatomy and disease, assisting clinicians in their diagnosis. Particularly, renal ultrasound is a first-line imaging technique due to its non-invasive nature and ability to show structural abnormalities, such as hydronephrosis or kidney stones. CT and MRI can similarly visualize the renal tissues better so as to evaluate tumors, cysts, and other complex conditions. By complementing initial clinical evaluation and laboratory examination, imaging plays a crucial role in establishing an overall profile of renal well-being and guiding future therapeutic interventions. Beyond their capacity for structural evaluation, imaging modalities make possible the assessment of renal perfusion and function. For instance, Doppler sonography is capable of measuring renal perfusion, showing valuable data on kidney vascularity and performance. This is particularly important in diagnosing conditions like renal artery stenosis, which can lead to secondary hypertension and chronic renal insufficiency. Furthermore, MRI has also been a powerful diagnostic tool for renal diseases, as it produces high-resolution images without exposing patients to ionizing radiation. Recent evidence suggests that MRI is also highly useful in evaluating the extent of renal injury in chronic kidney disease (CKD) and characterizing renal masses, thereby informing appropriate management strategies (Nakagawa et al., 2024). The addition of imaging in renal diagnosis enhances clinicians' ability to detect disease processes at various levels. Pathophysiologic understanding of renal illnesses continues to be sophisticated in nature; hence, correct diagnosis becomes necessary for effective management. As characterized in the literature, imaging modalities have become an essential part of this diagnostic conundrum, particularly in the evaluation of glomerular disease, where these diseases often present with nonspecific symptoms and laboratory findings (Festus et al., 2025). Combining laboratory studies with imaging workups gives a more comprehensive diagnostic strategy, allowing for an individualized treatment plan that considers each patient's nuances to their condition. Thus, the addition of sophisticated imaging technologies significantly supplements diagnostic accuracy and overall patient care in renal medicine. The integration of diagnostic strategies from several specialties, such as imaging, ultimately delivers better results in renal disease treatment and underscores the relevance of these technologies to clinical practice.

2.5. Advanced Diagnostic Tools

Advanced diagnostic technology has revolutionized the method of assessing renal function, providing higher precision in the diagnosis and care of kidney disease. Techniques such as imaging modalities, i.e., ultrasound and computed tomography (CT), enable clinicians to visualize renal structure and function better. Undoubtedly, CT scans have proven to be highly sensitive in assessing renal abnormalities and are more effective than traditional imaging methods. The association of such advanced imaging devices aids in determining the presence of structural changes, obstructions, or neoplasms, thereby informing the treatment plans. Advanced imaging not only facilitates early diagnosis but also enables further exploration of the pathophysiological processes underlying various renal conditions, ultimately leading to improved patient outcomes and justifying the need for timely intervention in chronic kidney disease (Liang et al., 2020). The discovery of biomarkers is another significant step toward developing imminent diagnostic tools for renal function testing. Novel biomarkers such as neutrophil gelatinase-associated lipocalin (NGAL) and kidney injury molecule-1 (KIM-1) have been promising in identifying acute kidney injury and chronic kidney disease before standard serum creatinine values. They can provide valuable insights into renal pathophysiology and response to treatment. Their application extends the diagnostic armamentarium, enabling a more advanced understanding of renal illness and wellness. Furthermore, integration of such biomarkers into clinical practice can enhance risk stratification along with personalized treatment regimens for the renal-compromised, thus treating individual patient needs more effectively (Cosentino et al., 2019). The adaptation of point-of-care testing (POCT) also reflects the trend toward more advanced diagnostic technology in nephrology. POCT enables the quick assessment of renal function, facilitating timely informed decisions by clinicians. Point-of-care technology for measuring serum creatinine or electrolyte levels enhances the speed and precision of renal evaluation. Access to real-time information facilitates instant clinical action, particularly in an acute environment where renal function plays a significant role in the patient's outcome. By improving access, ease, and timeliness of the data of diagnosis, POCT not only provides support for the early diagnosis of renal disorders but also makes it easier to constantly monitor renal patients with existing renal disorders. Consequently, these innovations in renal diagnostic equipment underscore the dynamism of nephrology practice and highlight the importance of integrating technology in patient care (Liang et al., 2020).

2.5.1. Kidney Biopsy Procedures

One of the most critical diagnostic techniques of evaluating renal pathology and function is the technique of kidney biopsy. The is applied to provide ultimate histological information that assists in making diagnoses for a number of renal diseases, including glomerulonephritis, nephrotic syndrome, and interstitial nephritis. A kidney biopsy typically involves the removal of a small sample of kidney tissue for microscopic examination, allowing clinicians to assess structural damage and inflammatory patterns. Indications for a kidney biopsy typically come up when non-invasive examinations fail to provide helpful information, hence the need for a more invasive procedure to verify underlying renal pathology. However, whether to proceed with a biopsy is based on careful observation of the patient's overall health and potential complications, and hence it is still a crucial part of renal diagnostic tests in clinical practice. Although kidney biopsies are safe overall, they are not complication-free. Most of them are minor, like abdominal pain, microscopic hematuria, but some, such as perirenal hematomas and bleeding, are serious. Research shows that an estimated 19.3% of patients will develop hematomas following a biopsy, and thus pre-procedure assessments are essential. For instance, patients with elevated pre-biopsy creatinine levels or hypertension tend to have complications, so they should be adequately screened before the procedure (Anvar et al., 2020). Physicians must remain vigilant, examining patients closely in the hours and days following the biopsy for any ill effects to reverse them promptly. Close observation serves to underscore the nuance and significance of patient selection and preparation in enhancing the safety of the kidney biopsy. A second crucial aspect of kidney biopsy is the use of genetic findings to inform the management of some conditions.

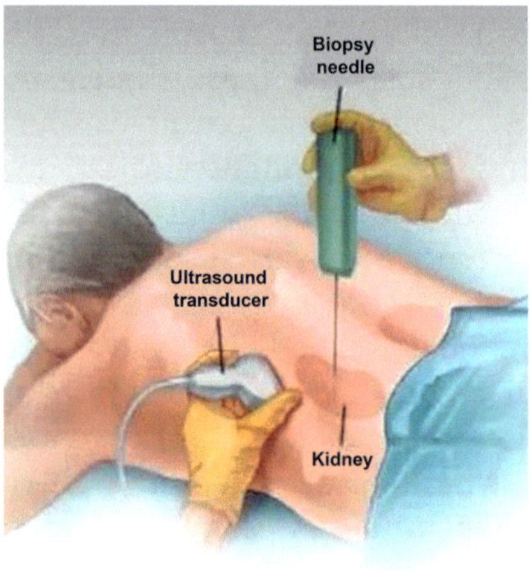

Figure 2.15. Kidney biopsy procedures.

Source: https://magicward.com/wp-content/uploads/2025/01/image-6.png.

This is particularly critical in cases where kidney injury is associated with inherited disorders, such as May-Hegglin anomaly (MHA). In patients with MHA, vascular complications of the procedure are augmented by chronic thrombocytopenia, which may rule out safe procedure performance (Matthew et al., 2024). These cases illustrate the interface between genetic assessment and decision-making at the time of the procedure in nephrology. Where biopsies cannot be done, other tests, including imaging scans and renal function tests, may become more critical in monitoring the condition. Lastly, the development of kidney biopsy techniques, coupled with advancements in genetic testing and patient care, is an essential element within the overall scheme of renal function testing and diagnosis (Figure 2.15).

2.5.2. Genetic Testing for Renal Disorders

With continuous advances in genetic testing, its role in diagnosing renal disorders has also become more prominent. Earlier, renal impairment was primarily assessed by biochemical studies and imaging techniques; however, with the inclusion of genetic assessment, there is a greater understanding of underlying causes. For instance, some inherited conditions, such as Alport syndrome and cystinosis, carry specific genetic mutations, for which selective testing is required for a definitive diagnosis. By identifying these genetic markers, clinicians cannot only make informed decisions about the best treatment options but also offer genetic counseling to affected families, thereby optimizing preventive interventions. This shift towards precision medicine emphasizes the importance of genetic testing in maximizing patient outcomes, particularly in cases where traditional diagnostic methods may be inadequate in determining the etiology of renal disease. With the advancement of genomics, the use of next-generation sequencing (NGS) has revolutionized the process of genetic testing for kidney disease. NGS facilitates the simultaneous screening of multiple genes, conserving time and cost compared to traditional single-gene testing. This is particularly useful for diseases with genetic heterogeneity. For instance, mutations in several genes can result in similar phenotypes, making diagnosis challenging. With methods like whole-exome sequencing, clinicians are able to identify a spectrum of mutations that make people susceptible to renal disease, as demonstrated in a number of studies on congenital kidney disease. In addition to enhancing the speed of diagnosis, this data enhances the genotype-phenotype correlation information, thus offering patients more targeted treatment options. The ongoing research and refinement of these methods have the potential to further expand the diagnostic frontiers. Furthermore, the relevance of genetic testing extends beyond simple diagnosis; it is an integral part of the successful management of renal diseases.

Inherited metabolic disorders such as tyrosinemia and cystic fibrosis often necessitate lifelong management plans that can be optimized based on genetic data. For example, understanding specific genetic mutations enables clinicians to regulate biochemical markers more effectively, as seen in the case of adjusting NTBC dosing based on blood levels of toxic metabolites. Not only does genetic testing reveal the diagnosis, but it also directs the patient's future treatment plan, promoting an anticipatory management approach. As renal genetics continues to advance, so will the sophistication of our diagnostic and treatment methods, ultimately improving quality of life for many people affected, as witnessed by the promising development observed in diseases resulting from specific gene mutations like those documented in N/A (2021), Garcia (2020) (Figure 2.16).

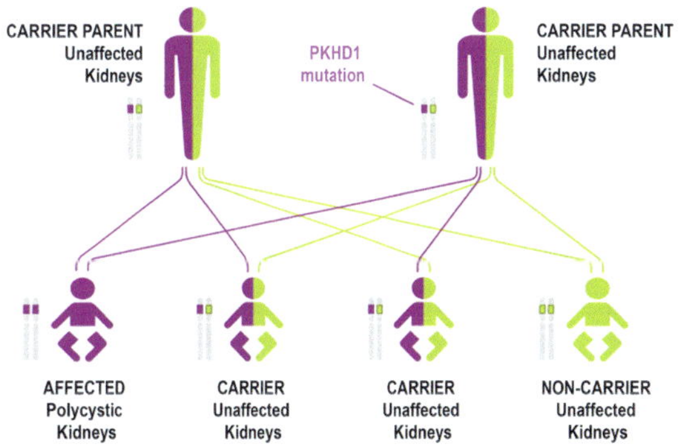

Figure 2.16. Genetic testing for renal disorders.

Source: https://pkdcharity.org.uk/images/pages/arpkd/arpkd-inheritance-diagram.svg.

2.5.3. Biomarkers in Renal Disease Diagnosis

The research into renal disease biomarkers has significantly altered the approach to renal function tests and diagnosis. The quantification of serum creatinine and estimated glomerular filtration rate (eGFR) was formerly employed to measure renal function. Although these measures are sensitive and specific in indicating kidney function, they are not satisfactory in that they fail to reveal prior kidney injury, a deficiency that results in a need for more sensitive and specific biomarkers. Recent studies have found evidence that biomarkers, such as ultrasonography-measured renal parenchymal thickness and serum creatinine, have a clear relationship with the progression of chronic kidney disease (CKD) (Ahmad et al., 2025).

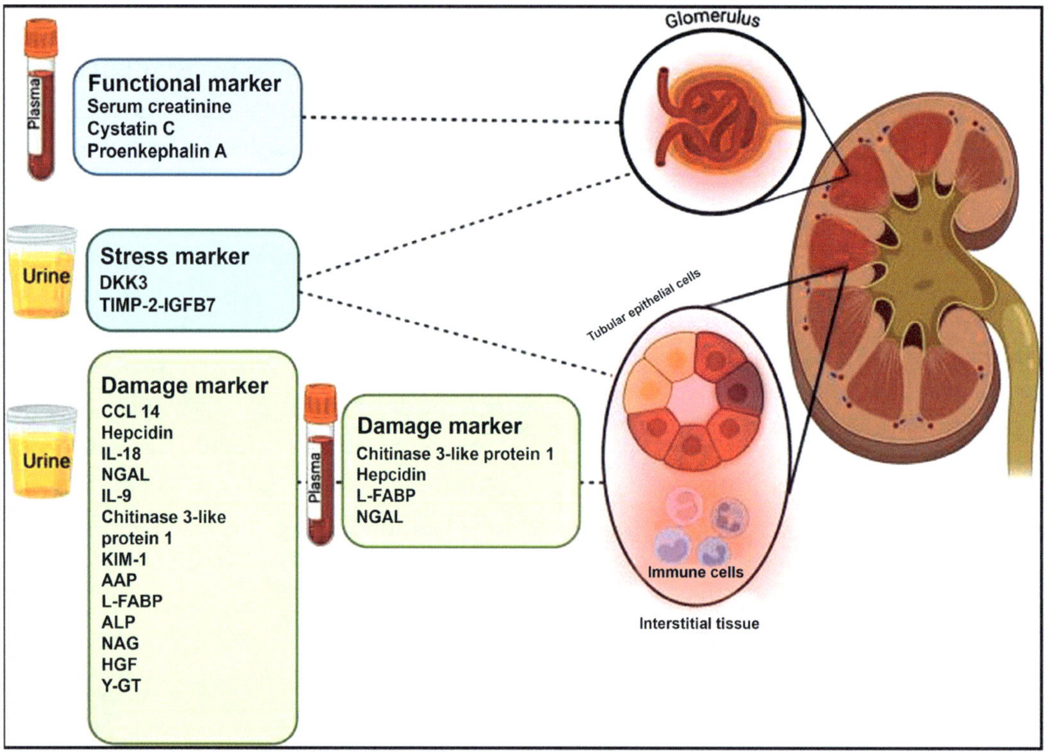

Figure 2.17. Biomarkers in renal disease diagnosis.

Source: https://media.springernature.com/lw685/springer-static/image/art%3A10.1186%2Fs13613-024-01360-9/MediaObjects/13613_2024_1360_Fig1_HTML.png.

This evidence warrants the integration of newer imaging technology with conventional blood testing, thereby enhancing the accuracy of renal disease diagnosis and enabling early treatment. Ultrasonography serves not only as a diagnostic imaging modality to quantify structural changes in the kidneys but also to evaluate renal parenchymal thickness, which reflects the health of the kidneys. In a case-control study, patients with CKD exhibited significantly reduced parenchymal thickness compared to controls, suggesting that this could be a promising biomarker (Ahmad et al., 2025). This non-imaging technology offers a cost-effective method of monitoring kidney health, particularly in at-risk groups of incipient CKD. Furthermore, the ability to measure renal parenchymal changes over time provides insightful data into disease progression, offering clinicians a dynamic view of kidney function that may otherwise go unnoticed through bloodwork. The combined use of ultrasonographic assessments with serum biomarkers provides an effective approach to early diagnosis of renal disease. As an adjunct to structural imaging, serum biomarkers have also been valuable in distinguishing the various forms of anemia that can be highly prevalent in renal disease diagnoses. For instance, the serum level of hepcidin is a significant determinant for discriminating iron deficiency anemia (IDA) from anemia of chronic disease (ACD), and both are highly prevalent in patients with renal impairment. The high specificity and sensitivity of serum hepcidin reveal the potential utility of the marker in the clinic, allowing nephrologists to limit their diagnostic target further. The combination of hepcidin assessment with routine renal function tests and imaging modalities may offer more accurate diagnoses and reduce the need for invasive strategies such as bone marrow biopsies. This broad-based strategy highlights the importance of biomarkers in enhancing the diagnosis and treatment of renal disease (Figure 2.17).

2.6. Limitations and Challenges of Renal Testing

Limitations and restrictions of renal testing are a significant factor in the diagnosis of renal disease in terms of efficiency and accuracy. The major limitation is the dependence on serum creatinine values and eGFR, which can be rendered unreliable due to several factors independent of renal function. Muscular mass, age, and hydration levels, for example, can distort these tests, leading to potential misdiagnosis or delayed treatment. Moreover, like in CKD research, this reliance on these conventional biomarker tests tends to overlook significant structural renal tissue changes capable of indicating the progression of disease (Ahmad et al., 2025). This drawback necessitates more generalized diagnostic modalities that optimize the balance between inter-patient heterogeneity and enhance renal function measurement accuracy in clinical environments. In addition, although ultrasonography is an advantageous non-invasive method for renal assessment, it has limitations. Dependence on operator ability and subjectivity of the ultrasound image may lead to differences in measurement of the kidneys, for instance, parenchymal thickness or renal pelvic diameter. For example, imaging diagnosis of disorders such as ureteropelvic junction obstruction (UPJO) largely relies on practitioner skill and technique (Mahasin et al., 2025). In addition, ultrasonically stratified renal status may result in over- or under-treatment if not supported by clinical findings in concordance with such imaging findings. Attention to these nuances is necessary for the development of an enhanced appreciation of ultrasound findings, ultimately resulting in improved patient care through the integration of various diagnostic methodologies. Other new diagnostic modalities, promising as they are, are often hindered by issues in application secondary to resource constraints and access limitations. For instance, advanced imaging techniques such as magnetic resonance imaging (MRI) or computed tomography (CT), although very informative, may not be available in all healthcare facilities, particularly in areas with limited resources. Unavailability hinders early renal condition diagnosis and complicates the reduction of health disparities across different populations. Accordingly, these restrictions need to be removed by collective efforts at the promotion of convergence of different renal test modalities so that medical professionals deliver renal diagnosis with precision as per the specific requirements of patients. Such an overall philosophy will prove essential in surpassing the present limitations and enhancing the efficacy of renal diagnostic modalities.

2.6.1. Factors Affecting Test Accuracy

Obtaining reliable test outcomes in renal function tests is influenced by a multitude of factors, ranging from procedural standards to the patients' inherent biological variation. The validity of such tests can be negatively impacted by factors such as the timing of sample collection, storage methodology, and analytical methods employed. For instance, serum creatinine levels, which are commonly used in estimating renal function, can be affected by patients' hydration state, muscle bulk, and even recent dietary intake. Such factors introduce a degree of imprecision into the interpretation of results, thereby hindering clinicians' ability to determine renal health properly. These factors need to be managed to enhance the precision of testing equipment, emphasizing the need for standardized testing procedures and comprehensive training for laboratory personnel to minimize variation in renal function testing. Additionally, the relationship between patient demographics and test reliability should not be overlooked. Age, sex, and previous medical history can all influence the interpretation of renal function tests. For example, older patients may have different baseline biomarker levels due to age-related physiological changes that affect the interpretation of results. Cheng et al. (2024) explain that acute kidney injury in geriatric patients is preceded by evolving prognostic indicators, and diagnostic criteria need to be adapted to properly diagnose elderly patients. Thus, the incorporation of demographic parameters into the assessment process not only aids personalized medicine but is crucial to optimizing patient outcomes with more precise diagnostic methods. Additionally, the integration of additional testing modalities can significantly enhance the precision of renal function assessment. As noted by recent studies, the inclusion of biomarkers such as tissue inhibitor of metalloproteinase-2 (TIMP-2) and insulin-like growth factor-binding protein 7 (IGFBP7) has the potential to improve predictive accuracy for renal outcomes in critically ill patients. Cheng et al. (2024) indicate evidence that the incorporation of these biomarkers along with established instruments, such as the Acute Physiology and Chronic Health Evaluation (APACHE II) score, is of greater predictive validity. This multi-factorial approach not only increases the diagnostic image but also reduces the false positive rate with standard tests. By embracing a more comprehensive approach that involves multiple biomarkers and clinical markers, healthcare providers can significantly increase the validity and credibility of renal function diagnoses (Figure 2.18).

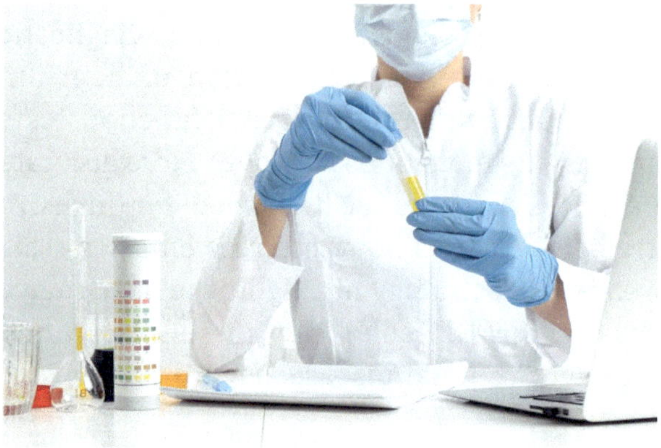

Figure 2.18. Accurate test for kidney function.

Source: https://cdn-jchih.nitrocdn.com/ytdfWkhjbUydjqTtHRyFWyUdfjAkmQbT/assets/images/optimized/rev-eed486f/abiscans.com/wp-content/uploads/2024/03/2149372015.jpg.

2.6.2. Interpretation Challenges in Diverse Populations

Interpretation of renal function tests is highly problematic in heterogeneous populations. Demographic heterogeneity based on age, sex, race, and ethnicity can influence the outcome of the tests and warrants careful interpretation and use of diagnostic tests. For instance, it has been found that estimates of glomerular filtration rate (GFR) tend to underestimate kidney function in certain ethnic groups, likely due to differences in body composition and muscle mass. Accordingly, clinicians must account for such differences to provide an accurate diagnosis and adequate treatment of renal disease. The need for nuanced interpretation renders the incorporation of population-specific data into renal diagnosis essential, allowing for individualized care that accommodates the diverse needs of various patient groups. Cultural competencies are also necessary for identifying the problems of interpretation related to renal function tests. Healthcare practitioners should recognize and value patients' cultural backgrounds, influencing their understanding of illness and health. For instance, certain cultures may hold peculiar beliefs about kidney disease, influencing whether they would agree to undergo screening or follow treatment recommendations. As patient-centered care is increasingly advocated, practitioners are advised to engage in active dialogue with patients to understand their backgrounds and likes. Incorporating these cultural variables into the interpretation of renal function tests will promote increased accuracy in diagnosis, patient and physician trust, and communication with improved outcomes. Blending advanced data analytics and machine learning techniques also offers remedies to these challenges of interpretation in differing populations. Using large datasets with diverse demographic and clinical histories will yield more robust, evidence-based predictive models to help improve the validity of renal function assessments. How this is presented in more recent discussions of machine learning in healthcare will be able to bring about improved decision-making by uncovering patterns and trends that might be lost on traditional models (Rajkomar et al., 2019). Nevertheless, the ethical concern of algorithm bias must be weighed carefully because diagnostic instruments should not unintentionally reinforce existing disparities in healthcare access. Thus, ongoing interprofessional cooperation between healthcare practitioners, data scientists, and ethicists is necessary to develop equitable diagnostic instruments that cater to the diverse needs of populations. This collaboration will enable technological advancements to enhance quality renal care access, rather than undermining it (Jean-Ricco et al., 2017).

2.6.3. Cost and Accessibility of Diagnostic Tools

The expense and accessibility of diagnostic tools for renal function evaluation are fundamental determinants that significantly influence patient outcomes and the deployment of healthcare resources. Advanced diagnostic imaging modalities, e.g., biomarkers and imaging devices, can provide valuable information about kidney health. Their expense, however, can be a limiting factor in their widespread use, particularly among resource-limited populations. Advances in new diagnostic technologies, such as nanotechnology-based methods, have shown promise in enhancing the specificity and sensitivity of renal function tests. Yet, the cost advantages of this innovation may deter its general application in clinical practice, especially in developing countries where there are few budgets for healthcare (Patra et al., 2018). The problem lies in balancing the need for the newest technologies with the background it takes to make them affordable and accessible to all patients. The second issue is to consider how to account for the impact of variation in the cost of diagnostic machinery on different populations. Patients, especially those in private insurance-based healthcare systems, may be exposed to prohibitively high out-of-pocket costs for new tests of renal function. This disparity can enhance existing health disparities, putting disenfranchised populations at greater risk of undertreated or undiagnosed renal disease. Moreover, patterns of referral and access to specialty testing vary significantly across geographic regions, affecting the timeliness and quality of patient care. Consequently, attempts to make renal diagnostics more affordable should focus on increasing accessibility and equitable provision throughout various health centers across different socioeconomic strata of the population (Fátima Cardoso et al., 2018). Lastly, while technological advancements in renal diagnostics hold the promise of greater effectiveness, they are not without concerns regarding cost and accessibility. For instance, utilization of overall renal function tests may require significant infrastructural expenditures from health facilities. Providers may also need training to interpret and make use of new diagnostics, again making them hard to utilize. Decision-makers and stakeholders in health must then work together to develop solutions to address these challenges, for example, by advocating for subsidies or insurance of critical diagnostic tests that can significantly influence patient management outcomes. The practical application of novel renal function diagnostic technologies in clinical practice not only relies on evidence of clinical utility but also on their accessibility to all individuals who need them (Patra et al., 2018) (Figure 2.19).

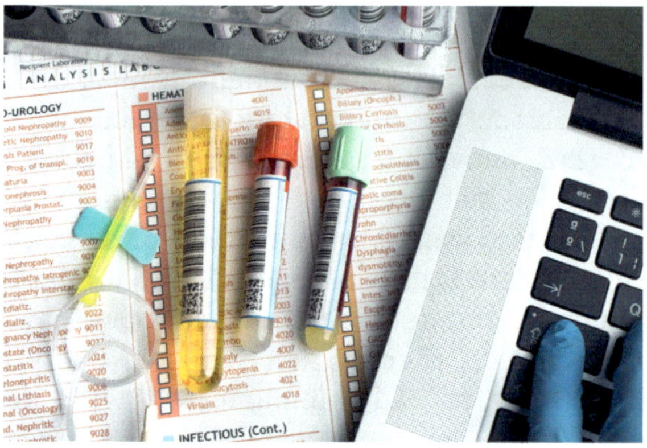

Figure 2.19. Cost and accessibility of diagnostic tools of renal function assessments.

Source: https://medlineplus.gov/images/KidneyTests_share.jpg.

SUMMARY

The measurement of renal function using various diagnostic tests is crucial for the successful management of kidney disease. The application of various imaging technologies, such as ultrasonography and renal scintigraphy, has enabled clinicians to more accurately assess renal status. As revealed by more recent studies, for instance, on renal pelvic diameter (RPD), the use of these techniques significantly increases the sensitivity and specificity of the diagnosis for diseases such as ureteropelvic junction obstruction (UPJO). Most importantly, highly significant results showed a notable RPD disparity in measures between normal and renal impairment patients, considering the potential of ultrasound as a primary diagnostic tool that, when coupled with other techniques, can provide more accurate readings for patients with renal complications at risk (Mahasin et al., 2025). Guiding practice and education for patients is also an area of investigation, including studies on dietary supplements such as creatine and their impact on renal function. Research on creatine supplementation has highlighted that concerns regarding its potential damage to renal function may be unfounded. With robust evidence lacking any relationship between creatine consumption status and renal function, as illustrated by the application of rigorous statistical methods such as Mendelian randomization, patients can be counseled to make evidence-based supplementation decisions. This can be applied to educate fitness enthusiasts and medical professionals about the importance of making decisions based on scientific facts and not anecdotal testimony (Zhou et al., 2024). The future of kidney diagnostics lies in further finer-tuning tests and the introduction of new technology that can accurately measure kidney function. Advancements in imaging technology and improved understanding of biochemical markers are essential in formulating more specific treatment procedures for patients with renal disease. Moreover, studies are constantly on the lookout for the safety of supplements and their effect on kidney function, which will facilitate better-informed health decisions by consumers. As the field of nephrology continues to evolve, there will be greater synergy between ancient empirical techniques and modern innovations as the solution to achieving optimal patient outcomes with less risk of kidney-associated complications. Bringing together research and diagnostics efforts places a high value on a whole-person approach to managing renal health.

Assessment of renal function is a crucial component of diagnosing and managing various medical conditions, particularly cardiovascular and renal disorders. Renal function tests, such as serum creatinine and eGFR, provide valuable information about the kidneys' capability to eliminate waste and maintain homeostasis. Additionally, understanding the bidirectional interaction between the heart and kidneys, particularly in conditions such as heart failure with preserved ejection fraction (HFpEF), is crucial. Recent studies highlight the significance of cardiorenal syndrome (CRS) in this context. Raised central venous pressure and activation of the RAAS are among the causes of deterioration in cardiac and renal function, which warrants extensive diagnostic investigations in edematous patients with cardiovascular comorbidities (Khandait et al., 2025). When evaluating renal function, it is essential to utilize a range of diagnostic tools in addition to routine serum markers. Biomarkers such as cystatin C, neutrophil gelatinase-associated lipocalin (NGAL), and kidney injury molecule-1 (KIM-1) are gaining recognition for their utility in detecting early renal impairment and risk stratification. The study in these biomarkers is further bringing attention to their potential in aiding diagnostic accuracy and prognostication in disorders such as CRS, where early recognition of renal impairment has a profound impact on clinical outcomes.

Furthermore, integrating the use of sophisticated imaging devices and cardiovascular biomarkers into routine practice would enable more nuanced exploration of the complex interdependencies between the heart and kidneys, and consequently, guide therapeutic interventions (Khandait et al., 2025). Therapeutic interventions for conditions like CRS and edema hinge upon a cooperative use of pharmacologic and nonpharmacologic approaches and each of the latter directed at addressing the underlying cause of renal dysfunction. The use of diuretics, particularly loop diuretics, is a cornerstone of edema treatment, facilitating the elimination of fluid and providing symptomatic relief. Adjuvant strategies, including patient education and global lifestyle modification, are equally as crucial in optimizing patient outcomes. Strategies that promote elevation of limbs, compression therapy, and dietary modification enable the prevention and management of edema, ultimately improving the quality of life for the group in question. The professional recommendations that emerge from initiatives like the Indian Edema Consensus emphasize the necessity of a stepwise approach to screening, diagnosis, and treatment, confirming the worth of an integrated model in optimizing renal function testing and therapy.

CLOSER LOOK

NEUTROPHIL GELATINASE-ASSOCIATED LIPOCALIN (NGAL)

NGAL, or lipocalin-2, is a small glycoprotein from the lipocalin superfamily and a critical protein of innate immunity, inflammation, and renal disease pathophysiology. It was initially reported in neutrophils, where it resides within specific granules and is released upon inflammation. NGAL sequesters siderophores—specifically, ferric siderophores—which are iron-binding molecules utilized by bacteria to sequester iron, thereby preventing bacterial growth. This antimicrobial function is a key aspect of NGAL's role in the body's primary defense against infection. Beyond its immunological function, NGAL has also emerged as a significant biomarker for acute kidney injury (AKI) and early kidney damage, with levels rising exponentially in the bloodstream and urine within hours of renal damage—far in advance of traditional markers such as serum creatinine.

NGAL is not only secreted by neutrophils but also by renal tubular epithelial cells, liver cells, and other tissues in conditions of cellular stress and injury. In normal physiology, blood and urine levels of NGAL are very low. With the insult to the kidneys from ischemia, nephrotoxins, sepsis, or inflammation, NGAL is rapidly induced, especially in the proximal tubules. This makes NGAL an effective early marker of AKI, allowing for intervention before irreversible renal injury. The rapid kinetics of NGAL's increase give it a distinct advantage over traditional kidney function markers, which can only rise after extreme nephron loss. This aspect is particularly valuable in intensive care and postoperative settings, such as cardiac surgery or transplantation, where renal function monitoring is crucial.

In addition to its role in AKI, NGAL has also been studied in chronic kidney disease (CKD), where it marks chronic tubular damage and disease progression. It participates in other disease pathologies, including cardiovascular disease, cancer, and metabolic disorders, due to its role in cell proliferation, apoptosis, and iron homeostasis. Elevated levels of NGAL have also been associated with more severe outcomes in heart failure and sepsis, and thus has been a potentially valuable prognostic indicator in several clinical conditions. NGAL has been found to regulate tissue remodeling and inflammation by binding to matrix metalloproteinase-9 (MMP-9), thereby stabilizing and enhancing MMP-9 activity. This binding enhances the breakdown of the extracellular matrix, which is vital in cancer metastasis and tissue injury repair.

Clinically, quantification of NGAL is gaining attention in laboratory diagnosis due to the availability of commercial assays for both plasma and urine specimens. Although it has not yet acquired a universal place in routine clinical practice, NGAL is becoming increasingly well valued for the purposes of early diagnosis, risk stratification, and monitoring of renal and systemic disease. The take-home message is that NGAL is an interdisciplinary protein with significant immunologic, iron homeostasis, and response to tissue injury functions. Its best-known clinical application is in the early detection of acute kidney injury, where it could improve patient outcomes through earlier treatment and diagnosis. Ongoing research continues to elucidate the function and utility of NGAL as a diagnostic and prognostic marker in medical conditions.

References

1. Su, L., Sheng, H., Li, X., Cai, Y., Mei, H., Cheng, J., Li, D., Lu, Z., Lin, Y., Chen, X., Peng, M., Huang, Y., Zhang, W., & Liu, L. (2024). Clinical and genetic analysis of methylmalonic aciduria in 60 patients from Southern China: a single center retrospective study. *Orphanet Journal of Rare Diseases, 19*(1). https://doi.org/10.1186/s13023-024-03210-0ACOG. (2019). *Obstetrics and Gynecology, 133*, 1–1. https://doi.org/10.1097/aog.0000000000003018 (accessed on 25th June 2025).
2. Ahmad, W., Mobeen, H., Shah, A. W. A., Mobeen, N., Rehman, A. U., & Bibi, A. (2025). Comparative ultrasound assessment of renal parenchymal thickness and renal function tests in chronic kidney disease. *Kashf Journal of Multidisciplinary Research*. https://www.semanticscholar.org/paper/924d4f8dc1574c82704467eced465bd4fffec21f (accessed on 25th June 2025).
3. Anvar, M., & Raghavendra, B. (2020). Hemodynamic assessment and study of bleeding complications following percutaneous renal biopsy in a tertiary care hospital. *Journal of Integrative Nephrology and Andrology, 7*, 41–46. https://www.semanticscholar.org/paper/4cf315927900f3d4a3894c52f8da10f22d0aca99 (accessed on 25th June 2025).
4. Babarinde, F. O., Ogwu, N. P., Babatunde, O. D., Babawale, E. A., Arrey Agbor, D. B., Afuh, R. N., Okoye, O. K., et al. (2025). Diagnostic approach to glomerular diseases. *International Journal of Surgery: Global Health, 8*. https://www.semanticscholar.org/paper/338f180124f182f0604eb9c35322348dd6bcd847 (accessed on 25th June 2025).
5. Bikbov, B., Purcell, C., Levey, A. S., Smith, M., Abdoli, A., Abebe, M., Adebayo, O., et al. (2020). Global, regional, and national burden of chronic kidney disease, 1990–2017: A systematic analysis for the Global Burden of Disease Study 2017. *The Lancet, 395*, 709–733. https://doi.org/10.1016/s0140-6736(20)30045-3 (accessed on 25th June 2025).
6. Campbell, S. C., Uzzo, R. G., Allaf, M. E., Bass, E. B., Cadeddu, J. A., Chang, A., Clark, P. E., et al. (2017). Renal mass and localized renal cancer: AUA guideline. *The Journal of Urology, 198*, 520–529. https://doi.org/10.1016/j.juro.2017.04.100 (accessed on 25th June 2025).
7. Cardoso, F., Senkus, E., Costa, A., Papadopoulos, E., Aapro, M., André, F., Harbeck, N., et al. (2018). 4th ESO–ESMO International Consensus Guidelines for Advanced Breast Cancer (ABC 4). *Annals of Oncology, 29*, 1634–1657. https://doi.org/10.1093/annonc/mdy192 (accessed on 25th June 2025).
8. Cheng, L., Jia, H., Zheng, X., Jiang, Y., Xin, X., & Li, W. (2024). Association between the levels of urinary cell cycle biomarkers and non-recovery of renal function among critically ill geriatric patients with acute kidney injury. *Renal Failure, 46*. https://www.semanticscholar.org/paper/6f1970395c1324a1ba3489a663a87cb4dc926ad2 (accessed on 25th June 2025).
9. Cosentino, F., Grant, P. J., Aboyans, V., Bailey, C. J., Ceriello, A., Delgado, V., Federici, M., et al. (2019). 2019 ESC guidelines on diabetes, pre-diabetes, and cardiovascular diseases developed in collaboration with the EASD. *European Heart Journal, 41*, 255–323. https://doi.org/10.1093/eurheartj/ehz486 (accessed on 25th June 2025).
10. Ding, Y., Liu, Y., Zhang, L., Deng, Y., Chen, H. L., Lan, X., Jiang, D., et al. (2023). Quantitative assessment of renal functions using ^{68}Ga-EDTA dynamic PET imaging in renal injury in mice of different origins. *Frontiers in Medicine, 10*. https://www.semanticscholar.org/paper/da186b49c1d746770bd3c8e8da4b87c3f2f60ec1 (accessed on 25th June 2025).

11. Dybiec, J., Frąk, W., Kućmierz, J., Tokarek, J., Wojtasińska, A., Młynarska, E., Rysz, J., et al. (2024). Liquid biopsy: A new avenue for the diagnosis of kidney disease: Diabetic kidney disease, renal cancer, and IgA nephropathy. *Genes, 15*. https://www.semanticscholar.org/paper/d42c587c5f2cc85debd2cab36d8a9817efaa8082 (accessed on 25th June 2025).

12. Garcia, C. A. (2020). Therapeutic approaches and development of genomic diagnostic tools for Usher syndrome. https://www.semanticscholar.org/paper/296d23a325c8063696551cccc36c26d2a774fb86 (accessed on 25th June 2025).

13. Ginsberg, D. A., Boone, T. B., Cameron, A. P., Gousse, A. E., Kaufman, M. R., Keays, E., Kennelly, M., et al. (2021). The AUA/SUFU guideline on adult neurogenic lower urinary tract dysfunction: Diagnosis and evaluation. *The Journal of Urology*, *206*, 1097–1105. https://doi.org/10.1097/ju.0000000000002235 (accessed on 25th June 2025).

14. Hassan, M. G., Elmahdi, T. S. A., Alotaibi, M., Fallatah, E., & Nasser, F. A. (2025). Accuracy of sonographic renal pelvic diameter in assessment of renal function among patients with ureteropelvic junction obstruction using scintigraphy as a gold standard. *International Journal of Medical Sciences*, *22*, 897–902. https://www.semanticscholar.org/paper/5ebd726711763ee5ffdb17930f43006cdd5c3e53 (accessed on 25th June 2025).

15. Humbert, M., Kovács, G., Hoeper, M. M., Badagliacca, R., Berger, R. M. F., Brida, M., Carlsen, J., et al. (2022). 2022 ESC/ERS guidelines for the diagnosis and treatment of pulmonary hypertension. *European Respiratory Journal*, *61*, 2200879–2200879. https://doi.org/10.1183/13993003.00879-2022 (accessed on 25th June 2025).

16. Isselbacher, E. M., Preventza, O., Black, J. H., Augoustides, J., Beck, A. W., Bolen, M. A., Braverman, A. C., et al. (2022). 2022 ACC/AHA guideline for the diagnosis and management of aortic disease: A report of the American Heart Association/American College of Cardiology Joint Committee on Clinical Practice Guidelines. *Circulation*, *146*. https://doi.org/10.1161/cir.0000000000001106 (accessed on 25th June 2025).

17. Khandait, H., Sodhi, S., Khandekar, N., & Bhattad, V. (2025). Cardiorenal syndrome in heart failure with preserved ejection fraction: Insights into pathophysiology and recent advances. *Cardiorenal Medicine*, *15*, 41–60. https://www.semanticscholar.org/paper/33f9e6850f6da869c61f0f6f1a18f21794e211e1 (accessed on 25th June 2025).

18. Kumaran, R., Abdalla, M. M. I., Caszo, B. A., & Somanath, S. (2025). Saliva urea nitrogen for detection of kidney disease in adults: A meta-analysis of diagnostic test accuracy. *PLOS One*, *20*. https://www.semanticscholar.org/paper/7ae4796a1b15eccdc6f9953849e8b2adab39320f (accessed on 25th June 2025).

19. Levin, A., Ahmed, S. B., Carrero, J. J., Foster, B. J., Francis, A., Hall, R. K., Herrington, W. G., et al. (2024). Executive summary of the KDIGO 2024 Clinical Practice Guideline for the evaluation and management of chronic kidney disease: Known knowns and known unknowns. *Kidney International*, *105*, 684–701. https://doi.org/10.1016/j.kint.2023.10.016 (accessed on 25th June 2025).

20. Liang, H., & Acharya, G. (2020). Novel coronavirus disease (COVID-19) in pregnancy: What clinical recommendations to follow? *Acta Obstetrician Et Gynecological Scandinavica*, *99*, 439–442. https://doi.org/10.1111/aogs.13836 (accessed on 25th June 2025).

21. Liu, J., & Qin, J. (2025). Computational modeling of network topology and molecular dynamics for the assessment of therapeutic potential of the *Astragalus membranaceus*–

Salvia miltiorrhiza drug pair in the treatment of chronic kidney and heart failure. *Iranian Journal of Kidney Diseases*, *19*(2), 69–83. https://www.semanticscholar.org/paper/c796fa923c1efc5a08c3fa79d853340d409813c3 (accessed on 25th June 2025).

22. Lurbe, E., Agabiti-Rosei, E., Cruickshank, J., Dominiczak, A. F., Erdine, S., Hirth, A., Invitti, C., et al. (2016). 2016 European Society of Hypertension guidelines for the management of high blood pressure in children and adolescents. *Journal of Hypertension*, *34*, 1887–1920. https://doi.org/10.1097/hjh.0000000000001039 (accessed on 25th June 2025).
23. Mach, F., Baigent, C., Catapano, A. L., Koskinas, K. C., Casula, M., Badimón, L., Chapman, M. J., et al. (2019). 2019 ESC/EAS guidelines for the management of dyslipidemias: Lipid modification to reduce cardiovascular risk. *European Heart Journal*, *41*, 111–188. https://doi.org/10.1093/eurheartj/ehz455 (accessed on 25th June 2025).
24. Manna, S., Chakrabarti, S., Singh, R., & Gambhir, I. (2025). Serum hepcidin level with iron profile assay might replace bone marrow iron study as a diagnostic tool for evaluation of anemia in elderly without chronic renal disease. *Journal of Family Medicine and Primary Care*, *14*, 356–362. https://www.semanticscholar.org/paper/6abea62e27d52a453221033e638aea0f686a26bd (accessed on 25th June 2025).
25. Martin, P., Gedroyc, W., Corbett, R., & Willicombe, M. (2024). #2115 Phase-contrast magnetic resonance imaging (PC-MRI) for quantification of volumetric flow in renal transplant arteries: An observational cohort study. *Nephrology Dialysis Transplantation*. https://www.semanticscholar.org/paper/dcffc4e6cc2ff35537454f09ccbfdf41032365e4 (accessed on 25th June 2025).
26. Massironi, S., Franchina, M., Ippolito, D., Elisei, F., Falco, O., Maino, C., Pagni, F., et al. (2024). Improvements and future perspective in diagnostic tools for neuroendocrine neoplasms. *Expert Review of Endocrinology & Metabolism*, *19*, 349–366. https://www.semanticscholar.org/paper/3f10150420340ad6993172c5de5552bfedea3ba8 (accessed on 25th June 2025).
27. Mathur, G., Wander, G., Joshi, S., Pal, J., Vora, A., Tiwaskar, M., Upadhyay, R., et al. (2024). Edema India: Executive summary of screening, diagnosis, and management of edema. *The Journal of the Association of Physicians of India*, *72*(7), 68–72. https://www.semanticscholar.org/paper/0f5d7a9dc408e2af30e9cd9592f180a86b377136 (accessed on 25th June 2025).
28. Minoo, F., Narimani, S., Mahdavi-Mazdeh, M., & Alamdari, A. (2024). The association of brain-dead donors' serum/urine NGAL with renal transplant function. *Journal of Renal Endocrinology*. https://www.semanticscholar.org/paper/4abdffac410db387304118932bcbc737b1656cb8 (accessed on 25th June 2025).
29. Nakagawa, S., Miyati, T., Ohno, N., Oda, Y., Kawano, K., & Kobayashi, S. (2024). Analyses of renal function using MRI in upright and supine positions. *Journal of Magnetic Resonance Imaging*, *61*. https://www.semanticscholar.org/paper/174f775d1648ef449cdeec8e12645d4e0d08aa9d (accessed on 25th June 2025).
30. Nguyen, M. D., Dileep, G., Quizon, M., Nguyen, V., Demirci, A. N., & Hanna, R. (2024). May-Haggling anomaly associated nephropathy: Case series. *SAGE Open Medical Case Reports*, *12*. https://www.semanticscholar.org/paper/0fb3be55eece445e3b46ff77f2d2a4a2f35d94d5 (accessed on 25th June 2025).

31. Patra, J. K., Das, G., Fraceto, L. F., Ramos Campos, E. V., Rodriguez-Torres, M. del P., Acosta-Torres, L. S., Díaz-Torres, L. A., et al. (2018). Nano based drug delivery systems: Recent developments and future prospects. *Journal of Nanobiotechnology, 16*. https://doi.org/10.1186/s12951-018-0392-8 (accessed on 25th June 2025).

32. Peterson, B. S., Trampush, J., Brown, M., Maglione, M., Bolshakova, M., Rozelle, M., Miles, J., et al. (2024). Tools for the diagnosis of ADHD in children and adolescents: A systematic review. *Pediatrics*. https://www.semanticscholar.org/paper/88685585a0fb4f39aa21a3acfcdbf33b6060238b (accessed on 25th June 2025).

33. Qahtani, S. A., Ismail, K. A., Hagag, H. M., Hulbah, M., Bakhuraysah, M., Johari, N. M., Alotaibi, S. M., et al. (2024). Relation between urine cytological findings and renal function in patients with kidney stones in Taif, Saudi Arabia. *Medicina, 60*. https://www.semanticscholar.org/paper/2c441ada9daa145f218fcf07360455f0fed5a5d5 (accessed on 25th June 2025).

34. Rajkomar, A., Dean, J. B., & Kohane, I. S. (2019). Machine learning in medicine. *New England Journal of Medicine, 380*, 1347–1358. https://doi.org/10.1056/nejmra1814259 (accessed on 25th June 2025).

35. Ricco, J. B., Bartelink, M. L., Björck, M., Brodmann, M., Cohnert, T., Czerny, M., De Carlo, M., et al. (2017). 2017 ESC guidelines on the diagnosis and treatment of peripheral arterial diseases, in collaboration with the European Society for Vascular Surgery (ESVS). *European Heart Journal, 39*, 763–816. https://doi.org/10.1093/eurheartj/ehx095 (accessed on 25th June 2025).

36. Schneider, B. J., Naidoo, J., Santomasso, B., Lacchetti, C., Adkins, S., Anadkat, M. J., Atkins, M. B., et al. (2021). Management of immune-related adverse events in patients treated with immune checkpoint inhibitor therapy: ASCO guideline update. *Journal of Clinical Oncology, 39*, 4073–4126. https://doi.org/10.1200/jco.21.01440 (accessed on 25th June 2025).

37. Sun, L., Xu, M., Deng, X., & Liu, X. (2025). Renal insufficiency caused by *TMEM216* gene mutation: Case report. *Frontiers in Medicine, 12*. https://www.semanticscholar.org/paper/2eca62b9c8a1947d79eaae1459901d5dd5dcac79 (accessed on 25th June 2025).

38. Wang, L., & Wang, X. (2024). Diagnostic value of multi-parameter ultrasound evaluation in sepsis complicated by acute kidney injury. *Renal Failure, 46*. https://www.semanticscholar.org/paper/673c87de0dfd6d9fa2fd06e3b7855297ea22e72e (accessed on 25th June 2025).

39. Williams, B., Mancia, G., Spiering, W., Agabiti Rosei, E., Azizi, M., Burnier, M., Clement, D. L., et al. (2018). 2018 ESC/ESH guidelines for the management of arterial hypertension. *European Heart Journal, 39*, 3021–3104. https://doi.org/10.1093/eurheartj/ehy339 (accessed on 25th June 2025).

40. XVth International Congress on Pediatric Laboratory Medicine, Munich, Nov 27–28, 2021; Poster presentation abstracts. (2021). *LaboratoriumsMedizin*. https://www.semanticscholar.org/paper/1e508cacc0e6af7159337d02518bb9de2b7d40e4 (accessed on 25th June 2025).

41. Zhou, B., Hong, M., Jin, L., & Ling, K. (2024). Exploring the relationship between creatine supplementation and renal function: Insights from Mendelian randomization analysis. *Renal Failure, 46*. https://www.semanticscholar.org/paper/882ea9348d9dd77797fb74e30e5bc28e7f59d34d (accessed on 25th June 2025).

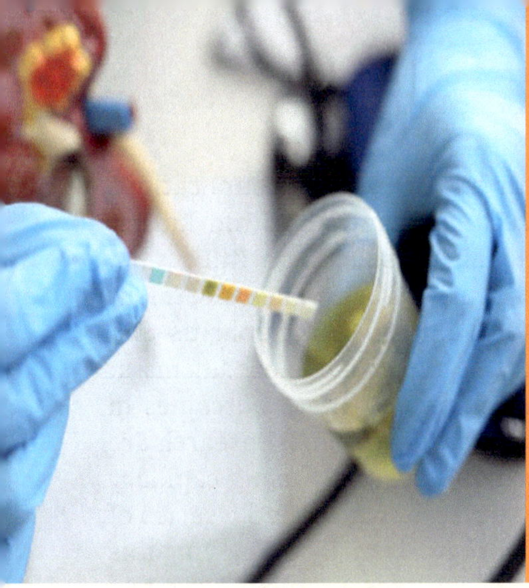

Chapter 3

GLOMERULAR DISEASES (GLOMERULONEPHRITIS)

Contents

Introduction

Glomerular disorders, and glomerulonephritis in particular, are a significant topic of research in the medical specialty of nephrology, attracting the attention of both scientists and doctors due to the complexity and varied presentation of these conditions. Glomerulonephritis is a collection of kidney conditions characterized by inflammation of the glomeruli, the essential renal filtering structures. Such conditions can be grouped based on etiology, pathophysiology, and clinical presentation and include primary and secondary manifestations of disease. Understanding glomerular diseases is essential not only for management and diagnosis but also for identifying the underlying biochemical and immunologic processes that cause renal dysfunction. With the increasing prevalence of non-communicable diseases and their complications, glomerular diseases are a newly emerging public health concern worthy of extensive research in both academic and clinical settings. One of the promising areas of research into glomerular diseases is the pathophysiological mechanism of sphingosine 1-phosphate (S1P) in kidney disease. This bioactive lipid has garnered interest with its far-reaching implications in cellular signaling processes that regulate inflammation and cell proliferation within kidney tissue. Specifically, studies have highlighted the modulation of signal transduction within renal glomerular and tubular cells by S1P, suggesting its utility as a therapeutic target for the treatment and management of glomerular disease, as well as conditions such as glomerulonephritis and diabetic nephropathy. Focus on S1P not only enhances insight into the molecular mechanisms at play but also opens new avenues for targeted therapies that would improve patient outcomes in these multifactorial conditions (Huwiler et al., 2013). Advances in urinary proteomics research are a paradigm shift in diagnostic and predictive assessment of glomerular disease. By using capillary electrophoresis coupled with mass spectrometry, researchers have successfully detected a series of urinary protein biomarkers associated with renal injury and disease progression. By employing this non-invasive technique, glomerular diseases can be diagnosed at an early stage, thereby improving clinical decision-making. Collagen fragments, serum albumin, and uromodulin have shown promise for enhanced sensitivity and specificity compared to traditional diagnostic methods. With the integration of urinary proteomics in the clinic, field development has the potential to transform our understanding and management of glomerulonephritis, leading to customized therapy and improved prognostication in these patients (Magalhães et al., 2016) (Figure 3.1).

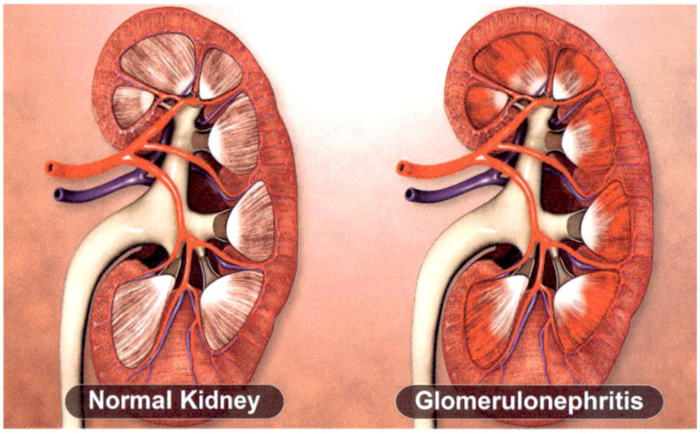

Figure 3.1. Glomerular diseases (glomerulonephritis).

Source: https://adultpediatricuro.com/wp-content/uploads/2020/01/glomerulonephritis-causes-symptoms-treatment-Omaha.jpg.

Definition of Glomerular Diseases

Glomerular diseases, also known as glomerulonephritis, are a group of diseases primarily affecting the glomeruli, the small filtering units of the kidneys. Glomerular diseases are characterized by glomerular inflammation and injury, resulting in alterations in kidney function. These changes in kidney function can be manifested clinically by proteinuria, hematuria, and acute or chronic renal injury. Glomerular diseases have a multifactorial cause; they can be triggered by infectious etiology, autoimmune disease, or secondary glomerulopathies resulting from systemic disease. Understanding the pathologic mechanisms of the diseases is critical to make accurate diagnoses and treat them appropriately, as variation in pathology oftentimes necessitates variation in therapy. Correct classification of the glomerular diseases is essential in order to guide clinical practice and institute appropriate therapeutic interventions. A proper evaluation would comprise histopathological examination of renal biopsies presenting with some patterns of injury deleterious to kidney function. Part of the prevalence and heterogeneity of these conditions has been highlighted in recent studies; for example, there was a Hong Kong prospective review that noted immunoglobulin A nephropathy as the most common form among patients with recurrent proteinuria. Of special interest, minimal-change nephrotic syndrome also accounted for a significant percentage of cases, supporting the importance of differential diagnosis within the context of clinical presentation (Chan et al., 1999). Finally, accurate classification not only assists in individualized therapeutic management but also in the understanding of disease prognosis and potential complications. In addition to the intricate nature of glomerular diseases, drug-induced kidney disease is a cutting-edge subject of interest within the specialty of nephrology. As practice in the clinics continues to change, more exposure to nephrotoxicity caused by various medications has been established. Recently, a panel developed standardized phenotypes of drug-induced kidney disease, categorizing cases based on clinical presentations such as acute kidney injury or particular glomerular damage. Through standardization of these phenotypes, researchers intend to develop a uniform system that assists clinicians in identifying and addressing drug-induced nephrotoxicity (Awdishu et al., 2015). Such standardization is warranted in an era characterized by an expanding arsenal of therapeutic drugs, where knowledge of drug mechanisms, risk assessment, and early treatment can minimize drug-induced glomerular damage very considerably.

Importance of Understanding Glomerulonephritis

It is vital to understand glomerulonephritis (GN) due to its variability in clinical manifestations and ultimate outcomes. GN is a collection of inflammatory kidney diseases that affect the glomeruli, which are essential kidney organs responsible for filtering the blood. Timely diagnosis and treatment significantly influence the development of disease since untreated or inadequately treated GN can lead to irreversible kidney damage and end-stage renal disease (ESRD). Furthermore, identifying the specific category of GN aids in selecting the appropriate therapeutic interventions. RPGN, for example, necessitates prompt intervention to minimize irreversible renal failure, highlighting the importance of effective clinical control based on accurate diagnosis and customized treatment protocols (Greenhall et al., 2015). The nuances of such conditions demand a deep appreciation not just by nephrologists but even by primary care providers who are involved in patient care and referral of patients with kidney-related complaints. The implications of an understanding of glomerulonephritis also involve the burden of healthcare that it imposes on patients and healthcare systems. Chronic primary glomerulonephritides (CPGN), for instance, might manifest as innocuous processes but have been found to pose a high risk of developing into ESRD, necessitating costly interventions such as dialysis or kidney transplantation. Not only do they augment the load on healthcare resources, but they also carry essential impacts on patients' quality of life as well as contribute to mortality (Bjørneklett et al., 2012). Moreover, recurrence of CPGN in transplanted kidneys also adds to patient complexity. Therefore, recognition of the possible courses of glomerulonephritis is essential for implementing preventive measures and mitigating the long-term complications of such diseases. Awareness of such medical as well as economic implications renders deep knowledge imperative for both patients and clinicians. Understanding glomerulonephritis allows healthcare practitioners to prioritize patient education and shared decision-making as primary considerations in treatment strategies. This realization is followed by a more forceful approach, with an emphasis on the importance of early diagnosis, lifestyle modifications, and adherence to treatment schedules. For example, for some forms of GN, patients can be educated about dietary modifications and blood pressure management to prevent exacerbation and progression towards ESRD. Furthermore, with the advancement of new research and clinical trials, updating knowledge about novel therapies and their effectiveness becomes an increasingly important task. As the existing literature has noted, the heterogeneity and complexity of GN require an evidence-based collaboration between patient and clinician that allows for individualized treatment planning and ultimately improves patient outcomes and quality of life associated with health (Bjørneklett et al., 2012). For these reasons, a knowledge of glomerulonephritis is a cornerstone of effective kidney disease management (Figure 3.2).

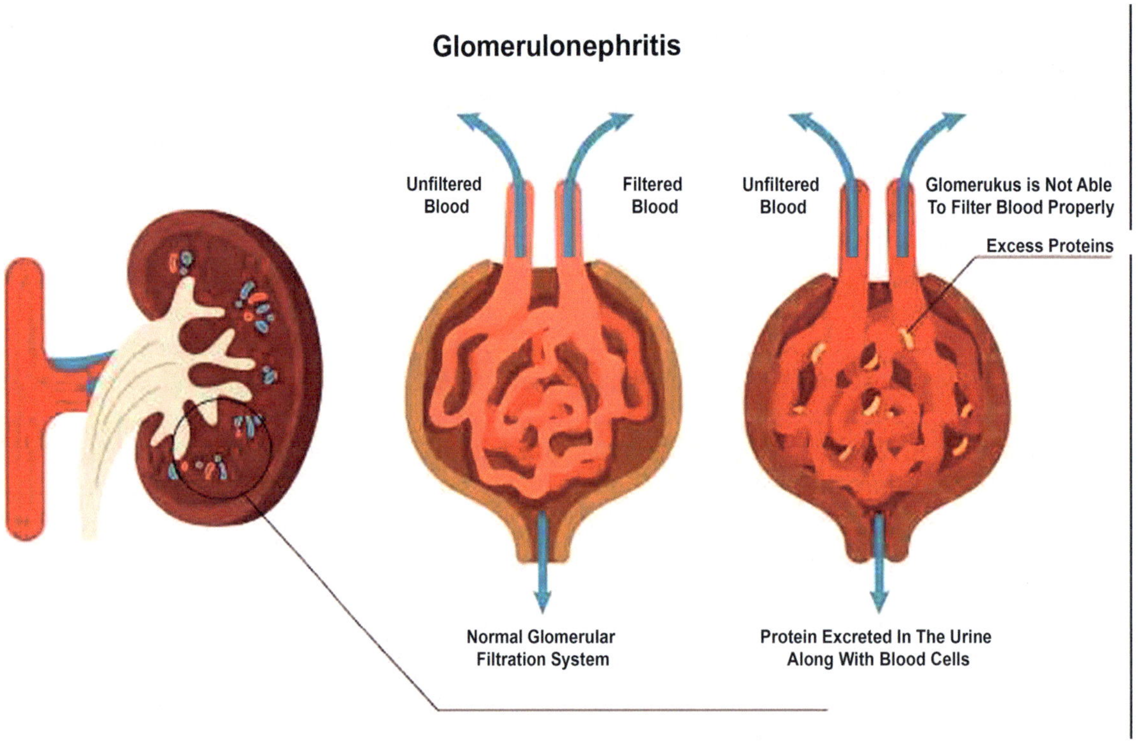

Figure 3.2. Understanding glomerulonephritis.

Source: https://www.carehospitals.com/ckfinder/userfiles/images/glomerulonephritis.webp.

3.1. Anatomy and Function of the Glomerulus

The glomerular structure, as an essential part of the kidney nephron, is the primary site for blood filtration. Its structure is made up of a capillary tuft covered by Bowman's capsule and has features that include a distinctive endothelial layer, glomerular basement membrane (GBM), and visceral epithelial cells named podocytes. The unique glomerular design permits the filtration barrier, which allows selectively water, ions, and small molecules but not larger proteins and blood cells. Filtration is responsible for maintaining fluid and electrolyte balance within the body and is essential in preventing the renal complications of most glomerular diseases. With the development of glomerular disease, such as glomerulonephritis, the function of this filtration device is compromised, and renal physiology is altered, resulting in various clinical presentations. In glomerulonephritis, the pathophysiologic changes in the glomerulus are typically due to inflammatory processes that disrupt its normal physiology and architecture. Abnormality may lead to abnormal functioning of the podocytes, which are crucial for maintaining glomerular filtration. Experiments indicate that during inflammatory conditions, such as in glomerulonephritis, podocytes exhibit migratory behaviors. Specifically, the motility proteins rise, allowing podocytes to leave their normal spatial configurations and thus contribute to crescent development under severe conditions. Such changes render it ever more challenging for the glomerulus to properly perform its filtering role, leading to impaired homeostasis and progression of kidney disease. Consequently, an understanding of glomerular anatomy and function is key where inflammatory disease impacts renal function. The glomerular filtration barrier, in turn, is made up basically of three layers: the fenestrated endothelium, the GBM, and the podocyte foot processes. All three are vital to preventing protein and blood cell loss into urine. When these architectures are disturbed, as is typically noted in glomerulonephritis, hematuria, and proteinuria may follow, causing further complications for the patient. Idiopathic nodular glomerulosclerosis, for example, exhibits a specific form of glomerular damage characterized by GBM changes and mesangial substance deposition. These alterations form the basis of the pathological profile of various glomerular diseases, underscoring the importance of familiarity with both the anatomy and the functional integrity of the glomerulus in their diagnosis and treatment. Appreciation of how glomerular diseases disrupt the anatomy and function of this critical organ relates to their broader implications for renal well-being and patient prognosis on a contextual basis (Salim et al., 2017; Besse-Eschmann et al., 2018) (Figure 3.3).

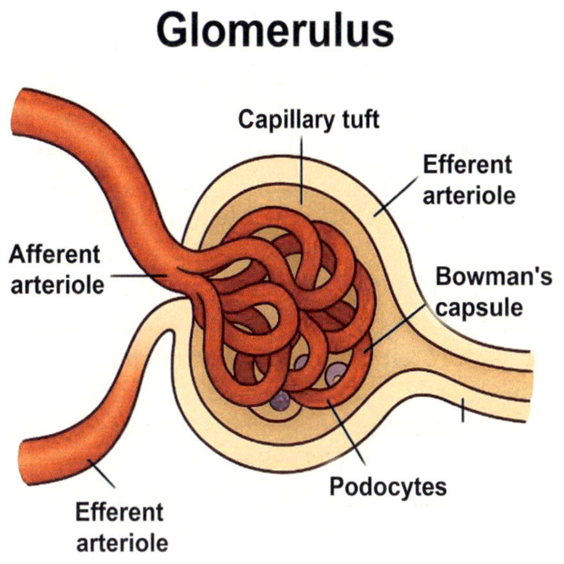

Figure 3.3. Anatomy and function of the glomerulus.

Source: https://gpatindia.com/wp-content/uploads/2025/04/ChatGPT-Image-Apr-4-2025-05_10_23-PM.png.

3.1.1. Structure of the Glomerulus

The glomerulus is a crucial renal structure that plays a vital role in the filtration process in the kidneys. As a capillary network, the glomerulus is encased with a Bowman's capsule, in which blood is filtered. Ultrafiltration begins here as the pressure from the blood pushes plasma through the walls of the capillaries, which are selectively permeable due to the fenestrae and glomerular basement membrane. This design allows for the filtration of larger molecules, such as proteins and red blood cells, while permitting smaller solutes, including ions and water, to pass through. The structural integrity of the glomerulus is thus vital to maintaining homeostasis in the body, underscoring its significance in glomerular disease processes such as glomerulonephritis, wherein structural changes can lead to severe clinical outcomes. The podocytes, specialized glomerular capillary-lined epithelial cells, are essential for guaranteeing glomerular filtration. Their foot processes interact to form filtration slits that further regulate permeability. Loss or damage of podocytes eliminates the filtration barrier, leading to increased protein permeability, a feature of various nephropathies. Recent research has highlighted the importance of examining the integrity of podocytes as an assessment of disease morbidity and the effectiveness of therapy. For instance, identifying urinary biomarkers that are specific to podocyte damage is possible for non-invasive disease screening. As discussed in the literature, these biomarkers provide valuable information about a patient's glomerular status, enhancing diagnostic and prognostic assessments and enabling early intervention against podocyte malfunction-derived diseases, such as glomerulonephritis (Sekulic et al., 2013). The glomerular structure is dynamically related to the clinical presentations that follow glomerular disease. Nephrotic syndrome with massive proteinuria, hypoalbuminemia, and edema illustrates the effects of alterations in glomerular permeability. Different grades of proteinuria could reflect various degrees of glomerular damage in this syndrome, demonstrating the quantitative nature of the underlying pathologic process (Michael et al., 1973). Since the glomerular structure fails due to injury or inflammation, the resultant disrupted filtration mechanism can lead to systemic effects, such as fluid overload and electrolyte imbalances. Understanding the intricate relationship between glomerular function, structure, and the physiological effects of glomerular disease is essential for designing specific therapeutic interventions and providing optimal patient care in glomerulonephritis (Figure 3.4).

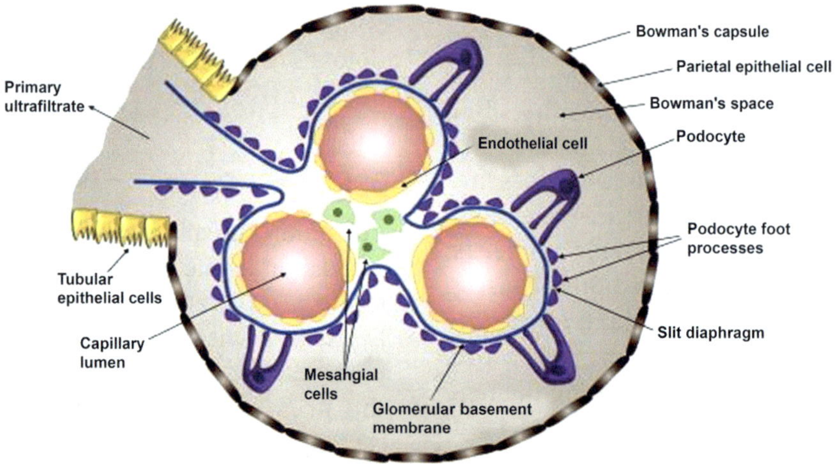

Figure 3.4. Glomerular structure.

Source: https://ars.els-cdn.com/content/image/1-s2.0-S1521661616301231-gr1.jpg.

3.1.2. Role in Filtration

The role of the glomeruli in the filtration process is pivotal to maintaining overall renal system homeostasis. Glomeruli are the initial line of defense that filter blood, allowing water, electrolytes, and molecular-weight solutes to pass through while excluding larger units such as proteins and blood cells. Selective filtration is crucial in preventing proteinuria, a hallmark of glomerular diseases such as glomerulonephritis. When structural or functional derangements occur in the glomeruli, as in the majority of nephritides, this delicate balance is disrupted, and extraneous material enters the filtrate. Therefore, awareness of the filtration mechanism and its application to diseased conditions enables the design of appropriate therapeutic measures for the recovery of glomerular function and renal salvage. In glomerular diseases, the integrity of the filtration apparatus is of prime concern. Damage to podocytes, endothelial cells, or the glomerular basement membrane will cause loss of this selectivity of permeability.

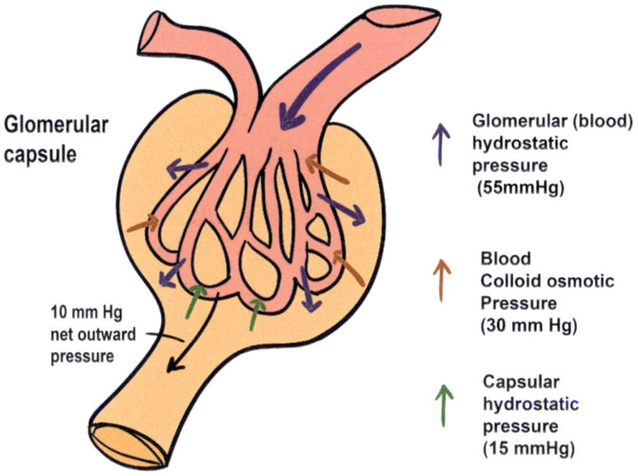

Figure 3.5. The role of the glomeruli in the filtration process.

Source: https://cdn.kastatic.org/ka-perseus-images/0e7bfc98302c3e45dc7ec73ab142566a57513ec3.svg.

Loss is typically accompanied by the production of nephrotic syndrome, manifested as loss of large quantities of protein in the urine, edema, and resultant secondary complications such as hypertension. The connection between endocrine function and renal function cannot be overlooked; diseases such as hypothyroidism have also been associated with nephrotic syndrome. As Barbano et al. (2017) explain, the relationship between nephrotic syndrome and thyroid dysfunction includes alterations in thyroid hormone metabolism due to elevated proteinuria. Thus, recognizing the multifaceted role of filtration in the case of glomerular disease can unveil avenues to effective management and treatment. The signal transduction pathways involved in mediating renal filtration are also significant to learn about in terms of glomerular disease development. Recent research has also demonstrated the relevance of sphingosine 1-phosphate (S1P) in modulating renal function and as a potential therapeutic application. S1P regulates cell signaling in glomerular and tubular cells, which may be involved in the pathogenesis of glomerulonephritis and other kidney diseases. As indicated in the study presented by Huwiler et al. (2013), modulation of S1P signaling has promising therapeutic potential. By addressing these pathways, scientists can design drugs that treat both the causes and symptoms of glomerular diseases in a similar manner. This integrated understanding of filtration, cellular signaling, and endocrine interaction may be a key to more efficient glomerular disease treatment, resulting in improved patient outcomes (Figure 3.5).

3.1.3. Importance in Kidney Function

The kidneys are responsible for maintaining homeostasis in the body, and their primary functions are closely tied to glomerular integrity. Glomeruli, tiny networks of capillaries contained within the kidneys, play a vital role in filtering blood such that the waste products are removed, but necessary substances such as proteins and electrolytes are retained. When glomerular function is compromised by glomerulonephritis, the filtering ability of the kidneys is compromised greatly. A reduction in this ability can lead to complications, such as an elevation in serum creatinine levels and alterations in electrolyte balance, further impairing renal function. Appreciation of the essential importance of glomerular filtration is vital to understanding the greater relevance of kidney diseases and their potential impacts on health overall, particularly in the context of the progressive nature of many glomerular diseases. Kidney function is more complex than filtration, with additional functions such as blood pressure regulation and the secretion of erythropoietin, a hormone critical to the production of red blood cells. Derangement of such functions, particularly in conditions such as diabetic kidney disease (DKD), can have secondary implications for overall health. Recent literature has been said to have unmasked heterogeneity in DKD, not only by varying degrees of albuminuria but also by nonalbuminuric renal impairment and advancing renal deterioration without albuminuria. Thus, patients are no longer always able to present with features classically, and therefore, early diagnosis and intervention plans become more challenging. An astute awareness of these pathways is essential for treating patients properly, particularly as modes of treatment evolve, emphasizing the importance of continuous education among healthcare professionals regarding new developments in treatment and their implications for kidney status (Barutta et al., 2019). In addition, the overlap between kidney function and systemic disease emphasizes the importance of early detection and ongoing management of glomerular disease. With continued research determining the pathophysiologic mechanisms underlying these conditions, it has become increasingly evident that early intervention has a significant impact on disease progression. For instance, new anti-hyperglycemic medications have been created that are specifically addressed to patients with compromised renal function, redrawing the treatment model for patients with diabetes and end-stage kidney disease. This progress reflects the need to integrate nephrology and comprehensive diabetes care in clinical practice, ensuring that patient management is holistic and supports optimal kidney function. Additionally, the importance of complete renal wellness on global quality of life underscores the pressing need for further research on identifying potential drug targets and biomarkers to mitigate the impact of glomerular diseases (Gutiérrez Rodríguez et al., 2019) (Figure 3.6).

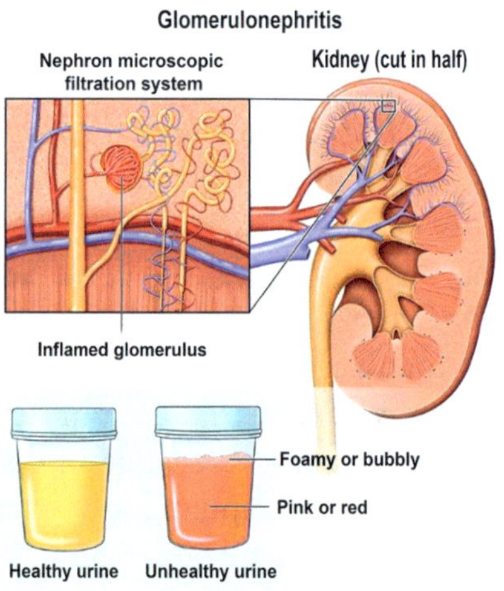

Figure 3.6. Glomeruli Importance in kidney function.

Source: https://my.clevelandclinic.org/-/scassets/images/org/health/articles/16167-glomerulonephritis.

3.2. Types of Glomerular Diseases

Of the other types of glomerular disease, the primary glomerulonephritides, such as Minimal Change Disease (MCD) and Focal Segmental Glomerulosclerosis (FSGS), are significant. MCD occurs predominantly in children and is diagnosed by the sudden onset of nephrotic syndrome with minimal changes under light microscopy. The pathogenic process is most often linked with abnormalities in the function of T-cells, leading to the secretion of substances that make the podocytes permeable. In contrast, FSGS can be a primary condition or secondary to numerous diseases, some of which include obesity and hypertension.

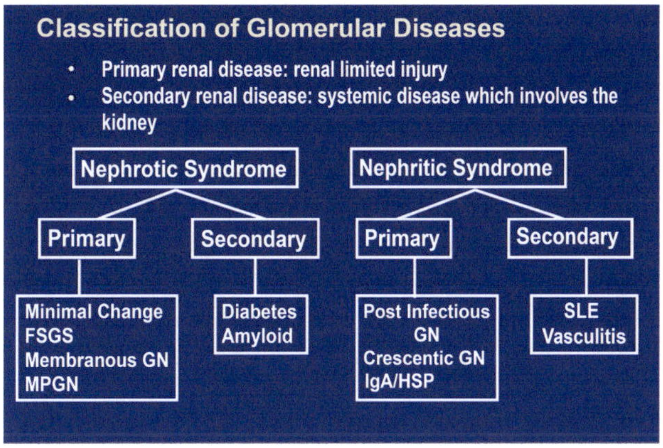

Figure 3.7. Types of glomerular diseases.

Source: https://pbs.twimg.com/media/BwgJfYxCEAA8rbK.jpg:large.

The pathologic feature of FSGS is the focal scarring of glomeruli, resulting in massive proteinuria and ultimately end-stage renal disease if left untreated. Both illustrate the heterogeneity of primary glomerular disease and highlight the need for individually tailored therapeutic interventions to reverse their effects on renal function. Secondary glomerular disease, which is frequently associated with systemic disorders, also requires individualized consideration due to its complexity and multifactorial etiology. Systemic lupus erythematosus (SLE) and diabetes mellitus appear in the glomeruli as a result of systemic inflammation or metabolic disarray. In SLE, lupus nephritis can result in immune complex deposition in glomeruli, resulting in severe renal impairment and necessitating aggressive immunosuppression. Diabetes mellitus is the principal cause of diabetic nephropathy, which is hyperglycemia-mediated damage to the glomerular filtration barrier. The progressive nature of these secondary glomerular diseases necessitates early identification and treatment to prevent irreversible damage, highlighting the importance of understanding their relationship with systemic health. Recent studies have also identified potential urinary biomarkers that can facilitate diagnosis and management, guiding clinical decision-making in nephrology (Magalhães et al., 2016). Furthermore, advances in medical science have expanded the scope of glomerular diseases, their diagnosis, and treatment. The development of novel biomarkers through urinary proteomics holds promise for enhancing the specificity and sensitivity of kidney disease assessment. Collagen fragments and uromodulin are among the biomarkers being investigated for their potential in characterizing mechanisms and disease progression. These findings underscore the need for ongoing research aimed at improving diagnostic accuracy and treatment regimens for patients with glomerulopathy (N/A, 2021). As nephrology continues to evolve, an integrated model that pairs progress in biomarker research with current clinical practice will prove invaluable in effectively tackling the complex nature of glomerular diseases. A greater focus will be placed on improving patient care and achieving optimal results through more personalized treatment approaches, which will require constant updating and access to resources by healthcare providers (Figure 3.7).

3.2.1. Primary Glomerulonephritis

Primary Glomerulonephritis constitutes a series of kidney diseases characterized by glomerular inflammation and damage, which are essential in blood filtration. The condition can manifest in varying forms like minimal change disease, focal segmental glomerulosclerosis, and membranous nephropathy with varying pathogenic mechanisms and manifestations. The etiology is likely to be idiopathic; however, secondary etiologies such as infections or systemic disease may also trigger glomerular injury. Understanding the pathophysiology is essential for clinicians to determine the appropriate treatment modalities and estimate patient prognosis. The clinical presentation is typically marked by proteinuria, hematuria, and edema, which can significantly contribute to the person's poor quality of life and compromised renal function. Early diagnosis and intervention are crucial in preventing disease progression and irreversible damage to the kidneys.

Treatment of primary glomerulonephritis varies slightly, depending on the subtype and severity of the illness. Corticosteroids and immunosuppressive agents, such as cyclophosphamide, are applied in the majority of instances to reduce inflammation and immune-related damage. New treatments, such as biologic agents, are being researched for their potential to offer more efficacy or less toxicity. As might be anticipated, patients with RPGN are faced with an emergent medical need since their renal function rapidly deteriorates and, if delayed, may lead to end-stage renal disease. Plasmapheresis and intense immunosuppression may be required measures to treat this ominous condition effectively, and ongoing research into the various causes of RPGN will enhance treatment strategies and patient outcomes.

The recent pathogenesis and treatment research on Primary Glomerulonephritis emphasize the importance of tailor-made treatment strategies. Cryoglobulinemia, for instance, often induced by infections such as hepatitis C, may cause extensive glomerular damage, thus underscoring the importance of specific interventions against both the underlying infection and its renal effects (Braun et al., 2007). The efficacy of more recently developed antiviral agents holds hope for secondary presentations of glomerular disease in the setting of such infection. Moreover, the paucity of robust clinical trials in RPGN is a significant issue; current guidelines for treatment rely on evidence from studies enrolling patients with less severe renal impairment (Greenhall et al., 2015). This highlights a need for larger cohort studies or biologic registries to validate therapeutic interventions in the management of advanced renal illnesses and enhance evidence-based practice among clinicians (Figure 3.8).

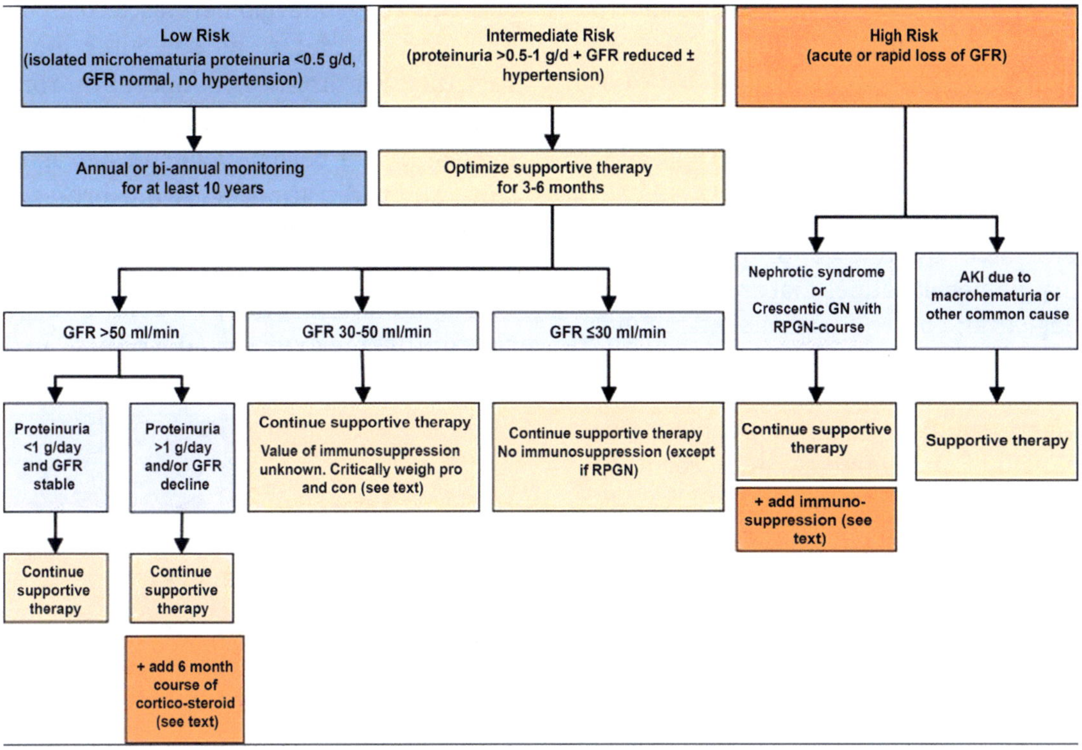

Figure 3.8. Primary glomerulonephritis.

Source: https://ars.els-cdn.com/content/image/1-s2.0-S2211913213000375-gr2.jpg.

3.2.2. Secondary Glomerulonephritis

Secondary glomerulonephritis is a form of renal inflammation that develops as a complication of systemic diseases, rather than as a primary disease within the kidneys. Infections, autoimmune diseases, and malignancies are common etiologies, underscoring the multi-etiological nature of the condition. For instance, viral infections, such as hepatitis C, may lead to cryoglobulinemia, which is an essential etiology of secondary glomerulonephritis and can progress to fulminant complications such as renal failure. The intricate interplay between systemic diseases and kidney involvement is why the need for multidisciplinary evaluation and management requires nephrologists to consider other organs in the presence of renal presentations in patients. Secondary glomerulonephritis pathophysiology is typically reflected by systemic diseases. For example, the deposition of immune complexes in autoimmune disease-related conditions, such as systemic lupus erythematosus, is responsible for initiating inflammatory reactions within the glomeruli and causing classic clinical syndromes. Vasculitides are also causative in secondary glomerulonephritis, where inflammation of blood vessels compromises renal perfusion and function. Multifactorial etiology necessitates proper investigative procedures to establish the etiology and design therapeutic measures accordingly, thereby improving patient outcomes. New treatment advances, particularly with the availability of targeted therapy for autoimmune disorders and viral infections, have been encouraging in managing secondary glomerulonephritis and arresting its progression. Ongoing research is transforming our understanding of secondary glomerulonephritis, paving the way for new treatment paradigms. Existing literature concurs with the understanding of the interface between glomerular disease and systemic disorders, guiding clinical practice and future research. Books such as "An Update on Glomerulopathies – Clinical and Treatment Aspects" provide insightful views into this emerging field, offering comprehensive overviews of primary and secondary glomerulopathies that are essential for nephrologists and other clinicians. Interestingly, these articles emphasize the importance of early detection and prompt treatment in preventing secondary glomerulonephritis from compromising renal function, underscoring the significance of ongoing education and research in this vital area of nephrology (Braun et al., 2007; N/A, 2021).

3.2.3. Hereditary Glomerular Diseases

Hereditary glomerular disease is a crucial subgroup of glomerulonephritis caused by genetic mutations that result in glomerular structural and functional abnormalities. It tends to manifest early in life and can result in progressive renal damage, giving rise to chronic kidney disease (CKD). The complex interaction between genes and renal function necessitates the importance of early diagnosis and careful management. Most relevantly, pathogenic variants in proteins that are instrumental to the structure of the glomerulus, such as nephrin or podocin, cause dysfunction in the filtration barrier.

These genetic processes not only predispose the patient to renal failure but also underlie a spectrum of renal manifestations, which are representative of a complete understanding in the context of hereditary glomerular disease. Hereditary glomerular disease pathogenesis is extremely heterogeneous, encompassing a range of structural and biochemical abnormalities. A range of genetic diseases, such as Alport syndrome and focal segmental glomerulosclerosis, illustrate how certain mutations can alter glomerular structure. For instance, in Alport syndrome, type IV collagen mutations lead to the breakdown of the glomerular basement membrane and greatly slow down filtration, allowing proteinuria to occur. This perturbation can potentially release a cycle of repeated damage and fibrosis that can culminate in CKD as outlined in the self-sustaining mechanisms described in recent studies (Benigni et al., 2007).

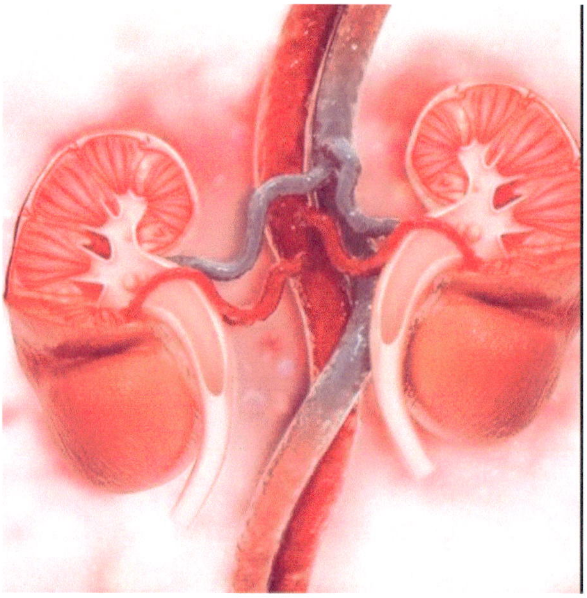

Figure 3.9. Mechanistic insights in hereditary kidney disease.

Source: https://www.frontiersin.org/files/special%20topics/44514/thumb_400.jpg.

These mechanisms are key to understanding, as they determine optimal treatment regimens that result in the reversal or arrest of progression to end-stage kidney disease. Hereditary glomerular diseases should be identified and classified to develop appropriate management plans and provide effective genetic counseling. The 2012 KDIGO CKD classification scheme offers a critical framework for determining the stages of kidney disease progression according to both the etiology and the level of proteinuria (Xasanova et al., 2024). Since hereditary glomerular diseases tend to cause early-onset CKD, earlier detection can significantly improve patient outcomes through intervention with such measures as specific therapies and lifestyle modification. Moreover, genetic diagnosis is even more critical in the diagnosis of these diseases, as it enables early treatment capable of preserving renal function and delaying the need for renal replacement therapies. This bimodal approach, which couples genetics with clinical management, is essential in reducing the effects of hereditary glomerular disease on patients and the healthcare system as a whole (Figure 3.9).

3.3. Pathophysiology of Glomerulonephritis

The pathophysiology of glomerulonephritis is multifaceted, comprising inflammation and damage to the glomeruli, the kidneys' primary filtering mechanisms. Glomerulonephritis can result from various etiologies, including both immunologic and non-immunologic causes. Immune processes are generally characterized by the deposition of immune complexes or antibodies within the glomerular tissue, leading to an inflammatory reaction that disrupts normal kidney function. Such an injury may lead to a range of clinical manifestations, including hematuria, proteinuria, and altered renal function.

The pathogenetic cascade triggered by these immune responses not only leads to edema and hypertension but also stimulates secondary pathologic mechanisms, culminating in impairment of the renal architecture and function altogether. In addition to the immunodysregulation, the impact on endocrine function has also come to be increasingly recognized in glomerulonephritis. For instance, thyroid dysfunction has been a serious complication of nephrotic syndrome, a well-known presentation of glomerulonephritis. Hypothyroidism may be caused by increased urinary excretion of thyroid hormones and binding proteins, as well as by changes in the metabolism of the hormones themselves resulting from severe proteinuria. These alterations are indicative of a potential nephroendocrine disease, and one that contributes to the patient's clinical complexity. Treatment protocols, including thyroid hormone replacement, are crucial for managing the disease and improving patient outcomes, underscoring the necessity for a comprehensive understanding of the pathophysiological interactions in glomerular disease (Barbano et al., 2017). Furthermore, recent evidence has demonstrated the etiological function of heparanase in the development of acute kidney injury (AKI), revealing its beta-defensive function in the pathogenesis of glomerular disease. As a heparan sulfate-degrading enzyme, heparanase is involved in the turnover of the extracellular matrix. It may intensify inflammatory reactions in renal tissues. Increased levels of heparanase have been associated with more severe tubular injury following ischemic insult, resulting in higher serum creatinine and blood urea nitrogen levels. Facilitating profibrotic and pro-inflammatory markers during such renal injuries is evidence of the enzymes' harmful effect. Interestingly, pharmacological heparanase inhibition has now also been viewed as a therapeutic option for enhancing renal impairment. This understanding of heparanases' function provides the avenue to continuing exploration of targeted therapy, having an enormous effect on the treatment of glomerulonephritis and other such renal pathologies (Abassi et al., 2017) (Figure 3.10).

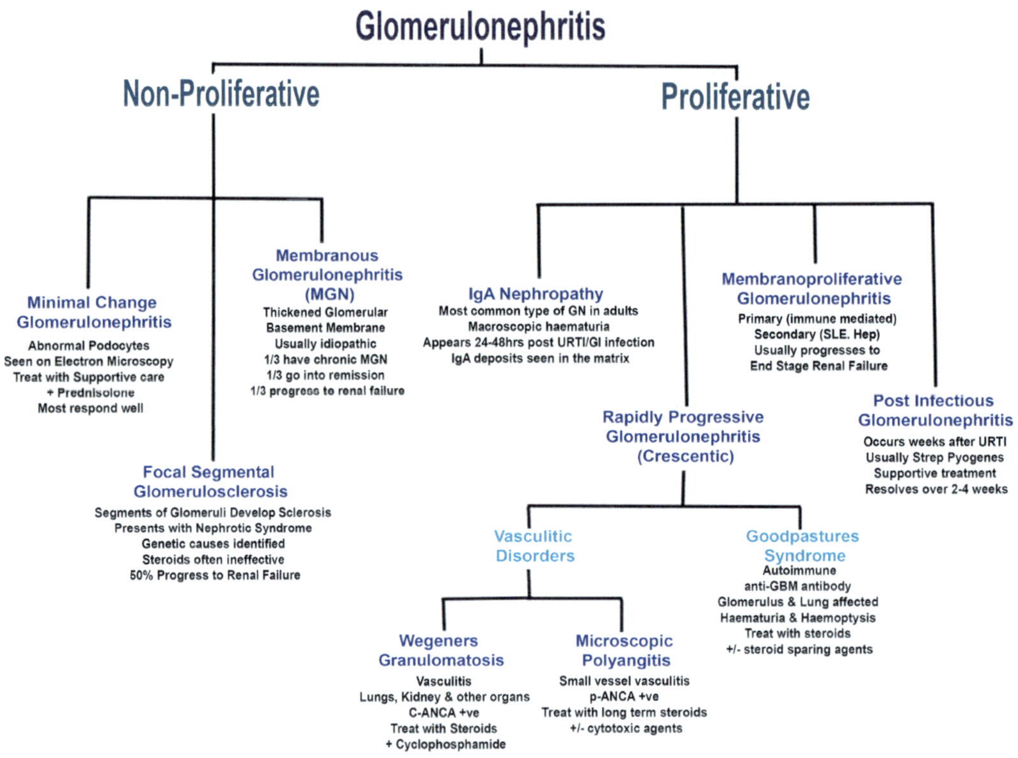

Figure 3.10. Pathophysiology of glomerulonephritis.

Source: https://i.pinimg.com/736x/52/1c/d2/521cd2aa7e0962309fcc88d42865d65e.jpg.

3.3.1. Immune Response Mechanisms

The mechanisms of the immune response in glomerular diseases, particularly glomerulonephritis, are a complex web of interactions among the various immune cells, chemokines, and cytokines. When the kidney is exposed to inflammation or injury, resident immune cells such as macrophages and dendritic cells become activated, leading to the secretion of pro-inflammatory cytokines. These cytokines then recruit other leukocytes to the site of injury and propagate the inflammatory response. This chemokine-directed immune cell recruitment subsequently propels the leukocytes out of the circulatory system into the renal parenchyma, where they may contribute to both protective immunity and tissue damage. The determination of the particular functions these immune components play within glomerular disease pathogenesis is critical to the determination of therapeutic regimens that may be modulated to regulate the immune system while preserving kidney function. The pathogenetic role of chemokines in glomerulopathies underscores their dual function of mediating renal inflammation, as well as possibly exacerbating it. Since chemokines orchestrate the leukocyte migration and activation, their expression profiles in the kidney can have a direct correlation to the degree of renal damage evident in glomerulonephritis. Experiments have shown that inhibiting chemokine activity can cause significant retardation of leukocyte infiltration and reduce renal injury. However, recent studies suggest that these treatments also have unforeseen consequences, demonstrating that inhibiting chemokine signaling can actually exacerbate inflammation under certain conditions. This foreboding paradox emphasizes the complexity of immune process workings in renal diseases. It necessitates a more harmonious approach in drug development, where the goal is to achieve an optimal balance between inhibiting inflammation and preserving immune function. Moreover, the impact of genetic models on knowledge regarding immune mechanisms of response in glomerular disease has greatly increased our understanding of glomerular pathologies. From genetically modified mouse models, researchers have studied the roles of single immune pathways in glomerulonephritis. For instance, the production and application of knock-out mice enable the examination of single-gene deficiencies that can reveal the critical roles that particular cytokines or chemokines play in the onset of disease. These models allow both mesangioproliferative and crescentic forms of glomerulonephritis to be investigated and lend considerable insight into the molecular mechanisms of these illnesses. Follow-up studies with such animal models not only support the mechanistic basis of immune responses in renal conditions but also allow for the identification of new therapeutic targets to improve clinical outcomes in patients with such conditions, closing the loop between bench findings and practical applications in the management of glomerular disease.

3.3.2. Inflammatory Processes

Inflammatory processes are central to the pathogenesis of glomerular disease, most notably in glomerulonephritis, where a deranged immune response causes tissue injury in the renal glomeruli. In each of these conditions, immune activation exacerbates inflammation by recruiting leukocytes and releasing pro-inflammatory cytokines and chemokines. These molecules not only facilitate leukocyte migration into injured tissues but also play a crucial role in amplifying inflammation. The correlation of the expression of these inflammatory mediators with renal injury severity suggests their significance in glomerular diseases. Notably, chemokines are involved in mediating the invasion of immune cells into the kidney, which can lead to repeated renal injury if not well-regulated, illustrating the delicate balance required in immune responses during inflammatory attacks (Abdi et al., 2004). The availability of certain signal molecules involved in inflammatory mechanisms further underscores their presence in glomerular disease. Such molecules include sphingosine 1-phosphate (S1P), which is identified as a critical molecule in renal glomerular mechanisms. S1P has been found to regulate multiple cellular functions, including cell survival, growth, and inflammation. S1P signaling modulation has been shown to significantly impact kidney function, with relevance to the progression of diseases such as diabetic nephropathy and glomerulonephritis. By modulating glomerular and tubular cells, S1P pathways are an attractive target for therapy because modulation of S1P-mediated signals can alter inflammatory responses and reverse renal injury. This highlights the necessity for further investigation into its actions and implications in kidney disease situations (Huwiler et al., 2013). Mechanisms of inflammation are not just an explanation of pathological signs but also encompass the therapeutic interventions that might mitigate renal damage. Targeting chemokines and their receptors has been explored as a therapeutic measure, though one that is difficult to implement based on the bidirectional function of these molecules to promote protective and harmful immune mechanisms. Therapies that modulate the inflammatory environment must be carefully tailored to avoid exacerbating renal damage. The potential for augmenting innate and adaptive immune capabilities by such intervention suggests restraint is required. Future studies will undoubtedly reveal more about how best to balance these therapeutic and disease-inducing characteristics of inflammation, potentially clearing the way for better management and therapeutic regimes for glomerular disease patients (Abdi et al., 2004) (Figure 3.11).

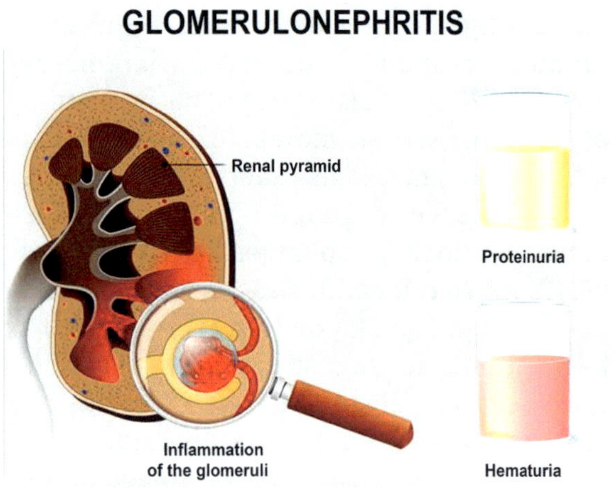

Figure 3.11. Inflammatory processes of glomerulonephritis.

Source: https://www.kidney.org/sites/default/files/glomerulonephritis.png.

3.3.3. Impact on Kidney Function

The impact of glomerular disease, particularly glomerulonephritis, on renal function is profound and far-reaching. Glomerular disease involves the glomeruli, the minute filtering structures of the kidney, and initiates a cascade of pathological mechanisms that disrupts proper renal function. Inflammatory responses typically play a role in glomerular damage, as evidenced by the accumulation of immune cells and the deposition of antibodies and pro-inflammatory cytokines. This inflammation can lead to a reduction in glomerular filtration rate (GFR), characterized by proteinuria, hematuria, and ultimately, renal failure if left uncorrected. Through examining the mechanisms underlying damage, researchers can gain valuable information about potential therapeutic targets for minimizing such effects and restoring kidney function. Moreover, new technological advancements in experimental nephrology have upgraded our understanding of the molecular mechanism of glomerular disease. Specifically, the use of genetically modified mouse models has allowed the study of the pathogenesis of many renal conditions. Knock-out mice have allowed scientists to study the role of individual genes in the development of renal disease and provide informative models that are able to model and situations in humans, such as crescentic glomerulonephritis and focal-segmental glomerulosclerosis. As mentioned in recent literature, care must be taken in consideration of the genetic strain of these models since it influences the severity and character of renal damage in experimental models (Anders et al., 2000). Better modeling not only promotes an understanding of the mechanisms of kidney failure but also serves as a platform for testing novel therapeutic interventions. The role of chemokines and their receptors in glomerular disease also complicates the scenario of renal function compromise. Chemokines play a crucial role in inflammatory processes, particularly in leukocyte recruitment into kidney tissues. Such activity leads to local damage, thereby potentially affecting the action of targeted therapy on chemokine activity. Yet, studies have shown that interference in chemokine pathways has paradoxical consequences in glomerular disease because blocking these signals would unintentionally worsen inflammation and ensuing renal damage. Analyzing the interactions among chemokines is crucial in developing effective therapies that minimize renal damage while minimizing undue side effects (Abdi et al., 2004). The duality of chemokine action highlights the need for a sensitive approach to therapeutic strategies aimed at preserving renal function in the context of glomerular disease.

3.4. Symptoms and Clinical Presentation

The clinical presentation and symptoms of glomerular diseases, i.e., glomerulonephritis, could primarily be based on the etiology and extent of kidney injury. The patients could initially have nonspecific signs and symptoms like malaise, fatigue, and anorexia. As the disease progresses, specific symptoms typically manifest. Common clinical presentations include hematuria, characterized by the presence of blood in the urine, which typically has a reddish or cola-colored appearance, and proteinuria, which is an abnormal presence of proteins in the urine. Both reflect altered glomerular function and are a cause for serious worry about kidney function. Swelling, or edema, typically occurs as a manifestation of the kidneys' diminished ability to control fluid balance, particularly in the extremities and face. Thus, timely detection of these symptoms is exceptionally critical for early medical intervention to prevent further renal damage. In some instances, glomerulonephritis can have extrarenal features comprising areas outside the urinary tract, which are evidence of pathophysiologic processes. Certain conditions, such as cryoglobulinemia, can manifest in the skin as cutaneous vasculitis, which can be either pre-renal or post-renal disease. This reidentification highlights the complexity of glomerulopathies and underscores the importance of a thorough evaluation of those presenting with unusual symptoms. Some secondary causes of glomerulonephritis, such as infections or autoimmune diseases, can further complicate the clinical presentation, resulting in a broad range of presentations. Hypertension, as a consequence directly related to renal impairment, is a significant presentation in others. Finally, awareness of the full spectrum of symptoms is crucial for accurate diagnosis and optimal management of glomerular disease, as early intervention can significantly influence patient prognosis (Braun et al., 2007). RPGN represents a catastrophic form of glomerular disease with sudden loss of renal function and crescentic injury to the glomerulus. Its presentation is by acute oliguria or anuria, indicative of acute renal failure, but with classical manifestations of glomerulonephritis. RPGN tends to be most commonly linked with the necessity of urgent evaluation and management to avoid sustained renal damage. Classical therapies employed in the situation have included glucocorticoids and immunosuppressive medications, such as cyclophosphamide, to reduce the pathogenetic inflammation. Despite improvements in treatment, the prognosis for individuals with severe disease remains precarious. The primary difficulty is that no randomized controlled trial has been conducted to specifically assess RPGN. Clinicians cannot base decisions regarding therapy solely on historical series and case reports. Multidisciplinary cooperation, such as the creation of biologic registries, may ultimately provide better insight into therapeutic efficacy in patients with crescentic glomerular damage (Greenhall et al., 2015) (Figure 3.12).

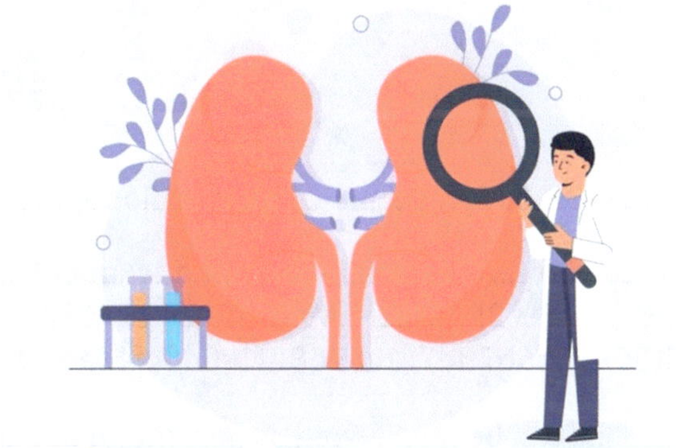

Figure 3.12. Clinical presentation of glomerular diseases.

Source: https://images.hindustantimes.com/img/2024/07/17/1600x900/kidney_1705573516844_1721194519676.jpg.

3.4.1. Common Symptoms of Glomerulonephritis

The clinical picture of glomerulonephritis is characterized by several signs and symptoms that reflect the pathological process of inflammation in the glomeruli. The most commonly seen symptoms are hematuria, or the presence of blood within the urine, which may make it red or tea-colored. This occurs due to damage to the glomerular capillaries, which causes extravasation of red blood cells into the urine. Proteinuria, or the presence of urinary protein, is often accompanied by hematuria and can result in frothy urine. Both of these are typical of the glomerular filtration barrier compromise, a characteristic of glomerular diseases. The severity and character of these findings may vary greatly in different individuals, typically related to the nature of the specific type of glomerulonephritis and the degree of kidney involvement. Identification of these symptoms is essential for early treatment and diagnosis. Moreover, glomerulonephritis patients may have severe fluid retention due to the impaired kidney capacity for excess water and sodium elimination.

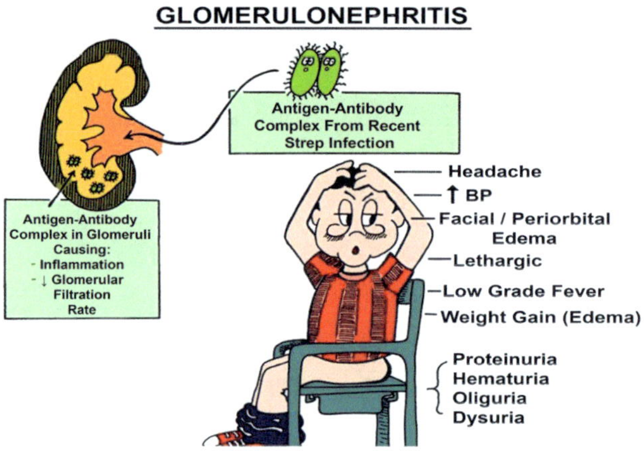

Figure 3.13. Symptoms of glomerulonephritis.

Source: https://external-content.duckduckgo.com/iu/?u=https%3A%2F%2Fi.pinimg.com%2Foriginals%2Ff5%2F02%2F14%2Ff50214a7e52bada4885a7dacaf05b1c1.jpg&f=1&nofb=1&ipt=c7bfefd85f60215a6b78d7c1c89b8df1c0d8cf42a488c6044d3f3235daff608f.

This can be manifested as peripheral edema, particularly of the ankles and feet, and hypertension resulting from volume overload. The combination of the symptoms not only signifies the deranged filtration processes but also contributes to the morbidity of glomerular diseases as a whole. The symptoms can, in some cases, advance to nephrotic syndrome, characterized by severe proteinuria, hypoalbuminemia, and enhanced edema. All of these clinical presentations signify the heterogeneity of glomerulonephritis, reflecting its capacity to evolve and become more severe into adverse renal conditions over time. Early diagnosis and treatment are necessary to minimize these risks. Additionally, because the condition is systemic in nature, glomerulonephritis can lead to issues beyond the kidneys, affecting other body systems. For instance, associated conditions like cryoglobulinaemia can worsen renal involvement and often accompany the root infections like hepatitis C. These infections may have classic clinical presentations, including dermatological rashes, arthralgia, and systemic weakness, revealing the multisystemic nature of the pathologic process. Furthermore, hypothyroidism, as a complication of nephrotic syndrome, reflects the endocrine ramifications of glomerular disease. The involvement of glomerular function in the performance of other body systems justifies the necessity of comprehensive clinical management for glomerulonephritis patients, including nephrological and systemic examinations, particularly when there is a change or worsening of symptoms (Braun et al., 2007; Barbano et al., 2017) (Figure 3.13).

3.4.2. Diagnostic Criteria

Diagnostic features of glomerular disease, particularly glomerulonephritis, require extensive knowledge regarding clinical presentation and laboratory findings. Extensive history and physical examination are crucial components, allowing clinicians to identify manifestations such as edema, hypertension, and unusual urine. Among the most significant laboratory investigations are typically urinalysis, serum biochemistry, and kidney function tests. For instance, a highly prominent increase in proteinuria is often an indicator of glomerular disease, and the urine protein-to-creatinine ratio is a simple and helpful measure for assessing protein loss. Additionally, the presence of hematuria and pathologic cellular components in urine can further refine the diagnostic approach. Identification of such clinical signs is imperative in directing future diagnostic workup to enable early and accurate detection of glomerular disease. Histopathologic examination remains a keystone of diagnosis for glomerulonephritis, providing irrefutable proof of inciting pathologies. Renal biopsy is frequently used to establish the inciting histopathologic changes that occur in kidney tissue. This diagnostic tool facilitates the distinction between various types of glomerulonephritis, including immune-mediated, infectious, and chemical-induced. For example, a study established that in protein-losing nephropathy secondary to Borrelia C6 antigen seroreactivity, distinctive clinicopathologic patterns were observed, including distinct blood cell changes and histopathologic features typical of immune-complex glomerulonephritis (RE G et al., 2019). The integration of these data supports the clear diagnosis, which leads to the development of specific therapeutic approaches. Additionally, clinicians should consider the overall systemic impact of glomerular diseases when making a diagnosis. Certain infectious conditions, such as coccidioidomycosis, have been linked to glomerular lesions suggestive of immune complex glomerulonephritis. In a large case series, renal impairment, biochemical findings, and a high prevalence of proteinuria were observed in dogs with coccidioidomycosis, highlighting the need to consider underlying infectious etiologies in patients with nephropathy (Mehrkens et al., 2016). The overlap between infectious and glomerular pathology justifies a multidisciplinary diagnostic approach, with the convergence of clinical, laboratory, and histopathological information to enhance patient treatment and management.

3.4.3. Importance of Early Detection

The significance of early diagnosis of glomerular diseases, that is, glomerulonephritis, cannot be overstated. Early diagnosis is also necessary in managing the progression of kidney decline and realizing better patient outcomes. Early detection of symptoms and etiology can lead to more effective intervention practices, allowing healthcare professionals to implement treatment regimens that can effectively reduce the threat of end-stage renal failure. For instance, secondary conditions such as cryoglobulinaemia, often induced by infections like hepatitis C, can manifest as glomerulonephritis with severe complications. Early diagnosis not only facilitates early initiation of appropriate antiviral therapies but also maximizes the quality of overall care for the patient's condition and minimizes the long-term effect on renal function (Braun et al., 2007). Additionally, the diagnosis and management of GPA underscore the importance of early diagnosis for glomerular disease. Both the upper respiratory tract presentation, if it occurs early, can potentially lead to misdiagnosis if properly investigated. Pathophysiology of GPA involves systemic vasculitis that affects the kidneys, and identification of evidence of nasal or sinus involvement has the potential for triggering early serology evaluation for anti-neutrophil cytoplasmic antibodies (ANCA). This aggressive approach is priceless, as delayed diagnosis results in renal impairment that vastly negates the prognosis, with a stark difference in survival rates based on renal status. Early detection thus serves to support a multidisciplinary approach crafted to avert the deleterious effects of the disease (Vincentiis et al., 2016). The additional integration of early detection strategies into daily healthcare practice demonstrates the importance of healthcare education and awareness. Increased patient and practitioner awareness of glomerular diseases can lead to heightened sensitivity to symptoms, resulting in earlier medical seeking. Educational initiatives that highlight risk factors, symptoms, and the importance of routine kidney function screenings can be key in reducing delayed diagnosis rates. Ultimately, these interventions may be linked with improved health outcomes and more cost-effective care associated with late disease onset. By focusing first on early detection, we can pave the way for a more efficient management landscape for glomerulonephritis and other associated disorders, thereby improving patient outcomes and experiences in a positive way (Figure 3.14).

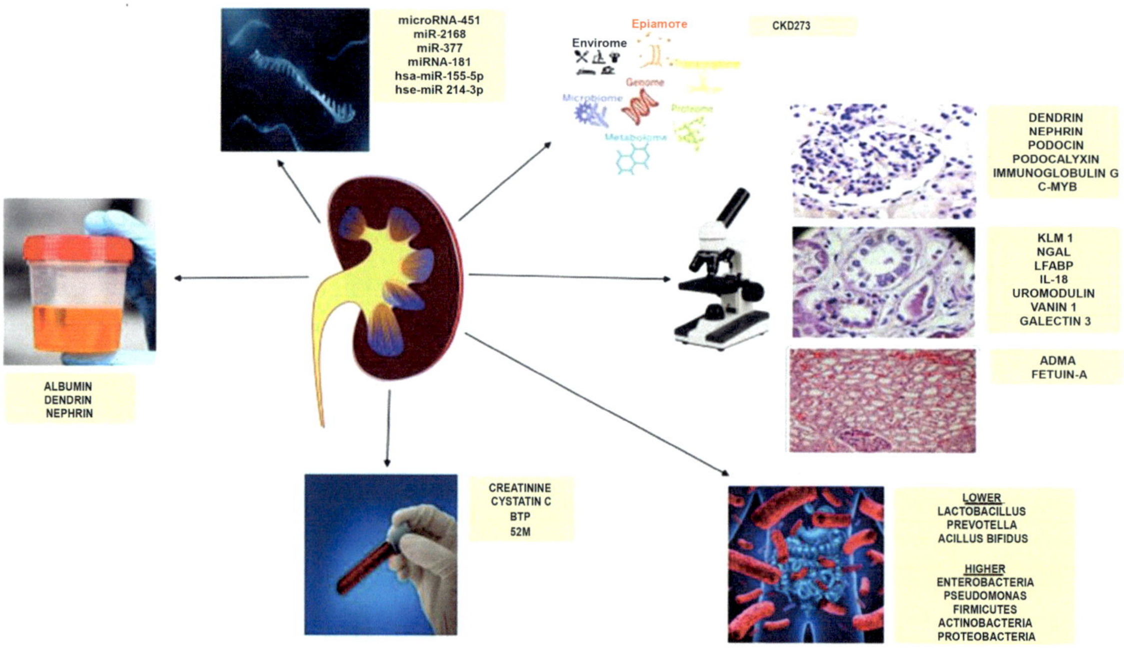

Figure 3.14. Early detection in glomerular diseases.

Source: https://www.mdpi.com/jpm/jpm-12-00548/article_deploy/html/images/jpm-12-00548-g001.png.

3.5. Diagnostic Methods

In the evaluation of glomerular diseases, particularly glomerulonephritis, a comprehensive approach is essential for determining and planning treatment effectively. Diagnostic procedures begin with a comprehensive history and physical examination of the patient, followed by a series of laboratory tests. Urinalysis is a significant element because it may detect proteinuria and hematuria, signs of dysfunctional glomeruli. Protein loss measurement, especially as indicated by the urine protein-to-creatinine ratio, provides a valuable index of disease severity. Clinical chemistries, such as serum creatinine and blood urea nitrogen, also alert the clinician to potential issues with renal function. Imaging techniques, such as ultrasound, enable structural abnormalities to be imaged and further refine the diagnostic picture and provide a definitive context of the patient's renal status. Histopathological examination is a cornerstone of the definitive diagnosis of several glomerulonephritides. The characteristics include the obtaining of renal biopsy tissue, usually by percutaneous needle biopsy, to assess the microscopic features of glomerular injury. The findings of the biopsy can be crucial in differentiating between primary and secondary causes of glomerular disease. In infections, such as those caused by the hepatitis C virus, histopathology reveals characteristic changes that may be informative for therapy. For instance, cryoglobulinemia, which is liable to cause both cutaneous vasculitis and glomerulonephritis, is best treated through this pathway, as it has a complex association with systemic diseases (Braun et al., 2007). Therefore, it is typically possible to obtain a renal biopsy only when non-invasive diagnostic methods are unable to delineate the pathogenetic mechanism of the disease. Recent studies underline the significance of correlating biochemical patterns with histopathology in order to enhance the diagnostic yield. A case in point is that in certain diseases, such as coccidioidomycosis, subtle biochemical alterations may initially be evident, yet ultimately become responsible for immune complex glomerulonephritis. This highlights the need for caution in managing patients who present with unusual symptoms, as renal undertones could be severe and underrecognized without thorough assessment (Mehrkens et al., 2016). Furthermore, newer biomarkers and genetic testing are increasingly being discussed, with potential to narrow down diagnostic techniques further. Such diagnostic advancements not only facilitate early intervention steps but also contribute to individualized treatment approaches, which improve patients' outcomes from glomerular diseases.

3.5.1. Urinalysis and Laboratory Tests

Urinalysis is a simple diagnostic method used in the investigation of a wide range of renal disorders, including glomerular conditions such as glomerulonephritis. At the bedside level, urinalysis enables the clinician to identify a wide range of abnormalities in the urine that may indicate underlying renal impairment. Parameters of investigation under the simple urinalysis include physical characteristics, chemical composition, and microscopic components. The presence of blood, protein, glucose, or white blood cells can indicate conditions such as glomerulonephritis, which, if left untreated, can lead to chronic kidney damage. Additionally, urinalysis can aid in monitoring disease progression and the effectiveness of therapeutic interventions. Knowledge of its limitations—i.e., false negative or positive results—reiterates the importance of supporting tests whenever the finding is abnormal. This critical analysis provides clinicians with an evidence base to make sound decisions about follow-up investigative avenues in the field of renal health (Hołownia et al., 2024). The clinical utility of urinalysis extends beyond initial screening, as it also involves monitoring existing renal illnesses, particularly glomerulonephritis. Serial urinalysis may detect changes in proteinuria or hematuria, which are crucial indicators of disease progression or improvement. Routine urine sediment examination helps identify pathognomonic cells or casts of a particular glomerular disease, making early intervention possible. Given its ease of execution and availability, urinalysis forms a cornerstone of the nephrologist's toolkit, useful in risk stratification of patients and guiding management strategies. Following the growth of knowledge in glomerular diseases, such as immune complex-mediated membranoproliferative glomerulonephritis (IC-MPGN) and complement 3 glomerulopathy (C3G), urinalysis becomes increasingly important in distinguishing between these conditions and thereby adding to diagnostic specificity (Bomback et al., 2025). Incorporating laboratory tests into urinalysis provides a more comprehensive means of diagnosing and treating glomerular disease. Advanced laboratory techniques, such as serologic assays and complement profiles, support urinalysis data and facilitate a deeper understanding of the disease processes involved in conditions like IC-MPGN and C3G. Such assays may detect underlying immunologic defects and help distinguish among clinically indistinguishable presentations, thereby allowing patients to be treated with tailored therapeutic regimens.

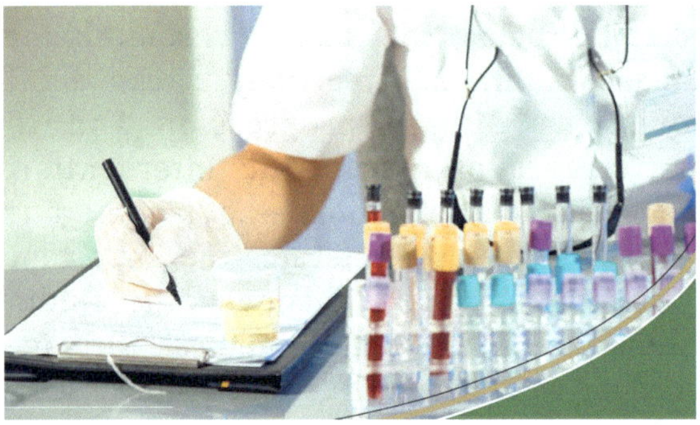

Figure 3.15. Urinalysis and laboratory tests.

Source: https://www.sweetcures.co.uk/cdn/shop/articles/Urine-Analysis_-Microscopic-_-Chemical-Examination.jpg?v=1632826752.

Multidisciplinary collaboration among nephrologists, laboratory staff, and general practitioners enhances the diagnostic procedure and optimizes outcomes in patients. Ultimately, urinalysis and laboratory integration encourage an interdisciplinary management style for glomerular disease, reiterating their vital contribution to contemporary clinical practice (Hołownia et al., 2024; Bomback et al., 2025) (Figure 3.15).

3.5.2. Imaging Techniques

Advanced imaging technologies play a pivotal role in the diagnosis and treatment of glomerular diseases in their assessment. High-resolution ultrasound (US) is employed as a first-line imaging technique due to its availability and lack of ionizing radiation. It is used in renal size, echogenicity, and anatomical anomaly identification, which are relevant in the diagnosis of glomerulonephritis among other disorders. Enhanced ultrasound techniques, such as Doppler imaging, can provide data on renal blood flow and reveal abnormalities that may be related to specific forms of kidney disease. Furthermore, contrast-enhanced ultrasound has emerged as an up-and-coming technique to image renal microvascular patterns, thus improving diagnostic quality and therapeutic intervention guidelines. A combination of these imaging methods assists in the clinical evaluation of patients with suspected glomerular disease because it offers a better perception of the disease mechanisms. CT and MRI are also valuable tools in the imaging arsenal of glomerular disorders. Computed tomography (CT) is particularly valuable when visualization of renal mass lesions or complications, such as urinary obstruction, is needed. In contrast, magnetic resonance imaging (MRI) offers better soft tissue contrast and can provide extensive functional information about renal perfusion and filtration. MRI has proven particularly valuable in describing renal pathological changes associated with glomerulonephritis. More sophisticated techniques, such as diffusion-weighted MRI, enable the measurement of cellularity, which can serve as an indicator of disease severity. Careful selection of imaging modality not only enhances the diagnostic phase but also influences therapy planning. Such imaging techniques, when properly utilized, are an invaluable component of the overall management of patients with glomerular diseases, providing essential information that facilitates directed therapeutic interventions. Furthermore, novel imaging technologies continue to redefine the approach to renal disease. Positron emission tomography (PET) and single-photon emission computed tomography (SPECT) are increasingly used to examine changes in kidney metabolism. PET imaging is a promising tool for assessing inflammatory foci in glomerular diseases and is therefore utilized by physicians to monitor disease progression and treatment response. Furthermore, future improvements in imaging contrast agents, particularly those that are specific to renal features, can offer enhanced diagnostic capability. The advances serve to underscore the value of integrating cutting-edge imaging technologies into clinical practice, improving the precision of diagnosis and intervention in glomerular disease. With the progression of science, these advances will be crucial in the delineation of the treatment of glomerulonephritis, eventually improving patient outcomes in this complex arena of renal health.

3.5.3. Kidney Biopsy

Kidney biopsy is an essential diagnostic tool in the diagnosis of glomerular disease, particularly glomerulonephritis. Through this technique, physicians can retrieve a specimen of kidney tissue, which can yield vital histopathological information about the underlying disease process. A case in point would be crescentic changes, which can indicate severe glomerular damage. By identifying the cellular makeup and structural soundness, a kidney biopsy allows differentiation between various types of glomerulonephritis, including rapidly progressive glomerulonephritis, which, if left untreated, can quickly lead to permanent kidney damage. The ability to recognize unique pathological findings not only aids in diagnosis but also informs treatment regimens individually tailored to the exceptional condition of each patient, thereby maximizing overall management of kidney disease. In the case of glomerular disease, not only does a kidney biopsy serve a diagnostic purpose, but it also has therapeutic implications. The histopathological data may directly influence treatment regimens, especially in RPGN. Early treatment is crucial since RPGN commonly presents with acute clinical conditions that require immediate therapeutic intervention to prevent irreversible renal damage. The mainstay traditional therapies include glucocorticoids and cyclophosphamide, but with advancements in medical technology, new therapies are being developed. Current evidence suggests the need for new management strategies that consider not only patient history but also biopsy results, which often identify previously undiagnosed renal pathologies, leading to more effective and personalized solutions for clinicians (Greenhall et al., 2015). Moreover, the use of kidney biopsy also involves understanding the etiology of secondary glomerulonephritis, for example, that associated with systemic diseases or infections. Cryoglobulinemia, which can frequently occur in hepatitis C virus infection, can induce vasculitis and glomerulonephritis and significantly affect patient prognosis. A biopsy provides valuable information on the underlying causes and mechanisms of renal injury and directs the selection of effective treatment. New antiviral therapy for hepatitis C offers a promising path for the therapy of cryoglobulinemic disorders and highlights the utility of biopsies in the development of effective management programs. By providing a basis for diagnosing the etiology of glomerular disease, renal biopsies not only direct clinical practice but also lead to new therapeutic modalities that treat the underlying causes rather than symptomatically manage them (Braun et al., 2007) (Figure 3.16).

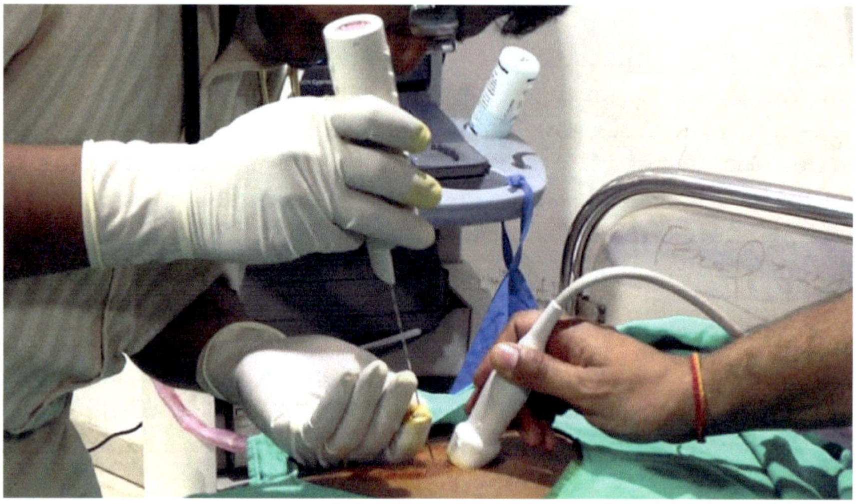

Figure 3.16. Kidney biopsy.

Source: https://flkidney.com/wp-content/uploads/Kidney-Biopsy-FKP-Comprehensive-Kidney-Care.jpg.

3.6. Treatment Options

Optimal management strategies for glomerular diseases, particularly glomerulonephritis, should be patient-specific, tailored to the underlying cause and disease severity. Immunosuppressive therapy is commonly employed in the management of autoimmune-mediated glomerulonephritis, where corticosteroids and cytotoxic drugs, such as cyclophosphamide, are used. These form the basis of the reduction in inflammation and nephrotoxicity. For patients with nephritic syndrome, initial management can include managing hypertension and fluid status since these factors may play an essential role in disease progression. This sort of holistic management is necessary, as it addresses symptomatic control and long-term kidney protection, ultimately benefiting the patient. For secondary etiologies, specific treatment can have dramatic results. For example, cryoglobulinemia, commonly seen in hepatitis C infections, is a clear indication of how antiviral treatments have become key therapeutic interventions. The incorporation of antiviral regimens can specifically treat the pathophysiological mechanisms underlying glomerulonephritis. As noted in recent reviews, these novel antiviral treatment strategies offer a potential for causal therapy in cryoglobulinemia, thereby making conventional immunosuppressants comparatively effective only in symptom and complication control, but not in addressing the underlying cause of the disease (Braun et al., 2007). Novel therapeutic strategies are also targeting the function of leukocytes in the progression of glomerular disease. Experiments have established that infiltrating leukocytes play a significant role in renal injury. Thus, inhibition of chemokine receptors, particularly CCR1, is a potential candidate for intervention. By inhibiting the processes that facilitate leukocyte adhesion and migration into renal tissues, it is possible to prevent injury even at advanced stages of chronic kidney disease. Clinical investigation of CCR1 small molecule antagonists suggests significant potential in promoting renal health, with promise for advancing therapeutic models in glomerulonephritis and chronic kidney disease a reality (Anders et al., 2005).

3.6.1. Pharmacological Interventions

Pharmacotherapy plays a significant role in the management of glomerular diseases, particularly glomerulonephritis. Therapy is directed towards the modulation of the mechanisms of pathophysiology behind the injury of glomeruli and subsequent CKD. The principal classes of pharmacological agents are angiotensin-converting enzyme inhibitors (ACEi) and angiotensin receptor blockers (ARBs), which efficiently reduce proteinuria and prevent disease progression by alleviating glomerular pressure. Recent studies have established that ACEi remains effective in altering the glomerular molecular profile, leading to favorable changes in cellular pathways that control extracellular matrix production, which could bring new insights into the treatment sphere for glomerular diseases (Huwiler et al., 2013). In addition to ACEi, new targets such as sphingosine 1-phosphate (S1P) have promising avenues for pharmacological modulation. S1P receptors also play a role in the immune response and fibrosis within the kidney, and therefore hold potential for a dual-purpose function that is beneficial to patients with glomerular disease. With research uncovering the complexity of S1P-mediated signaling among renal cell types, particularly glomerular and tubular cells, there is potential for developing agents that can activate or inhibit these processes, providing a tailored form of treatment (Huwiler et al., 2013). Thus, the discovery of and characterization of these molecular targets' function in renal pathology significantly enhances the armamentarium of drugs for the therapy of glomerular disease. Furthermore, ongoing investigations into individual genes, such as Rarres1 and NPR3, are beginning to elucidate the mechanism of pharmacologic response at the molecular level. These observations suggest that personalized medicine can become a viable approach to treating glomerulonephritis, with individualized genetic fingerprints informing the choice and dosage of pharmacological agents. For instance, inhibition of NPR3 has yielded variable but promising renoprotective effects in preclinical models of glomerular injury, suggesting that selective interventions can mitigate injury and enhance renal function (Dabaghie et al., 2023). As our understanding of gene expression and its contribution to drug response improves, the future of pharmacologic intervention in glomerular disease will increasingly rely on a precision medicine strategy that maximizes benefit for patients affected (Figure 3.17).

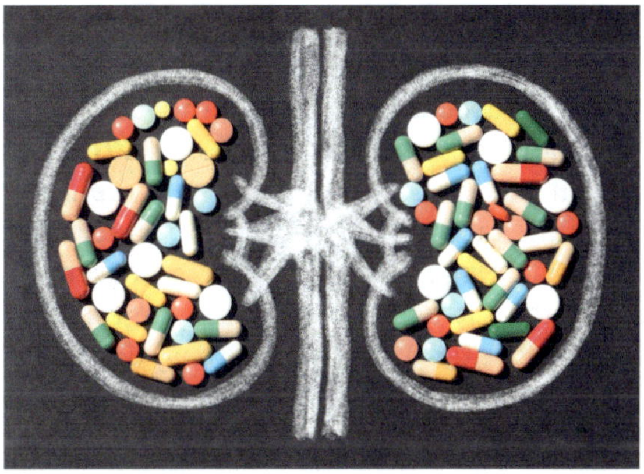

Figure 3.17. Pharmacological Interventions in managing glomerular diseases.

Source: https://www.nps.org.au/assets/NPS/images/Kidney-medicines.jpg.

3.6.2. Lifestyle Modifications

Lifestyle modification constitutes the cornerstone of therapy of glomerular disease, such as glomerulonephritis of various forms. By following a healthier lifestyle, patients can have excellent control of their disease progression and quality of life. Dietary modifications, including limiting salt intake and restricting protein, are significant since they prevent hypertension and reduce renal load. This has a specific application for patients with chronic kidney disease (CKD), with elevated protein levels exacerbating kidney function decline. A review considering dietary regimes in adults with CKD identifies the appropriateness of specific nutritional strategies, with certain dietary modifications potentially having positive health effects without causing harm (Campbell et al., 2015). These modifications not only address physical health but also extend to behavioral modifications, including regular exercise and quitting smoking, which contribute to enhancing patient well-being. In addition to dietary modification, regular exercise is also an essential lifestyle modification for patients suffering from glomerulonephritis. Exercise has been found to improve cardiovascular health, which is an additional benefit since patients with glomerular disorders are typically at risk for cardiovascular morbidity. Adequate levels of physical exercise may also help with weight control and overall metabolic well-being, an essential factor in preventing additional kidney damage. Additionally, research has proven that structured exercise programs will improve mental wellness, reducing depression and anxiety commonly seen in patients with chronic illness. The KDIGO Clinical Practice Guideline emphasizes that multidimensional approaches, including lifestyle modification along with pharmacological therapy, can provide a comprehensive management plan for glomerular diseases (Adler et al., 2021). Thus, incorporating exercise into daily life is a crucial part of optimizing the health outcomes for these patients. Lastly, lifestyle modification should also comprise mental health counseling and education. Chronic illnesses like glomerulonephritis can evoke tremendous psychological distress, and so effective mental health management is equally important. Education programs, support groups, and counseling can equip patients with the skills needed to cope with their condition and make lifestyle changes more effectively. Such interventions can provide an optimal climate in which patients feel empowered to make the changes in their lives. Moreover, awareness of their disease can lead to increased compliance with therapeutic regimens, thereby improving clinical outcomes. Thus, an integrated strategy involving diet, physical, and mental changes becomes imperative in the total management of glomerular diseases, showing the interconnected role of lifestyle determinants and renal function.

3.6.3. Dialysis and Transplantation

The course of chronic primary glomerulonephritides (CPGN) can progress to the serious state of end-stage renal disease (ESRD), necessitating therapy with dialysis or kidney transplantation. Although such therapy exists, it is not without its limitations; both therapeutic modalities can significantly impact a patient's quality of life and survival. Dialysis, for instance, while lifesaving, often demands a fair amount of lifestyle alteration, like adhering to nutritional restrictions and regular attendance in clinics, which can impose emotional and physical stress on patients. Moreover, the economic burden of long-term dialysis can be economically crippling, resulting in added expenses on individuals and healthcare systems. On the other hand, transplantation will yield a more permanent solution but is also associated with the risk of organ rejection and related immunosuppressive therapy complications, which can expose patients to significant long-term health risks, including malignancies and infections (Bjørneklett et al., 2012). Kidney transplant is a significant advancement in the treatment of ESRD due to glomerular diseases, and enables patients to regain independence and a degree of normalcy in life. The success of transplantation is also intimately related to the etiology of kidney failure, particularly the type of glomerular disease the patient suffers from. Some diseases, such as membranous nephropathy or IgA nephropathy, have a high likelihood of recurrence after transplantation, which can compromise the function of the allograft [1]. Strong pre-transplant evaluation protocols and careful patient selection are thus essential to achieve optimal results. Moreover, management of potential recurrence and immunosuppression protocols are significant factors that lead to transplant survival and patient outcome. Ongoing research on the long-term effect of various glomerular diseases on transplant outcomes remains critical in optimizing the treatment protocols (Bjørneklett et al., 2012). Patients with glomerular disease require a multidisciplinary approach, involving not only nephrologists but also transplant surgeons and immunologists. This collaboration is crucial in addressing the complications associated with treating CPGN and acquiring ESRD. Tailored treatment based on the specific type of lupus nephritis and the individual case of the patient is advised by today's guidelines. The incorporation of sophisticated monitoring and timely intervention strategies can halt the progression of kidney disease, thus avoiding or delaying dialysis and transplantation. With further research advances delineating prognostic variables and response to therapies, it will be increasingly possible to afford targeted treatments that can improve patient outcomes as well as reduce the incidence of ESRD as a result of glomerular diseases. Open communication within the medical community will drive innovative solutions to the current challenges faced by patients with such disabling diseases.

SUMMARY

Glomerular disease, and glomerulonephritis in particular, demonstrates the complexities of renal pathology and its far-reaching effects on patient health. A detailed understanding of the disease processes is necessary, as it determines explicitly the treatment modality and patient care guidelines. The new advances in diagnostic methods, including the application of urinary proteomics, have unveiled new possibilities in the discovery of biomarkers indicative of disease progression. The benefit of such biomarkers is that they can provide more precise measurements, thereby allowing more accurate prognosis and tailor-made therapy. Last but not least, long-term research funding is needed to fully elucidate the complex biological pathways involved in glomerular diseases, which underscores the necessity of introducing new diagnostic equipment into the clinic. The best management of glomerulonephritis is multidisciplinary, synthesizing various treatment modalities within disease-specific categories. Divergent guidelines across different jurisdictions are harmonized to streamline care and maximize patient outcomes with this condition. The personalized induction and maintenance therapy, in particular for different histological classes, emphasizes the concept of personalized medicine in nephrology. As documented in the current literature, the heterogeneity of response to interventions such as corticosteroids and immunosuppressants necessitates ongoing evaluation and re-optimization of treatment protocols. Consequently, general guidelines of therapy, including those discussed in Bajema et al. (2015), provide clinically relevant information that guides health practitioners in making informed decisions regarding the management of patients based on patient-specific characteristics. Lastly, the progress in understanding and managing glomerular disease is robust but ongoing. The advancement in diagnostic techniques, for instance, the exploration of urinary proteomics, is considerable towards the realization of a more comprehensive understanding of disease mechanisms and patient needs (Magalhães et al., 2016). Despite these advancements, there are still strong calls to explore the underlying pathophysiology further, investigate new modalities for treatment, and develop long-term patient management strategies. By encouraging interdisciplinary cooperation among researchers, clinicians, and patients, the nephrology community can maximize the efficiency of treatments and ultimately provide individuals with glomerulonephritis improved quality of life. It is essential that the collective here continues to pave the way toward more efficient and individualized therapeutic regimens.

A thorough understanding of glomerular disease involves an appreciation of the various mechanisms underlying such disease, and of first importance is an understanding of the role of chemokines in inflammatory reactions. Chemokines are small signaling proteins that induce the migration of immune cells towards the site of inflammation, and they are essential in glomerulonephritis. However, recent studies demonstrate that chemokine expression within renal tissue does not necessarily reflect expected functional outcomes. A discrepancy such as this is of critical importance in posing questions regarding the mechanisms of renal leukocyte infiltration, specifically why chemokine antagonism should lead to only partial reductions in renal inflammation. These open questions serve to illustrate the complexity of renal chemokine biology and highlight the need for continued investigation of putative therapeutic strategies that will render chemokine antagonists more effective in treating kidney diseases, such as glomerulonephritis (Anders et al., 2010). The second significant consideration to keep in mind is the use of urinary proteomics for the diagnosis and monitoring of glomerular disease progression. As urine is a readily accessible fluid for identifying biomarkers, advances in mass spectrometry have led to the discovery of promising urinary protein biomarkers. These biomarkers, such as fragments of collagen, serum albumin, and uromodulin, have tremendous potential in presenting information about the pathophysiology of diseases. The increased sensitivity and specificity of these biomarkers relative to traditional diagnostic methods encourage more informed clinical decision-making processes. Thus, urinary proteomics may provide a better understanding of glomerulonephritis, ultimately leading to improved diagnosis and prognosis, and demonstrating how patient care can be enhanced through modified therapeutic approaches (Magalhães et al., 2016). Overall, studies on glomerular disease, and indeed glomerulonephritis, comprise a multifaceted landscape in which chemokine-induced inflammation and newer technologies, such as urinary proteomics, intersect. Understanding the roles of chemokines not only informs on the inflammatory cascades that underlie such illnesses but also on novel avenues for therapeutic intervention. Concurrently, proteomic analysis of urine provides opportunities for identifying biomarkers that facilitate substantially improved monitoring and treatment of kidney disease. Overall, these considerations highlight the need to implement new research technologies in clinical practice to maximize diagnosis and treatment planning, thereby avert the formation of glomerular diseases and further improve patient outcomes.

CLOSER LOOK

NEPHROTIC SYNDROME

Nephrotic syndrome is a clinical syndrome with a typical set of features that are representative of severe impairment of the glomerular filtration barrier in the kidney. The usual features include excess loss of protein (typically over 3.5 g/day), low albumin levels, generalized edema, and hyperlipidemia. It results from glomerular injury, the small kidney vessels that filter out waste and excess substances from the blood but retain essential proteins. When the barrier is disrupted, immense amounts of protein, mainly albumin, leak into urine. The ensuing low serum albumin level reduces plasma oncotic pressure, leading to interstitial fluid infiltration and resulting in generalized edema. As a replacement for the loss of protein, the liver . This increase in lipoprotein production, in turn, results in elevated levels of triglycerides and cholesterol, ultimately leading to hyperlipidemia, a condition commonly observed in such patients.

Nephrotic syndrome is either primary (idiopathic) or secondary. Kidney-related primary etiologies are characterized by conditions such as minimal change disease, focal segmental glomerulosclerosis (FSGS), and membranous nephropathy. A kidney biopsy diagnoses these conditions. Minimal change disease typically occurs in children and is characterized by normal glomeruli on light microscopy, but with effacement of podocyte foot processes on electron microscopy. FSGS and membranous nephropathy are more prevalent in adults and may progress to chronic kidney disease unless treated optimally. Secondary nephrotic syndrome arises as a complication of systemic conditions such as diabetes mellitus, systemic lupus erythematosus, infections (e.g., hepatitis B or C, HIV), and use of certain drugs or toxins. In diabetic nephropathy, e.g., prolonged hyperglycemia leads to progressive glomerular damage and proteinuria.

The nephrotic syndrome has more than edema and proteinuria as a clinical presentation. They are at risk of infection due to urinary loss of immunoglobulins and complement proteins, as well as thromboembolic events secondary to urinary loss of antithrombin III and other anticoagulant proteins. Malnutrition, anemia, and acute renal injury are other complications. Diagnosis is generally done on clinical findings aided by laboratory tests in the form of urinalysis with proteinuria, blood tests indicating low serum albumin, hypercholesterolemia, and, rarely, renal biopsy for the measurement of underlying disease.

Treatment of nephrotic syndrome consists of treatment of the underlying cause, reduction of proteinuria, and suppression of symptoms. Corticosteroids are commonly used, especially in minimal change disease, but immunosuppressive agents such as cyclosporine, tacrolimus, or cyclophosphamide may be used in steroid-resistant nephrotic syndrome. Diuretics for edema control, ACE inhibitors or ARBs for the reduction of proteinuria and maintenance of renal function, and statins for lipid control are also part of the treatment regimen. Anticoagulants may be necessary in high-risk patients for thrombosis. Dietary modification, such as salt restriction and a proper intake of proteins, is equally important.

REFERENCES

1. Abassi, Z., Hamoud, S., Hassan, A., Khamaysi, I., Nativ, O., Heyman, S. N., Muhammad, R. S., Ilan, N., Singh, P., Hammond, E., Zaza, G., Lupo, A., Onisto, M., Bellin, G., Masola, V., Vlodavsky, I., & Gambaro, G. (2017). Involvement of heparanase in the pathogenesis of acute kidney injury: nephroprotective effect of PG545. *Oncotarget*, *8*(21), 34191–34204. https://doi.org/10.18632/oncotarget.16573Abdi, R., Anders, H. J., Bruhl, H., Burne-Taney, M. J., Feng, L., et al. (2004). Identifying chemokines as therapeutic targets in renal disease: Lessons from antagonist studies and knockout mice. https://core.ac.uk/download/16432527.pdf (accessed on 25th June 2025).
2. Abdul Salim, S., Fülöp, T., Hamrahian, S. M., Mollaee, M., et al. (2017). Idiopathic nodular glomerulosclerosis in a chronic marijuana user: A case report and review of the literature. https://core.ac.uk/download/155271521.pdf (accessed on 25th June 2025).
3. Adler, S. G., Barratt, J., Bridoux, F., Burdge, K., et al. (2021). Executive summary of the KDIGO 2021 guideline for the management of glomerular diseases. https://core.ac.uk/download/479497730.pdf (accessed on 25th June 2025).
4. Anders, H. J., & Ninichuk, V. (2005). Chemokine receptor CCR1: A new target for progressive kidney disease. https://core.ac.uk/download/16432945.pdf (accessed on 25th June 2025).
5. Anders, H. J., & Schlöndorff, D. (2000). Murine models of renal disease: Possibilities and problems in studies using mutant mice. https://core.ac.uk/download/16432493.pdf (accessed on 25th June 2025).
6. Anders, H. J., Sayyed, S. A., & Vielhauer, V. (2010). Questions about chemokine and chemokine receptor antagonism in renal inflammation. https://core.ac.uk/download/16432498.pdf (accessed on 25th June 2025).
7. Awdishu, L., Cerda, J., Chakaravarthi, R., Davenport, M., et al. (2015). Phenotype standardization for drug-induced kidney disease. https://core.ac.uk/download/323065889.pdf (accessed on 25th June 2025).
8. Bajema, I. M., Bertsias, G. K., Boumpas, D. T., Gordon, C., et al. (2015). Lupus nephritis management guidelines compared. https://core.ac.uk/download/77009956.pdf (accessed on 25th June 2025).
9. Barbano, B., Cianci, R., Di Mario, F., Gigante, A., et al. (2017). Hypothyroidism and nephrotic syndrome: Why, when and how to treat. https://core.ac.uk/download/132156565.pdf (accessed on 25th June 2025).
10. Barutta, F., De Nicola, L., Di Paolo, S., Gesualdo, L., et al. (2019). Diabetic kidney disease: New clinical and therapeutic issues. Joint position statement of the Italian Diabetes Society and the Italian Society of Nephrology on "The natural history of diabetic kidney disease and treatment of hyperglycemia in patients with type 2 diabetes and impaired renal function." https://core.ac.uk/download/231749247.pdf (accessed on 25th June 2025).
11. Benigni, A., Boonstra, A., Cases, A., Katz, A., Nishiyama, A., Eddy, A. A., Fogo, A. B., et al. (2007). Mechanisms of progression of chronic kidney disease. https://core.ac.uk/download/pdf/7772867.pdf (accessed on 25th June 2025).
12. Besse-Eschmann, V., Endlich, K., Endlich, N., Le Hir, M., et al. (2018). Alterations of podocytes

in a murine model of crescentic glomerulonephritis. https://core.ac.uk/download/159150961.pdf (accessed on 25th June 2025).

13. Bjørneklett, R. O. (2012). Long-term prognosis in chronic primary glomerulonephritis's. https://core.ac.uk/download/30897668.pdf (accessed on 25th June 2025).
14. Bomback, A. S., Charu, V., & Fakhouri, F. (2025). Challenges in the diagnosis and management of immune complex-mediated membranoproliferative glomerulonephritis and complement 3 glomerulopathy. https://core.ac.uk/download/655063048.pdf (accessed on 25th June 2025).
15. Bowman, S. J., Giles, I. P., Ioannou, Y., Rahman, A., et al. (2005). Review of presentations at the 6th European Lupus Meeting 3–5 March 2005. https://core.ac.uk/download/1669257.pdf (accessed on 25th June 2025).
16. Braun, G. S., Horster, S., Ihrler, S., Schmid, H., et al. (2007). Cryoglobulinemic vasculitis: Classification and clinical and therapeutic aspects. https://core.ac.uk/download/12175185.pdf (accessed on 25th June 2025).
17. Campbell, K. L., Craig, J. C., Johnson, D. W., Maggo, J., et al. (2015). Dietary patterns for adults with chronic kidney disease. https://core.ac.uk/download/196602465.pdf (accessed on 25th June 2025).
18. Chan, D. T. M., Chan, K. W., & Cheng, I. K. P. (1999). Clinical and pathological characteristics of patients with glomerular diseases at a university teaching hospital: 5-year prospective review. https://core.ac.uk/download/37889943.pdf (accessed on 25th June 2025).
19. Dabaghie, D. (2023). Identification of genes and pathways involved in the development and progression of glomerular diseases. https://core.ac.uk/download/555550331.pdf (accessed on 25th June 2025).
20. De Vincentiis, M., De Virgilio, A., Fusconi, M., Gallo, A., et al. (2016). Clinic manifestations in granulomatosis with polyangiitis. https://core.ac.uk/download/74319070.pdf (accessed on 25th June 2025).
21. De Vincentiis, M., De Virgilio, A., Fusconi, M., Gallo, A., et al. (2017). Sialendoscopic management of autoimmune sialadenitis: A review of literature. https://core.ac.uk/download/98339930.pdf (accessed on 25th June 2025).
22. Goldstein, R. E., Grauer, G. F., Kalish, R. A., Levy, S., Levy, S. A., Rolla, D., & Scorpio, D. G. (2019). Differences in clinicopathologic variables between *Borrelia* C6 antigen Sero reactive and *Borrelia* C6 seronegative glomerulopathy in dogs. https://core.ac.uk/download/323071861.pdf (accessed on 25th June 2025).
23. Greenhall, G. H. B., & Salama, A. D. (2015). What is new in the management of rapidly progressive glomerulonephritis? https://core.ac.uk/download/29416059.pdf (accessed on 25th June 2025).
24. Gutiérrez Rodríguez, A. (2019). Diagnosis of some diseases through biomarkers. https://core.ac.uk/download/288157992.pdf (accessed on 25th June 2025).
25. Hołownia, W., Krzesłowska, W. J., Pytel, P., Szewczyk, M., et al. (2024). Urinalysis in primary care doctor practice. https://core.ac.uk/download/613193044.pdf (accessed on 25th June 2025).
26. Huwiler, A., Koch, A., & Pfeilschifter, J. M. (2013). Sphingosine 1-phosphate in renal diseases. https://core.ac.uk/download/16515935.pdf (accessed on 25th June 2025).

27. Magalhães, P., Mischak, H., & Zürbig, P. (2016). Urinary proteomics using capillary electrophoresis coupled to mass spectrometry for diagnosis and prognosis in kidney diseases. https://core.ac.uk/download/74362547.pdf (accessed on 25th June 2025).

28. Mehrkens, L. R., Mohr, F. C., & Sykes, J. E. (2016). Clinicopathologic and histopathologic renal abnormalities in dogs with coccidioidomycosis. https://core.ac.uk/download/323070128.pdf (accessed on 25th June 2025).

29. Michael, A. F., McLean, R. H., Roy, L. P., Westberg, N., et al. (1973). Immunologic aspects of the nephrotic syndrome. https://core.ac.uk/download/pdf/82779108.pdf (accessed on 25th June 2025).

30. N/A. (2021). An update on glomerulopathies. https://core.ac.uk/download/478123386.pdf (accessed on 25th June 2025).

31. Pichler Sekulic, S., & Sekulic, M. (2013). A compendium of urinary biomarkers indicative of glomerular podocytopathy. https://core.ac.uk/download/28947337.pdf (accessed on 25th June 2025).

32. Xasanova, N. Q. (2024). Prevalence and risk factors of chronic kidney disease. https://core.ac.uk/download/651276960.pdf (accessed on 25th June 2025).

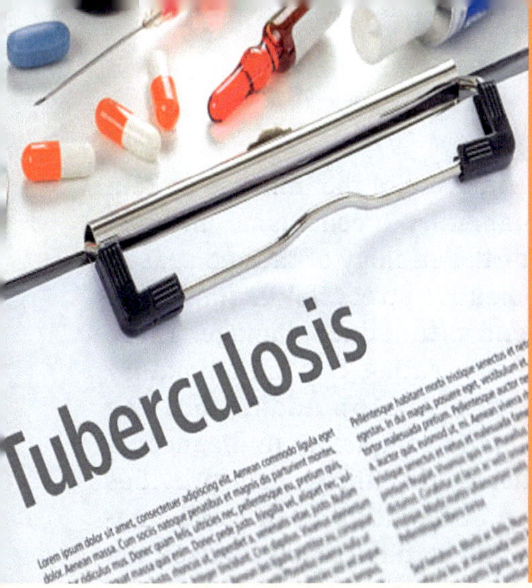

Chapter 4

TUBULOINTERSTITIAL DISEASES

Contents

Introduction

The tubulointerstitial diseases are a heterogeneous collection of renal diseases that predominantly affect the kidneys' tubules and interstitial tissue. The illnesses may be caused by a wide range of etiologies, including autoimmune reactions, infections, toxins, and metabolic dysfunction. Pathophysiology would most frequently involve inflammation and multifactorial host-environment interaction. On most occasions, tubulointerstitial disease is capable of leading to significant kidney damage. It carries consequences for overall health, as well as a sense of urgency surrounding early detection and treatment. The multifactorial etiology of such conditions needs to be understood since early treatment is capable of impeding the progression of kidney injury as much as improving the patient's prognosis. As we examine the mechanisms underlying the particular etiologies of tubulointerstitial diseases, it is essential that they share common mechanisms for producing renal damage and influencing the prognosis of recovery with proper therapeutic intervention. Although in discussing tubulointerstitial diseases, one should take note of the very rare but very important vital role of the immune system in their pathogenesis. Recent studies have highlighted that inflammatory mechanisms, in most cases caused by immune dysregulation, are primarily responsible for the etiology of these diseases. Exaggerated generation of reactive oxygen species and resultant oxidative stress, for example, are often accompanied by a defective antioxidant response and are central to kidney damage. These alterations can be observed in many tubulointerstitial conditions, indicating that inflammatory processes are at the core of their pathophysiology (Osorio-Alonso et al., 2016). Additionally, the interaction between renal inflammation and autoimmunity confirms the complexity in diagnosing and managing these conditions. Understanding of such mechanisms of pathogenesis provides insights into therapeutic targets as well as the importance of close observation to prevent long-term loss of renal architecture. New diagnostic and therapeutic approaches have revolutionized the therapy of tubulointerstitial diseases. Advances in biomarker science and imaging techniques have enhanced the ability to diagnose the incidence and distribution of renal damage, allowing for more customized treatment regimens. The application of immunotherapeutic and theoretical concepts to practice is a breakthrough in the management of these diseases. For example, the utilization of targeted immunosuppression and the development of novel agents that minimize oxidative stress have the potential to introduce a new era of hope for sufferers. Secondly, the fact that tubulointerstitial disease and metabolic syndromes are interrelated has created new opportunities for the comprehensive management strategies incorporating both renal function and metabolic disorders (Aga Khan University Hospital, 2015). As studies continue to grow in these frontiers, it is imperative for researchers and clinicians to stay updated with the changing evidence that can potentially lead to improved outcomes in these recalcitrant disorders (Figure 4.1).

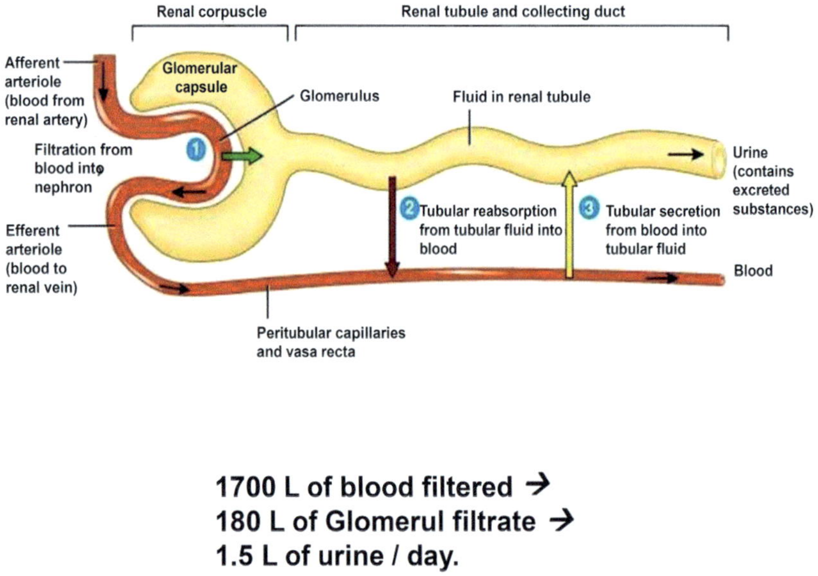

Figure 4.1. Tubulointerstitial diseases of the kidney.

Source: https://external-content.duckduckgo.com/iu/?u=https%3A%2F%2Fimage2.slideserve.com%2F4752965%2Fslide6-l.jpg&f=1&nofb=1&ipt=de729aab18f8948c357ee03adbc755456aa56516035cdb0e1309a8a6029a242e.

Definition of Tubulointerstitial Diseases

Understanding the definition of tubulointerstitial diseases enables one to comprehend their impact on kidney function. Tubulointerstitial diseases basically attack the tubules and interstitial kidney tissues, leading to functional disturbance with potential progression to chronic kidney disease. Pathology of tubulointerstitial disease could have various inflammatory and fibrosing processes secondary to a range of etiologic conditions, including infections, autoimmune disorders, and toxic exposure. These conditions, noteworthy to consider, can also manifest through many clinical presentations, such as alterations in urine output, electrolyte imbalance, and hypertension, all of which need a thorough clinical workup for definitive diagnosis and treatment. Distinguishing between glomerular disease and tubulointerstitial disease is necessary; both conditions are characterized by kidney impairment, but the latter specifically accounts for the injury that occurs within the tubular and interstitial areas, thereby highlighting distinct therapeutic and prognostic factors. Presentation and diagnosis of tubulointerstitial diseases can be complex and multifactorial. Diagnostic approaches can include urinalysis, imaging studies, and renal biopsies, and can yield classic findings such as interstitial inflammation or fibrosis. For instance, acute interstitial nephritis is typically linked with drug reactions or infection, which is characterized by urinary white blood cell elevation and renal inflammatory responses. For presentation of acute interstitial nephritis, refer below. Conversely, chronic types can develop slowly, leading to widespread scarring and tubular atrophy, rendering cases like those complicated for treatment. The observation that the extent of renal damage corresponds with clinical results emphasizes the importance of early identification and intervention. Additionally, pathologies such as ANCA-associated renal vasculitis demonstrate how these diseases mirror systemic diseases, and a thorough understanding of the mechanisms underlying them is required for the development of effective treatment strategies as well as improved patient prognoses (Eri et al., 2017). Recent research has only begun to explore the function of circulating fibrocytes in the progression of tubulointerstitial disease. These bone marrow-derived fibrocytes are involved in the fibrogenic processes of chronic kidney disease. They can differentiate into fibroblasts and, as such, are a potential source of renal fibrosis, an ubiquitous consequence of tubulointerstitial disease. It has been found that levels of circulating fibrocytes rise in direct proportion to the severity of renal fibrosis and thus could be used as markers for disease progression (Fici et al., 2014). Identification of the function of such cellular processes not only enhances the definition of tubulointerstitial disease but also offers new avenues for therapeutic regimens. With the identification of specific pathways involved in fibrosis, medical therapies can be further refined to target these processes, thereby rendering patients with tubular and interstitial kidney disease better outcomes.

Importance of Understanding Tubulointerstitial Diseases

The knowledge of tubulointerstitial disease not only plays a crucial role in appropriate diagnosis but also in suitable management of chronic kidney disease. Fibrosis of the renal tubulointerstitium is a hallmark that defines tubulointerstitial diseases through the supranormal deposition of extracellular matrix in the interstitium of the kidneys. The process is particularly relevant since it constitutes a unifying mechanism for many kidney disorders, which underscores the importance of detecting the earliest signs of tubulointerstitial injury. Through extensive research and clinical observation, medical professionals can better identify proactive treatments that target the fundamental fibrotic processes. This data can then ultimately enhance patient outcome and inform the development of novel therapies for chronic kidney disease, a disease increasingly prevalent among humans as well as companion animals like cats, where Elliott et al. (2015) provide an insightful understanding of the mechanisms responsible for renal injury. Second, the incorporation of experimental models has transformed the molecular knowledge of tubulointerstitial diseases. Gene-targeting strategies and the generation of knock-out mice allow for the study of renal disease pathogenesis under standardized conditions. Importantly, models with manifestations of tubulointerstitial disease provide scientists with a means to study the processes of renal injury and fibrosis in detail. Understanding the genes involved in these conditions is essential to the design of targeted therapy that can efficiently reverse renal damage. Further, as the literature has demonstrated, attention to the genetic constitution of the model systems is vital to ensure that the findings are not only valid but also reproducible. As with Anders et al. (2000), such developments provide a promising avenue of research into potential interventions for human renal disease. The growing recognition of the importance of understanding tubulointerstitial diseases also forms a framework for interprofessional approaches in both research and clinical practice. Knowledge from basic and translational studies is converted into clinical guidelines, allowing the formulation of a more integrated care approach in treating patients. Through collaboration among researchers, pathologists, and nephrologists, healthcare systems are able to enhance their capabilities towards earlier diagnosis and treatment of such complicated diseases. Additionally, the cooperative comprehension of tubulointerstitial disease molecular mechanisms creates an avenue for new therapies tailor-made for each patient's requirements. As a combination, these initiatives aim not only to enhance the efficacy of therapy but also to further advance the understanding of kidney disease and health, ultimately improving both animal and human health, as proposed in the ongoing research ons renal fibrosis and its relevance (Figure 4.2).

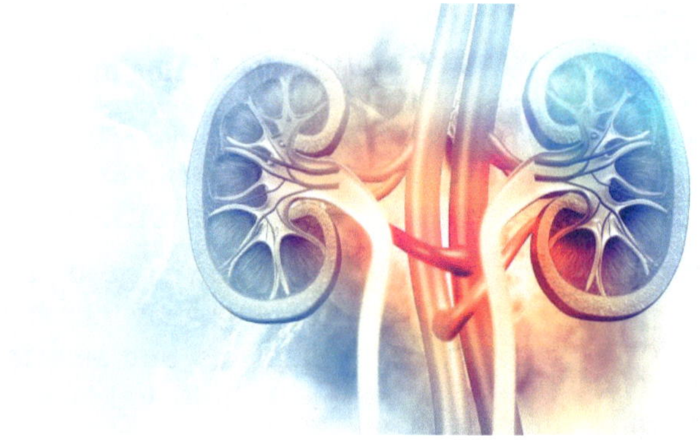

Figure 4.2. Understanding tubulointerstitial diseases.

Source: https://stgaccinwbsdevlrs01.blob.core.windows.net/newcorporatewbsite/blogs/october2023/detail-main-Tubulointerstitial-Nephritis.jpeg?w=828&q=75.

4.1. Anatomy and Physiology of the Kidney

The anatomy of the kidney is a complex structure well-adapted to facilitate efficient filtration and homeostasis. The kidney is composed of approximately one million functional units called nephrons, which consist of glomeruli and tubules. The glomerulus serves as a filter that allows water, electrolytes, and waste products to pass while retaining larger molecules such as proteins and blood cells. Upon filtration, the filtrate flows into the proximal tubule, where there is massive reabsorption of required substances, including glucose, amino acids, and bicarbonate. The tubules vary in shape and length, with the loop of Henle and collecting ducts playing critical roles in concentrating urine and regulating water balance. With their intricate organization, the kidneys are well-adapted to control fluid balance, electrolyte homeostasis, and the excretory elimination of metabolic waste, setting the stage to understand how tubulointerstitial diseases can disrupt these life-supporting processes. Physiologically, the kidneys perform their life-sustaining functions due to a delicate balance of cell-to-cell communication and biochemical interactions. However, in tubulointerstitial diseases, this balance is disrupted, and inflammation and fibrosis of the renal interstitium occur. Inflammatory responses involve mobilization of leukocytes and other inflammatory cells to the affected area, which may add to damage of the kidney over time. As inflammatory mediators accumulate, they can stimulate renal fibroblast activation and ensuing fibrosis, which contributes to the impairment of nephron function. The role played by the interstitium in this case is critical, as it ensures the structural integrity of the nephron and facilitates communication between the vasculature and renal parenchyma. Through studies of the cellular and molecular underpinnings of tubulointerstitial disease, the significance of maintaining kidney health and preventing progression to chronic kidney disease is set. Recent studies have begun to demystify the mechanisms of lymphatic biology, which was discovered to have a central role in renal homeostasis and injury reaction. The recently formed lymphatic vessels, or neolymphangiogenesis, are generated in inflammation and provide a pathway for drainage of excess interstitial fluid and immunocompetent cells. This compensation process is critical, as it regulates the state of fluid overload that occurs during renal inflammation, thereby preventing further injury and fibrosis. Both the accumulation of inflammatory cells and their eventual resolution through lymphatic drainage are mediated by a cooperative interaction between adhesion molecules and chemotactic cytokines. As highlighted in more recent research, understanding these lymphatic pathways is essential for the development of targeted therapy approaches to tubulointerstitial disease and for potentially influencing patient prognosis and outcome in diseases such as multiple myeloma, where tubulointerstitial fibrosis plays a primary role in renal injury (Bonani et al., 2017; Ayati et al., 2018).

4.1.1. Structure of Nephrons

The nephron is the functional and structural unit of the kidney and is responsible for fluid and electrolyte balance regulation. Composed of many components, every nephron begins with a renal corpuscle, which is made up of the glomerulus and Bowman's capsule. The glomerulus, a network of capillaries, carries out the process of blood filtration, allowing water, ions, and small molecules to pass into the renal tubule while retaining larger proteins and blood cells. Following the glomerulus, the filtrate flows into the proximal convoluted tubule, where reabsorption of essential materials occurs, preparing the fluid for further processing in the nephron. The intricate nephron structure places a strong focus on its vital role in maintaining homeostasis of the organism. It bears witness to the significance of its architectural integrity in the context of tubulointerstitial disease. The nephron structure not only facilitates effective reabsorption and filtration but also plays a crucial role in modulating the renal interstitial environment. The tubule's components, which are the loop of Henle, the distal convoluted tubule, and the collecting duct, are involved in the concentration of the urine and in electrolyte balance. Abnormalities in nephron structure, resulting from pathological conditions such as tubulointerstitial fibrosis, may compromise these functions. For instance, extracellular matrix deposition in the renal interstitium during chronic kidney disease harmfully impacts nephron function through compromising the delicate balance essential for efficient reabsorption of water and solutes. Such a change is significant in defining the path of renal diseases, particularly those with abnormalities like multiple myeloma, impacting not just nephron structure but also patient prognosis (Ayati et al., 2018).

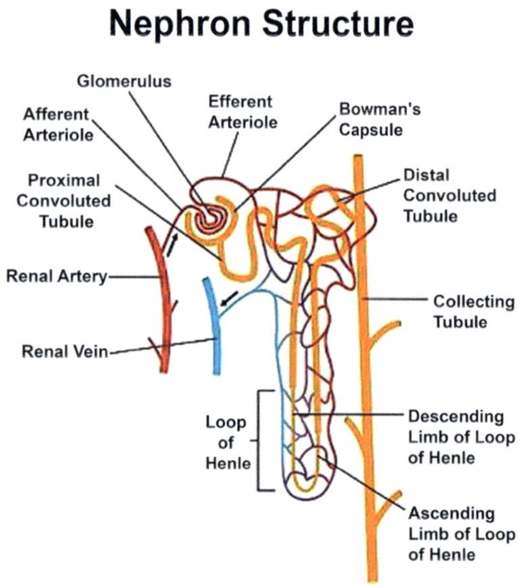

Figure 4.3. Nephron structure.

Source: https://www.science*Source:*com/pix/250/2500927_t.jpg.

Furthermore, nephron integrity has ramifications beyond renal filtration to encompass systemic well-being. When tubulointerstitial disease leads to renal fibrosis, the resultant loss of functional nephrons deprives the organism of its ability to remove waste, resulting in systemic manifestations such as fluid overload and electrolyte disturbances. In feline models of chronic kidney disease, the most frequent diagnosis points in the direction of renal tubulointerstitial fibrosis, which best illustrates the compelling necessity to understand the underlying pathophysiological mechanisms at play (Elliott et al., 2015). Such understanding not only assists in the quest for potential therapeutic targets but also guides approaches toward preventing the progression of kidney diseases. Therefore, the structure of the nephron becomes a critical central point in discussing the pathogenesis of tubulointerstitial diseases and its implications for renal wellness in general (Figure 4.3).

4.1.2. Role of Tubules and Interstitium

The nephron tubules play a vital role in the reabsorption and secretion of materials, thereby impacting renal function and overall homeostasis. The tubules, comprising both proximal and distal segments, are designed to reclaim essential solutes and water from the filtrate, along with the ejection of waste products. In tubulointerstitial diseases, alterations in tubular function can have significant clinical consequences, including metabolic disturbances and water overload. For instance, reduced expression of crucial endocytic transporters, such as megalin and cubilin, has been linked to diabetic nephropathy, underscoring the tubules' role in chronic kidney disease pathophysiology. This derangement can synergistically exacerbate tubular injury and interstitial fibrosis, ultimately leading to progressive renal impairment and underscoring the importance of targeted therapeutic interventions in maintaining tubular integrity (Bahamonde et al., 2017). Interstitium, a connective tissue surrounding tubules and glomeruli, is no less a party to renal pathophysiology, particularly regarding inflammation and immunity. Histopathological examination frequently reveals that interstitial cells, like T lymphocytes and macrophages, are dominant in tubulointerstitial diseases and are responsible for renal damage. It has been proven that such inflammatory cells modulate renal function by the production of cytokines and mediators, leading to the dissemination of tissue injury and fibrosis. In lupus nephritis, for example, there is a high concentration of T lymphocytes and monocyte/macrophages, which correlates with the level of chronic damage and can be utilized as a means of predicting disease progression. Such an association demonstrates that the interstitium is not merely a passive matrix but is itself an active effector of renal inflammation, facilitating the interaction between immune activation and tissue damage (Alexopoulos et al., 1990). Clarification of the intricate interactions between interstitium and renal tubules is crucial to unraveling the pathogenesis of tubulointerstitial disease. Tubular reabsorptive dysfunction can trigger a cascade of interstitial changes, like inflammation and fibrosis, that subsequently diminish the tubular function and set up a vicious cycle of renal injury. Interstitial inflammation, conversely, can cause damage to the tubules, disrupting the renal structure and increasing susceptibility to injury from various stimuli. Preservation of the tubule-interstitium integrity is imperative to prevent the progression of chronic kidney disease. Therefore, therapeutic approaches specifically designed to address these intricate interactions can potentially modulate the pathological effects of tubulointerstitial disease, underscoring the critical roles that each element plays in maintaining healthy kidneys and regulating kidney disease (Figure 4.4).

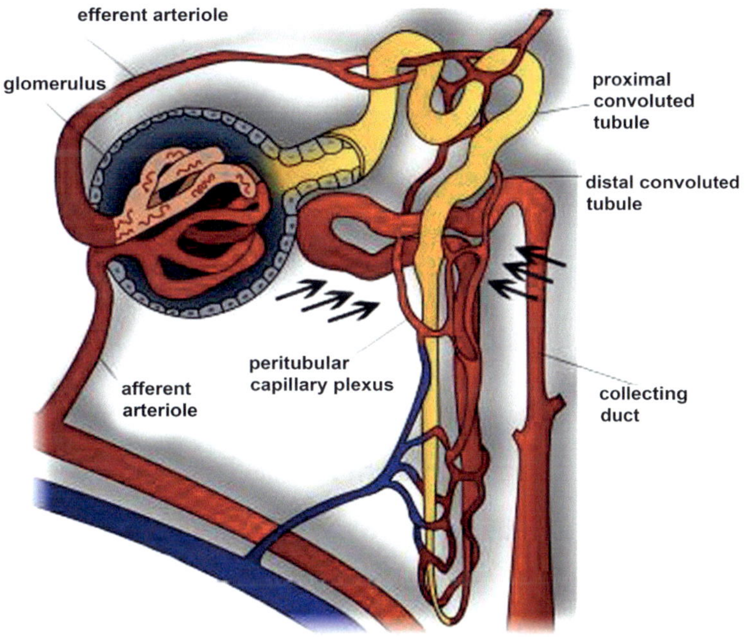

Figure 4.4. Role of tubules and interstitium.

Source: https://ars.els-cdn.com/content/image/3-s2.0-B978012380928510003X-f03-10-9780123809285.jpg.

4.1.3. Importance of Tubulointerstitial Function

The tubulointerstitial component of the kidney plays a focal role in homeostasis, primarily through its involvement with the processes of reabsorption, secretion, and repair. Normal tubulointerstitial function ensures the efficient reabsorption of essential solutes and water from the filtrate, which is crucial for maintaining electrolyte balance and blood volume. Furthermore, the interstitium also offers structural support for renal tubules, facilitating interaction between blood vessels and tubular cells. When the function of the tubulointerstitial apparatus is impaired, as in most renal diseases, the consequences are dire, leading to chronic kidney disease (CKD). For instance, tubular atrophy and interstitial fibrosis have been identified as critical markers that are associated with renal dysfunction, indicating the need to preserve tubulointerstitial integrity to prevent further progression of kidney disease, such as CKD, particularly in feline populations with renal fibrosis as a common pathological manifestation (Elliott et al., 2015).

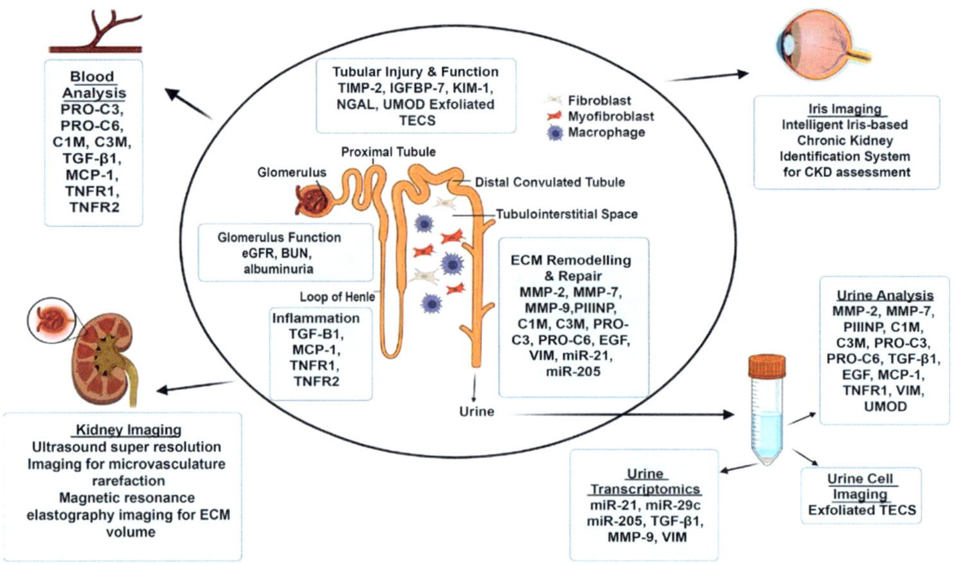

Figure 4.5. Importance of tubulointerstitial function.

Source: https://physoc.onlinelibrary.wiley.com/cms/asset/4d064727-9e90-4dc8-a560-6a2b8bb08fcc/tjp15620-fig-0001-m.jpg.

Its second important role is the efficacy of protein reabsorption by transporters in the tubules of the kidney, particularly in the proximal tubule. Studies have indicated that reduced megalin and cubilin expression, two important endocytic transporters, have been linked to tubulointerstitial damage in disease states early in the disease process, for example, in diabetic nephropathy (DN). The abnormal functioning of these transporters can lead to a significant reduction in protein reabsorption, further exacerbating tubulointerstitial damage and initiating a vicious cycle of deterioration. This interaction is meant to illustrate how tubulointerstitial dysfunction can trigger a cascade of pathological events leading to chronic fibrosis and impaired renal function. The findings highlight the need for therapeutic agents targeting tubulointerstitial integrity to reduce the disease burden of conditions like DN and promote the recovery of renal function towards normalcy (Bahamonde et al., 2017). Moreover, the tubulointerstitial microenvironment is not a passive bystander in renal pathologies; rather, it has an active contribution in the inflammatory response frequently observed in kidney disease. Inflammatory mediators and fibrogenic factors are profoundly active in the tubulointerstitial compartment, regulating both mechanisms of tissue damage and tissue repair. When kidneys are subjected to insults, such as hypoxia or nephrotoxins, the interstitium reacts by initiating mechanisms of inflammation and fibrosis. This reaction, adaptive initially, can become maladaptive and lead to chronic injury unless inhibited. It is vital to appreciate the dynamics of the tubulointerstitium while formulating therapies aimed at the resolution of inflammation and fibrosis. Thus, preservation of tubulointerstitial function not only aids in a rapid resolution of acute kidney injuries but also potentially avoids long-term functional damage, which again highlights the importance of this renal segment toward the overall health of the kidney (Figure 4.5).

4.2. Classification of Tubulointerstitial Diseases

The classification of tubulointerstitial disease is crucial for understanding its pathophysiology, diagnosis, and management strategies. Tubulointerstitial diseases are broadly categorized into infectious, inflammatory, and fibrotic processes. Tubulointerstitial infections typically refer to viral or bacterial infections that directly attack the renal interstitium, thereby inducing an inflammatory response. Concurrently, inflammatory diseases can be caused by autoimmune disease processes or be secondary in relation to systemic illnesses, such as lupus erythematosus, and lead to tubulointerstitial nephritis. These are significant to clinicians because they guide diagnostic approaches and treatment attempts, which are critical for managing renal well-being and preventing chronic kidney disease (CKD) or end-stage renal failure. A key component of tubulointerstitial disorders is renal fibrosis, a condition characterized by the overproduction of fibroblasts and the inappropriate deposition of extracellular matrix within the renal interstitium. It is typically the eventual outcome of various insults and forms an important pathway through which kidney damage is manifested. Notably, renal tubulointerstitial fibrosis has been described as the unifying pathological feature of many underlying diseases, diabetes and hypertension, and is most evident in chronic kidney disease progression. Interestingly, in cats, renal fibrosis and impairment are related to each other, bringing focus to the research of mediators and mechanisms.

In particular, progress in renal fibrosis holds promise for new avenues of intervention to potentially halt the progression of tubulointerstitial disease, as this pathological process remains a significant area of research in nephrology (Elliott et al., 2015). Chronic allograft nephropathy (CAN) serves as an excellent example of the multifactorial nature of tubulointerstitial disease among transplant recipients, where the interstitial compartments of the kidneys are compromised due to several determinants of transplantation. Research in CAN has provided insights into the biological processes underlying renal fibrogenesis, which are core to the mechanisms of transplant failure. Despite progress with immunosuppressive drugs, CAN remains a leading cause of renal transplant loss, highlighting the need for further investigation in prevention. Moreover, the definition of some therapeutic targets is now essential since the present complexity of the fibrosis process is considered the key to improving graft survival and patient outcome in renal transplant recipients.

The ongoing research of these pathologies demonstrates how classification, pathophysiology, and therapy continue to evolve dynamically in tubulointerstitial diseases (Haylor et al., 2014) (Figure 4.6).

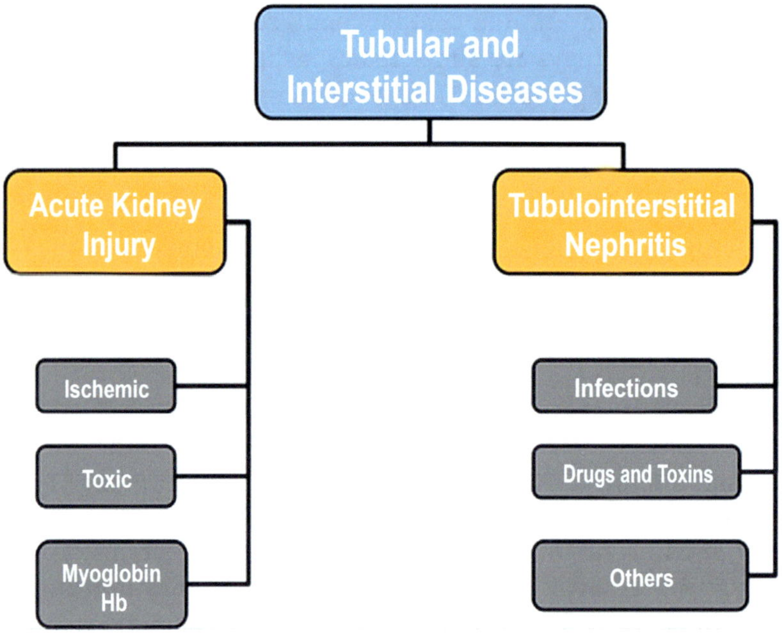

Figure 4.6. Classification of tubulointerstitial diseases.

Source: https://o.quizlet.com/nsQK7mW7BEoyi63hUKd3iQ.png.

4.2.1. Acute Tubulointerstitial Nephritis

Acute Tubulointerstitial Nephritis (ATIN) is characterized by inflammatory changes in the kidney's interstitium, which can lead to severe renal impairment. The etiopathogenesis of ATIN is complex, with multiple etiologies extending from drug hypersensitivity to infection. Drugs, particularly non-steroidal anti-inflammatory drugs (NSAIDs), antibiotics, and certain diuretics, have been primarily implicated in precipitating this syndrome. Apart from the pharmacologic precipitants, other systemic diseases like autoimmune diseases can also manifest with acute tubulointerstitial injury. Its presentation can include elevated serum creatinine, electrolyte imbalance, and hematuria, and underlines the relevance of early diagnosis and treatment. Early diagnosis of the disorder is crucial, for if it occurs late, it can lead to irreversible renal damage, emphasizing the need for clinicians to have a high degree of suspicion of ATIN in the patient with acute renal impairment. Infectious etiologies also play a role in the development of acute tubulointerstitial nephritis. For instance, leptospirosis, a zoonotic disease, presents with a typical triad of presentation, including fever, jaundice, and acute renal failure, typically implicating more widespread systemic illness. The renal picture of leptospirosis is predominantly one of tubulointerstitial nephritis, which identifies the infectious etiology for most cases of ATIN. Research has discovered that the interaction of Leptospira outer membrane proteins with renal tubular cells can induce an inflammatory response via Toll-like receptors, causing damage to the tubules and ultimately leading to dysfunction. This indicates the inherent nature of ATIN, as it can occur not only from the usual toxicological exposures but also through systemic infection, necessitating multimodal treatment regimens and an understanding of the underlying renal inflammation mechanism. Integrative treatment of Acute Tubulointerstitial Nephritis is important because the disease can be one of several syndromes, such as tubulointerstitial nephritis and uveitis (TINU) syndrome. TINU syndrome is a rare but significant presentation that is linked to autoimmune conditions, based on case reports in patients with relapsing polychondritis. Effective management of ATIN, particularly when it is associated with systemic diseases, necessitates a coordinated, multidisciplinary effort not only focused on renal inflammation but also on control of the attendant disease process. This can include immunosuppressive therapy when autoimmune mechanisms are implicated, and careful monitoring of renal function and supportive care. With approximately 200 cases of TINU documented and other potential complications of ATIN, ongoing research into its pathophysiology and treatment remains crucial for maximizing patient outcomes (Yang et al., 2007; Sierra et al., 2017) (Figure 4.7).

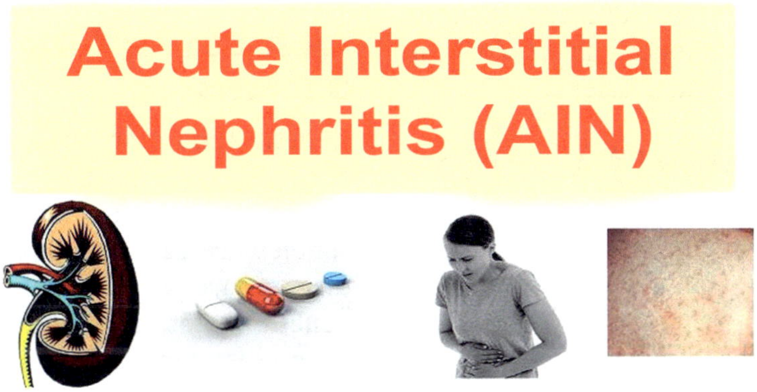

Figure 4.7. Acute interstitial nephritis (AIN).

Source: https://i.ytimg.com/vi/1tTlEQlJ-NY/hq720.jpg?sqp=-oaymwEhCK4FEIIDSFryq4qpAxMIARUAAAAAGAElAADIQj0AgKJD&rs=AOn4CLDTyQif5tlWX4HtqCem4KwPhqoMsw.

4.2.2. Chronic Tubulointerstitial Nephritis

Chronic Tubulointerstitial Nephritis (CTIN) is one of the leading causes of tubulointerstitial disease, through the progressive inflammation and fibrosis of the renal interstitium. Unlike its acute versions, which could be reversible on timely intervention, chronic nephritis can lead to irreversible loss and end-stage renal disease if left untreated. Pathologies of CTIN are multifactorial, most prominently caused by prolonged exposure to nephrotoxins, autoimmune conditions, and certain infections. With the sinister character of the onset of disease, patients may present with nonspecific symptoms such as fatigue, malaise, and urinary disturbances, posing early diagnosis as an issue. Protracted impairment of renal function typically occurs before the initiation of definitive therapy, highlighting the need for health practitioners to observe the subtle presentation of this condition. There has been research that established an association between Chronic Tubulointerstitial Nephritis and systemic disease, including Sjögrens syndrome and lupus erythematosus. In some cases, one of the most significant characteristics will be immune complex deposition in the interstitium; nevertheless, these events occur without glomerular participation, which is relatively rare in clinical practice. In an attempt to make the complex relationship more understandable, a case report described a patient with renal insufficiency due to an atypical immunological reaction in CTIN. Increased autoantibodies will complicate the clinical presentation, and a thorough investigative process is necessary to rule out overlapping syndromes. Chronic renal impairment can also lead to systemic manifestations, demonstrating how extra-renal features may be dependent upon one another in chronic inflammatory kidney disease like CTIN (Azevedo et al., 2015). Management of Chronic Tubulointerstitial Nephritis usually involves addressing the underlying etiology in an attempt to prevent future disease.

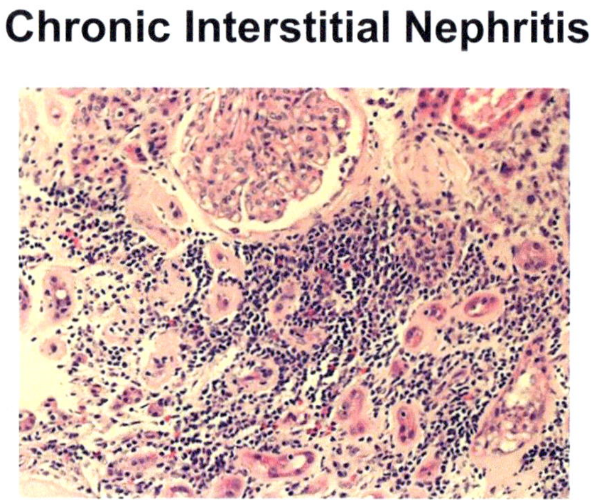

Figure 4.8. Chronic interstitial nephritis.

Source: https://external-content.duckduckgo.com/iu/?u=http%3A%2F%2Fmedia.renalandurologynews.com%2Fimages%2Fdsm%2Fch5842.fig1.jpg&f=1&nofb=1&ipt=a0ad05dbd6f101a0912d6ec645db623095a41866c41e879ed347f8e4ff559bbf.

As an example, withdrawal from offending agents such as certain drugs can prove to be essential in reversing the disease process, although it may not always be achievable. For instance, in patients with TINU syndrome, treatment with corticosteroids can effectively manage inflammation and prevent further kidney damage (Sierra et al., 2017). Notably, prompt diagnosis and personalized treatment regimens not only alleviate symptoms but also preserve renal function, thereby enhancing patient outcomes. Interestingly, as knowledge concerning CTIN continues to broaden, it becomes increasingly clear that both genetic susceptibility and environmental stimuli have a remarkable influence on the course of this disease, underlining the need for further research in this complex area (Figure 4.8).

4.2.3. Genetic Tubulointerstitial Disorders

Genetic tubulointerstitial diseases represent a multifactorial family of kidney diseases in which both the kidney interstitium and tubules are affected. Genetic tubulointerstitial diseases are generally connected with inherited genetic mutations that disrupt normal kidney functions, leading to compromised kidney health. Pathophysiology is typically a spectrum of abnormalities, ranging from reduced tubular reabsorption to architectural changes in the renal interstitium. Some genes have been identified through studies as contributing to tubulointerstitial dysfunction, and a genetic predisposition has been emphasized in such disorders. Understanding these genes plays a critical role in supporting early diagnosis and therapy, in line with existing efforts to assess therapeutic modalities aimed at preventing the progression of tubulointerstitial disease. Evidence exists that many genetic disorders of the kidney express themselves as tubulointerstitial disease, and molecular genetics plays a key role. For instance, advances in genomic studies have provided information about genes that are predominantly expressed in renal tissues. Notably, such a study as that by Anders et al., (2010) provided a large dataset elucidating genes with known function in glomerular and tubulointerstitial function. The study is pivotal to breaking down the complexity involved in genetic tubulointerstitial disease, revealing new molecular mechanisms not known to be associated with kidney pathology. These observations identify potential areas for the identification of biomarkers that may allow earlier diagnosis and more individualized treatment protocols in individuals affected by the condition. Furthermore, genetic tubulointerstitial disorders interdigitate importantly with systemic conditions such as diabetes mellitus, one of the leading etiologies of chronic kidney disease. The interaction between the underlying genetic predispositions and environmental determinants, such as blood glucose level, highlights the multifactorial etiology of these diseases. Evidence suggests that certain genetic predispositions may exacerbate renal impairment; however, specific interventions, such as zinc supplementation, have been shown to reduce oxidative stress and glomerular injury in diabetic patients, as reported by Fernando et al. (2015). This means that knowledge of genetic predisposition provides not only a pathophysiological explanation but also a blueprint for creating targeted treatment approaches and lifestyle modifications to sustain renal function in individuals at risk of tubulointerstitial disease (Figure 4.9).

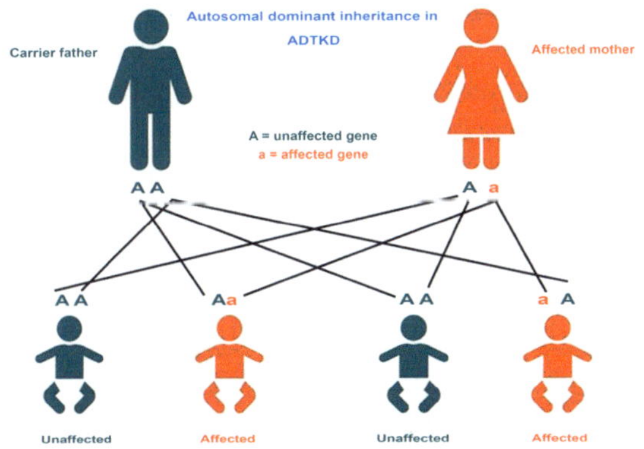

Figure 4.9. Genetic tubulointerstitial disorders.

Source: https://kcuk.cdn.ngo/media/images/ADTKD_-_inheritance_diagram.width-700.png.

4.3. Etiology of Tubulointerstitial Diseases

The pathogenesis of tubulointerstitial disease is multifactorial and dependent on a myriad of intrinsic and extrinsic variables that result in dysfunction of the renal interstitial tissue. The most frequent cause of acute tubulointerstitial nephritis (TIN) is an immune response to drugs or infections, resulting in inflammation and injury within the interstitium of the kidneys. As an example, administration of certain drugs has been known to trigger a hypersensitivity reaction, resulting in acute renal failure. Infectious agents can also invade the kidney, resulting in acute inflammatory alterations that involve the invasion of renal cells, tubular damage, and ultimately, loss of renal function. Such situations emphasize the importance of early diagnosis and treatment, particularly given that most patients present with a high percentage of late-stage disease, rendering efficient management decisions difficult, as demonstrated in research establishing the heterogeneity of underlying etiologies of acute and chronic TIN (Butler-Dawson et al., 2019). Chronic tubulointerstitial diseases typically arise from prolonged exposure to toxic products, metabolic disorders, and systemic diseases. These diseases, such as hypertension and diabetes mellitus, are responsible for chronic fibrotic change in the interstitium of the kidney and result in chronic kidney disease (CKD). Recurrent inflammation, recurrent hemodynamic changes, and resultant structural modifications of the interstitium and tubules typically define pathophysiologic mechanisms. Environmental determinants such as heat stress and dehydration are also significant risks for chronic interstitial nephritis. Butler-Dawson et al. (2019) describe the association between rising global temperature and renal function, emphasizing the contribution of heatacclimatized conditions to induce recurring episodes of inflammation and renal injury, particularly in vulnerable populations. Such chronic insults can finally lead to widespread fibrosis and loss of functional nephron mass, emphasizing the importance of addressing underlying etiologies in prevention and treatment strategies. Finally, genetic predispositions and inherited disease states are typically the underlying causes of tubulointerstitial diseases. As an example, familial nephronophthisis and medullary cystic disease are the genetic etiology of chronic interstitial nephritis in children, and they are the most common. The pathologic findings of these genetic diseases typically exhibit a homogeneous inflammatory response and structural changes, as can be demonstrated in studies of kidney biopsies from affected individuals. These familial syndromes highlight the absolute need for genetic screening and counseling in patients with a history of kidney disease in the family, enabling early diagnosis and potentially proactive treatment. Secondarily, familiarity with the specific genetic underpinnings can guide tailoring of therapeutic regimens, with the potential to ultimately improve patient prognosis and retard the progress of the disease in the afflicted (Babaheidarian et al., 2015).

4.3.1. Infectious Causes

Tubulointerstitial disorders, which affect the interstitium and renal tubules, can be triggered by a wide range of infectious agents, resulting in a profound impact on kidney function. The diseases are most often the result of viral, bacterial, or parasitic infections, which cause inflammation and subsequent renal impairment. Notably, the Human Immunodeficiency Virus (HIV) can induce a range of renal abnormalities in infected individuals. Studies have pointed out that HIV-infected patients present with varied renal pathologies, like tubulointerstitial nephropathy, which highlights the intricacy of kidney diseases related to infectious etiologies. Further, renal biopsies are performed in a small number of such patients, which adds to the difficulty in managing and diagnosing such infection-induced renal diseases and because of mounting HIV and renal disease, knowing such facts is crucial in setting up proper treatment protocols to avoid renal deterioration in such affected populations (Carvalho et al., 2011). Other than HIV, other causes of infections also lead to tubulointerstitial diseases. For instance, bacterial infections such as pyelonephritis act directly on the renal interstitium, causing inflammation that can proceed to scarring and chronic renal damage. Infections caused by viral pathogens, such as cytomegalovirus (CMV) and Epstein-Barr Virus (EBV), have also been linked to renal injury, particularly in immunocompromised patients. The difficulty with managing these types of tubulointerstitial diseases is early detection and subsequent therapeutic strategies that take into account the infectious etiology. Because these diseases can sometimes occur silently, as in the case of pediatric uveitis, medical treatment providers must be careful to search for patients with signs of renal involvement (Foster et al., 2014). Carefulness is essential in limiting long-term complications and achieving maximum optimal patient outcomes. Infectious causes of tubulointerstitial diseases must be researched not only for diagnosis but also to ensure proper and timely treatment. The identification of certain infections is followed by specific therapeutic regimens that can help improve morbidity associated with renal disease. For instance, HIV-associated renal disorders must be treated with caution and may include antiretroviral therapy, among other supportive treatments, to address renal insufficiency. In pyelonephritis, too, early antibiotic application is necessary to prevent further extensive renal injury. Further investigation into the implications of infectious agents on renal pathology is necessary to improve diagnostic criteria and treatment protocols, particularly for high-risk groups. By gaining a deeper understanding of these infectious causes, healthcare systems can be better prepared to address the complexities of tubulointerstitial disease, ultimately improving patient outcomes and care (Carvalho et al., 2011) (Figure 4.10).

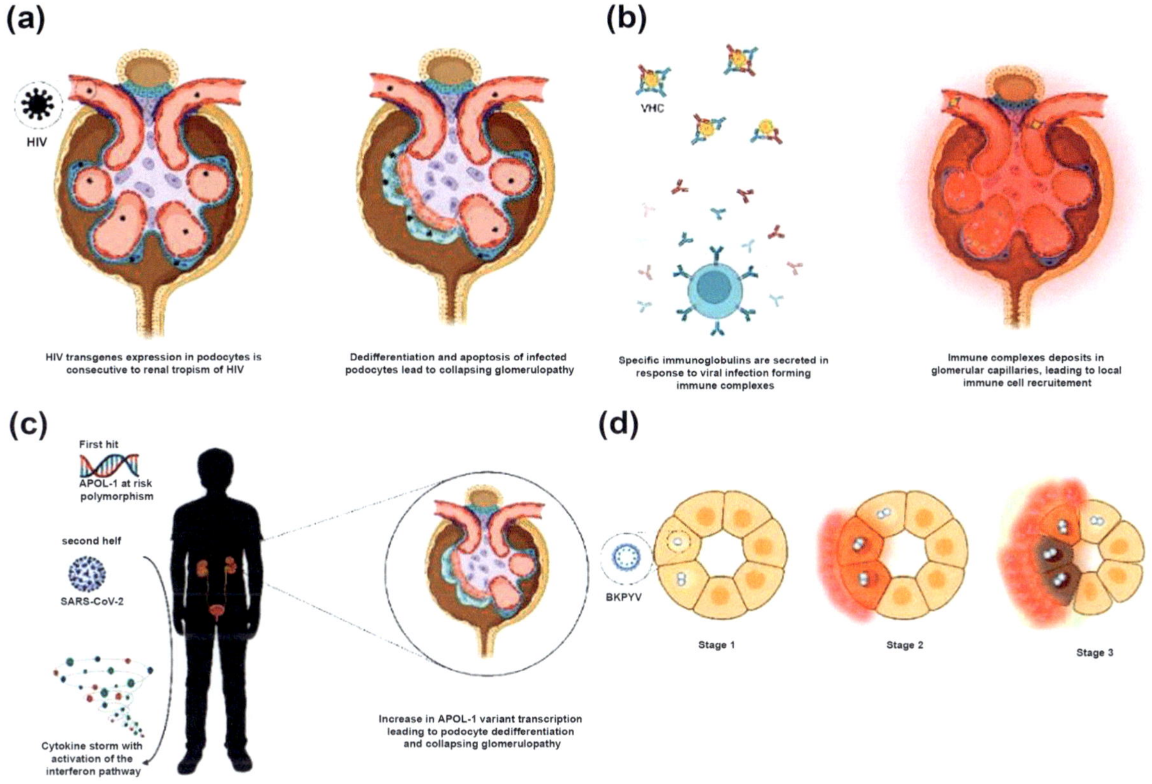

Figure 4.10. Infectious causes of tubulointerstitial diseases.

Source: https://pub.mdpi-res.com/ijms/ijms-23-12014/article_deploy/html/images/ijms-23-12014-g001.png?1665382685.

4.3.2. Drug-Induced Causes

The link between tubulointerstitial disease and drug-induced disease is increasingly recognized in the context of renal health. A variety of drugs, including non-steroidal anti-inflammatory drugs (NSAIDs), antibiotics, and certain chemotherapeutic drugs, have been known to cause interstitial nephritis, an inflammation of the renal interstitium. Inflammation may lead to altered renal function and has been linked to the use of drugs that induce hypersensitivity reactions. The clinical picture may include acute renal failure and associated symptoms; therefore, early diagnosis is necessary to prevent long-term effects. Ultimately, awareness of these drug-induced causes is essential for clinicians as it can significantly influence both treatment strategies and patient prognosis in individuals with renal impairment. Pathogenesis of drug-induced tubulointerstitial disease may be multi-factorial and most often involves direct nephrotoxicity and immune-mediated injury. Some drugs can cause cellular senescence, resulting in cell cycle arrest irreversibly and the release of pro-inflammatory factors. This leads to the formation of the senescence-associated secretory phenotype (SASP), which causes the maintenance of renal injury through additional inflammation and fibrosis of the renal interstitium. Detection of this intricate drug-renal cell response is critical in the treatment of drug-induced renal diseases. A deeper understanding of cellular senescence mechanisms can also inform therapeutic measures to prevent or mitigate renal damage, a fascinating area for future inquiry and treatment in nephrology. In view of the complex multiplicity of drug-induced tubulointerstitial disease, preventive and therapeutic approaches demand cautious review. Techniques include careful observation of renal function in drug-nephrotoxic patients and identification of alternative treatment strategies when necessary. The focus has become increasingly on comprehension and identification of potential therapeutic agents capable of intervening in the pathogenetic events of chronic allograft nephropathy, an important and significant cause of renal transplant failure. Of special concern, nonetheless, with advances in immunosuppression therapy, chronic allograft nephropathy remains a clinical issue, requiring new strategies to account for the role of drug-induced etiology in the progression of renal disease. By furthering our understanding and targeting these mechanisms, there is potential for improved outcomes in patients with drug-induced tubulointerstitial diseases (Haylor et al., 2014; Alpini et al., 2020) (Figure 4.11).

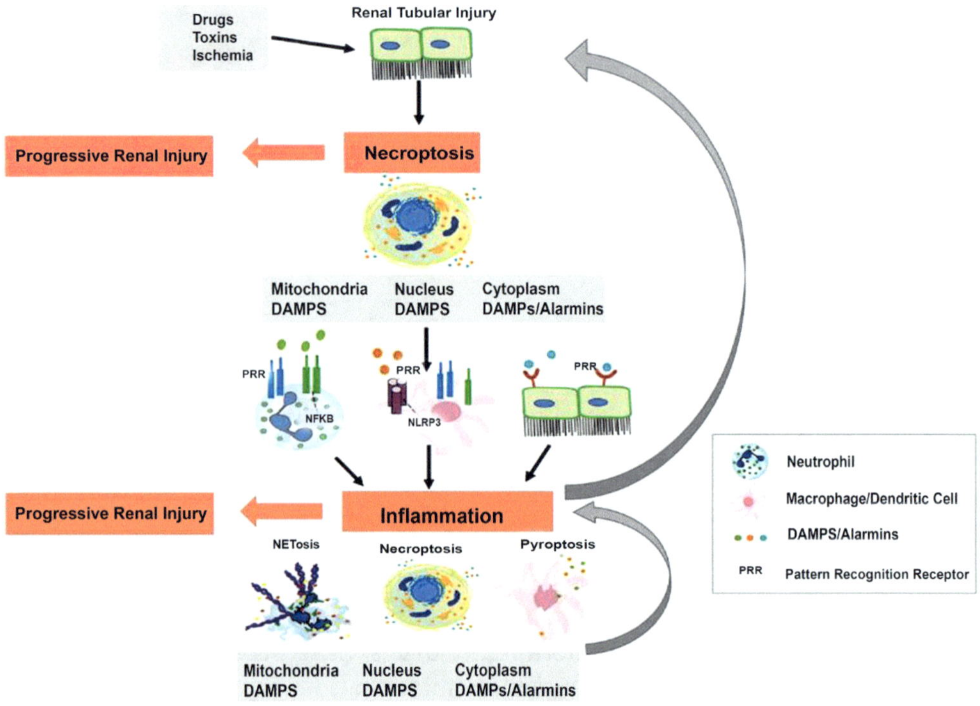

Figure 4.11. Drug-induced tubulointerstitial nephritis.

Source: https://media.springernature.com/lw1200/springer-static/image/art%3A10.1007%2Fs00467-019-04207-9/MediaObjects/467_2019_4207_Fig2_HTML.png.

4.3.3. Autoimmune and Systemic Diseases

Autoimmune and systemic disorders represent a significant field of interest for the study of tubulointerstitial diseases since they are capable of inducing complicated pathology that impairs renal function. Autoimmune diseases occur when the body's own immune system attacks the body's own tissues, resulting in inflammation and damage. In particular, systemic lupus erythematosus (SLE) and vasculitis have been observed to have renal manifestations, often leading to tubulointerstitial disease. These systemic disorders can cause acute or chronic tubulointerstitial nephritis, characterized by inflammation and fibrosis of the renal interstitium. The genetic predisposition of these diseases, combined with environmental triggers, makes it challenging to appreciate the mechanisms by which they affect kidney function. It is essential to understand the pathophysiology by which autoimmune diseases affect renal function in order to develop effective treatment regimens and improve outcomes in patients. Research has shown certain autoimmune conditions, such as Sjögrens syndrome and relapsing polychondritis, to present unique difficulties in the context of tubulointerstitial disease. The combination of autoimmune presentation and renal disorder requires multimodal diagnostic and treatment strategies. A specific example is the tubulointerstitial nephritis and uveitis (TINU) syndrome, which has been labeled an inflammatory oculorenal syndrome of infrequent occurrence associated with autoimmune disease. As noted in recent literature, TINU syndrome can be related to acute bilateral uveitis and tubulointerstitial nephritis complicating the clinical picture (Sierra et al., 2017). Diagnosis of these syndromes is very important because it will cause a lot of morbidity if it is not diagnosed and treated promptly. Moreover, the interplay between autoimmune diseases and the development of chronic kidney disease justifies more research in this area. Animal models have proven to be highly valuable in elucidating the mechanisms of kidney injury in autoimmune and systemic diseases. Genetically altered mice, particularly those with targeted gene deletions and specific mutations, have enabled the investigation of how immune dysregulation leads to tubulointerstitial disease. Current murine models have the potential to replicate a variety of human renal pathologies, including those associated with autoimmune conditions such as lupus nephritis and IgA nephropathy (Anders et al., 2000). Understanding the genetics of these entities will enhance our understanding of the disease mechanisms involved and inform the development of targeted therapies. As experimental nephrology advances, there remains much possibility to explore where autoimmune disease and tubulointerstitial nephropathy overlap, ultimately striving to improve therapeutic outcomes in patients afflicted by them.

4.4. Pathophysiology of Tubulointerstitial Diseases

The pathophysiology of tubulointerstitial disease is characterized by a complex interaction between several cellular and molecular pathways that lead to causative renal injury. Most of such entities commonly arise as a result of renal tubular and interstitial injury caused by multiple possible reasons, including autoimmune disorders, metabolic disturbances, and nephrotoxicity. The primary damage typically triggers an inflammatory response. This triggers the activation of various immune cells, such as macrophages and lymphocytes, involved in the continuation of tissue damage. The inflammatory condition not only exacerbates existing damage but also creates a suitable environment for fibrosis, as activated myofibroblasts produce greater numbers and lay down extracellular matrix constituents. This leads to terminal scarring of the kidney tissue. Clarifying these underlying processes is crucial in the development of targeted treatment protocols to halt or reverse the disease process. The consequences of diabetic nephropathy (DN) are a classic example of the possible severe renal compromise resulting from tubulointerstitial dynamic alterations. Studies indicate that the diminution of the expression of transporters, including megalin and cubilin, in the tubules is strongly associated with diabetic renal dysfunction. This decrease in protein reabsorption transporters is related to increased tubulointerstitial damage and fibrosis formation, suggesting that early tubulointerstitial changes are key in the pathogenesis of DN. As observed with the use of animal models, loss of such transporters resulted in impaired urinary protein reabsorption and thus worsened renal outcomes. These observations confirm the essential role of the tubulointerstitial compartment in maintaining kidney function and highlight the pathogenic implications of its failure, underscoring the urgency for interventions targeting these pathways with greater precision (Bahamonde et al., 2017). New research has explored the therapeutic value of novel metabolites of dietary fatty acids, and particularly omega-3 polyunsaturated fatty acids. Research has indicated that metabolites such as 19,20-EDP have potent protective effect against tubulointerstitial models of renal fibrosis. Acting via mechanisms such as inhibiting epithelial-to-mesenchymal transition (EMT) and modulating inflammatory responses, the metabolites reversed fibrosis and restored renal structure and function. In animal experiments, treatment with 19,20-EDP resulted in reduced expression of fibrotic markers and preservation of renal tubular integrity, indicating a potential therapeutic avenue for tubulointerstitial diseases. By leveraging the distinct biological actions of these metabolites, future treatments will not only avert renal damage but also promote repair mechanisms in the tubulointerstitial space, again emphasizing the role of cellular signaling pathways in the treatment of kidney disease (Hammock et al., 2016).

4.4.1. Mechanisms of Injury to Tubules

The pathophysiology of tubule damage in tubulointerstitial disease is complex and involves a multitude of interconnected processes that result in cellular damage and renal impairment. In diabetic nephropathy, a reduction in the expression of critical transport proteins, such as megalin and cubilin, can be observed. These proteins play a central role in protein reabsorption, particularly in the form of albumin. Decreased expression of such transporters has been linked with increased tubulointerstitial injury, including fibrosis, thickening of the tubular basement membrane, and increased metalloprotease activity in tubular cells. This results in a pathological cycle in which abnormal reabsorption of proteins enhances tubulointerstitial damage, which highlights the importance of such transport mechanisms in maintaining renal health (Bahamonde et al., 2017). Recognition of these processes is vital for the development of therapeutic interventions aimed at preventing early diabetic nephropathy injury. A second important characteristic of tubule injury mechanisms is the role played by inflammatory processes, which are often activated in response to an underlying disease process. In multiple myeloma, myeloma cells have been shown to interact with renal fibroblasts and free light chains, triggering tubulointerstitial fibrosis. The fibrotic changes that accompany them not only interfere with the tubular structure itself but also support a chronic inflammatory environment that perpetuates renal injury. Mathematical modeling of such interactions provides insight into the mechanisms of the tubule injury and fibrosis. Quantitative approaches like these can be valuable in determining the specific interactions that exacerbate kidney damage, thereby informing potential therapies for patients with multiple myeloma and associated kidney failure (Ayati et al., 2018). In addition to inflammation and metabolic pathways, oxidative stress is also a significant contributor to injury pathways affecting the renal tubules. Enhanced ROS production can lead to cellular apoptosis and further disrupt the normal interstitial space. Oxidative stress, as previously described, aggravates tubular cell structural integrity and promotes the recruitment of inflammatory cells, resulting in a vicious cycle of injury and repair that typically becomes deranged. Antioxidant protocols incorporated may be beneficial in reversing oxidative damage and improving prognosis in tubulointerstitial disease. Building on our understanding of these mechanisms is crucial to the development of targeted interventions, with the ultimate aim of restoring tubule function and inducing renal preservation in affected patients. As studies further reveal the complexities of these injury mechanisms, clinicians become increasingly skilled at designing therapeutic regimens that specifically address the etiology of renal dysfunction (Figure 4.12).

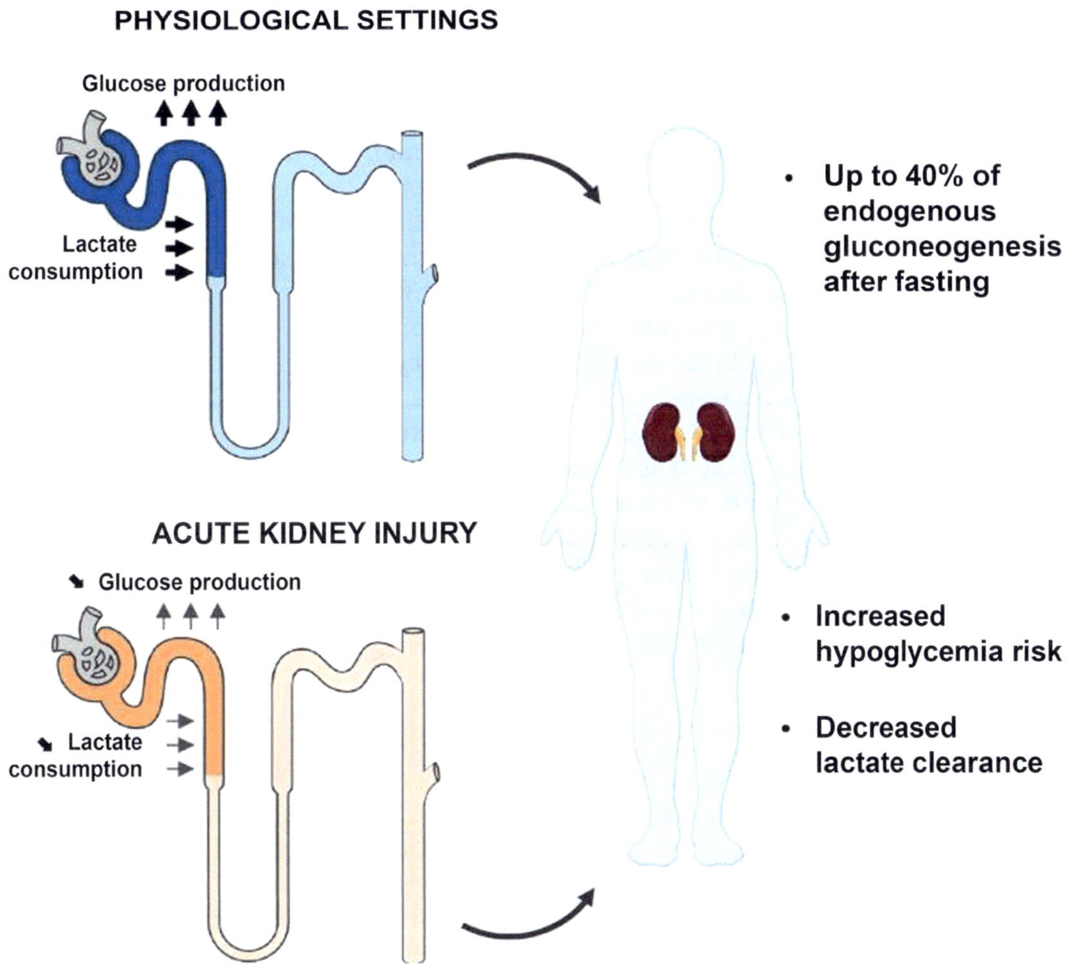

Figure 4.12. Metabolic mechanisms of acute proximal tubular injury.

Source: https://media.springernature.com/lw1200/springer-static/image/art%3A10.1007%2Fs00424-022-02701-y/MediaObjects/424_2022_2701_Fig3_HTML.png.

4.4.2. Role of Inflammation in Disease Progression

Inflammation is a key component of the pathogenesis of tubulointerstitial diseases as a cause and consequence of renal damage. The kidneys, being highly vascular organs, respond to damage and insults by mounting an inflammatory cascade triggered by various reasons, including infections, toxins, or autoimmune diseases. Cytokines and chemokines are the choreographers behind this inflammatory response, conducting the immigration of immune cells to the damaged site. Specifically, chemokines permit leukocyte trafficking, which, if poorly regulated, can exacerbate local tissue damage. While inflammation may serve a temporary protective role by removing pathogenic agents and initiating repair, chronic inflammation can lead to structural changes and functional impairment of renal tissue, contributing to the progression of tubulointerstitial kidney diseases. A key aspect of understanding the pathophysiology of inflammation in tubulointerstitial disease is its relationship with renal fibrosis. Prolonged inflammation leads to the accumulation of extracellular matrix constituents, ultimately to renal tubulointerstitial fibrosis, a pathologic hallmark of end-stage kidney disease. Renal fibrosis is characterized by a widespread scarring process that disrupts the fine balance between tissue repair and breakdown, commonly causing irreparable injury. As explained in existing research, cross-talk between fibrotic pathways and inflammatory mediators is essential, as it suggests potential therapeutic interventions for managing chronic kidney disease (CKD). Such an understanding of this pathologic process enables the availability of targeted intervention options to interrupt the cycle of fibrosis and inflammation that underlies the progression of kidney disease (Elliott et al., 2015). Furthermore, the intricate interplay of immune mechanisms involved in kidney inflammation offers opportunities for novel therapies. Although anti-inflammatory agents have shown promise in preclinical models, their clinical effectiveness is at best context-dependent and inconsistent. Researchers have focused increasing attention on blocking certain chemokines as a mechanism to engineer the modulation of kidney inflammation (Abdi et al., 2004). However, more recent evidence indicates that these interventions can be detrimental, such as in the case of exacerbating renal inflammation in some pathologies. Hence, it is critically important to gain a clear understanding of the dual role of inflammation in both healing and damaging kidney tissues, in order to devise effective therapies for the future. By elucidating the mechanisms involved in inflammation and its effect, it is possible to design a therapy that adequately retards disease progression without the loss of kidney functional integrity.

4.4.3. Consequences of Tubulointerstitial Damage

Tubulointerstitial injury has profound implications for renal function and overall well-being. The interstitium and tubules are crucial in the process of homeostasis, particularly in regulating electrolyte balance, acid-base status, and waste excretion. Tubulointerstitial damage can invalidate these processes and result in acute and chronic renal failure. For example, acute tubular necrosis may result from a multitude of insults, leading to acute kidney injury characterized by a reduced glomerular filtration rate (GFR) and subsequent electrolyte disturbances. In addition, chronic injury can lead to a stepwise reduction in renal function, frequently leading to end-stage renal disease, which would require dialysis or transplantation. The frequency of such effects underscores the need for early detection and control of tubulointerstitial disorders to prevent long-term damage to kidney health. Damage to the tubulointerstitium also has far-reaching systemic effects beyond the renal system. One of the most important is the formation of enhanced vulnerability to cardiovascular conditions, as kidney impairment is so intimately connected with cardiac status. The change in renal function can cause hypertension through several mechanisms, such as volume expansion and augmentation of the renin-angiotensin-aldosterone system (RAAS) activity. Further, chronic kidney disease (CKD) has been associated with vascular stiffness and left ventricular hypertrophy, contributing to cardiovascular risk. Additionally, the pro-inflammatory environment of tubulointerstitial damage, as seen in diseases such as diabetic nephropathy, can contribute to atherosclerosis and negatively impact vascular integrity. In light of these outcomes, tubulointerstitial health is not only crucial for the maintenance of kidney function but also for overall cardiovascular risk control. The role of environmental influences in exacerbating tubulointerstitial damage cannot be overstated, particularly in the context of global warming and associated heat stress. Acute kidney injury can be caused by heat through dehydration and inflammation resulting from heat exposure. Evidence supports that long-term exposure to high temperatures severely increases the risk of heat-induced kidney disease, which may aggravate existing kidney disease and lead to chronic kidney disease. These environmental aspects again highlight interaction between external factors and renal function, indicating a need for interventional strategies focused on hydration and ecological adaptations to avoid kidney damage. The multifaceted consequences of tubulointerstitial damage necessitate joint efforts to understand both intrinsic and extrinsic mechanisms, which will be followed by new therapeutic approaches to counteract these problems (Butler-Dawson et al., 2019; Arribas et al., 2010) (Figure 4.13).

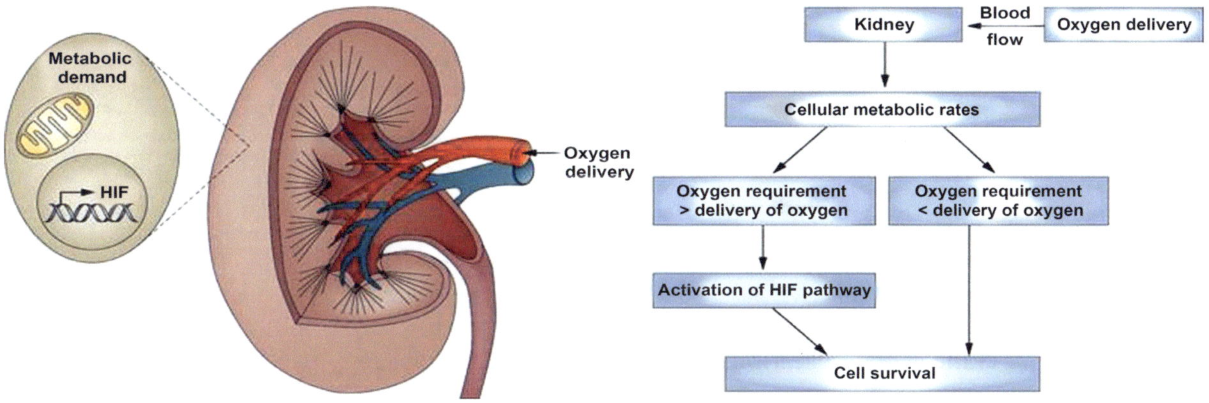

Figure 4.13. Tubulointerstitial damage.

Source: https://media.springernature.com/full/springer-static/image/art%3A10.1038%2Fnrneph.2010.124/MediaObjects/41581_2010_Article_BFnrneph2010124_Fig1_HTML.jpg.

4.5. Clinical Manifestations

The clinical presentation of tubulointerstitial diseases varies greatly with the etiology and degree of renal involvement. Tubulointerstitial diseases are often accompanied by nonspecific malaise, weakness, and fatigue, which can make diagnosis difficult. Renal dysfunction is a characteristic feature of tubulointerstitial diseases, as evidenced by elevated serum creatinine levels and reduced glomerular filtration rates. Patients may also experience electrolyte abnormalities, particularly in potassium and phosphate levels, due to disrupted tubular function. These abnormalities can lead to additional symptoms such as muscle cramping and bone pain. In some cases, renal imaging tests may reveal structural changes; however, these do not correlate with the severity of renal impairment, further highlighting the subtlety of diagnosing and treating these disorders. Yet another clinically significant category of presentations comes under the context of specific syndromes of tubulointerstitial disorders. TINU syndrome, for example, although rare, illustrates how the renal and ocular systems can be concurrently involved by inflammatory processes. This kind of syndrome is more prevalent in young female patients and is often related to autoimmune diseases, infection, or certain drugs.

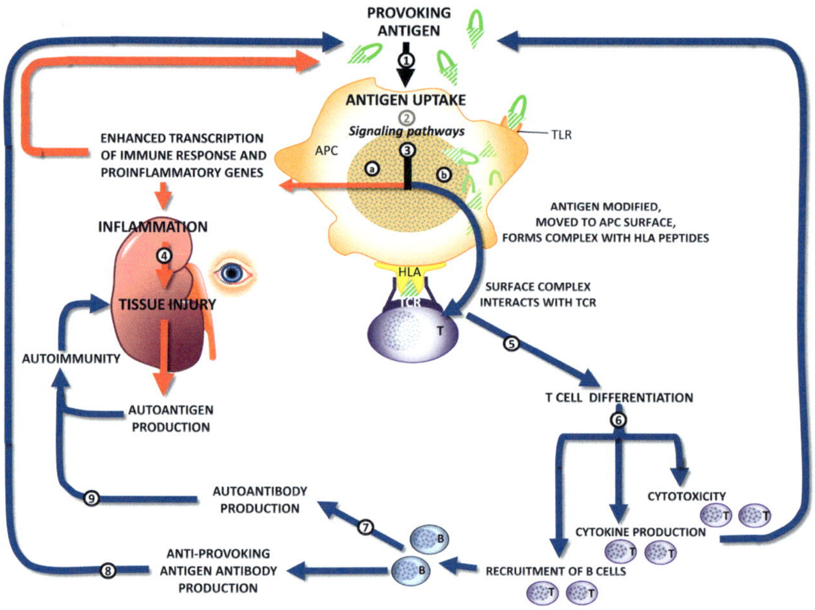

Figure 4.14. The clinical manifestations of tubulointerstitial diseases.

Source: https://external-content.duckduckgo.com/iu/?u=https%3A%2F%2Fels-jbs-prod-cdn.jbs.elsevierhealth.com%2Fcms%2Fattachment%2Fbee38e54-54d4-455b-b325-a68ba568b15a%2Fgr2_lrg.jpg&f=1&nofb=1&ipt=16735227d02d3fd37c13a24f2d1169eae9442fa5956ce3f97898b8afba3cb773.

A case report documented a patient with relapsing polychondritis who came with repeated episodes of bilateral uveitis along with tubulointerstitial nephritis, demonstrating the significance of clinicians being attentive to such associations. The occurrence of TINU syndrome underscores the importance of early diagnosis and management of comorbid symptoms in maintaining renal function, preventing permanent kidney damage, and preserving visual health in affected individuals (Sierra et al., 2017). Also of note is another disease that presents with the appearance of a tubulointerstitial disease, namely immunoglobulin G4-related disease (IgG4-RD). This is a systemic inflammatory illness with diverse clinical presentations, as it affects various organs, including the kidneys. Specifically, renal manifestation in patients with IgG4-RD may appear as tubulointerstitial nephritis with widespread lymphoplasmacytic infiltration and fibrosis. Physicians can identify increased serum

IgG4 concentrations, but such an increase is not permanent in all patients. Histopathological examination has a tendency to reveal storiform fibrosis and obliterative phlebitis, which are definitive in making a specific diagnosis. Glucocorticoids are the primary treatments, with other immunosuppressive drugs used in patients who relapse (Macchiorini et al., 2014). Knowledge of and early recognition of the clinical manifestations of IgG4-RD are crucial for its proper management and avoidance of renal sequelae (Adelheid et al., 2014) (Figure 4.14).

4.5.1. Symptoms of Tubulointerstitial Diseases

The symptom presentation of tubulointerstitial diseases is typically indicative of intrinsic renal dysfunction and may be highly varied based on the chronicity and severity of the disease. Patients may have a wide array of nonspecific symptoms, including fatigue, malaise, and anorexia; thus, early diagnosis is challenging. One of the typical presentations of such illnesses is the exhibition of renal concentrating impairment, leading to hyperuricemia, secondary nocturia, and polyuria. As renal function worsens, symptoms such as hypertension become apparent, compounded by the retention of metabolic waste. This spectrum of clinical presentations necessitates efficient clinical evaluation to distinguish these symptoms from those of other renal disease syndromes, thereby providing appropriate management and intervention for patients. Electrolyte disturbances are another significant symptom of tubulointerstitial diseases, which can lead to severe metabolic derangements. The patients may present with hypokalemia, hyperkalemia, or hyponatremia based on the tubulointerstitial pathology and its impact on tubular function. These imbalances can culminate in clinical complications like weakness of muscles, cardiac arrhythmias, and neurological symptoms, ultimately affecting quality of life as a whole. Additionally, the presence of proteinuria, although less severe than in glomerular conditions, can be observed, alerting healthcare providers to the underlying renal impairment. The impact of such symptoms is both physical and psychological; hence, constant monitoring and management are necessary. Treatments for these electrolyte disturbances need to be effectively integrated into the overall management plan to avoid chronic kidney damage and to improve patient outcomes. Tubulointerstitial patients also have more severe cases, such as acute kidney injury (AKI) or chronic kidney disease (CKD), which are irreversible conditions of deterioration in renal function. The connection between diabetes mellitus and renal failure brings this problem to attention, with chronic kidney disease itself causing nearly 44% of new diagnoses in the United States, sustaining the long-term consequences of neglected diseases (Fernando et al., 2015). Furthermore, markers of inflammation and other diagnostic indicators, including Plasma Neutrophil Gelatinase-Associated Lipocalin (NGAL), have been instrumental in identifying acute kidney injury resulting from tubulointerstitial diseases (Aga Khan University Hospital, 2015). Early diagnosis and early treatment interventions are crucial in preventing the development of end-stage renal disease and managing associated symptoms. Multidisciplinary care is often necessary to address the complexities of these symptoms and their underlying causes in an effective manner.

4.5.2. Diagnostic Approaches

The diagnosis of tubulointerstitial disorders must be approached with a multi-dimensional approach, keeping in view the complexities of renal pathology. Traditional methods, such as renal biopsies, provide valuable histological information but are fraught with significant risks and limitations. These intrusive procedures cannot be realistically repeated for continuous follow-up. While trying to overcome these limitations, scientists are now considering non-invasive diagnostic procedures. These methods include new imaging technologies and biomarker research, which can provide data on the renal interstitium's health without the requirement of biopsies. New technologies, such as high-throughput gene expression profiling, also support the understanding of the molecular mechanisms underlying tubulointerstitial diseases, rendering it feasible to differentiate among various etiologies based on distinctive gene expression profiles. The integration of these advances holds the promise of much enhanced diagnostic precision, eventually leading to more targeted therapeutic strategies for affected patients. This is supported by the potential of proteomics in non-invasive diagnosis of renal transplant rejection, highlighting its relevance to tubulointerstitial disease. While conventional diagnosis remains strongly reliant on invasive procedures, proteomic examination of urine and blood represents a compelling alternative option.

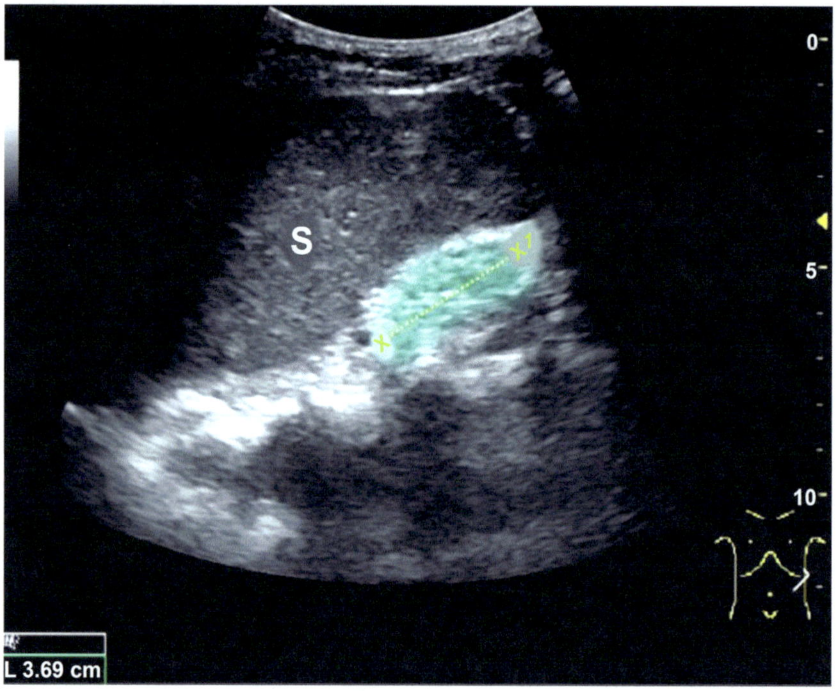

Figure 4.15. The diagnosis of tubulointerstitial diseases.

Source: https://media-us.amboss.com/media/views/62cd6332790d74.46761389.jpg.

A thorough review of 29 studies between the years 2003 highlights the advances towards the identification of individual proteins as biomarkers for acute and chronic rejection, showing how similar techniques can be used in diagnosing tubulointerstitial disease. Utilizing the specificity of these biomarkers, medical practitioners can obtain timely and accurate diagnoses, thereby improving clinical outcomes. However, the inherent shortcomings and limitations, such as protein expression variation and standardization essential for assay purposes, indicate a necessity for ongoing research for further development of these non-invasive techniques. The future of diagnostic techniques in tubulointerstitial diseases is bright with ongoing advancements in genomics and proteomics. As highlighted by glomerular gene expression data, identification of novel transcripts associated with kidney health can also inform the development of precision therapies for tubulointerstitial disease (Anders et al., 2010). Second, the exploration of non-invasive biomarkers would bridge the practice gap by providing clinicians with actionable information at minimal risk to the patient (Gwinner et al., 2016). Through continued research, the combination of these approaches can drive a paradigm shift in both the diagnosis and treatment of tubulointerstitial disease, thereby enhancing the quality of care for those afflicted with it. The recognition of the potential impact of these methodologies is crucial for advancing patient outcomes and renal pathophysiology in general (Figure 4.15).

4.5.3. Laboratory Findings and Imaging Techniques

The diagnosis of tubulointerstitial diseases often needs the combination of imaging modalities and laboratory data to establish a firm diagnosis. Laboratory tests are helpful by providing information regarding the functional status of the kidneys while revealing subtle pathophysiologic mechanisms. For instance, serum creatinine and blood urea nitrogen (BUN) levels are typically elevated, indicating impaired renal function. Additionally, urinalysis may reveal pathological characteristics, such as proteinuria or hematuria, indicating interstitial inflammation or renal tubular injury. Conditions such as IgG4-related disease, a type of tubulointerstitial disease, may reveal elevated serum IgG4 levels, although this is not definitive (Adelheid et al., 2014). Collectively, these laboratory findings represent an underlying paradigm for explaining the specific pattern of tubular and interstitial disease in which the patient will be at risk. Imaging modalities complement laboratory investigations by providing a visual image of renal architecture and abnormalities related to tubulointerstitial disease. Ultrasound is most frequently used as the initial imaging study due to its accessibility and ability to detect renal enlargement or echogenic kidney abnormalities that may indicate inflammation or fibrosis. More sophisticated imaging studies, such as magnetic resonance imaging (MRI) and computed tomography (CT), are more likely to yield more sensitive data about the renal architecture, with evidence of scarring, vascular abnormalities, or even infiltrative diseases, such as in IgG4-related disease. For instance, storiform fibrosis and obliterative phlebitis, as described in the histopathology, may also be accompanied by specific imaging findings that aid in diagnosis (Adelheid et al., 2014). Thus, both laboratory and imaging modalities must be used in a multidisciplinary diagnostic approach to effect proper assessment and management of these complex disorders. In addition to routine laboratory and imaging studies, some biomarkers and advanced techniques are increasingly being incorporated in the workup for the diagnosis of tubulointerstitial diseases. These include cytokine and chemokine analysis that can assist in elucidating the inflammatory process within the renal interstitium. Recent studies suggest that measuring renal biomarkers may be able to differentiate between tubulointerstitial diseases and non-tubulointerstitial diseases, as well as between various subtypes of IgG4-related disease (Adelheid et al., 2014). Additionally, novel imaging technologies like functional MRI and renal scintigraphy will allow real-time measurement of renal perfusion and function, which can prove to be priceless in estimating the severity and volume of tubulointerstitial disease. Combined, these lab advances and imaging tools not only enhance diagnostic precision but also inform therapeutic regimens, paving the way for more precise treatment options for the investigation of tubulointerstitial disease.

4.6. Treatment and Management

Treatment and management of tubulointerstitial disease are multifactorial in nature, focused on the etiology as well as on the kidneys' functional preservation. A central position is occupied by nutritional therapy and individualized nutritional change, particularly in those conditions related to chronic kidney disease (CKD). Due to the etiological heterogeneity of tubulointerstitial diseases, a thorough understanding of each patient's individual condition, including dietary and risk factors, is essential. Studies have indicated that dietary changes can significantly impact disease progression, improving patient outcomes by achieving symptom relief and reducing the metabolic stress imposed on kidney function. Collaboration among medical professionals, such as nephrologists, dietitians, and primary care providers, is crucial in developing effective therapies and delivering comprehensive patient care. The integration of information from other areas of research, including animal studies on protective mechanisms in kidney disease, can yield new management strategies with potential clinical applications (Arnold et al., 2018). Pharmaceutical management has evolved to the extent that best medical therapy is now the first-line treatment for disorders like ischemic nephropathy caused by atherosclerotic renal artery stenosis. Current recommendations favor a conservative approach, with a focus on renal protection and blood pressure management, over interventional methods. RAAS-blocking agents are primarily responsible for mitigating the drastic pathophysiologic consequences of renal hypoperfusion. Antihypertensives not only have their direct effect in lowering blood pressure but also possess intrinsic cardio- and renoprotective actions, especially vital in high-risk patients. Continuous research into the intricate dynamics of these pharmacological agents enhances our understanding of their efficacy in preventing renal damage, as well as corresponding cardiovascular events, supporting a systematic approach to treating tubulointerstitial diseases (Barbano et al., 2016). Aside from pharmacotherapy and dietary control, new modalities, including biologics and regenerative therapies, are being explored as potential future treatment strategies for tubulointerstitial diseases. Regenerative medicine, through the body's own repair mechanisms, can potentially provide new avenues for restoring kidney function or preventing further injury in patients with diseased kidneys. Research into stem cell therapy and tissue engineering approaches demonstrates the potential of such technologies to alter the disease course significantly. A combination of emerging therapies with current treatments can provide a more integrated approach, addressing both the acute disease signs and the chronic patient health. An integrative approach that combines traditional therapies with cutting-edge research can maximize outcomes and improve welfare in patients with tubulointerstitial diseases, ultimately advancing patient care and nephrology (Arnold et al., 2018).

4.6.1. Pharmacological Interventions

Treatment of tubulointerstitial disease often requires a multidimensional approach, including pharmacological therapy targeted at reducing inflammation and fibrosis. The most interesting strategy is possibly with the use of angiotensin receptor blockers (ARBs) and angiotensin-converting enzyme (ACE) inhibitors, which have been shown to possess antiproteinuric effects in various conditions of the kidneys. In particular, studies on Alport syndrome show that these agents, in addition to repressing proteinuria, also inhibit cytokine and collagen synthesis, thereby decreasing tubulointerstitial inflammation and fibrosis. The pathophysiology of action of this drug illustrates the potential of these agents as treatments for chronic diseases leading to end-stage renal disease, such as the progression of tubulointerstitial disease. However, long-term effectiveness and safety in children are areas that require further study, and the cautious nature of modern therapeutic strategies, as characterized in clinical trials (Gross et al., 2009), is evident here. In addition to RAAS blockers, immunosuppressive agents have recently become included in therapy for inflammatory tubulointerstitial nephropathies. Cyclosporine, for instance, is known to lower proteinuria in certain diseases but at the cost of nephrotoxic side effects that make it cumbersome to give, particularly in children. While short-term benefits may be evident, long-term dangers necessitate a judicious evaluation of each patient's case. What is also increasingly being realized is the role of newer therapeutic drugs in handling oxidative stress in chronic kidney disease. Notably, antioxidant therapy protocols, including vitamin D supplementation and pharmacological treatment of hyperuricemia, have been proposed as strategies for reducing oxidative damage and improving renal function (Osorio-Alonso et al., 2016). These therapies underscore the need for individualized pharmacologic treatment based on the distinct pathophysiological mechanisms in each of the tubulointerstitial diseases. Finally, ongoing studies of novel and combination therapies promise improved pharmacologic management of the tubulointerstitial diseases. Among the lines of hope are plant-derived antioxidants and other therapeutic interventions aimed at enhancing the antioxidant protection of the kidneys with minimal risk of conventional medication. There is also evidence to suggest that diabetic nephropathy will have a response to the use of non-insulin-dependent antidiabetic drugs, which can be used to improve metabolic control while simultaneously treating kidney disease. Such a multi-faceted approach not only aims to control current symptoms but also seeks to slow the progression of kidney disease longitudinally. With the pharmacological management scenario still evolving, it is increasingly essential to have an objective assessment of the safety and efficacy of these treatments, thereby emphasizing the importance of properly conducted clinical trials that yield unequivocal evidence for their use (Osorio-Alonso et al., 2016) (Figure 4.16).

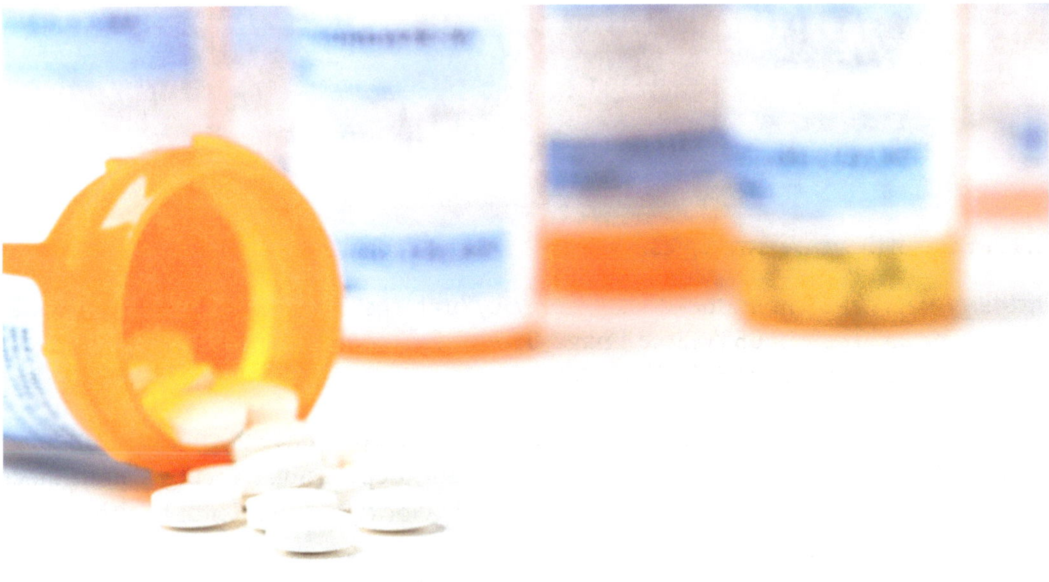

Figure 4.16. Pharmacological interventions of tubulointerstitial diseases.

Source: https://external-content.duckduckgo.com/iu/?u=https%3A%2F%2Fildeducation.ucsf.edu%2Fsites%2Fg%2Ffiles%2Ftkssra1111%2Ff%2Fwysiwyg%2Fmedications.jpg&f=1&nofb=1&ipt=9b84c2bedbbbf2b9f514ffa599563115d93180d487fa20aa956bcb294445485f.

4.6.2. Supportive Care Strategies

Treatment of tubulointerstitial diseases is a multifaceted process where measures of supportive care are the primary response to avoid further progression of disease and handle patient outcomes. Supportive care may range from optimizing fluid balance to correcting electrolyte imbalances because patients suffering from such diseases develop changes in renal dysfunction that lead to systemic complications. Constant monitoring of renal values and early interventions, such as fluid overload with diuretics or individualized dietary modification, is the solution. These not only stabilize the kidney function but also alleviate symptoms and enhance the quality of life in patients suffering from tubulointerstitial diseases. By addressing these supportive needs, clinicians can create a more comprehensive treatment plan that addresses both the short-term and long-term problems posed by these conditions. Pain control and psychosocial support are also fundamental components of supportive care for patients with tubulointerstitial diseases.

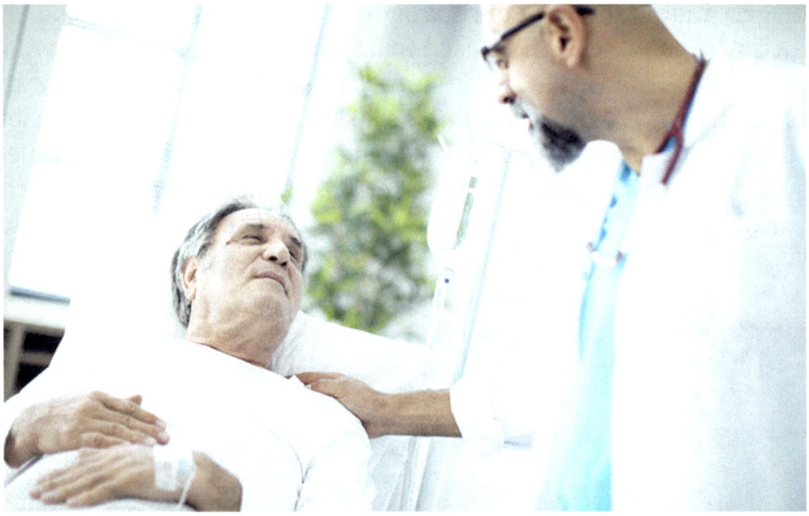

Figure 4.17. Supportive care strategies.

Source: https://external-content.duckduckgo.com/iu/?u=https%3A%2F%2Fmascc.org%2Fwp-content%2Fuploads%2F2022%2F05%2Fscc_image_01.jpg&f=1&nofb=1&ipt=990ca5a7d18be5d90ae3fcab535f0956fb000c3606392e74892d5b1fe80fb763.

The chronic nature of these conditions often results in the presence of chronic pain and varying levels of psychological disturbance, including anxiety and depression. Having a multidisciplinary team, which includes pain management specialists, social workers, and mental health professionals, can be invaluable in addressing both the physical and psychological aspects of pressure. Additionally, educating patients about their condition and involving them in planning their own care can enhance compliance and satisfaction. With evidence-based support from current literature, an understanding of the interaction between a patient's physical and mental well-being can potentially result in enhanced recovery and a favorable prognosis for tubulointerstitial diseases. Advances in studies aid in improving supportive care interventions, particularly for the post-acute kidney injury scenario, wherein patients are at higher risk for chronic kidney disease progression. Recent studies have illuminated the complex interaction between cellular integrity in tubules and interstitial spaces, which is significant in bringing targeted supportive interventions. In the case of fibrosis, as defined by Budd et al. (2017), understanding how tubular epithelial cells and interstitial mesenchymal cells function enables clinicians to intervene proactively in managing emergent complications of acute events. Likewise, understanding the effects of endotoxemia on renal function and the risk of renal fibrosis, as investigated in Brienza et al. (2014), means that interruption of the culpable inflammatory processes may be an essential aspect of supportive treatment. Under such circumstances, certain maneuvers that act to reverse such pathologic processes can dramatically enhance patients' long-term survival (Figure 4.17).

4.6.3. Importance of Early Detection and Intervention

Early treatment and diagnosis of tubulointerstitial disease are essential in avoiding long-term consequences, including chronic kidney disease (CKD). Since the kidneys play a crucial role in handling critical functions, the condition of the tubulointerstitial compartment is essential to the overall health of the kidneys. Late diagnosis of the diseases could lead to irreparable damage, necessitating more aggressive and less effective treatment measures in the future. The identification of risk factors through wise clinical assessments and owner-provided data, such as that identified in geriatric cat studies, highlights the need for routine monitoring. For instance, dental disease and vaccination are highly predictive indicators of azotemic CKD development, which suggests that an early health management plan could enable better early detection and management (Abraham et al., 2016). Early therapy drastically alters the disease's course, thereby rendering intense follow-up a priority for high-risk groups. In addition, the relationship between early diagnosis and improved patient outcomes cannot be stressed enough, particularly in the context of tubulointerstitial diseases. It appears from evidence that renal AA-amyloidosis can develop insidiously, as exemplified by symptomatic presentation in the presence of nephrotic-range proteinuria up to two years before the demonstration of a decline in glomerular filtration rate (GFR) (Amann et al., 2012). That period is significant; early diagnosis and treatment can lead to reduced morbidity with these conditions. Healthcare providers must provide a top priority to screening in high-risk populations, such as lifestyle issues, such as intravenous drug use, because early intervention can change the course of illness. Therefore, implementing standard screening procedures and educating patients about the early signs can enable intervention at an early stage, ultimately preserving kidney function and improving quality of life in patients affected by tubulointerstitial diseases. Apart from the tangible clinical benefits, early diagnosis also serves to maximize healthcare resource utilization by mitigating the burden on healthcare systems. In the case of earlier diagnosis and treatment of tubulointerstitial diseases, there is a significantly reduced need for greater use of more resource-hungry care and hospital stays, which are also costly. With the transition towards value-based care within the healthcare landscape, earlier intervention is increasingly associated with more comprehensive public health efforts. Besides this, as the pathological mechanisms of the pathogenetic process of tubulointerstitial kidney diseases are increasingly deciphered by research, clinicians will be able to individualize preventive action more effectively, thereby accentuating the value of multidisciplinary collaboration in early diagnosis. With comprehensive intervention involving regular assessment, patient education, and targeted intervention tactics, healthcare systems can maximize patients' overall outcomes without escalating costs associated with managing complex diseases (Amann et al., 2012; Abraham et al., 2016) (Figure 4.18).

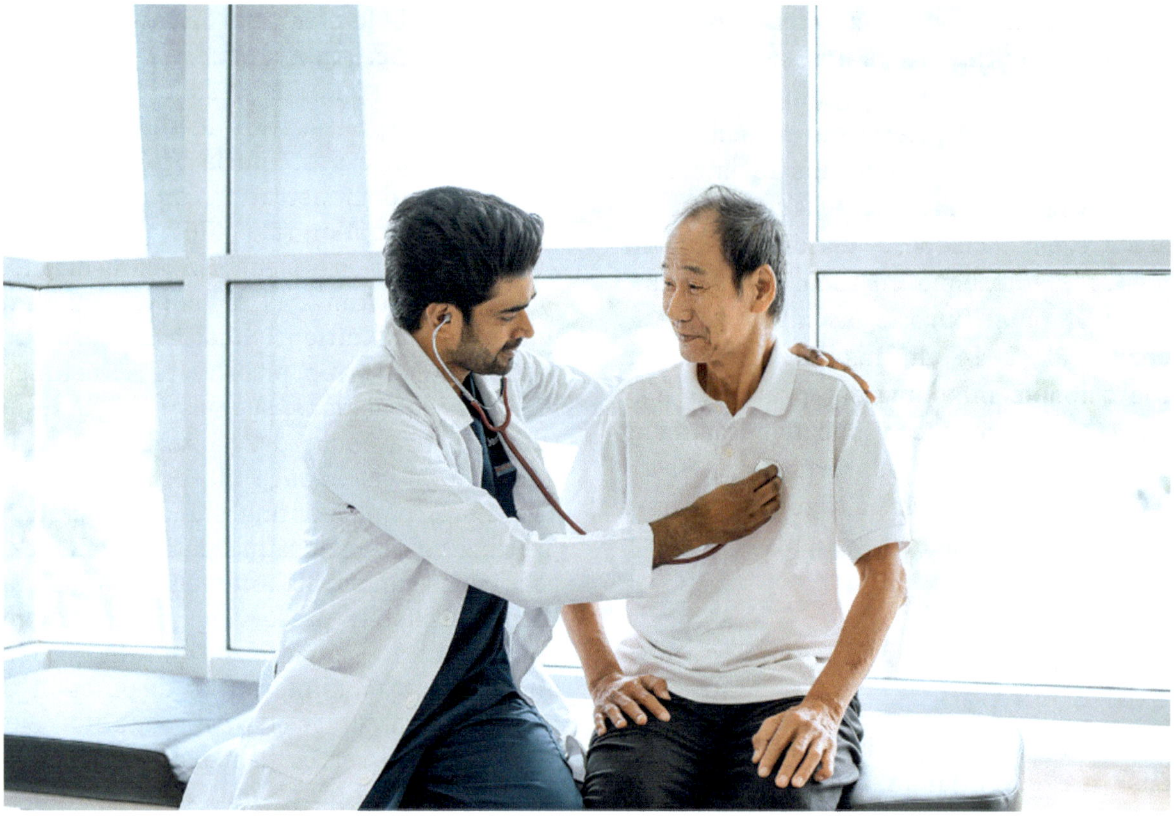

Figure 4.18. Early detection and intervention.

Source: https://external-content.duckduckgo.com/iu/?u=https%3A%2F%2Fwww.chenmed.com%2Fsites%2Fdefault%2Ffiles%2F2024-01%2FThe%2520Role%2520of%2520Primary%2520Care%2520in%2520Early%2520Detection%2520and%2520Intervention%2520for%2520Seniors.jpg&f=1&nofb=1&ipt=ae165e900addf859e359fef950e20fc6cfbb2b5faba325b1c54213d47f63029f.

SUMMARY

In studying tubulointerstitial disease, it is essential to acknowledge the multifactorial pathogenesis of these diseases, as they often overlap with glomerular disease and more diffuse kidney pathology. The complexity of renal interstitial injury thus highlights the precarious balance between heterogeneous pathological reactions, like inflammation and fibrosis. Research has developed to highlight the communication within the renal microenvironment, detailing how tubular and interstitial cells communicate in the context of injury and repair. The compounding nature of these diseases necessitates multidimensional evaluation and management. Clarification of the underlying molecular events, with a focus on those disclosed in such experiments as the identification of glomerulus-enriched genes, is crucial to determine effective targeted treatments that can potentially significantly improve patient prognosis (Anders et al., 2010). The inflammatory components, which play pivotal roles in the pathogenesis of tubulointerstitial diseases, must not be overlooked. As leukocytes infiltrate kidney tissue, immune cell accumulation is associated with the production of chemokines that induce renal damage. Stimulation of these inflammatory mechanisms by selective chemokine receptor antagonists has been a productive treatment approach. In a significant breakthrough, it has been shown that blockade of receptors such as CCR1 can effectively inhibit leukocyte recruitment and reduce kidney injury even in advanced disease. These discoveries suggest the potential for novel therapies that not only alleviate the symptoms of renal failure but also actively disrupt the processes that lead to disease progression (Anders et al., 2005). In summary, tubulointerstitial diseases are multifactorial and require consideration of both pathophysiologic and therapeutic factors. There should be future research directed to elucidate the multifactorial nature of these diseases, along with the discovery of novel biomarkers for early diagnosis. Furthermore, the integration of new therapies targeting inflammatory pathways holds promise for a brighter future in terms of more efficient control mechanisms. Through the expansion of knowledge regarding interstitial kidney disease and the formulation of new therapeutic regimens, healthcare providers can enhance patient care and outcomes in this severely impacted group of patients with chronic kidney diseases. Enhancing treatment techniques will likely be a function of cross-talk between basic research and clinical practice, providing opportunities for continued advances within this critical subdomain of nephrology.

Pathophysiologic mechanisms behind tubulointerstitial diseases require a critical comprehension, as well as their associated renal tissue pathological alterations. Tubulointerstitial diseases focus on the renal tubules and interstitial compartments of the kidneys, resulting in extreme changes in the function and structure of the kidneys. Cellular senescence is a critical component of diseases that involve end-stage cell cycle arrest and contribute to the scarring and degeneration of renal tissue. The senescence-associated secretory phenotype (SASP) is also significant due to the secretion of pro-inflammatory cytokines and other molecules that have the potential to exacerbate kidney damage and promote the development of renal dysfunction. This diminished cellular function highlights the importance of exploring therapeutic approaches to inhibit cellular senescence and SASP, thereby reversing the detrimental effects of tubulointerstitial diseases on long-term kidney health (Alpini et al., 2020). Beyond cellular senescence, manifestations of renal transplant rejection are another significant issue in the context of tubulointerstitial diseases. episodes. Rejection episodes can dramatically compromise allograft function and survival, and risk not only jeopardizing the transplanted kidney but also the general condition of the patient. Early treatment and diagnosis are essential in addressing rejection, but are not practically feasible utilizing traditional allograft biopsies for continuous monitoring. This limitation has prompted researchers to investigate proteomics as a potential means of non-invasive diagnosis. Through the analysis of urine and blood, proteomic techniques aim to identify unique biomarkers of acute and chronic rejection, revealing a considerable body of work in this field (Gwinner et al., 2016). The utilization and application of these diagnostic technologies can enhance patient prognosis and direct therapy in the management of tubulointerstitial disease. Last but not least, the integration of findings in different studies on tubulointerstitial disease provides a wide range of the multifaceted nature of the disease. The relationship between cell activity, immunological responses, and renal function is a reflection of the complexity in diagnosing and treating renal pathology effectively. Considering key points relevant to tubulointerstitial disease necessitates an interdisciplinary approach that incorporates basic research as well as clinical application. Future research should aim to refine non-invasive diagnostic methods, and new therapeutic agents should focus on refining these methods while critically examining the flaws and limitations of current approaches. The ultimate goal in the long run is to maximize patient treatment and tailor-directed therapies according to the specific needs of patients with tubulointerstitial disease, in order to preserve the kidney as well as overall health.

CLOSER LOOK

DIABETIC NEPHROPATHY (DN)

DN or diabetic kidney disease is the most serious microvascular complication of type 2 diabetes mellitus and type 1 diabetes mellitus. It is an insidious nephropathy that occurs due to chronic hyperglycemia and leads to structural as well as functional changes of the kidneys, eventually leading to chronic kidney disease (CKD) and, in advanced stages, to end-stage renal disease (ESRD). DN is defined by a progressive rise in urinary excretion of albumin (first microalbuminuria and then macroalbuminuria), decreasing glomerular filtration rate (GFR), increased blood pressure, and histologic alterations such as thickening of the glomerular basement membrane, expansion of the mesangium, nodular glomerulosclerosis (Kimmelstiel-Wilson nodules), and fibrosis of the tubulointerstitium. It is the major etiology of renal failure worldwide and also carries a high risk for cardiovascular disease, and so is a priority target in the management of diabetic patients.

The pathogenesis of diabetic nephropathy involves a complex interaction between metabolic and hemodynamic mechanisms. Hyperglycemia continuously activates several destructive mechanisms, including the polyol pathway, advanced glycation end-product (AGE) formation, and increased oxidative stress, all of which cause glomerular damage. Activation of protein kinase C and the renin-angiotensin-aldosterone system (RAAS) by hyperglycemia also increases inflammation, fibrosis, and vasoconstriction, further diminishing kidney function. Hemodynamically, hyperfiltration and early glomerular hypertension cause mechanical stress on the glomerular capillaries, which accelerates the progression of nephropathy. Apart from genetic susceptibility, other risk factors are hypertension, dyslipidemia, and smoking that impact the progression and development of DN.

Clinically, diabetic nephropathy is usually asymptomatic in its initial stage. The earliest detectable sign is microalbuminuria, i.e., the excretion of 30–300 mg of albumin per day in the urine. It may progress untreated to macroalbuminuria (greater than 300 mg/day), decreased GFR, and ultimately ESRD requiring dialysis or renal transplant. Albuminuria screening and estimation of GFR must be routinely performed in every patient with diabetes to detect DN early and initiate proper treatment promptly. The diagnosis is frequently clinical, based on the grounds of diabetes, chronic albuminuria, and deteriorating renal function. A renal biopsy is usually not needed unless there are unusual features suggesting a possible alternative diagnosis.

Management of diabetic nephropathy focuses on achieving strict glycemic control, controlling blood pressure, and inhibiting the RAAS. Strict control of blood sugar by insulin or oral hypoglycemic agents can slow the development and progression of DN. Angiotensin-converting enzyme inhibitors (ACEIs) or angiotensin receptor blockers (ARBs) are considered first-line treatments because they lower intraglomerular pressure and reduce albuminuria. Dietary sodium restriction, weight loss, and smoking cessation are necessary lifestyle modifications. More novel drugs, such as SGLT2 inhibitors and GLP-1 receptor agonists, hold promise in preventing kidney disease progression and reducing cardiovascular risk in individuals with diabetes. Management of lipids with statins should also be employed to reduce cardiovascular morbidity. Regular monitoring of renal function and albuminuria is essential for assessing the impact of treatment and determining disease progression.

References

1. Vielhauer, V., Eis, V., Schlöndorff, D., & Anders, H. (2004). Identifying Chemokines as Therapeutic Targets in Renal Disease: Lessons from Antagonist Studies and Knockout Mice. *Kidney & Blood Pressure Research*, *27*(4), 226–238. https://doi.org/10.1159/000079867Abraham, L. A., Adams, V. J., Bang, K. M., Bartlett, P. C., Boor, P., Brown, C. A., Chambrone, L., et al. (2016). Risk factors for development of chronic kidney disease in cats. https://core.ac.uk/download/36779272.pdf (accessed on 25th June 2025).
2. Aga Khan University Hospital, Karachi. (2015). *LABRAD*, *41*(2). https://core.ac.uk/download/47263391.pdf (accessed on 25th June 2025).
3. Aguilar Sierra, M., & Lonngi, M. (2017). Tubulointerstitial nephritis and uveitis syndrome: Case report and review of the literature. https://core.ac.uk/download/86436302.pdf (accessed on 25th June 2025).
4. Alexopoulos, E., Hartley, B. R., Seron, D., Cameron, S., et al. (1990). Lupus nephritis: Correlation of interstitial cells with glomerular function. https://core.ac.uk/download/pdf/82072233.pdf (accessed on 25th June 2025).
5. Alpini, G., Chen, R., Francis, H., Glaser, S., et al. (2020). The emerging role of cellular senescence in renal diseases. https://core.ac.uk/download/299809015.pdf (accessed on 25th June 2025).
6. Amann, K. U., Betz, C., Bickel, M., Büttner, M., et al. (2012). Renal AA-amyloidosis in intravenous drug users – A role for HIV-infection? https://core.ac.uk/download/14527288.pdf (accessed on 25th June 2025).
7. Anders, H. J., & Ninichuk, V. (2005). Chemokine receptor CCR1: A new target for progressive kidney disease. https://core.ac.uk/download/16432945.pdf (accessed on 25th June 2025).
8. Anders, H. J., & Schlöndorff, D. (2000). Murine models of renal disease: Possibilities and problems in studies using mutant mice. https://core.ac.uk/download/16432493.pdf (accessed on 25th June 2025).
9. Anders, H. J., Cohen, C. D., Edenhofer, I., Eichinger, F., et al. (2010). Systematic analysis of a novel human renal glomerulus-enriched gene expression dataset. https://core.ac.uk/download/12175685.pdf (accessed on 25th June 2025).
10. Arnold, W., Johnson, R. J., Kuro-o, M., Lanaspa, M. A., et al. (2018). Novel treatment strategies for chronic kidney disease: Insights from the animal kingdom. https://core.ac.uk/download/150600152.pdf (accessed on 25th June 2025).
11. Arribas, I., Bosch, R. J., Bover, J., Esbrit, P., et al. (2010). A transgenic mouse model for studying the role of the parathyroid hormone-related protein system in renal injury. https://core.ac.uk/download/8472187.pdf (accessed on 25th June 2025).
12. Ayati, B. P., Holstein, S. A., & Walk, J. C. (2018). Modeling the effects of multiple myeloma on kidney function. http://arxiv.org/abs/1602.03214 (accessed on 25th June 2025).
13. Azevedo, A., Carvalho, F., Fernandes, V., Ferreira, M., et al. (2015). Nefrite túbulo-intersticial hipocomplementémica idiopática. https://core.ac.uk/download/71739069.pdf (accessed on 25th June 2025).

14. Babaheidarian, P., Hooman, N., Koochak, A., Mehrazma, M., et al. (2015). Clinicopathological findings in pediatric tubulointerstitial nephritis: Iranian experience. https://core.ac.uk/download/483636723.pdf (accessed on 25th June 2025).

15. Bahamonde, J., Ezquer, F., Ezquer, M., Giraud Billoud, M., et al. (2017). Tubulointerstitial injury and proximal tubule albumin transport in early diabetic nephropathy induced by type 1 diabetes mellitus. https://core.ac.uk/download/159301014.pdf (accessed on 25th June 2025).

16. Barbano, B., Cianci, R., Coppolino, G., Di Mario, F., et al. (2016). Pharmacological effects of RAAS blockade in ischemic nephropathy. https://core.ac.uk/download/74319200.pdf (accessed on 25th June 2025).

17. Bertolotto, M., Cantisani, V., & Kim, S. H. (2021). Ultrasound of the kidneys and adrenal gland. https://core.ac.uk/download/480000127.pdf (accessed on 25th June 2025).

18. Bonani, M., Seeger, H., & Segerer, S. (2017). The role of lymphatics in renal inflammation. https://core.ac.uk/download/85216959.pdf (accessed on 25th June 2025).

19. Brienza, N., Castellano, G., Crovace, A., Di Palma, A., et al. (2014). Endothelial dysfunction and renal fibrosis in endotoxemia-induced oliguric kidney injury: Possible role of LPS binding protein. https://core.ac.uk/download/pdf/54176063.pdf (accessed on 25th June 2025).

20. Budd, D. C., Formentini, I., Hartmann, G., Meier, D., et al. (2017). From acute injury to chronic disease: Pathophysiological hypothesis of an epithelial/mesenchymal crosstalk alteration in CKD. https://core.ac.uk/download/85220110.pdf (accessed on 25th June 2025).

21. Butler-Dawson, J., Diaz, H. F., Garcia, G., Hernando, L., et al. (2019). Climate change and the kidney. https://core.ac.uk/download/322973173.pdf (accessed on 25th June 2025).

22. Carvalho, D., Carvalho, F., Ferreira, A. C., Galvão, J., et al. (2011). Renal pathology in Portuguese HIV-infected patients. https://core.ac.uk/download/71736827.pdf (accessed on 25th June 2025).

23. Elliott, J., Jepson, R. E., Lawson, J. S., Syme, H. M., et al. (2015). Renal fibrosis in feline chronic kidney disease: Known mediators and mechanisms of injury. https://core.ac.uk/download/36777966.pdf (accessed on 25th June 2025).

24. Fernando, J., & Zhou, S. (2015). The role of zinc in renal pathological changes in diabetic status. https://core.ac.uk/download/130975189.pdf (accessed on 25th June 2025).

25. Fici, P. (2014). Circulating fibrocytes, their role in renal fibrosis and molecular pathways involved: Possible biomarkers of fibrogenesis in chronic kidney disease. https://core.ac.uk/download/76519594.pdf (accessed on 25th June 2025).

26. Foster, C. S., Freitas-Neto, C. A., & Wentworth, B. A. (2014). Management of pediatric uveitis. https://core.ac.uk/download/28950356.pdf (accessed on 25th June 2025).

27. Gross, O., & Kashtan, C. E. (2009). Treatment of Alport syndrome: Beyond animal models. https://core.ac.uk/download/pdf/82768863.pdf (accessed on 25th June 2025).

28. Gwinner, W., Husi, H., Marx, D., Metzger, J., et al. (2016). Proteomics for rejection diagnosis in renal transplant patients: Where are we now? https://core.ac.uk/download/46559952.pdf (accessed on 25th June 2025).

29. Hammock, B. D., Khan, M. A. H., Imig, J. D., Lee, C. R., et al. (2016). Novel omega-3 fatty acid epoxygenase metabolite reduces kidney fibrosis. https://core.ac.uk/download/323070320.pdf (accessed on 25th June 2025).

30. Haylor, J., & Shrestha, B. M. (2014). Biological pathways and potential targets for prevention and therapy of chronic allograft nephropathy. https://core.ac.uk/download/42138051.pdf (accessed on 25th June 2025).

31. Imai, E., Hirayasu, K., Naoki, M., Saito, C., Tsunoda, R., Usui, J., Yamagata, K., et al. (2017). Anemia is an essential complication of ANCA-associated renal vasculitis: A single center cohort study. https://core.ac.uk/download/145225260.pdf (accessed on 25th June 2025).

32. Osorio-Alonso, H., Pedraza-Chaverri, J., Scholze, A., Sánchez-Lozada, L. G., et al. (2016). New pathogenic concepts and therapeutic approaches to oxidative stress in chronic kidney disease. https://core.ac.uk/download/pdf/50717190.pdf (accessed on 25th June 2025).

33. Wöhrer, A., Oppl, B., Pieringer, H., Parzer, I., Zwerina, J., & Reis, P. (2014). IgG4-related disease: An orphan disease with many faces. https://core.ac.uk/download/pdf/81907024.pdf (accessed on 25th June 2025).

34. Yang, C. W. (2007). Leptospirosis renal disease: Understanding the initiation by Toll-like receptors. https://core.ac.uk/download/pdf/82165021.pdf (accessed on 25th June 2025).

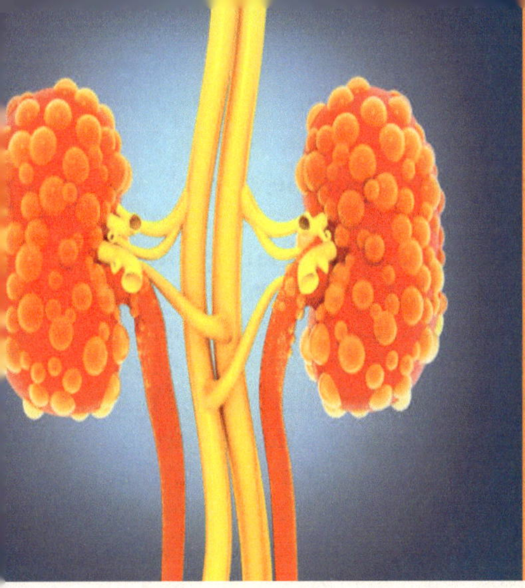

Chapter 5

POLYCYSTIC KIDNEY DISEASE AND CONGENITAL DISORDERS

Contents

Introduction

Polycystic kidney disease (PKD) manifests as a significant genetic disorder with a substantial effect on kidney function and general health, in the form of numerous fluid-filled cysts that impair kidney function. PKD can also be classified into two broad categories: Autosomal Dominant PKD (ADPKD) and Autosomal Recessive PKD (ARPKD), each of which has distinct genetic causes and clinical manifestations. PKD is not an isolated disease but one of a spectrum of congenital conditions, and in etiology, the expression of a complicated interaction between mutation and developmental abnormality. As the World Kidney Day campaign dictates, awareness and early detection of renal pathology in children are of primary importance, especially since congenital malformations are responsible for most kidney disease in children and evolve into long-term health conditions such as CKD (Schaefer et al., 2016). The intricacy of PKD thus serves as a stepping stone for the disclosure of genetic determinants of disease and the path of health from early life onwards. The pathogenesis of PKD and its association with other congenital conditions illustrate a fundamental aspect of the science of medicine, particularly genetics and developmental biology. Ciliopathies, for example, have risen to the center stage of research due to their role in kidney disease, revealing how genetic defects in ciliary proteins lead to heterogeneous phenotypes like PKD. Recent research indicates that alterations in ciliary function are linked not just with renal pathology but also with other systemic symptoms, such as retinal degeneration and skeletal dysplasias (Gherman et al., 2011). The multi-modal significance of these observations calls for an entire paradigm to study PKD as genotypic distinction may lead to diverse clinical expressions. In addition, this study expands the conversation regarding signal transduction mechanisms by which dysfunctional cilia suppress critical pathways, further perpetuating PKD and related disorders. Lastly, the implications of PKD extend beyond clear renal impact to influence more general categories of patient well-being and quality of life. Because of its genetic basis, this disease presents unique challenges within the realm of genetic counseling and patient care. The need for early diagnosis, as emphasized during efforts such as World Kidney Day, underscores the importance of integrating awareness programs into medical practice to maximize outcomes for those affected. Furthermore, awareness regarding causes at a genetic level provides hope for targeted interventions and therapies that may suppress or relieve the disease process. As investigators delve further into the genetic basis of PKD and associated congenital disorders, there is hope that advances in personalized medicine will translate into effective solutions that improve the quality of life for everyone affected by these complex genetic diseases.

Definition of Polycystic Kidney Disease (PKD)

PKD is a group of inherited disorders characterized by the formation of numerous cysts in the kidneys, which can lead to a gradual loss of kidney function and other manifestations of the disease. Autosomal dominant polycystic kidney disease (ADPKD) and autosomal recessive polycystic kidney disease (ARPKD) are the most common forms of PKD. ADPKD has a relatively later age of onset and a more insidious course of renal failure. In contrast, ARPKD usually becomes evident in infancy, typically with associated severe liver and biliary tree disease. This correlates with the highly variable clinical presentation and outcome of PKD and necessitates careful patient management plans that take into account both renal and extrarenal features. The underlying genetic mechanisms of PKD result from mutations in specific genes that play a role in the proper functioning of cilia and renal epithelial cells. In ADPKD, mutations in PKD1 or PKD2 genes affect the typical architecture and function of renal tubules, leading to cyst development and aberrant cell proliferation. In contrast, ARPKD is, overall, associated with mutations in the PKHD1 gene, which encodes fibrocystin, a protein involved in regulating ciliary function. Primary ciliary pathology underlies the pathogenesis of both PKD disorders. It is a fundamental concept for the more general subject of the ciliopathies, which include a vast group of genetic diseases due to dysfunctional cilia. The treatment and diagnostic implications are profound, given the complex interaction of genes and their role in the etiology of PKD. The knowledge of ciliopathies enlarges the basis of diseases like PKD, illustrating the interrelatedness of the various organ systems, which can be impacted by cystic alterations. For instance, in ARPKD, disruption of cilia also leads to hepatic development defects, including in conjunction with biliary atresia, an inflammatory and obstructive condition of the bile ducts culminating in fibrosis. The overlap suggests a multidisciplinary diagnostic and treatment approach, particularly because effective monitoring and intervention can significantly improve the quality of life in affected individuals. With progressive research, the focus on functional classification of ciliopathies, rather than strict clinical criteria, may provide a more nuanced understanding of PKD, thereby optimizing therapeutic interventions to address both its specific renal and systemic components (Blair-Reid et al., 2010; Mitchison et al., 2016) (Figure 5.1).

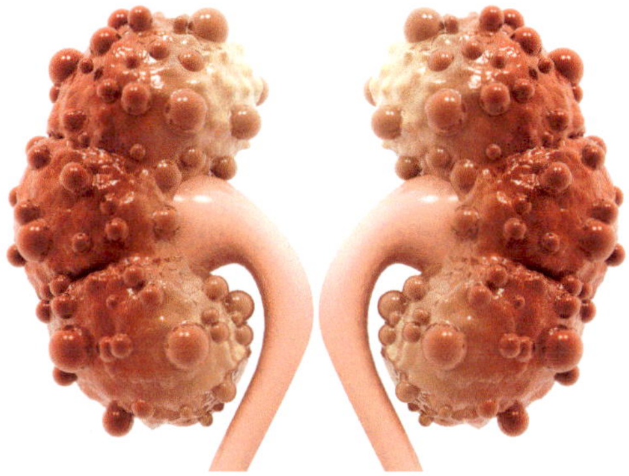

Figure 5.1. Polycystic kidney disease (PKD).

Source: https://external-content.duckduckgo.com/iu/?u=https%3A%2F%2Fassets-global.website-files.com%2F6318d21d08c6e801ac5b6254%2F636b0cd7dff0c353903c9c2b_pkd1920.webp&f=1&nofb=1&ipt=0d07e5fe56823bf03a8f53ece1642e4e31a6ab999ba29bcf708fb34f1a48a807.

Overview of Congenital Disorders

Congenital disorders represent a general group of abnormalities at birth, often due to genetic mutations, environmental factors, or both. The disorders can affect all systems in the body and have effects that will not present until adulthood. Of all the broad categories of genetic disorders, polycystic kidney disease (PKD) stands out due to its vast impact on kidney function and overall health. Autosomal dominant PKD, in particular, is a classic case of one genetic mutation potentially leading to far-reaching systemic effects, serving as an indication of the importance of early diagnosis and treatment regimens for congenital disorders. The diverse manifestations of congenital diseases underscore the importance of continued research, which elucidates their etiology and advances molecular genetic progress that could enable targeted therapies and novel treatments. Among the congenital disorders, the pathophysiology of polycystic kidney disease and other such diseases is highly interwoven with abnormalities in cell structures known as cilia. Cellular signaling and homeostasis are functions of primary cilia, and mutations in the genes associated with these organelles can lead to a range of ciliopathies, such as PKD. For instance, mutations in the PKHD1 gene have been associated with autosomal recessive polycystic kidney disease, which is also linked to biliary atresia. The association is indicative of a common pathway where tubulomorphogenesis and epithelial cell growth dysregulation take place due to the malfunctioning of cilia. With the use of high-resolution imaging techniques, our understanding of cilia's roles in normal development and disease has been greatly increased, as evidenced by ultrastructural analyses that study ciliary function across various patient groups (BA A et al., 2017). Congenital conditions' impacts are not only experienced at the individual level but are also hugely challenging for healthcare systems and communities. For any inherited condition, like PKD, early diagnosis through prenatal screening and genetic counseling can fundamentally alter patient trajectories. Early treatment enables the implementation of management strategies that can prevent complications and improve quality of life. Furthermore, understanding of the intersecting pathways of different congenital diseases—such as the intersection between PKD and biliary atresia via ciliary dysfunction—can lead to prolonged therapeutic maneuvers that address multiple conditions simultaneously. Continued research, particularly in the areas of genetic causation and cellular processes, will be necessary to develop new therapies and improve the quality of treatment for individuals with congenital disorders (Blair-Reid et al., 2010) (Figure 5.2).

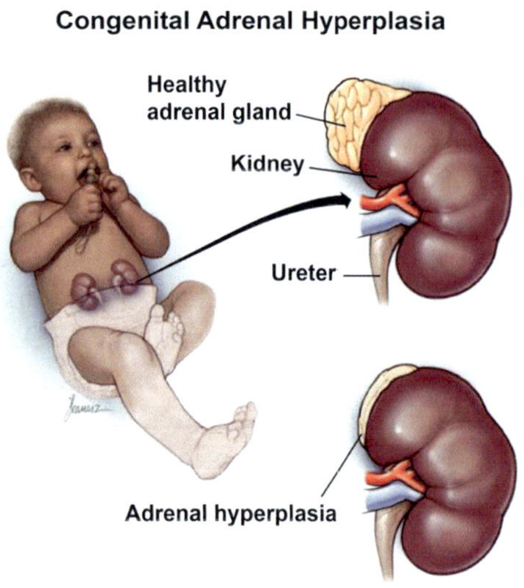

Figure 5.2. Overview of congenital disorders.

Source: https://my.clevelandclinic.org/-/scassets/images/org/health/articles/17817-congentital-adrenal-hyperplasia.

Importance of Studying the Relationship Between PKD and Congenital Disorders

The research of polycystic kidney disease (PKD) in conjunction with congenital conditions is essential for a variety of reasons, primarily for early intervention and diagnosis purposes. Congenital abnormalities, especially those that manifest while the fetus is developing, account for a high percentage of long-term health complications experienced by infants and toddlers. Taking into consideration how PKD may interact with these congenital abnormalities can lead to enhanced surveillance methods for high-risk patients. For example, research has been conducted to indicate that infants with specific congenital defects have a predisposition towards developing long-term health complications later in life, including the onset of chronic kidney disease (CKD) (Schaefer et al., 2016). The early detection of such a relationship can allow medical intervention at the right time, promoting patient outcomes and quality of life. Additionally, the association of PKD with congenital disease highlights the interplay between genetic and environmental factors in the pathogenesis of renal disease. Investigating these associations may provide insight into the heritability of kidney disease and its relationship with other congenital malformations, which is relevant to family planning and genetic counseling. These investigations are essential for healthcare practitioners with the mandate to treat patients throughout their life cycle, who may present different risks based on their family history and congenital diseases. As highlighted in ongoing research, understanding the interaction between chronic conditions, such as diabetes, and congenital diseases can help support improved healthcare outcomes through targeted interventions (Bolt et al., 2015). This cross-disciplinary approach fosters an integrative system that informs clinical care and public health policy. Furthermore, inquiry into the connection between PKD and congenital disease is very enlightening about long-term care of those who are affected. CKD caused by congenital disease presents challenges unique to the condition, and individualized management plans are needed to deal with both renal and overall health. With an understanding of the intricate relationships between PKD and congenital disease, clinicians can be better equipped to institute more effective screening strategies and treatment interventions tailored to the individual needs of each patient. Furthermore, early detection-based and multidisciplinary approaches can significantly affect the disease course pathway, possibly reducing the CKD burden on the population. The need to intervene in these converging domains of research is also underscored by the requirement to equip healthcare systems with the knowledge necessary to effectively care for patients with such complex health profiles (Schaefer et al., 2016).

5.1. Types of Polycystic Kidney Disease

Polycystic kidney disease (PKD) is a hereditary disease in which numerous cysts form on the kidneys, which gradually impair their function. Autosomal dominant polycystic kidney disease (ADPKD) and autosomal recessive polycystic kidney disease (ARPKD) are the two most prominent types of PKD. ADPKD is more common and typically occurs during adulthood and may not be symptomatic until individuals are in their 30s or 40s. This type is caused by mutations in either the PKD1 or PKD2 genes, leading to cysts and renal enlargement. Hypertension is frequently present in patients, and they eventually develop chronic kidney disease (CKD). Awareness of these two distinct genetic causes is crucial for clinicians because it determines the treatment and prognosis of the individuals involved, mainly because renal failure can cause significant morbidity and may need renal replacement therapies. On the other hand, the presentation of ARPKD is somewhat different, in that the disorder is an advanced renal disease that typically presents in infancy and early childhood. Characterized by large, echogenic kidneys, ARPKD often presents prenatally via ultrasound when oligohydramnios is present.

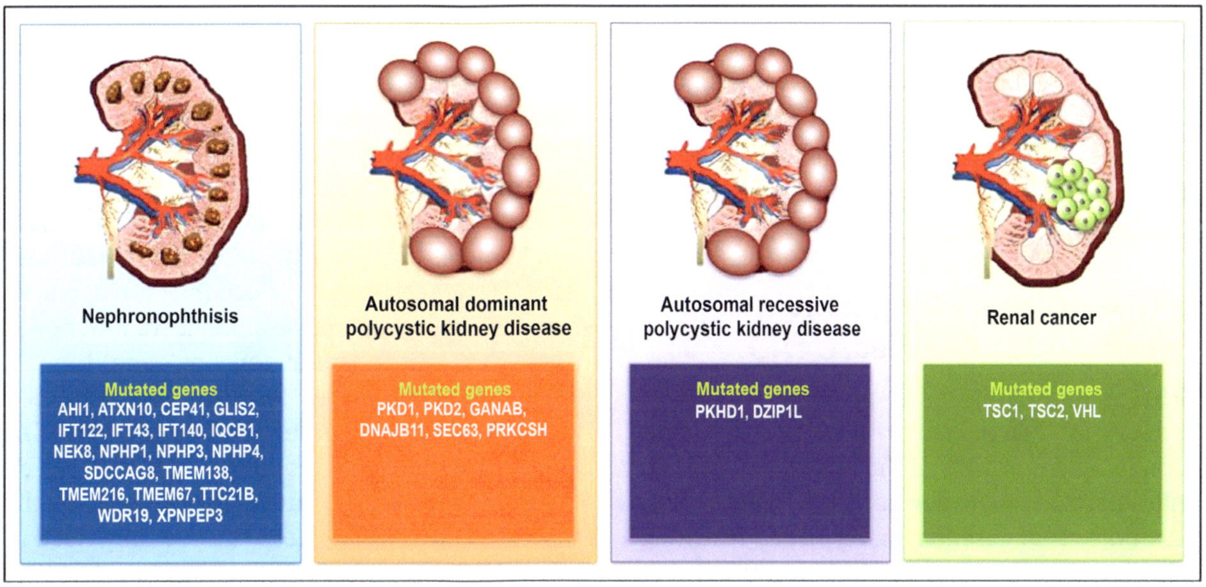

Figure 5.3. Types of polycystic kidney disease.

Source: https://external-content.duckduckgo.com/iu/?u=https%3A%2F%2Fpub.mdpi-res.com%2Fdiagnostics%2Fdiagnostics-10-01099%2Farticle_deploy%2Fhtml%2Fimages%2Fdiagnostics-10-01099-ag.png%3F1608217534&f=1&nofb=1&ipt=f01be0daef1a93dbe6ef651cd855a412799c35ed31783f939d60064caf988511.

The clinical presentation extends beyond renal abnormality, as the disease also creates severe hepatic disease, such as congenital hepatic fibrosis. This condition requires multidisciplinary treatment of the patient by collaboration with specialists such as pediatric nephrologists and hepatologists in order to manage adequately. ARPKD has a tremendous impact on quality of life and requires active monitoring of kidney and liver function, thereby making early identification and intervention strategies a necessity for affected families, according to Guay-Woodford et al. (2014). While each individual presentation of PKD comes with its own unique challenges, they are all part of the larger category of renal diseases characterized by cyst formation. What is significant is that treatment of PKD entails a consolidated approach that not only addresses renal well-being but also possible systemic expressions. For example, children with ARPKD might need to address additional complications, including neurocognitive dysfunction, as shown by current studies. Therefore, management strategies often employ a multidisciplinary approach involving a broad range of healthcare providers to provide comprehensive support that extends beyond the renal aspect of the disease. The identification of genetic susceptibilities and multisystem involvement encapsulates the essence of PKD within the larger category of congenital disease, as emphasized by Schaefer et al. (2016) (Figure 5.3).

5.1.1. Autosomal Dominant Polycystic Kidney Disease (ADPKD)

ADPKD is one of the most prevalent inherited disorders of renal function with significant morbidity and mortality in those affected. ADPKD is characterized by the development of numerous cysts in the renal parenchyma, typically resulting in chronic deterioration of renal function over many years. ADPKD is primarily caused by mutations in two essential genes, PKD1 and PKD2, which encode proteins involved in renal tubular cell function. Interestingly, although ADPKD often presents in adulthood, the disease might show aspects of premature onset in some cases, emphasizing the complex genetic control over its presentation and inheritance characteristics. Clarification of the genetic basis of ADPKD is vital for diagnosis and genetic counseling since the disease shows high expressivity and penetrance variability between members of a family, complicating patients' management. Recent advances in genetic studies have been driven by a deeper understanding of the heterogeneous phenotypes of ADPKD. Of particular interest is the increasing recognition of phenocopies, or clinically indistinguishable diseases from ADPKD, and the importance of differential diagnosis for cystic kidney disease. This heterogeneity requires an increased range of genetic tests, including next-generation sequencing techniques, to ensure optimal diagnostic accuracy. By enabling the concurrent assessment of multiple genes of potential significance, clinicians are more prone to interpret variants and avoid potential misdiagnoses correctly. In addition to identifying typical mutations, the use of these advanced techniques also enables the exploration of potential epigenetic and environmental factors that may influence the disease course and clinical presentation, thereby informing patient-specific management regimens. The push toward accurate genetic delineation is essential for both treatment planning and empowering concerned families through informed reproductive choice mechanisms (Bergmann, 2014). Therapeutically, ADPKD has seen the introduction of tolvaptan, the first FDA-approved pharmacologic treatment with a specific indication for delaying renal function impairment from the disease. The treatment does have limitations, however, including modest efficacy and considerable side effects, which can adversely affect the patient's quality of life. Consequently, there is a pressing need for novel therapies that more effectively treat the underlying pathophysiology of ADPKD. Current studies are exploring a range of treatments, from mammalian target of rapamycin inhibitors to novel strategies targeting renal cyst metabolism and inflammation. The systemic effect of such interventions remains one of the biggest hurdles, as many of the molecular targets for ADPKD are critical in other organs too. This suggests the potential for developing targeted treatments that minimize extrarenal effects, thereby enhancing the management of ADPKD in a chronic context (Bourgeois et al., 2018) (Figure 5.4).

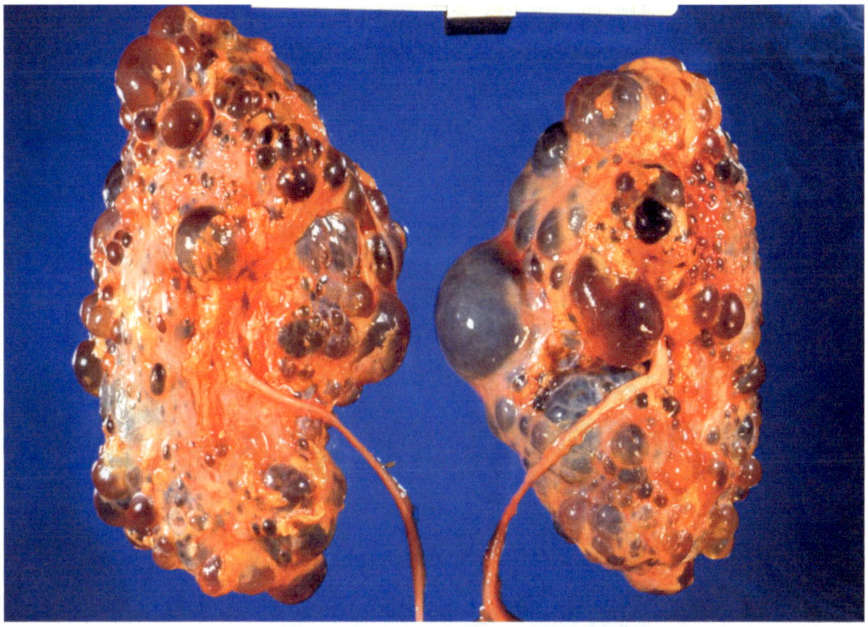

Figure 5.4. Autosomal dominant polycystic kidney disease (ADPKD).

Source: https://upload.wikimedia.org/wikipedia/commons/2/2c/Polycystic_kidneys%2C_gross_pathology_CDC_PHIL.png.

5.1.2. Autosomal Recessive Polycystic Kidney Disease (ARPKD)

Autosomal recessive polycystic kidney disease (ARPKD) is a genetic condition that primarily affects kidney development, resulting in the formation of numerous cysts within the kidneys. The condition has cystic dilatation of the collecting ducts, which leads to severe kidney damage and can cause hypertension and renal failure during infancy and childhood. The genetic cause of ARPKD is most commonly associated with mutations in the PKHD1 gene, which encodes fibrocystin, a protein implicated in the regulation of tubular cell function and the maintenance of renal architectural integrity. As ARPKD arises at an early age, early treatment and diagnosis are critical to control of symptoms and maximization of prognosis in affected individuals. The multifactorial nature of the disease is one of the reasons why studying its pathogenesis and cellular mechanisms is crucial for understanding its clinical presentation (Bergmann, 2014). Studies on the genetic cause of ARPKD provide an indication of the disease's complexity, particularly in differentiating it from other forms of polycystic kidney disease. ADPKD and ARPKD share identical phenotypic manifestations but differ significantly in their patterns of inheritance and clinical presentation. Recent evidence suggests that the recessive form may be associated with other ciliopathies, a group of conditions resulting from defective cilia function that are responsible for diverse renal pathologies. Identification of additional mutations and complex interactions between these diseases has made accurate genetic diagnosis a vital component of patient management and family counseling. Advances in next-generation sequencing technologies have been instrumental in this endeavor, enabling the more accurate identification of pathogenic variants that may be overlooked by conventional methods (Avner et al., 1996). The therapeutic care of ARPKD employs a multidisciplinary approach focused on alleviating symptoms and improving the quality of life for patients. The initial treatments may include controlling blood pressure, monitoring renal function, and providing supportive therapy tailored to the patient's needs. Notably, renal replacement treatments such as dialysis or transplantation may become necessary as the disease progresses, particularly because most children experience a significant decline in renal function during childhood. Additionally, ongoing research into newer therapeutic regimens holds promise for future treatment of ARPKD. Knowledge of the molecular and genetic basis of diseases, nevertheless, presents opportunities for targeted therapy that may potentially not only improve outcomes but also offer therapeutic directions for disease modification. This integrated approach highlights the compelling need for further research into the complexities of ARPKD as part of a broader understanding of polycystic kidney diseases and congenital disease (Bergmann, 2014) (Figure 5.5).

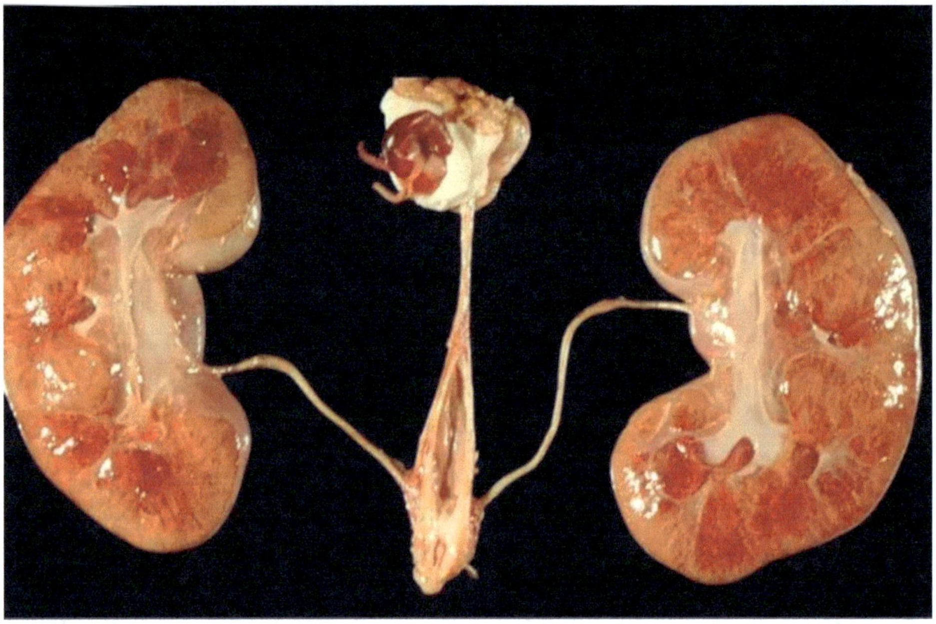

Figure 5.5. Autosomal recessive polycystic kidney disease (ARPKD).

Source: https://www.webpathology.com/_next/image?url=https%3A%2F%2Fd3cyex60hhnlth.cloudfront.net%2Ffit-in%2F650x650%2Ffilters%3Aformat(webp)%2Fcase%2Fdetail_images%2Fcystic-diseases-of-kidney_1731943040.jpg&w=1920&q=75.

5.1.3. Other Rare Forms of PKD

The pathogenesis of PKD encompasses other uncommon forms that differ from the well-defined autosomal dominant and recessive forms. Some of these are congenital conditions, such as dilatation of the bile duct (CDD) in utero, which, despite being predominantly hepatobiliary, often presents concomitantly with renal malformations. The condition of CDD is characterized by stasis of bile, which, depending on the extent and complications, can result in severe implications. Genetic studies indicate that de novo variants implicate multi-gene interactions. Mutations that have been found are connected with epithelial and connective tissue disorders, suggesting a widespread genomic contribution to congenital malformations, like those in PKD scenarios. This heterogeneity at the genetic level implies that patients can carry several mutations responsible for different manifestations of the disease, further indicating that PKD is not just a solitary defect but rather part of a complex fabric of genetics, similar to what was identified among a subset of rare genetic presentations involving biliary and kidney anatomy (Campbell et al., 2016). Further investigation into the genetic etiology of PKD reveals ciliopathy associations, a recently emerging class of diseases that disrupt ciliary function. They demonstrate inherent resemblance to PKD, particularly in the presence of cyst formation within the kidneys. Defective ciliary signaling affects cellular processes such as developmental patterning and homeostasis, thereby establishing a pathophysiologic commonality with PKD. Recent focus on ciliopathies has identified numerous genes associated with these disorders, which often exhibit variable phenotypes depending on the nature of the mutations. As PKD is increasingly recognized as belonging to this broad spectrum, there is a need to explain how genes involved in ciliopathies influence kidney development and cystogenesis. This kind of knowledge not only enhances diagnostic criteria but also informs potential therapeutic approaches, suggesting the need for interdisciplinarity within genetic studies in both domains (Gleeson et al., 2011). In addition to this, diagnosis and therapy for such uncommon types of PKD demand a multiprofessional approach because the intersection of genetics and the environment can make clinical situations more complex. For instance, features in both PKD and CDD patients may overlap such that distinguishing diagnostic features requires extensive assessment. Clarifying the shared pathways and genetic interactions may not only improve the detection of rare variants but also enable the development of targeted therapies that address the fundamental processes. With the progress of research, the integration of genetic testing together with comprehensive phenotypic assessments is key to unraveling the complexities of such diseases. This comprehensive approach sets the path for precision medicine, through which tailored treatment regimens can be developed, ultimately enhancing patient care and outcomes for individuals affected by uncommon forms of PKD and other inherited diseases (Gleeson et al., 2011; Campbell et al., 2016).

5.2. Genetic Basis of Polycystic Kidney Disease

The genetic etiology of polycystic kidney disease (PKD) reveals a complex interplay between environmental and genetic susceptibility. Primarily, PKD is classified into two predominant types: Autosomal Dominant PKD (ADPKD) and Autosomal Recessive PKD (ARPKD), both associated with mutations in unique genes. In ADPKD, mutations in the PKD1 or PKD2 genes are responsible for the formation of cysts, with the PKD1 gene mutation being responsible for most cases. Conversely, ARPKD is primarily caused by mutations in the PKHD1 gene, which are central to the proper development of the kidneys. Furthermore, studies suggest that PKD may not be solely governed by genes; environmental factors, as evidenced by inbred mouse lines with varying susceptibility to drug-induced PKD, illustrate the multi-factorial composition of the disease (Blecher et al., 1990). Understanding this genetic framework is crucial for identifying individuals at risk and developing targeted therapeutic interventions. Murine models have significantly contributed to elucidating the genetic basis of PKD, reflecting both the conditions phenotypic variability and its underlying mechanisms. Several models, including the Han:SPRD-CY rats, replicate the histopathological characteristics of human PKD, particularly in ARPKD. The identification of the wpk mutation in these rats is an excellent model for disease study. This mutant presents with nephromegaly, hypertension, and early cystic formation, all of which are nearly identical to those in humans but without the biliary tract disturbances of ARPKD. Although the mapped genetic loci on the rat chromosome show variations from human genes, the renal features common to both highlight the significance of such models in disease pathology and pharmacological research (Dokkum et al., 2000). Murine studies thus not only enhance our knowledge of genetics but also yield promising lines of future therapeutic study. The utility of genetic research also extends to enhancing screening and management strategies for PKD. Since early diagnosis has a significant impact on patient management and outcomes, identifying the specific genetic variants involved in PKD enables targeted genetic screening. Those with a familial history of PKD may be assisted by genetic counseling, which helps estimate risk in offspring. Understanding the polygenic involvement in PKD, as revealed by various studies, can help health practitioners monitor and manage their patients effectively. Furthermore, the revelations of genetic research pave the way to gene-targeted therapies that could potentially change disease progression. Advances toward gene therapy and CRISPR technology have hopeful potential for treating PKD at its roots, setting the stage for a new paradigm in the treatment of congenital diseases like PKD. Interpreting this genetic information into clinical care has significant potential for improving patient outcomes and individualized treatment (Figure 5.6).

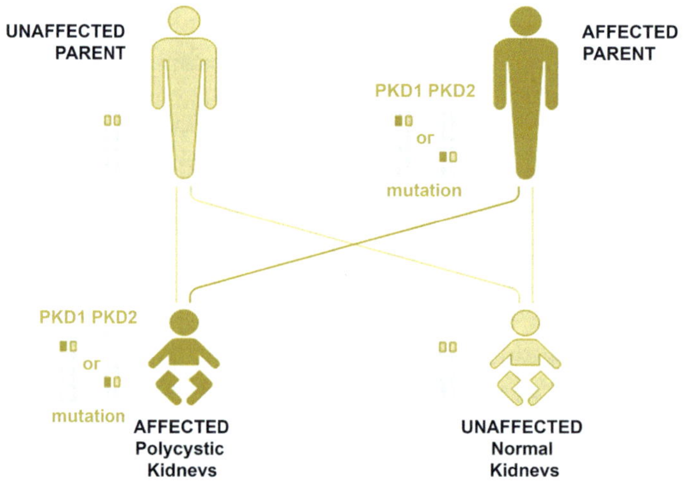

Figure 5.6. Genetic basis of polycystic kidney disease.

Source: https://pkdinternational.org/images/pages/adpkd-inheritance-diagram.svg.

5.2.1. Inheritance Patterns of PKD

Understanding the pattern of inheritance of Polycystic Kidney Disease (PKD) is critical in genetic counseling and family management of the patient. PKD is predominantly in two forms: Autosomal Dominant PKD (ADPKD) and Autosomal Recessive PKD (ARPKD). ADPKD is responsible for approximately 90% of cases and is typically associated with variable penetrance, meaning that not all individuals carrying the mutation will be affected. This form is caused by mutations in either the PKD1 or PKD2 genes, of which the former is associated with more severe manifestations of the disease. ARPKD, however, usually presents in childhood and is caused by mutations of the PKHD1 gene. The differentiation between the two forms is not only theoretical; knowledge of the modes of inheritance allows the clinician to organize a surveillance strategy for affected families and generations of carriers accordingly. Besides, atypical patterns of inheritance complicate the clinical presentation of PKD. Even though ADPKD and ARPKD are the predominant forms, genetic studies indicate that mutations leading to cystic kidney diseases may also a contribution in a system of intricate interactions. For instance, PKD1 and PKD2 may have dosage-sensitive effects leading to variability in clinical manifestations. Additionally, several other disorders, known as phenocopies, present similarly to PKD but result from mutations in different genes. Some ciliopathies, like nephronophthisis and Bardet–Biedl syndrome, can have the presentation of cyst formation, hence complicating clear-cut diagnoses without thorough genetic testing. Therefore, proper genetic diagnosis takes center stage in determining the nature of the condition, as well as providing treatment to patients and their families accordingly (Bergmann, 2014). New genetic techniques, particularly next-generation sequencing, have revolutionized the approach to diagnosing PKD and related diseases. Such technology enables the simultaneous examination of many genes, a factor that significantly enhances the detection rates of disease-causing variants among individuals with cystic kidney disease presentations. Several reports, for example, have demonstrated that comprehensive genetic analysis can resolve challenging cases, as in instances where unusual inheritance is suspected. In one classic case, a child presented with the rare association of Caroli disease, cystic dysplasia, and situs inversus, ultimately caused by a homozygous NPHP3 gene mutation, presenting an atypical presentation of a ciliopathy with autosomal recessive inheritance (Belli et al., 2018). Thus, understanding the vagaries of PKD inheritance patterns is not only crucial for accurate diagnosis but also dictates the treatment plan and risk assessment for affected families (Figure 5.7).

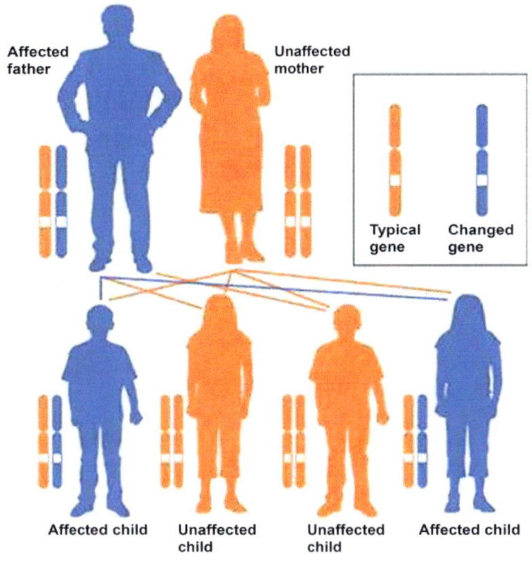

Figure 5.7. Inheritance patterns of PKD.

Source: https://www.mayoclinic.org/-/media/kcms/gbs/patient-consumer/images/2013/11/15/17/37/r7_autosomaldominantthu_jpg.jpg.

5.2.2. Role of PKD1 and PKD2 Genes

The PKD1 and PKD2 genes play central roles in the pathogenesis of autosomal dominant polycystic kidney disease (ADPKD), which is the most common inherited cause of kidney failure in both children and adults. Mutations of the PKD1 gene account for approximately 85% of ADPKD, while mutations of PKD2 result in an attenuated phenotype that typically develops later in life. The proteins encoded by these genes, polycystin-1 and polycystin-2, are essential for the formation and maintenance of renal tubules and for signaling pathways that regulate renal growth and function. Dysfunctions of these pathways lead to the development of renal cysts, a hallmark feature of PKD, which, with time, can impair kidney function. Thus, understanding the molecular mechanisms by which these genes contribute to disease pathology is crucial for the development of targeted treatments and improvements in patient outcomes (Bergmann, 2014). In contrast to the autosomal dominant form of the disease, autosomal recessive polycystic kidney disease (ARPKD) generally results from mutations in the PKHD1 gene, but PKD1 and PKD2 can also exhibit patterns of recessive inheritance in rare instances. The phenotypic variability of such mutations complicates the performance of diagnostic tests and underscores the importance of advanced genetic testing strategies. New technologies, such as next-generation sequencing (NGS), have revolutionized the identification of mutations in these genes, enabling more accurate diagnosis in patients with cystic kidney disease and associated symptoms. The consistency of NGS platforms has enabled the detection of numerous previously uncharacterized mutations, thereby broadening the genetic map of PKD. This advancement in genetic analysis underscores the importance of incorporating cutting-edge technology to inform clinical management and genetic counseling practices in affected individuals and families (Bergmann, 2014). The implications of PKD1 and PKD2 gene mutations extend not only to the health conditions of an individual but also to public health concerns and healthcare resources. Since PKD is a frequent cause of end-stage renal disease, the economic burden of treating the condition is significant. Early detection through genetic testing can enable better control of the disease and potentially delay its onset, potentially delaying the progression to end-stage renal insufficiency, thereby enhancing quality of life and reducing healthcare costs. Furthermore, identification of specific mutations in these genes enables high-risk families to make informed reproductive choices. As research continues to illuminate the complexities of PKD, including the interaction between these genes and other environmental factors and genes, the focus will likewise increasingly be on personalized medicine approaches that optimize therapeutic gain in patients with polycystic kidney disease (Minardi et al., 2017) (Figure 5.8).

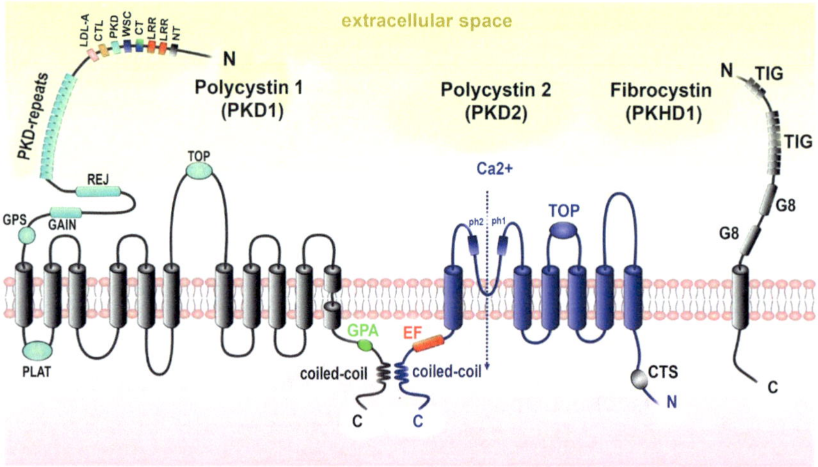

Figure 5.8. Role of PKD1 and PKD2 genes.

Source: https://www.frontiersin.org/files/Articles/693130/fphys-12-693130-HTML/image_m/fphys-12-693130-g002.jpg.

5.2.3. Genetic Mutations Associated with PKD

The molecular geography of PKD is a complex interplay of mutations that have a significant impact on the pathogenesis of the disease. Autosomal Dominant PKD (ADPKD) and Autosomal

Recessive PKD (ARPKD) are two dominant forms of PKD with characteristic genetic mutations. In ADPKD, the most common mutations occur in the PKD1 and PKD2 genes, which encode proteins whose standard structure and function are essential for normal kidney function and epithelial cell structure. These mutations disrupt cellular processes responsible for maintaining renal architecture, leading to cyst formation and progressive renal impairment. Identification of these mutations offers key insight into the molecular pathogenesis of PKD and lays the groundwork for future target therapy, establishing the value of continued genetic research within this field. Recent advances in genetic screening and whole-exome sequencing have also revealed a broad spectrum of genetic variations that cause PKD, including de novo mutations and variant alleles in multiple genes. A number of these genes have been linked to other developmental disorders, so understanding the broader implications of genetic mutations in PKD is essential. For instance, patients are found to be harboring mutations in several evolutionarily conserved genes both leading to cystic and extra-renal phenotypes, according to studies. This encounter suggests that the polygenic cause of the majority of PKD cases indicates the condition may arise from the accumulation of mutations, rather than a single gene mutation, as genetic heterogeneity for congenital dilatation of the bile duct, as reported in the literature, suggests (Campbell et al., 2016). Besides simple diagnosis, the clinical significance of these genetic mutations extends beyond providing a diagnosis, affecting patient treatment and family counseling. In ARPKD, mutations are early in life and lead to severe multisystem pathology, including congenital hepatic fibrosis and respiratory distress due to kidney enlargement. Early multidisciplinary management is thus indicated, with efforts needing to be coordinated among nephrologists, geneticists, and other specialists to address the broad spectrum of related medical issues that are encountered (Guay-Woodford et al., 2014). Families are also faced with significant decision-making regarding genetic testing and counseling for associated risks. Understanding of the complex genetic history of PKD thus not only enhances clinical practice but also supports critical debate on implications for individuals and their families, highlighting the close linkage between congenital disease and genetics.

5.3. Symptoms and Diagnosis of PKD

PKD also encompasses a diverse set of symptoms that can have a direct and severe impact on an individual's lifestyle. Flank or abdominal pain is among the classic signs of PKD because of the formation of cysts in the kidneys that press against surrounding tissues. Hypertension, hematuria, and recurrent urinary tract infections are other classic signs. Fatigue also occurs in patients, which can be disabling and detract from their overall health and well-being. It was found in a study that severe fatigue due to such individuals caused advanced complications of polycystic liver disease, adding to the clinical picture of the PKD patients (Gordon et al., 1990). Because symptoms are unpredictable and can mimic those of other conditions, they can hinder diagnosis and treatment, making awareness crucial in epidemiological situations. Diagnosis of PKD is based on a combination of clinical evaluation, family history, and imaging techniques. The approach initially involves ultrasound scanning, which identifies the presence of multiple cysts in the kidneys and confirms the advancement of the disease. For individuals with indeterminate imaging results or unusual presentations, newer imaging modalities, such as Magnetic Resonance Imaging (MRI) and Computed Tomography (CT) scans, may be utilized. Genetic testing has become increasingly important in diagnosing PKD, particularly for early-onset or atypical presentations. As PKD can present differently in various individuals, identifying associated genes, such as PKD1 and PKD2, is critical for achieving an accurate diagnosis and management (Bergmann, 2014). Not only does this genomic approach aid in diagnosis, but it also enhances genetic counseling for the relatives. Such a complexity of PKD presentations warrants a comprehensive approach to diagnosis as well as management. Clinicians must consider differential diagnoses because other cystic kidney disorders can present in the same way. Autosomal recessive polycystic kidney disease (ARPKD) and certain ciliopathies can mimic the symptoms of PKD; thus, proper diagnosis is crucial (Bergmann, 2014). Next-generation sequencing technology is now increasingly useful for differentiation between PKD and other diseases that resemble it, allowing researchers and clinicians to sequence several genes simultaneously. These advances in technology enable improved comprehension of the genetic component of cystic kidney diseases and therefore improved diagnostic precision as well as specific therapeutic measures. The synergy approach of imaging, genetic analysis, and careful patient history facilitates improved PKD management, which in turn translates into better patient outcomes and a higher quality of life (Figure 5.9).

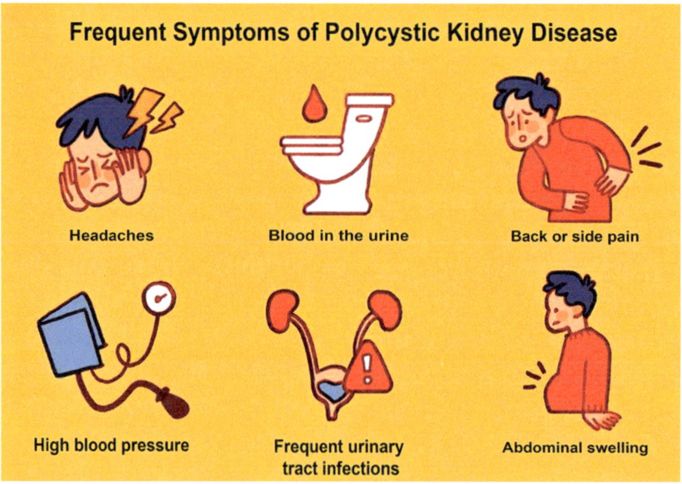

Figure 5.9. Symptoms and diagnosis of PKD.

Source: https://www.verywellhealth.com/thmb/TjiNPzq2-uyjQgJyG5sCwMCTkFo=/1500x0/filters:no_upscale():max_bytes(150000):strip_icc()/polycystic-kidney-disease-signs-symptoms-and-complications-5204728-Final-44f1e1e2faaf4c5a937146f13dc9d938.jpg.

5.3.1. Common Symptoms of PKD

PKD is characterized by the growth of multiple cysts in the kidneys and eventually severe complications. One of the most frequent among these symptoms is hypertension, found in nearly 60-70% of all patients suffering from the disease. High blood pressure in PKD patients is a result of the increased renal volume and changed renal hemodynamics caused by the expanding cysts. Moreover, flank pain or discomfort, most often resulting from the compressive action of enlarging cysts on neighboring structures, may appear as the disease progresses. Such discomfort may, in some cases, escalate to more severe abdominal pain, which indicates potential complications like cyst rupture or pyelonephritis. It is essential, thus, to have early recognition of such symptoms to initiate proper management protocols and improve the quality of life in patients. With the advancement of PKD, secondary symptoms may develop, significantly contributing to the patient's health. One of these symptoms is hematuria, or the presence of blood in the urine, resulting from the rupture of cysts or destruction of the renal vascular system. Such a symptom is frightening and an indicator of the presence of complications that need to be addressed immediately. Besides, patients also experience recurring urinary tract infections (UTIs) as urinary urgency, frequency, and pain. UTIs are typically related to the structural changes in the renal environment resulting from cyst formation. The interplay between the symptoms, particularly hypertension, and hematuria, points towards careful clinical monitoring and laboratory-guided management since the presentation may mimic renal impairment and deterioration of kidney disease. In addition, PKD may result in complications beyond the kidneys, affecting overall health and organ function. Extrarenal manifestations include liver cysts, which occur in a high percentage of patients, as well as pancreatic and splenic cysts, although these are usually not symptomatic. These cysts, however, may lead to hepatic complications such as pain and liver dysfunction. Others will also evolve cardiovascular complications, such as the risk of an aneurysm, which highlights the systemic nature of the disease. Psychiatric disturbances, such as depression and anxiety, can arise secondary to the chronic nature of symptoms and the distress of having a progressing disease. Including collaborative care that addresses both physical and psychological needs is also vital in enhancing the wellbeing of patients with PKD, as well as adopting holistic treatment approaches beyond nephrology (Gleeson et al., 2011; Bergmann, 2014).

5.3.2. Diagnostic Imaging Techniques

The employment of imaging diagnostic techniques plays a crucial role in the diagnosis and management of PKD and other congenital disorders. These imaging modalities, including ultrasound, computed tomography (CT), and magnetic resonance imaging (MRI), play a vital role in detecting kidney cysts, estimating their size and number, and assessing kidney function. Ultrasound, being the most commonly employed initial imaging modality of choice, is non-invasive, devoid of ionizing radiation, and highly effective in revealing cystic formation in the kidneys. Studies have shown that the early manifestations of polycystic kidney disease can be identified using ultrasound, making it a valuable tool for screening susceptible individuals and informing clinical judgments (Bergmann, 2014). Additionally, advanced imaging modalities such as MRI provide accurate cross-sectional images of the kidneys, enabling clinicians to visualize complex anatomical structures and associated vascular defects commonly seen in congenital abnormalities. CT scanning is another essential diagnostic imaging technique applied to outline renal anatomy and assess the severity of polycystic kidney disease. CT scanning provides higher resolution than ultrasound; however, due to the application of ionizing radiation in CT scanning, proper caution should be exercised, particularly in children. For ambivalent or conflicting ultrasound results in patients, CT may resolve complicated cysts that may mimic PKD or provide other diagnoses and enhance the precision of genetic counseling and treatment plans. Furthermore, the utilization of three-dimensional imaging modalities allows for more precise impressions of the architectural changes in the kidney, thereby optimizing patient-specific treatment regimens. This three-dimensional imaging modality also helps in the recognition of potential complications of PKD, say as renal failure or hypertension, which also needs multidisciplinary management of the patient in the case of congenital disease (Bergmann, 2014). Next-generation sequencing technologies are also revolutionizing diagnostic applications for PKD, especially when the traditional methods are unfruitful. Combining the imaging findings and genetic analysis raises the diagnostic yield and aids in clarifying indeterminate presentations of the disease. For instance, identification of mutations in the PKD1 or PKD2 genes, coupled with correlating these findings with imaging, provides invaluable information about the severity and progression of the disease. In addition, the ability to identify phenocopies of PKD through the use of advanced genetic testing further supports the importance of an integrated evaluation strategy that incorporates both imaging and genetic techniques. As more loci are identified for cystic kidney diseases, reliance on advanced diagnostic imaging in combination with genetic data will be crucial in enabling more accurate diagnoses, informed prognostication, and improved patient management for patients afflicted with both polycystic kidney disease and congenital cystic disease (Figure 5.1).

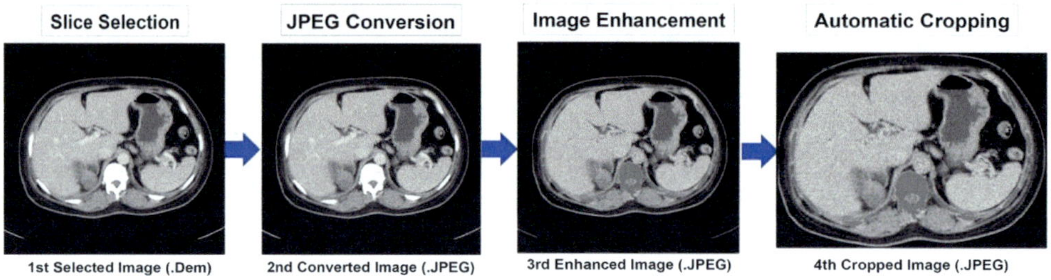

Figure 5.10. Diagnostic imaging techniques of PKD.

Source: https://www.mdpi.com/diagnostics/diagnostics-10-01113/article_deploy/html/images/diagnostics-10-01113-g004.png.

5.3.3. Laboratory Tests for Kidney Function

An understanding of kidney function is essential in the diagnosis and management of conditions such as polycystic kidney disease (PKD) and other congenital disorders. Tests of kidney function typically include estimation of serum creatinine, blood urea nitrogen (BUN), and measurement of the glomerular filtration rate (GFR). The tests provide significant information regarding the effectiveness with which the kidneys clear the waste products from the blood. Elevated serum creatinine and BUN levels can be indicative of impaired renal function, particularly relevant in patients with PKD because the disease usually leads to chronic deterioration of kidney function. Early detection of such findings can enable proper intervention, which reduces the impact of the disease on kidney function and overall health. In addition to serum creatinine and BUN, a urine examination also plays a significant role in assessing kidney health. A urinalysis can reveal various abnormalities, including protein, blood, or abnormal cellular casts that indicate underlying pathology such as nephron injury or cystic disease progression. Patients with PKD are closely monitored for urinary protein concentration, as proteinuria is a sign of kidney injury and a marker of disease progression. Interpretation of such testing results enables clinicians to develop management plans tailored to the individual. Furthermore, detection of declining kidney function through laboratory testing can guide the need for more invasive therapy or planning for a kidney transplant in patients with advanced complications of such diseases as PKD and associated liver diseases (Gordon et al., 1990). An accurate genetic diagnosis is crucial for the treatment of polycystic kidney disease and for understanding its impact on kidney function. Genetic analysis enables the identification of mutations in PKD genes, such as PKD1 and PKD2, with widespread implications for prognosis and disease management. The advent of next-generation sequencing has allowed for the ability to detect these mutations better. It has increased knowledge regarding renal cyst diseases, allowing for more specific diagnoses, which is crucial for effective clinical management (Bergmann, 2014). With the integration of laboratory findings and genetic data, healthcare providers can more effectively assess kidney function and provide comprehensive treatment to patients, thus improving outcomes in those afflicted with polycystic kidney disease and associated congenital conditions (Figure 5.11).

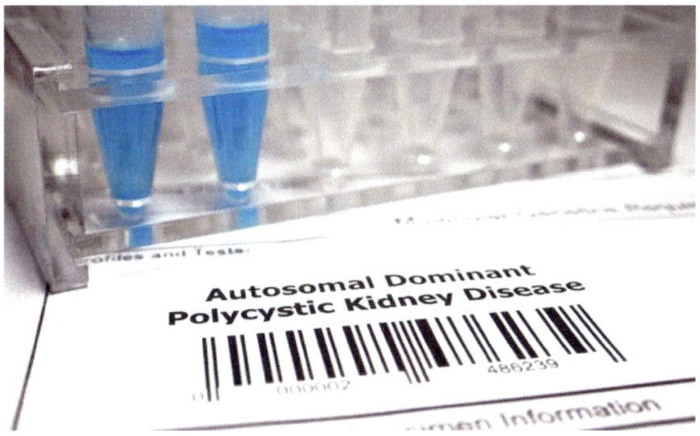

Figure 5.11. Laboratory tests for kidney function of PKD.

Source: https://mumcdnstorage.blob.core.windows.net/dwnews/2020/05/Autosomal-Dominant-Polycystic-Kidney-Disease-e1655152391353.jpg.

5.4. Congenital Disorders Related to PKD

The link between congenital conditions and Polycystic Kidney Disease (PKD) is becoming increasingly recognized as a significant area of research to pursue. PKD, particularly its autosomal dominant variant (ADPKD), has identified new avenues to research not only its specific renal issues but also its relationship with larger congenital conditions. Genetic research has established that PKD mutations overlap with those found in numerous other congenital conditions. For instance, recent evidence suggests correlations between congenital epithelial tissue disorders and mutations common among ADPKD patients. Such findings suggest a genetic cause of these disorders, characterized by complex interactions of multiple genes, a concept supported by recent studies in the involved fields, including those on congenital dilatation of the biliary tract and other structural abnormalities (Campbell et al., 2016). Moreover, genetic and phenotypic heterogeneity in PKD patients also has implications beyond renal function. Heterogeneity that is genetic in congenital diseases related to PKD suggests that more than a single implicated gene has the capacity to regulate not only kidney development but also affect other organ systems. Recent studies have identified a series of de novo variants that can lead to varied developmental complications, suggesting that mutations related to PKD may manifest in a range of congenital defects, including those affecting the biliary and liver systems. Such findings are groundbreaking, especially given that scientists are researching the relationship between ADPKD cystogenesis and resultant developmental complications in other organ systems (Gabow et al., 1991). Understanding these relationships can inform clinical management strategies and prevention strategies in high-risk individuals. An understanding of congenital disorders in relation to PKD also holds therapeutic implications. The genetic knowledge gleaned from observing congenital disorders related to PKD can be used to guide the development of targeted therapies that attempt to restore or modify the underlying genetic defect. With increased awareness of PKD's genetic landscape, it can also assist in the identification of susceptible individuals so that preliminary interventions can be made to avert catastrophic results typical of this disorder. Precise genetic mutations would be utilized to create interventions, bringing hope for individualized medicine solutions in the treatment of congenital diseases related to PKD. The intersection of PKD gene discoveries and associated congenital anomalies represents a critical step towards maximizing clinical outcomes and quality of life in affected patients across different organ systems (Campbell et al., 2016) (Figure 5.12).

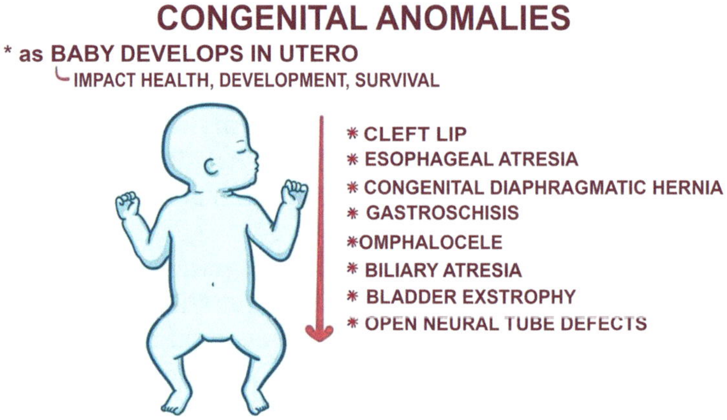

Figure 5.12. Congenital disorders related to PKD.

Source: https://external-content.duckduckgo.com/iu/?u=https%3A%2F%2Fosmose-it.s3.amazonaws.com%2FbcSAJX3gTrSDjk-Yg4SkvCGyQ_u-CZ2y%2F_.jpg&f=1&nofb=1&ipt=4935ce52ce44fe292999c72e0b375db7327c3075781ede0d735db9589f38cb21.

5.4.1. Overview of Congenital Disorders

Congenital disorders are a collective group of disorders that are found at birth and in the majority of cases, are caused by genetic faults or environmental factors during fetal life. The disorders can affect any part of the body, and in all their different forms, can express organ structural changes, metabolic imbalances, or chromosomal abnormalities. The earlier they are diagnosed, the better, as congenital disorders can significantly impact the child's growth, development, and well-being. For instance, congenital anomalies of the kidney, such as renal agenesis and dysplasia, are more susceptible to acquiring chronic kidney disease (CKD) in their later years. Screening those who are susceptible, particularly children who have experienced high-risk factors at birth, can help lead to early interventions and better outcomes. Effective monitoring procedures can help healthcare providers identify early warning signs of kidney disease and initiate the proper treatment techniques, ultimately enhancing the quality of life for those afflicted with it (Schaefer et al., 2016). The intricate relationship between congenital disorders and genes is highlighted by diseases such as Nephronophthisis (NPHP), which are predominantly inherited and lead to end-stage renal disease in childhood. This autosomal recessive disease manifests in symptoms like nocturia and polyuria, which reflect a defect in the concentrating ability of the urine. Renal ultrasound may reveal features such as corticomedullary cysts and increased echogenicity, which can further aid in diagnosis. Importantly, NPHP usually has extrarenal manifestations, particularly retinal degeneration, further complicating patient management. Genetic testing has also gained increasing application for diagnostic confirmation and reduced reliance on invasive methods, such as renal biopsy. As our knowledge of NPHP and other genetic diseases increases, so too should our strategies for screening and treating these conditions in affected families (Eley et al., 2011). A comprehensive understanding of the overall context of congenital disease, particularly that of renal pathology, requires an interdisciplinary approach that unites genetics, pediatrics, and patient advocacy. Public awareness and education about these disorders can be an essential consideration for improving early detection rates as well as access to health services for everyone. According to World Kidney Day campaigns, there is a need for collaboration among health professionals in promoting awareness and utilizing effective treatment strategies for congenital kidney disorders. The disparities in the availability of care must be addressed to offer interventions required by children with congenital anomalies, regardless of socioeconomic status or place of residence. Complete management regimens, including genetic counseling and supportive care, can potentially facilitate the best outcomes for these vulnerable populations (Schaefer et al., 2016).

5.4.2. Specific Congenital Disorders Associated with PKD

The overlap between polycystic kidney disease (PKD) and congenital illnesses reveals significant understanding of the genetic and phenotypic complexities of the conditions. A case in point is the ciliopathies group of diseases, which encompasses a group of genetic ailments involving ciliary dysfunction. The overlapping clinical presentation of these conditions, including renal cysts, neurological impairment, and skeletal abnormalities, suggests a broader spectrum of systemic involvement. A number of studies have recognized ciliopathies as the result of a cluster of gene mutations in cilia structure and function, which suggests that these genes are involved in complicated developmental associations. This shared pathophysiology suggests that PKD is not merely a standalone renal disease, but rather a part of a larger framework of congenital defects governed by ciliary biology (Gleeson et al., 2011). Hence, the detection of complex phenotypes associated with PKD can enable researchers and clinicians to treat and study these conditions more effectively. Amongst all the congenital anomalies related to PKD, congenital dilatation of the bile duct (CDD) is a comparatively rare but dangerous condition. Occurring sporadically, CDD is typically found in Asian patients and has been characterized as being related to severe complications due to bile impaction. Exome sequencing analyses reveal pathogenic de novo variants in several genes that regulate epithelial and connective tissue formation, indicating a multifactorial genetic etiology for this disorder. Detection of recurrent mutations in developmental disease as well as biliary carcinoma-associated genes suggests an interaction between these genetic factors and CDD's disease pathogenesis. Notably, CDD depicts how congenital disorders might overlap with PKD through shared genetic pathways, strongly highlighting the interconnected nature of the conditions and promoting further insight into the possible shared etiology (Campbell et al., 2016). In addition to ciliopathies and CDD, several other congenital disorders have associated relationships with PKD that also highlight the importance of genetic screening among patients. For instance, conditions such as renal agenesis and syndromic disorders such as the Bardet-Biedl syndrome have been reported to be co-occurring with PKD features. Such associations primarily result from mutations within the genes involved in kidney development, leading to malformations that express or co-occur with cystic transformation, a characteristic of PKD. Given that these conditions directly relate to each other, it becomes essential to understand their complex relationship for effective diagnosis and treatment planning. The study of the genetic links between such disorders not only helps establish the genetic etiology of PKD but also defines the need for managing patients with such complex presentations in a multidisciplinary manner. By expanding the remit of studies into coexisting congenital disorders, we derive valuable lessons in the broader implications of PKDs and their therapeutic management in the future (Figure 5.13).

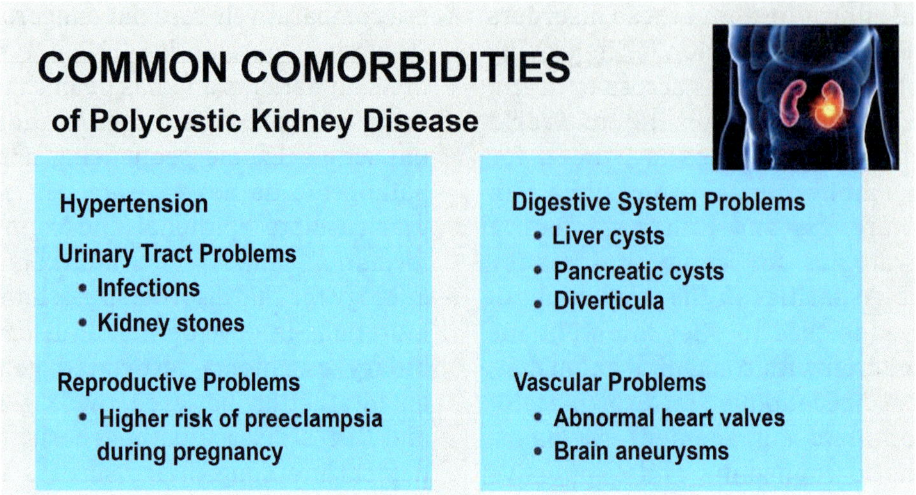

Figure 5.13. Specific congenital disorders associated with PKD.

Source: https://images.ctfassets.net/222znibi5gto/4Kh1b8EZHAlIHqG58bhAh/2add3c4064010cfa81ee0bcb230de7fb/Draft_ADPKD_Comorbitities-2.png.

5.4.3. Impact of PKD on Congenital Disorder Outcomes

The association of polycystic kidney disease (PKD) with congenital disorders reflects a complex interplay of genes that regulate kidney development and function. PKD, a genetic disorder characterized by the expansion of fluid-filled cysts within the kidneys, has been associated with a variety of congenital malformations, most significantly organ laterality-related ones. One of the most significant aspects of this association is the fact that illnesses like PKD can predispose one to a wide range of unfavorable outcomes involving congenital abnormalities. Children whose development is impacted by PKD are generally predisposed to be at higher risk for CKD and secondary complications throughout their early years. Early intervention and monitoring in these cases are essential to improve health trajectories because established treatments are available to cope with the consequences of CKD if they are identified early (Schaefer et al., 2016). PKD's impact on outcomes of congenital disorders significantly goes beyond the development of diseases like biliary atresia splenic malformation (BASM), which shows renal and hepatic development interrelationship. Research highlights that infants with biliary atresia tend to exhibit defects of laterality, which have been found linked with PKD variants. The observation of bi-allelic and heterozygous variants in BASM patients of PKD1L1 indicates that PKD-associated genetic factors not only cause damage to the kidney but also affect other organ systems, particularly the liver (Alonso et al., 2019). This connection points towards the necessity for proper clinical evaluation in the affected subjects since the prevalence of such genetic defects calls for a multidisciplinary treatment plan in addressing the diverse presentation of congenital malformations. A concern regarding the implications of PKD to congenital diseases involves a specific approach towards pediatric care, taking into account the long-term potential consequences related to congenital anomalies in children. Because some children born with congenital malformations like those due to PKD may subsequently experience severe sequelae impairing kidney function in adult life, it is crucial to take steps to follow them up regularly and intervene early (Schaefer et al., 2016). Children need to be offered resources for facilitating health equity, particularly among underrepresented groups. Genetic advances and diagnostic techniques will be critical in demystifying the interconnection between PKD and other congenital conditions, ultimately dictating individualized treatment protocols and prognostic outcomes for those afflicted.

5.5. Treatment Options for Polycystic Kidney Disease

The complexity of managing polycystic kidney disease (PKD) calls for a multi-angled approach tailored to patient-specific demand and the extent of disease. Pharmacotherapy is primarily aimed at managing hypertension, the shared condition among PKD patients. Blood pressure control is of great importance as it can reverse the development of renal injury. Physicians commonly use medications such as angiotensin-converting enzyme (ACE) inhibitors or angiotensin receptor blockers (ARBs). Not only do these agents decrease blood pressure, but they also exert renal protective actions by lowering proteinuria and slowing the deterioration of renal function. As PKD progresses, the effective treatment of associated symptoms becomes increasingly important, with ongoing monitoring and adjustments to treatment regimens to ensure optimal patient outcomes. In addition to drug therapy, modification of lifestyle is a vital component of the overall management strategy of PKD. Patients are generally advised to adopt dietary interventions that emphasize reduced salt intake and hydration, which help reduce hypertension and maintain renal function. Exercise is also encouraged, as it can help manage blood pressure and overall well-being. Smoking cessation is also strongly advised owing to the high cardiovascular risk associated with PKD. The inclusion of these lifestyle changes can significantly augment the efficacy of medical therapies and contribute toward better management of the disease's complications in the long term, thereby focusing attention on the importance of an integrated approach to treatment. Apart from pharmacologic and lifestyle management, new therapies are being explored to hold out the promise of better outcomes in PKD patients. One of the therapeutic approaches with promise is the administration of vasopressin V2 receptor antagonists, which, in clinical trials, have been shown to slow renal cyst expansion and preserve kidney function. Gene therapy methods that block the molecular pathways leading to PKD are another area under investigation by researchers. Such novel approaches reflect a shift towards more customized medicine, with the potential to rechannel the disease process at the cellular level. With each advancement in new therapies, patients and providers must stay informed about ongoing research and emerging treatment options that hold promise for improving quality and extending renal function in patients with PKD (Figure 5.14).

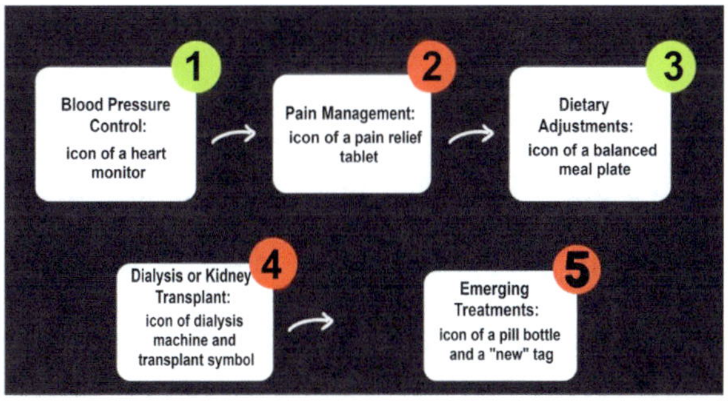

Figure 5.14. Treatment options for polycystic kidney disease.

Source: https://vshospitals.b-cdn.net/wp-content/uploads/2024/11/Polycystic-Kidney-Disease-Treatment-vs-1024x671.webp.

5.5.1. Lifestyle Modifications and Management

Successful management of PKD involves a multifaceted approach that emphasizes lifestyle changes as well as medical treatment. As patients deal with the intricacies of this chronic and increasingly debilitating disorder, incorporating specific lifestyle adjustments can dramatically affect health outcomes. Fundamental changes involve the institution of a well-balanced diet with a focus on low-sodium, nutrient-dense foods, along with sufficient hydration. These nutritional changes can potentially maintain kidney function and control related symptoms. Secondly, weight control is crucial since obesity exacerbates complications in PKD. Exercise not only aids in weight control but also significantly contributes to overall cardiovascular health, a valuable consideration for patients with PKD, as they have an elevated risk of cardiovascular issues. Involvement in preventive health behaviors and vigilant monitoring of symptom tracking ensures that patients are actively engaged in their care process, thereby enhancing their quality of life (Kent et al., 2017).

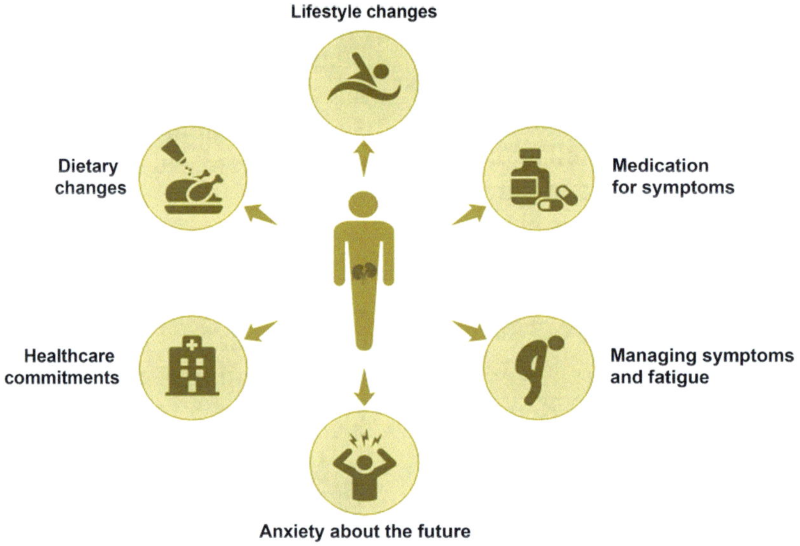

Figure 5.15. Lifestyle modifications and management treatment for polycystic kidney disease.

Source: https://pkdinternational.org/images/pages/managing-pain.svg.

Beyond what they consume, the psychological and social dimensions of coping with PKD cannot be avoided. Patients usually encounter emotional and psychological challenges that accompany carrying a chronic disease. Involvement in support groups can provide a common experience and sharing of coping strategies, so that patients do not feel isolated. Furthermore, educating patient about PKD can give individuals control to make informed decisions about their health. This involves understanding the semantics of taking medicine and visiting the doctor frequently to monitor kidney function and detect any adverse trends early. A coordinated, patient-focused strategy that addresses both physical and mental well-being can significantly improve patient outcomes and satisfaction with treatment (Baron et al., 2016). Therefore, addressing the determinants of lifestyle and mental illness is a priority in the global management of PKD. Other than diet and psychosocial interventions, other lifestyle modifications are crucial in the efficient management of PKD. Decreasing alcohol intake and preventing smoking are essential because both can harm kidney function. The patients also need to take measures to cope with other potential health complications, such as high blood pressure and diabetes, with active measures such as sticking to medication and periodic check-ups. For instance, keeping blood pressure under control is particularly important because it can lower the risk of complications from PKD. Additionally, individuals are encouraged to maintain ongoing communication with medical professionals to tailor lifestyle guidance to their personal situations. This cooperative paradigm aligns with contemporary models of care that adopt a shared decision-making philosophy, thereby promoting more tailored management regimens. Ultimately, the adoption of these lifestyle changes not only manages PKD but also improves overall health outcomes (Kent et al., 2017) (Figure 5.15).

5.5.2. Pharmacological Treatments

The pharmacology of treating PKD has come a long way in recent years, with the addition of tolvaptan to the approved list by the FDA in 2018. Tolvaptan is a vasopressin receptor antagonist, the first to be employed pharmacologically for the specific purpose of slowing autosomal dominant polycystic kidney disease (ADPKD). Though of clinical use, tolvaptan has demonstrated only limited efficacy and is accompanied by side effects that negatively influence patient compliance and quality of life. As the literature has demonstrated, there is a critical need for the development of more effective and safer treatments. Future treatments and improvements can include new approaches, such as targeting the mammalian target of rapamycin signaling pathways, which may provide new avenues for managing ADPKD in an efficient and effective manner without compromising patient health (Bourgeois et al., 2018). In children, too, managing hypertension is extremely crucial since it is associated with chronic kidney disease and its effect on cardiovascular function in the long term. The pharmacological treatment of hypertension in children requires a systematic process, with diagnosis based on the use of normative tables of blood pressure. Following identification, a clinical evaluation is necessary to determine the presence of comorbidities or target organ injury. Then, clinicians should initiate personalized care regimens featuring therapeutic lifestyle change together with, if required, pharmacologic treatment targeted to the child's health requirements. Such a holistic treatment tends to neutralize hypertension's deleterious effects, supporting overall kidney well-being in the management of congenital diseases such as PKD (Bruyne et al., 2014).

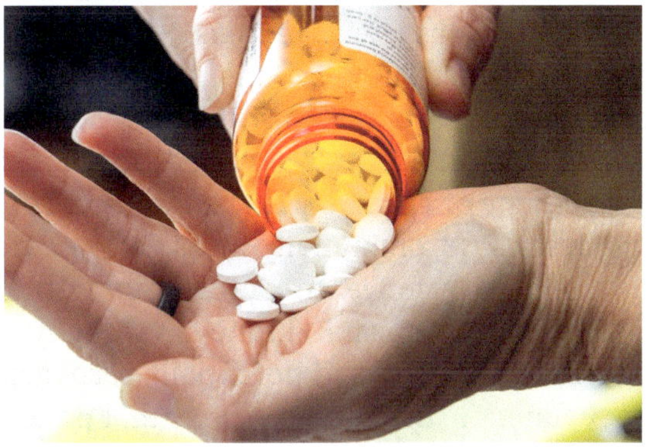

Figure 5.16. Reduction in risk of hemodialysis in patients with ADPKD treated with tolvaptan.

Source: https://mumcdnstorage.blob.core.windows.net/dwnews/2019/05/5.22-rheum-photo-e1558540929739.jpg.

Recent advances in PKD research have also highlighted the importance of exploring novel pharmacological interventions for tissue-targeted therapies. This is intended to reduce the systemic side effects of drugs that are generally effective by developing agents that can specifically target renal cysts. The novel therapeutic modalities that may be envisioned include small molecules and monoclonal antibodies, which will provide therapy directly to the involved tissues without affecting adjacent healthy organs. Moreover, interventions such as dietary interventions are also being tested as effective pharmacologic measures to control symptoms and slow the course of the disease.

With the increasing use of pharmacotherapy, it has the potential to significantly contribute to improving the quality of life for patients with polycystic kidney disease and congenital disorders through individualized and targeted therapies (Bourgeois et al., 2018) (Figure 5.16).

5.5.3. Surgical Interventions and Kidney Transplantation

Surgical interventions are of paramount significance in the management of polycystic kidney disease (PKD) complications, particularly in those patients with extensive morbidity and renal function impairment. For surgical interventions, renal cyst decortication has been proven to be an acceptable intervention in the management of chronic pain that is caused by renal cysts. It is a minimally invasive operation that aims to remove the cyst wall without destroying the normal kidney parenchyma, hence reducing pain and potentially recovering kidney function. Evidence confirms that patients with uncontrollable pain that is not responsive to conservative treatment are more likely to find relief after decortication, which accounts for its status as an effective treatment for symptomatology due to PKD (Bacallao et al., 2015). Furthermore, laparoscopic techniques have been developed that optimize recovery time and minimize postoperative complications, enhancing this procedure for both the surgeon and the patient. With further development of PKD, a kidney transplant typically becomes the definitive therapy, especially when end-stage renal disease (ESRD) is attained. Surgical expertise in nephrectomy is crucial when patients need to undergo transplantation since the removal of the diseased kidneys may facilitate the surgical intervention as well as minimize the risk of post-transplant complications. In cases where bilateral cystic distortions are severe, nephrectomy also provides relief from chronic pain and recurrent infections, thereby improving the quality of life for such patients. Surgical transplantations have made significant advancements, with improvements in immunosuppressive therapies positively enhancing graft survival (Bacallao et al., 2015). Timing of kidney transplant is also essential; early transplant has better long-term graft function and can reduce the pre-transplant need for hemodialysis (Bacallao et al., 2015). Multifactorial congenital disorders such as Caroli's disease further indicate the intricacies of surgical procedures in the broader context of polycystic disorders. For liver involvement, treatment such as liver resection or transplantation may be warranted. The surgical interventions are designed to decrease recurrent infection, such as cholangitis, and improve the patient's quality of life. The extent of liver surgery is typically based on a complete understanding of the interaction between kidney and liver dysfunction in patients with congenital disorders. Thus, coordination of surgical care between more than one organ system is necessary for maximum management, particularly as intervention therapy becomes more advanced with the increased potential for treating patients with complex presentations from polycystic kidney disease and related conditions (Figure 5.17).

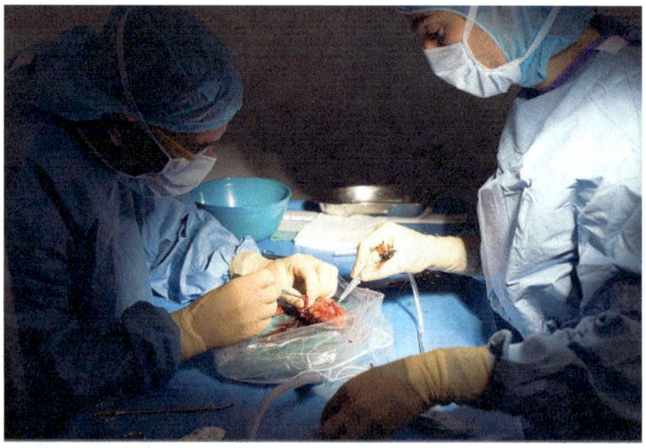

Figure 5.17. Surgical interventions and kidney transplantation for polycystic kidney disease.

Source: https://clf1.medpagetoday.com/assets/images/resource-center/kidney%20transplant%20(1).jpg.

5.6. Research and Future Directions

The study of PKD and associated congenital disease is being revolutionized by developments in genetic science and an expanding body of knowledge about disease processes. Future research avenues are expected to focus on elucidating the genetic mutations associated with specific forms of PKD, particularly in underprivileged communities such as those in the MENA region. Modern research suggests that genetic heterogeneity, particularly due to consanguinity, may affect the frequency and manifestation of these diseases. As noted in Bourke et al. (2017), autosomal recessive polycystic kidney disease (ARPKD) is much more frequent in such locations, where intense region-based genetic screening and intervention methods that account for local genetic diversity are highly recommended. This particular strategy can promote early diagnosis, thereby improving patient management and outcomes, and ultimately leading to the development of personalized therapeutic protocols. Additionally, the research is increasingly addressing the interaction between environmental and neurological factors in ARPKD patients. The condition-related susceptibilities tend to develop early in life, which causes neurocognitive impairment, a concern as observed in Bourke et al. (2017). Future epidemiologic and clinical research ought to aim at investigating the neurodevelopmental progression of children with ARPKD, particularly how it is related to associated health complications such as liver disease and hypertension. By focusing on interdisciplinary studies that link nephrology, neurology, and psychology, we can gain pivotal knowledge on how these co-occurring conditions impact health outcomes. This approach is likely to facilitate the establishment of integral intervention models that not only address renal wellness but also foster intellectual and psychosocial development among children with the condition. Clinical research is also necessary to address gaps in management systems and healthcare services among patients with PKD, especially in areas with high levels of ARPKD incidence. As noted, most MENA patients with ARPKD present in advanced disease stages, which leads to less-than-optimal outcomes and necessitates more timely therapeutic intervention (Elgebaly et al., 2024). The future focus in this area should include establishing best practice guidelines and unified care pathways to enable earlier detection and care. Additionally, collaborative research efforts can streamline data collection and reporting in clinics, facilitating a greater understanding of disease progression and treatment efficacy. By establishing an environment that fosters research collaboration among various healthcare stakeholders, the path to improved care for PKD patients and individuals with associated conditions can be significantly enhanced.

5.6.1. Current Research Trends in PKD

Trends in PKD research reveal a multiaxial model of its etiology and course. Current investigation has provided evidence for an essential role of genetic factors, together with environmental factors, in establishing susceptibility to PKD. There is robust evidence to suggest that PKD shows varying patterns in various inbred strains, based on thresholds of genes and environmental triggers. For instance, one study of hydrocortisone acetate administration revealed that different strains exhibited corresponding levels of cystic development, suggesting an interplay between genetic predispositions and environmental factors that impacts the severity of PKD. Such findings underscore the advantage of a multifactorial approach to studying the disease, which enables the identification of targeted therapy based on patients genetic backgrounds and their specific physiological responses (Blecher et al., 1990). Yet another significant area of ongoing research explores the molecular mechanisms of cystogenesis. Investigations have concentrated on the role of fluid dynamics in nephric systems, a critical function that such systems play in the genesis and progression of cysts. Recent studies comparing excretory systems in widely divergent species revealed high evolutionary conservation, enhancing our understanding of kidney pathologies. For example, planarian studies have developed a model that closely mimics some of the features of human PKD, thereby advancing our understanding of the mechanisms involved in cystogenesis. RNA-directed genetic interference has shown that alterations in flow sensing can result in the formation of tubular cysts, mimicking the features of vertebrate CKD. This new trend in research seeks to demonstrate the potential of using less complex models to study complex kidney diseases, potentially leading to breakthroughs in therapy and prevention (Alexander et al., 2015). Moreover, advancements in genetic and gene-editing technologies have revolutionized the landscape of PKD research. Techniques such as CRISPR-Cas9 allow researchers to replicate some PKD-associated genes, obtaining valuable insights on the pathways of cell division and differentiation within the kidney. The technology enables the precise identification of gene function and the discovery of new therapeutic targets. While researchers continue to unravel the genetics of PKD, the prospects for personalized medicine become increasingly tangible. The use of genetic profiling for clinical care can potentially enhance the management of PKD by ensuring tailored interventions that consider special genetic vulnerabilities. Overall, these avenues of research project a symbiotic relationship among genetics, molecular biology, and the generation of therapeutic agents against polycystic kidney disease with promise for better clinical results and a more profound understanding of congenital conditions (Blecher et al., 1990; Alexander et al., 2015) (Figure 5.18).

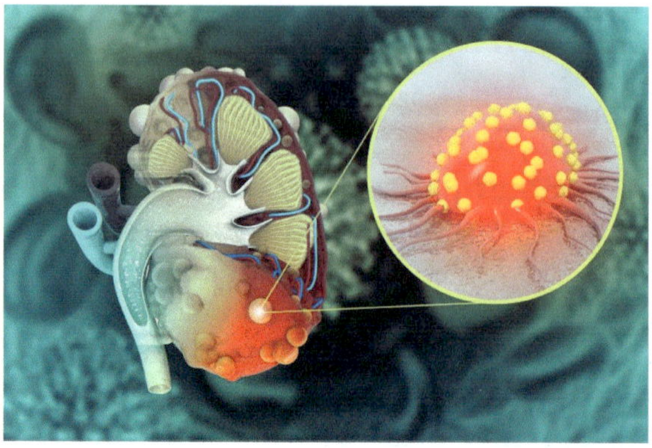

Figure 5.18. Current research trends in PKD.

Source: https://www.drugtargetreview.com/wp-content/uploads/shutterstock_2308899035-750x500.jpg.

5.6.2. Advances in Genetic Therapies

The arena of genetic therapies for diseases such as polycystic kidney disease (PKD) and other birth defects is evolving at a dizzying rate, offering hope to patients and their families. Gene editing technologies, such as CRISPR-Cas9, have revolutionized the approach to genetic illnesses by making precise alterations at the DNA level possible. With this precision comes the promise of cures for diseases previously viewed as chronic or intractable. While scientists investigate the intricacies of genetic expression and inheritance in diseases like polycystic kidney disease, there is a developing interest in not just correcting genetic mutations but also in correcting the mechanisms behind disease progression. Some potential avenues include the development of targeted therapies that utilize these innovative technologies to specifically address the genetic defect causing PKD, thereby enhancing patients' quality of life. Furthermore, subsequent studies have revealed the potential effect of gene therapy not only on the progression of polycystic kidney disease but also on concomitant comorbidities, which are frequently comorbid with congenital disease. Another significant pharmacological breakthrough in managing autosomal dominant polycystic kidney disease (ADPKD) is the development of tolvaptan, which has been found to offer modest benefits in halting disease progression, albeit with certain side effects (Bourgeois et al., 2018). The study of gene therapy can potentially revolutionize outcomes by going directly to the causative genes responsible for developing and growing kidney cysts. With advanced genetic modifications, researchers are exploring methods that not only help reduce symptoms of PKD but also prevent renal failure. These techniques underscore the importance of ongoing research into genetic therapies as a viable long-term treatment option for congenital kidney conditions. In addition to gene editing and targeted therapies, the integration of personalized medicine in the treatment of PKD is another significant advancement in genetic therapies. With genomic information specific to the patient, healthcare providers can tailor treatments to match individual profiles, potentially making therapeutic approaches more effective. As the understanding of PKD's genetic etiology improves, it becomes more feasible to construct individualized treatment schedules that are directed not only at the genetic mutations themselves but also at the metabolic and environmental triggers of kidney disease. Investigations funded by a variety of health programs continue to attempt to elucidate the multifaceted involvement of genes in kidney disease, paving the way for new therapeutic strategies. In general, advances in gene therapies represent a novel paradigm for understanding and intervening in congenital diseases, as exemplified by PKD, with future possibilities for more efficient and tailored treatments (Schaefer et al., 2016) (Figure 5.19).

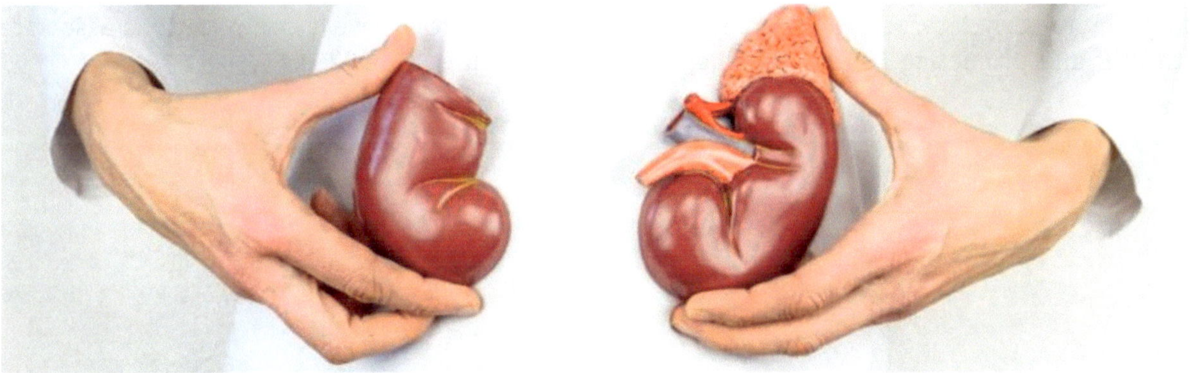

Figure 5.19. Advances in genetic therapies in PKD.

Source: https://www.genesispub.org/resource/images/articles/image566.jpg.

5.6.3. Potential for Early Intervention and Prevention

The potential of early intervention and prevention for PKD and congenital disorders is increasingly recognized in medicine. Detection of PKD at an earlier stage can potentially allow earlier therapeutic interventions to slow disease progression and enhance quality of life. Developing imaging and genetic screening technologies enables medical practitioners to detect kidney abnormalities at an earlier stage, thereby creating a time window for intervention before the development of serious complications. For instance, monitoring blood pressure and renal function among individuals with a family history of PKD can lead to the implementation of preventive interventions aimed at mitigating these impacts, thereby emphasizing the ultimate significance of heightened awareness and preventive care among vulnerable populations. Such an addition not only averts the progression to more severe symptoms but is also in accordance with broader public health goals, encouraging families to engage in active health assessment and intervention as stipulated in current guidelines (Agabiti-Rosei et al., 2016). Engaging in preventive care is indispensable since it directly addresses the evolving role of CKD in PKD. With projections that CKD may be one of the leading causes of morbidity by the year 2040, specific prevention strategies are essential (Andreoli et al., 2020). Primary prevention, in this case, would be geared toward altering risk factors such as hypertension and diabetes—both of which are prevalent among individuals with PKD. Educating young adults and teenagers who present with risk factors for regular renal function screening would enable practitioners to identify any abnormal progression at an early stage. Education regarding lifestyle modifications, including dietary changes and physical activity, can be incorporated into patient care plans to aid in kidney function. Such preventive measures not only address individual outcomes but also help lower healthcare costs associated with end-stage renal failure and complications. The role of policy in the formation of a culture of prevention cannot be overstated, particularly with PKD and congenital illness. There is a pressing need for government and institutional policies to sustain education and awareness programs targeting kidney well-being. The current healthcare systems lack in-depth strategies explicitly aimed at CKD prevention. By prioritizing treatment screening, management, and education policies, significant progress in public health can be achieved. Inter-sectoral coordination among the policymaking sector, the healthcare sector, and the education sector can create a scenario in which preventive measures are integrated into community practices. These collaborative efforts can enhance the identification of individuals at risk and promote early intervention, thereby preventing the onset of severe complications associated with PKD and promoting proactive kidney health (Andreoli et al., 2020).

SUMMARY

The interaction between PKD and congenital disease underscores the complexity of genetic influences on renal pathology. This study shows that some syndromic disease states, such as biliary atresia splenic malformation (BASM), share genetic predispositions with PKD, that is, with variants of the PKD1L1 gene involved in ciliary function and determination of laterality. The detection of bi-allelic and heterozygous BASM patient variants highlights the need to continue refining genetic screening methods in pediatric populations. With this effort comes an assurance of enhanced diagnostic precision and a deeper understanding of disease mechanisms, thereby enabling more effective management strategies for those affected (Alonso et al., 2019). Additionally, the findings on Townes-Brocks syndrome (TBS) demonstrate how congenital illness can manifest as a single renal condition and complicate precise diagnosis and treatment. The progression from seemingly benign cystic kidneys in infancy to end-stage renal failure (ESRF) emphasizes that extra-renal manifestations must be recognized in congenital syndromes. Genetic testing, as depicted in TBS, is not only but also necessary for diagnosis, family planning, and prognostic counseling. These findings underpin a robust, multi-disciplinary approach to treating patients with PKD and congenital illness to help healthcare providers identify hidden syndromic relationships that might otherwise remain undiagnosed (Bian et al., 2016). The generalizability of the findings has implications for both clinical practice and the performance of future genetic studies. Clinicians' appreciation of PKD/congenital disease correlations can enhance patient screening activities, leading to earlier intervention and detection. Additional research into shared pathways of inheritance can also provide insight into novel therapeutic targets, with the potential for more effective therapies. As our understanding of these complex relationships deepens, it becomes increasingly clear that a collaborative approach, encompassing geneticists, nephrologists, and pediatric specialists, is essential in navigating the multifaceted nature of polycystic kidney disease and its related congenital disorders. Ultimately, ongoing research will be crucial in uncovering the full spectrum of genetic influences that contribute to these conditions, thereby paving the way for advancements in medical care and improved patient outcomes.

The complexity of Polycystic Kidney Disease (PKD) and its association with congenital conditions demonstrates a complex model of renal pathology. The crucial aspect of PKD revolves around inherited determinants that are important in the development of renal cysts, which are basically fluid-filled pouches within kidney tissue. The contrast between autosomal dominant and autosomal recessive PKD reveals the genetic heterogeneity and clinical relevance to the patient. Apart from this, research has suggested the implication of certain cystoproteins that are localized at the cilia centrosome complex (CCC), which may be underlying pathways to cyst development. This not only clarifies the mechanism of PKD pathophysiology but also raises questions fundamentally about treatment options, particularly in children whose disease could follow uniquely from adult-type disease (Loftus et al., 2012). Aside from genetic predisposition, presentation of PKD is precisely influenced by its association with other congenital defects. Many PKD patients also have associated developmental abnormalities in different organ systems, which contribute to the intricacy of diagnosis and management. For instance, other organs such as the liver or pancreas may have concurrent structural abnormalities, which require extensive patient assessment to initiate timely interventions. The correlation of PKD with other congenital diseases makes it even more challenging to treat patients, as practitioners must handle a greater variety of symptoms and potential complications. Thus, integrating knowledge of PKD with other congenital diseases becomes essential to achieve optimal patient outcomes and tailor treatment methods according to the patient's overall condition profile (Alexander et al., 2015). The ongoing exploration of the molecular etiology of PKD and related congenital diseases remains essential to treatment advances in the future. Present research is geared toward an understanding of the evolutionary conservation of renal systems across species, with insight from simpler models like planarians informing a greater sense of human disease. Experiments have demonstrated that cystogenesis processes are not only preserved but also exhibit a profound evolutionary connection, which may hold the key to novel therapeutic interventions. Through the utilization of the advantage of genetic modeling and manipulation in invertebrate systems, researchers can further understand etiology in CKD, moving towards targeted interventions. This line of research promises to dramatically change PKD treatment, ushering in the practice of evidence-based medicine in harmony with the complexity of congenital disease (Loftus et al., 2012).

CLOSER LOOK

NEPHRONOPHTHISIS (NPHP)

NPHP is a rare, hereditary kidney disease that is the most common genetic cause of end-stage renal disease (ESRD) in children and teenagers. It is characterized by chronic tubulointerstitial nephritis with progressive impairment of renal function, typically without overt proteinuria or hematuria in the early stages. The pathognomonic pathological features are disruption of tubular basement membranes, tubular atrophy, interstitial fibrosis, and corticomedullary cyst formation. NPHP is a ciliopathy, a group of disorders caused by defects in the structure or function of primary cilia, microtubule-based organelles present on nearly all cells, including those of the renal tubular epithelial cells. Mutations in more than 20 genes (termed NPHP genes) have been reported, with NPHP1 being most commonly implicated. These genetic defects lead to ciliary signaling and function, compromising cellular homeostasis in the kidney and other body systems, resulting in both renal and extrarenal features.

Clinically, NPHP is of three forms based on the age of onset: infantile, juvenile, and adolescent/adult. The juvenile form is the most common and typically occurs at an age of 4 to 12 years with the following manifestations: polydipsia, polyuria, retardation of growth, anemia, and fatigue due to progressively diminishing concentrating ability and renal function deterioration. The kidneys are usually small or of normal size, in contrast to the large kidneys of polycystic kidney disease. Cysts are typically present at the corticomedullary junction in advanced cases. Most patients are diagnosed only after they have developed ESRD, often less than 20 years of age. The infantile type of presentation is more severe and may present within the first year of life with rapid progression to renal failure. In contrast, the adolescent type remains asymptomatic until late in the teenage years or early twenties.

Most importantly, NPHP is a multisystem disorder in the majority of cases. An estimated 10–20% of patients have features other than within the kidneys, specifically of the eyes (retinal degeneration leading to Senior-Løken syndrome), liver fibrosis, skeletal deformity, and neurological abnormality. The presence of these features often relates to which gene is mutated. For instance, mutations in NPHP5 are strongly associated with retinal involvement. Given its genetic etiology and heterogeneity, diagnosis typically involves genetic testing, particularly in the case of a family history of premature renal disease. A kidney biopsy can reveal histologic features, but genetic confirmation is essential to provide correct classification and counselling.

There is no established curative treatment for nephronophthisis. The therapy is supportive, consisting of fluid and electrolyte management, anemia management, and preparation for renal replacement therapy such as dialysis or a kidney transplant. With no effective treatments to halt the disease process, early detection is vital so that intervention and genetic counseling may be initiated early. Research further enhances the knowledge of molecular methods in ciliary defects with a view to developing future targeted therapy.

References

1. Mitchison, H. M., & Shoemark, A. (2017). Motile cilia defects in diseases other than primary ciliary dyskinesia: The contemporary diagnostic and research role for transmission electron microscopy. *Ultrastructural Pathology*, *41*(6), 415–427. https://doi.org/10.1080/01913123.2017.1370050Agabiti-Rosei, E., Cruickshank, J. K., Dominiczak, A., Erdine, S., et al. (2016). 2016 European Society of Hypertension guidelines for the management of high blood pressure in children and adolescents. https://core.ac.uk/download/46165193.pdf (accessed on 25th June 2025).
2. Alexander, R., Alvarado, A., Lakshmanaperumal, N., McClain, J., et al. (2015). Stem cells and fluid flow drive cyst formation in an invertebrate excretory organ. https://core.ac.uk/download/46961575.pdf (accessed on 25th June 2025).
3. Alonso, E. M., Berauer, J. P., Bezerra, J. A., Bull, L., et al. (2019). Identification of *PKD1L1* gene variants in children with the biliary atresia splenic malformation syndrome. https://core.ac.uk/download/187423807.pdf (accessed on 25th June 2025).
4. Amante, M., Cassini, E., Duek, F., Garay, A., et al. (2007). Bile duct cyst type V (*Caroli's disease*): Surgical strategy and results. https://core.ac.uk/download/pdf/82500028.pdf (accessed on 25th June 2025).
5. Andreoli, S., Fung, W. W. S., Garcia-Garcia, G., Hradsky, M., et al. (2020). Kidney health for everyone everywhere–From prevention to detection and equitable access to care. https://core.ac.uk/download/548660494.pdf (accessed on 25th June 2025).
6. Avner, E. D., Bryda, E. C., Christine, B., Collier, J., et al. (1996). Evidence that two phenotypically distinct mouse *PKD* mutations, *bpk* and *jcpk*, are allelic. https://core.ac.uk/download/pdf/82153387.pdf (accessed on 25th June 2025).
7. Bacallao, R. L., Bahler, C. D., Shumate, A. M., Sundaram, C. P., et al. (2015). Management of pain in autosomal dominant polycystic kidney disease and anatomy of renal innervation. https://core.ac.uk/download/46961575.pdf (accessed on 25th June 2025).
8. Baron, D. A., Bergman, P. J., Bryan, J. N., Calvet, J. P., et al. (2016). A One Health overview, facilitating advances in comparative medicine and translational research. https://core.ac.uk/download/323068355.pdf (accessed on 25th June 2025).
9. Belli, D., Birraux, J., Bottani, A., Calinescu-Tuleasca, A., et al. (2018). *Caroli* disease, bilateral diffuse cystic renal dysplasia, situs inversus, postaxial polydactyly, and preauricular fistulas: A ciliopathy caused by a homozygous *NPHP3* mutation. https://core.ac.uk/download/159147697.pdf (accessed on 25th June 2025).
10. Bergmann, C. (2014). *ARPKD* and early manifestations of *ADPKD*: The original polycystic kidney disease and phenocopies. https://core.ac.uk/download/pdf/81853221.pdf (accessed on 25th June 2025).
11. Bian, F., Gale, D., Jiang, G. R., Lin, M., et al. (2016). Delayed diagnosis of Townes–Brocks syndrome with multicystic kidneys and renal failure caused by a novel *SALL1* nonsense mutation: A case report. https://core.ac.uk/download/81675732.pdf (accessed on 25th June 2025).
12. Blair-Reid, S. A. (2010). An investigation of the ciliary protein *PKHD1* in cyst development in liver disease: Clues to the pathogenesis of biliary atresia. https://core.ac.uk/download/75865.pdf (accessed on 25th June 2025).

13. Blecher, S. R., Cole, D. E. C., Crocker, J. F. S., Digout, J. A., et al. (1990). Glucocorticoid-induced polycystic kidney disease—A threshold trait. https://core.ac.uk/download/pdf/82438068.pdf (accessed on 25th June 2025).

14. Bolt, D. M., Fink, J., Greenlee, R. T., Magnan, S., et al. (2015). The relationship of individual comorbid chronic conditions to diabetes care quality. https://core.ac.uk/download/323070914.pdf (accessed on 25th June 2025).

15. Bourgeois, B. C., Kruger, S. L., Shillingford, J. M., Torres, V. E., et al. (2018). Emerging targeted strategies for the treatment of autosomal dominant polycystic kidney disease. https://core.ac.uk/download/323063067.pdf (accessed on 25th June 2025).

16. Bourke, B., Knaus, U., & Stenke, E. (2017). Risk factors for neurocognitive functioning in children with autosomal recessive polycystic kidney disease. https://core.ac.uk/download/304663490.pdf (accessed on 25th June 2025).

17. Burity, J., Fonte, I. B. da, & Melo, P. B. de. (2014). Radiological Society of North America (RSNA) 3D printing Special Interest Group (SIG): Guidelines for medical 3D printing and appropriateness for clinical scenarios. https://core.ac.uk/download/212867900.pdf (accessed on 25th June 2025).

18. Campbell, D., Cheng, G., Cherny, S. S., Chung, B. H., et al. (2016). Genetic study of congenital bile-duct dilatation identifies de novo and inherited variants in functionally related genes. https://core.ac.uk/download/77601212.pdf (accessed on 25th June 2025).

19. De Bruyne, P., & Vande Walle, J. (2014). Management of hypertension in children and adolescents. https://core.ac.uk/download/55853879.pdf (accessed on 25th June 2025).

20. Eley, L., Hynes, A. M., Sayer, J. A., Simms, R. J., et al. (2011). Nephronophthisis: A genetically diverse ciliopathy. https://core.ac.uk/download/83940589.pdf (accessed on 25th June 2025).

21. Elgebaly, A., Elgebaly, A., Salman, M. A., Salman, A., et al. (2024). Epidemiology and outcomes of pediatric autosomal recessive polycystic kidney disease in the Middle East and North Africa. https://core.ac.uk/download/615274665.pdf (accessed on 25th June 2025).

22. Gabow, P. A. (1991). Polycystic kidney disease: Clues to pathogenesis. https://core.ac.uk/download/pdf/82604050.pdf (accessed on 25th June 2025).

23. Gherman, A., Noor, A., den Hollander, A. I., Masyuk, A. I., Barakat, A. J., Ross, A. J., et al. (2011). Ciliopathies: An expanding disease spectrum. https://core.ac.uk/download/pdf/8567519.pdf (accessed on 25th June 2025).

24. Gleeson, J. G., & Lee, J. E. (2011). A systems-biology approach to understanding the ciliopathy disorders. https://core.ac.uk/download/323066742.pdf (accessed on 25th June 2025).

25. Gordon, R., Mieles, L., Reyes, J., Starzl, T. E., et al. (1990). Liver transplantation for polycystic liver disease. https://core.ac.uk/download/12204466.pdf (accessed on 25th June 2025).

26. Guay-Woodford, L. (2014). Autosomal recessive polycystic kidney disease: The prototype of the hepato-renal fibrocystic diseases. https://core.ac.uk/download/230852283.pdf (accessed on 25th June 2025).

27. Kent, A., Ong, A. C. M., de Coninck, B., Clément, D., Peters, D., Levtchenko, E., Van Poppel, H., et al. (2017). European ADPKD Forum multidisciplinary position statement on autosomal dominant polycystic kidney disease care. https://core.ac.uk/download/146491236.pdf (accessed on 25th June 2025).

28. Loftus, H., & Ong, A. C. M. (2012). Cystic kidney diseases: Many ways to form a cyst. https://core.ac.uk/download/30270688.pdf (accessed on 25th June 2025).

29. Minardi, R. (2017). Dominant and recessive polycystic kidney disease: A novel molecular diagnostics approach based on next-generation sequencing. https://core.ac.uk/download/86546591.pdf (accessed on 25th June 2025).

30. Mitchison, H. M., & Valente, E. M. (2016). Motile and non-motile cilia in human pathology: From function to phenotypes. https://core.ac.uk/download/226596058.pdf (accessed on 25th June 2025).

31. Schaefer, F., Ingelfinger, J. R., & Kalantar-Zadeh, K. (2016). Averting the legacy of kidney disease: Focus on childhood. https://core.ac.uk/download/pdf/81549064.pdf (accessed on 25th June 2025).

32. van Dokkum, R. P. E., Goedbloed, M. A., Guay-Woodford, L. M., Herck, L., et al. (2000). New rat model that phenotypically resembles autosomal recessive polycystic kidney disease. https://core.ac.uk/download/19185843.pdf (accessed on 25th June 2025).

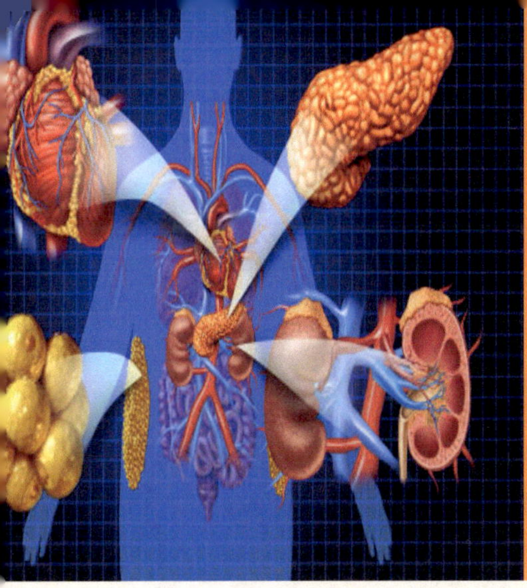

Chapter 6

HYPERTENSIVE AND DIABETIC NEPHROPATHY

Contents

Introduction

Hypertensive and diabetic nephropathy development has turned into an acute problem of contemporary medicine, becoming a kind of interface between two chronic conditions with a broad impact on renal function. Hypertension, a state of elevated blood pressure, is a severe threat to kidney function, as persistent pressure may damage the glomeruli and subsequently lead to reduced renal function. At the same time, diabetes mellitus has become more and more associated with nephrotoxic manifestations of the disease, manifested primarily in diabetic nephropathy. The dualism complicates the clinical situation, as patients typically present with combined risk factors and pathophysiological processes. Knowledge of the interaction between diabetes and hypertension is crucial for the formulation of effective prevention and targeted treatment, particularly with the prevalence of these diseases globally. A systematic examination of the molecular and physiological changes responsible for the development and exacerbation of renal complications has addressed it. Recent studies in the field of kidney function have identified urinary proteomics as a potential field for monitoring and detecting kidney conditions, such as hypertensive and diabetic nephropathy, in patients. This new approach makes use of urinary protein analysis in the detection of kidney disease biomarkers with greater sensitivities in diagnosis than traditional methods. Studies have demonstrated that urinary protein markers, including collagen peptides, serum albumin, alpha-1-antitrypsin, and uromodulin, serve as disease progression markers, shedding valuable light on the pathophysiology of nephropathy. The advent of non-invasive techniques revolutionizes renal health screening, which has the potential to advance clinical decision-making and enable health professionals to initiate interventions closer to the onset of the disease process. Ironically, the integration of these advanced diagnostics into primary practice may radically change management dogma for individuals living with these highly entangled conditions (Magalhães et al., 2016). The public health consequences of diabetic and hypertensive nephropathy necessitate urgent heed, considering the growing rate of hypertension in children and youths. As science continues to grow, guidelines for hypertension management in young individuals accentuate awareness and preventive measures in curbing such ailments collectively. Hypertension not only signifies potential cardiovascular risk but also has a direct association with renal impairment; hence, early treatment is critical. Current evidence supports the use of a multidisciplinary assessment and management plan involving lifestyle modifications, drug therapy, and ongoing monitoring of renal function. By developing a multidimensional strategy for treating hypertensive and diabetic nephropathy, healthcare systems can mitigate the long-term effects of these conditions, thereby reducing the burden on affected populations while enhancing overall public health benefits (Agabiti-Rosei et al., 2016) (Figure 6.1).

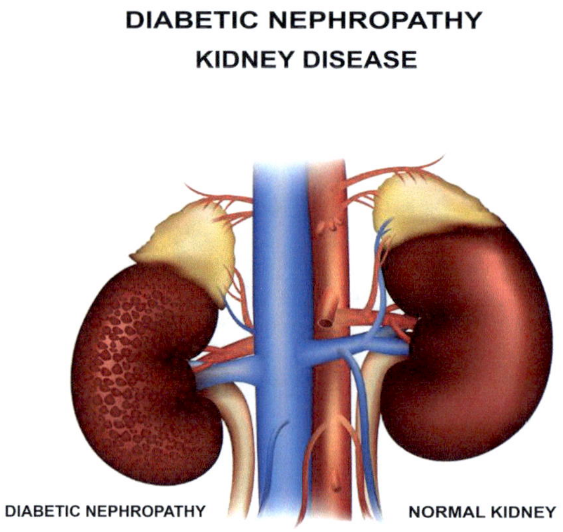

Figure 6.1. Diabetic nephropathy.

Source: https://external-content.duckduckgo.com/iu/?u=https%3A%2F%2Fmantracare.org%2Fwp-content%2Fuploads%2F2021%2F07%2FDiabetic-Nephropathy.jpg&f=1&nofb=1&ipt=cfb37760058f3ced3ea812e93990c004690f7593bcfcc5eeeb6d32dbe49b288b.

Definition of Hypertensive Nephropathy

Hypertensive nephropathy is a form of kidney damage that results from longstanding high blood pressure. It is a crucial pathophysiologic link between the hypertension process and renal impairment since chronic blood pressure exposure leads to structural changes as well as functional changes within the kidney. The resultant cascade includes glomerulosclerosis, a mechanism that causes scarring and hardening of the glomeruli, which are the functioning filtration units of the kidney. Over a period of time, the progressive damage can result in impaired renal function, which eventually results in chronic kidney disease (CKD). The dynamic between hypertension and nephropathy is also supported by epidemiological studies that indicate a high susceptibility of kidney disease among patients with chronic hypertension, justifying early diagnosis and treatment to prevent inevitable damage. Clinical presentation of hypertensive nephropathy shares overlapping features with that of chronic kidney disease, such that diagnosis and treatment become challenging. It is characterized by a slow decline in glomerular filtration rate (GFR) and proteinuria, which indicates damage to the kidneys. The involvement of a combination of several factors, including the duration of hypertension and predisposing genetic factors such as the APOL1 gene variants, also makes it a complex condition to diagnose and treat. Research demonstrates that people who possess specific APOL1 variants exhibit increased vulnerability to CKD, and this supports the need for knowledge of genetic risk factors among populations with hypertensive nephropathy.

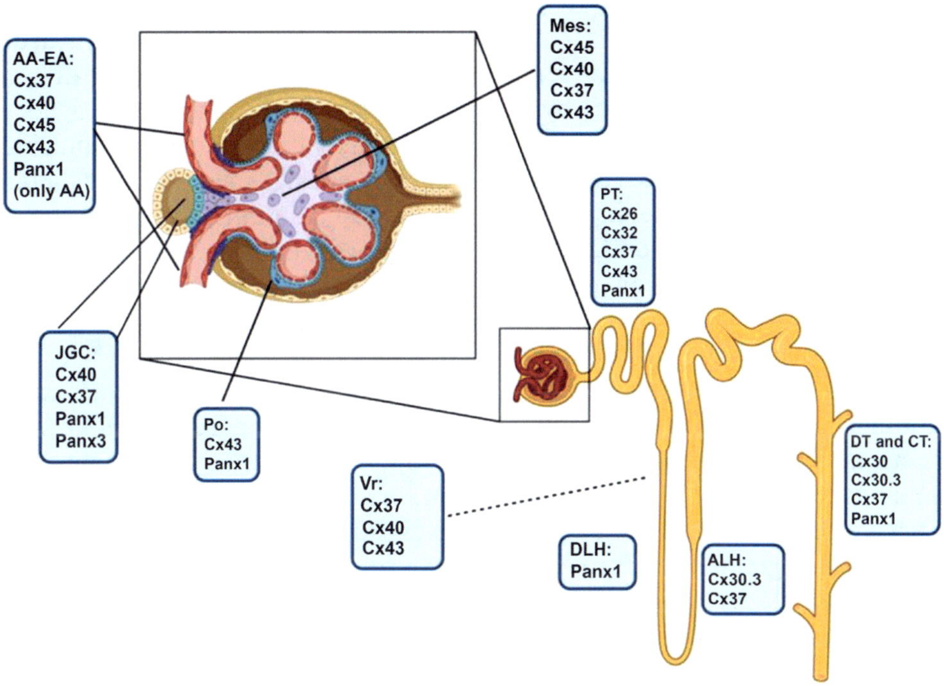

Figure 6.2. Hypertensive nephropathy.

Source: https://external-content.duckduckgo.com/iu/?u=https%3A%2F%2Fencyclopedia.pub%2Fmedia%2Fitem_content%2F202212%2F63a5196721c52ijms-23-15936-g004.png&f=1&nofb=1&ipt=cc3994c4d2010958d3929eb6ff1a7fa5c1fac0f61b8d1086fdd7bdaddcc91522.

As clinicians look to ways in which they can prevent this condition, acknowledging the multifactorial etiology of kidney injury from hypertension becomes critical in-patient management. In addition, the management of hypertensive nephropathy must be conducted by a multidisciplinary team, which includes strict control of blood pressure and frequent monitoring of kidney function. Antihypertensive treatments, especially those aimed at the renin-angiotensin-aldosterone system, have been promising in preserving renal function. Lifestyle modifications, including dietary regimen and weight control, also play an essential role in determining the course of the disease. Gender differences between the sexes in the prevalence and control of hypertensive nephropathy also reflect larger trends in health inequality, illuminating differences in treatment compliance and risk factors for hypertension between population groups. Such differences, as highlighted by more contemporary research, require tailored management approaches to optimize effective control among population groups, thereby reducing the overall outcome of patients with both hypertensive and diabetic nephropathy (Hinstersteiner et al., 2013; Bild et al., 2015) (Figure 6.2).

Definition of Diabetic Nephropathy

Diabetic nephropathy is a significant renal diabetic complication characterized by a progressive decline in renal function owing to persistent hyperglycemia and resultant pathophysiologic events. Diabetic nephropathy, as a microvascular complication of both type 1 and type 2 diabetes, is manifested as an increase in albuminuria excretion and a decrease in GFR. Clinically, it is present with an incipient pattern of increased albuminuria, which will often appear before any measurable decline in renal function. The pathophysiological processes implicated in diabetic nephropathy include hyperglycemia-induced glomerular hypertension leading to glomerulosclerosis. In addition, the condition places a patient at risk for further complications like cardiovascular disease and end-stage renal disease, highlighting the need for early detection and management in preserving renal function in the patient. The relationship between glycemic control and diabetic nephropathy remains the focus of attention in investigations, demonstrating the impact of diabetes control on long-term renal outcomes. A direct correlation between elevated HbA1c and nephropathy progression indicates that optimal blood glucose control is crucial in preventing renal complications. Higher glycemic variability—a surrogate of poor diabetes control—has been implicated as the cause of the development and progression of renal complications based on research findings. In the meta-analysis, it was found that increased HbA1c variability was significantly associated with an increased risk of diabetic nephropathy in diabetic patients, which suggests the need for interventions aimed at normalizing glucose levels. As a result, successful policy interventions towards achieving stable glycemic control have the potential to prevent or postpone the onset of diabetic nephropathy. Therefore, timely and effective interventions are essential to achieve stable glycemic control. Additionally, patient education regarding diabetic nephropathy risk and its implications is a crucial component of overall diabetes care. Patients with diabetes must be educated about kidney health, including the importance of regular screening for albuminuria and kidney function tests. Modifiable risk factors such as obesity, inactivity, and dietary habits can also play a significant role in the development of diabetic nephropathy. Encouraging changes in lifestyle, like increased physical activity and dietary nutritional habits, can be employed as protective measures. For this purpose, healthcare professionals must emphasize early intervention and regular follow-up to ensure proper management of diabetes. In this manner, the occurrence of renal complications can be significantly reduced, and patient outcomes overall are enhanced, in essence addressing the twin risk that is posed by diabetic and hypertensive nephropathy.

Importance of Studying These Conditions

The rising prevalence of diabetic and hypertensive nephropathy underscores the imperative for research on these conditions in contemporary medicine. Hypertension and diabetes are the most common etiologies of chronic kidney disease (CKD) and have a profound impact on patient morbidity and mortality. Understanding the pathogenesis of these conditions can facilitate early diagnosis and intervention, prompting alterations in disease trajectories and improved patient outcomes. Through identification of risk populations, renal function may be screened for and preventive interventions initiated. Early intervention can significantly cut down on the handicaps of CKD, including the emergence of end-stage renal disease that is costly to treat via dialysis or transplantation. Besides, recent evidence highlights the potential of novel biomarkers in diagnosing and treating diabetic kidney disease (DKD), emphasizing the need for future studies. According to recent results, proteomic biomarker investigations have been categorized as a potentially desirable target area for future development in clinical practice. The biomarkers not only reflect the underlying (patho)physiological mechanisms of DKD, but also pave the way for personalized medicine strategies. By employing rigorous validation and harmonization between industry and academia, clinicians canto identify better patients who are at higher risk and provide tailored therapy. The implementation of these newer biomarker strategies may revolutionize patient care by enabling improved monitoring of disease and treatment response, thereby directly addressing the issues posed by hypertension and diabetes in nephrology (Heerspink et al., 2016). In addition to enhancing clinical outcomes, studying hypertensive and diabetic nephropathy enhances our understanding of the broader implications for the global healthcare system. The impact of these conditions is not confined to individual patients alone, resulting in excessive healthcare costs and resource allocation challenges. With the growing global population of older adults and the rising prevalence of obesity, hypertension, and diabetes, the burden of renal disease is likely to rise further, contributing to the renal disease burden. Through research at conferences such as the South African Renal Congress, scientists will be able to provide crucial information that guides future care standards and policy-making. The importance of conducting this research, therefore, lies not only in improving current patient care but also in preparing health systems for future challenges arising from hypertensive and diabetic nephropathy (Davies et al., 2024).

6.1. Pathophysiology of Hypertensive Nephropathy

The pathophysiology of hypertensive nephropathy is significantly complex and is marked by multifaceted interactions among various systemic signaling pathways. Central to the process lies the role of the renin-angiotensin-aldosterone system (RAAS), which plays a regulatory role in blood pressure and fluid balance. In conditions of hypertension, elevated levels of angiotensin II are responsible for glomerular hypertension and hyperfiltration and lead to renal injury. Stimulation of the AT1 receptor leads to vasoconstriction and increased vascular permeability, which can result in further damage to renal tissue. The long-term effects of hypertension extend beyond hemodynamics; they induce cellular adjustments that alter the function of epithelial, endothelial, and immune cells, triggering inflammatory responses that augment kidney damage. This interaction of altered signaling pathways leads to the development of hypertensive nephropathy, underscoring the interplay between hemodynamics and cellular disease (Eckardt et al., 2019). Apart from hemodynamic changes, the biochemical milieu of hypertensive nephropathy is also important in renal damage. Enhanced oxidative stress is a hallmark of the disorder, where reactive oxygen species (ROS) disrupt cellular signaling and facilitate fibrotic mechanisms in the kidneys. It exacerbates inflammation and induces apoptosis in renal cells, particularly those of the proximal tubule, thus impairing renal function with time. Furthermore, the fibrogenic committee, particularly transforming growth factor-beta (TGF-β), is induced as a result of chronic injury, leading to the deposition of extracellular matrix and renal fibrosis. These molecular alterations accentuate the pathophysiological transition from compensatory towards maladaptive mechanisms, which eventually drive chronic kidney disease progression in hypertensive patients (Eckardt et al., 2019). The overlap of diabetic nephropathy with hypertensive nephropathy only serves to increase pathophysiological complexity. Type 1 Diabetes (T1D) patients have heightened susceptibility to renal injury, often exacerbated by concomitant hypertension. Diabetic nephropathy is characterized by specific renal changes, including glomerular hyperfiltration and alterations in the glomerular basement membrane composition. Recent evidence suggests that urinary microRNAs are valuable markers for such diseases, reflecting the underlying molecular dysregulation leading to renal disease development. For instance, the distinctive urinary microRNA profiles of patients with diabetes at various stages of nephropathy reveal extensive gene expression dysregulation, involving growth factor signaling and renal fibrosis processes. Understanding these cross-talking pathways not only enhances our knowledge about hypertensive nephropathy but also guides one towards possible therapeutic interventions for the treatment of both diabetic and hypertensive nephropathy complications of the kidney (Figure 6.3).

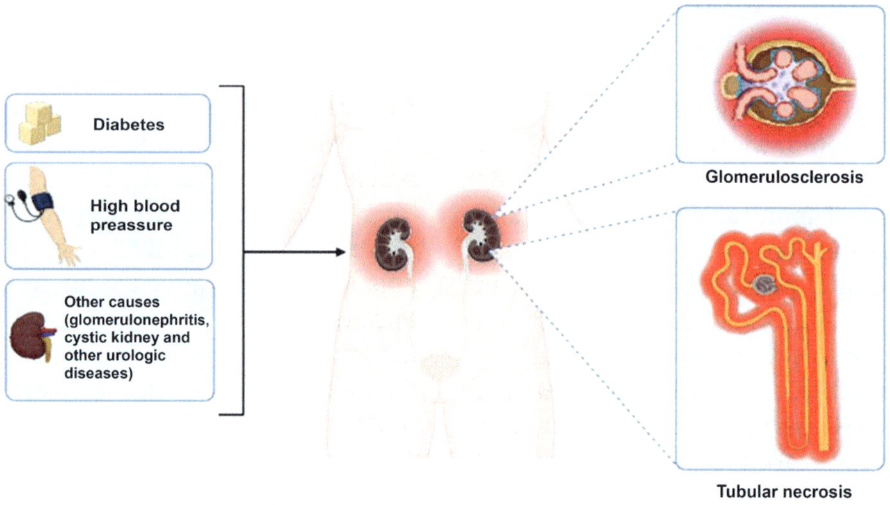

Figure 6.3. Pathophysiology of hypertensive nephropathy.

Source: https://encyclopedia.pub/media/item_content/202212/63a5190e9be64ijms-23-15936-g001.png.

6.1.1. Mechanisms of Hypertension Affecting Kidney Function

Hypertension is a central factor in the development and progression of kidney disease, primarily through several interconnected mechanisms. Elevated blood pressure leads to overloading of the renal vasculature, endothelial dysfunction, vascular remodeling, and ultimately nephron damage. The renin-angiotensin-aldosterone system (RAAS) is central to it all, where enhanced production of angiotensin II leads to arterial vasoconstriction, increased glomerular filtration pressure, and resultant glomerulosclerosis. Such a cascade may trigger a self-sustaining cycle, with renal damage caused by hypertension also further augmenting the hypertensive state by inducing renal ischemia and releasing other pro-inflammatory mediators. An understanding of these mechanisms is essential for planning therapeutic interventions that can effectively ameliorate renal damage in patients with hypertensive nephropathy, emphasizing the need to address the RAAS and its downstream effects on renal function (Eckardt et al., 2019). For diabetic nephropathy, the cross-talk between diabetes and hypertension highly complicates renal outcomes. Hyperglycemia secondary to diabetes can induce augmented oxidative stress and inflammation that exacerbate vascular changes, enhancing hypertension. Studies indicate that angiotensin II not only mediates hemodynamic actions but also affects cellular processes of inflammation, fibrosis, and apoptosis in the kidney.

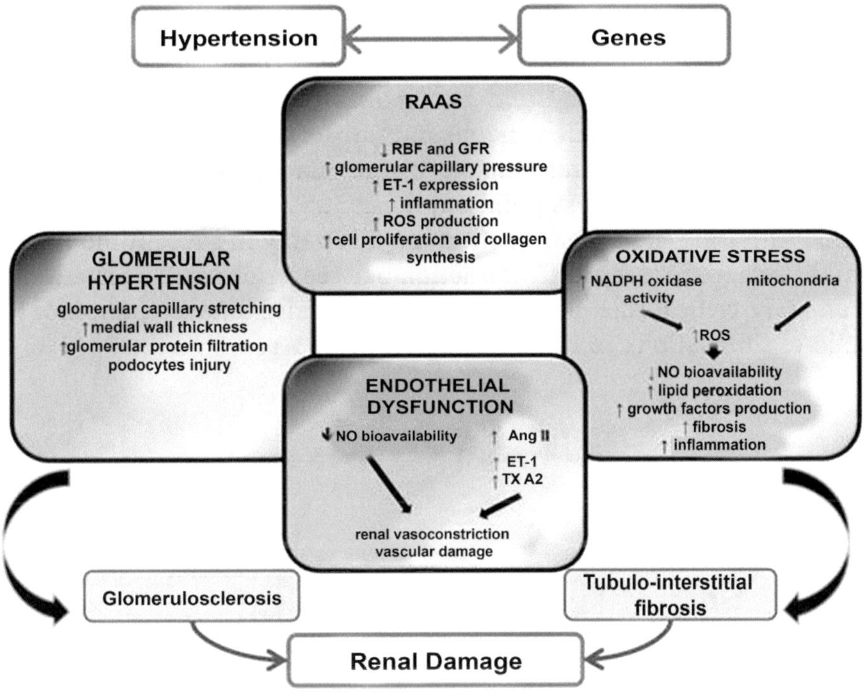

Figure 6.4. Mechanisms of hypertension affecting kidney function.

Source: https://media.springernature.com/full/springer-static/image/art%3A10.1038%2Fjhh.2013.55/MediaObjects/41371_2014_Article_BFjhh201355_Fig1_HTML.jpg.

Additionally, the activation of pro-fibrotic pathways, such as TGF-β signaling, contributes to the progression of kidney injury. The divergent response of the kidney to these insults is designed to highlight the critical need for specially formulated therapies. For instance, therapies that are specifically targeted at opposing the hypertensive effect on renal function will be more protective against the twin threat posed by hypertension and metabolic diabetes, promoting overall renal integrity (Eckardt et al., 2019). In describing pharmacologic modalities for management of diabetic nephropathy with hypertension, the employment of angiotensin receptor blockers (ARBs) is particularly pertinent. Evidence suggests that a subgroup of ARBs, i.e., candesartan, has renoprotective actions by modulating the protective arm of the RAAS, i.e., the angiotensin-converting enzyme 2 (ACE2) pathway. Surprisingly, intermediate doses of candesartan have been reported to be helpful in reducing renal tubular injury and albuminuria, extremely valuable markers of kidney function. In contrast, ultra-high dosing causes unanticipated renal injury, illustrating the complexity of controlling hypertension in patients with diabetes. This complex understanding of dosing and its effects further reinforces the need to tailor treatment regimens to prevent renal injury, in addition to managing blood pressure (Figure 6.4).

6.1.2. Role of Renal Blood Flow and Glomerular Filtration

RBF control is closely linked to the maintenance of GFR, which is essential for optimal renal function. During hypertension, systemic blood pressure changes can induce renal blood vessel hypertrophy and structural remodeling, compromising their ability to respond to physiological demands. This compromise may also exacerbate kidney damage through mechanisms such as increased glomerular capillary pressure and hyperfiltration. As outlined in recent studies, activation of the renin-angiotensin-aldosterone system also makes this one more difficult, contributing to glomerular hypertension with subsequent nephron injury. The dynamic interaction of rising renal perfusion pressure and renal structural damage further underscores the contribution of RBF to hypertensive nephropathy. These factors point out the central role of renal blood flow in preserving renal integrity and facilitating the development of nephropathy in susceptible individuals (Eckardt et al., 2019). In diabetic nephropathy, the interaction between glomerular filtration and renal blood flow plays an even more critical role. Diabetes can compromise autoregulation of GFR, making the kidneys vulnerable to fluctuations in renal perfusion pressure.

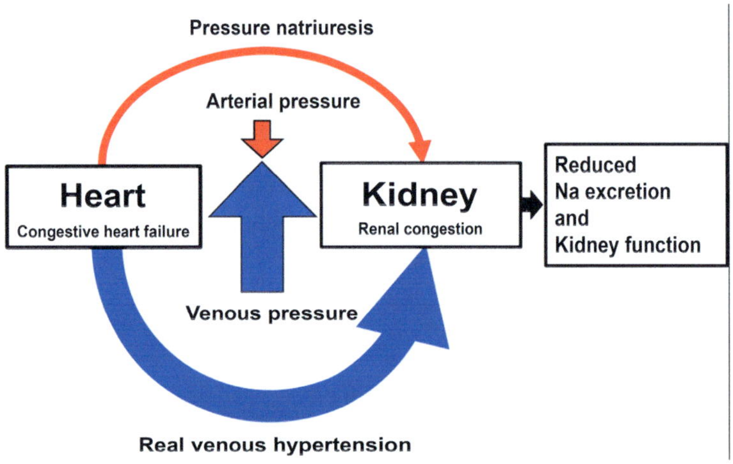

Figure 6.5. Renal venous hypertension to the regulation of pressure natriuresis in heart failure.

Source: https://media.springernature.com/full/springer-static/image/art%3A10.1038%2Fs41440-023-01512-7/MediaObjects/41440_2023_1512_Figa_HTML.png.

Pharmacologically induced hypotension can also decrease GFR, as in studies on non-diabetic nephropathy patients. In these patients, albuminuria and GFR showed significant and opposite correlations following decreases in blood pressure, indicating the susceptibility of autoregulatory mechanisms in deranged renal systems. Cessation of autoregulation is an essential element of diabetic nephropathy, indicating the significance of RBF for the maintenance of GFR. The decrease not only raises the risk for nephropathic progressive kidney disease but also emphasizes the necessity for interventions aimed at maintaining renal function in diabetes treatment (Christensen et al., 1999). The findings have important implications when considering therapeutic intervention for diabetic and hypertensive patients with nephropathy. Optimal management requires a subtle balance between providing adequate renal blood flow and avoiding excess filtration pressure. Therapies targeting the renin-angiotensin-aldosterone system may mitigate some of the pressures on the kidneys, but must be administered cautiously to avoid further compromising renal blood flow autoregulation. Lifestyle interventions, such as dietary modification and blood pressure control, can also contribute to improved renal outcomes by preserving RBF and GFR. Subsequent research must focus on delineating the optimal ways to optimize renal perfusion and filtration for the purpose of halting the progression of nephropathy before initiating permanent damage. Understanding such dynamics will be paramount in developing comprehensive care approaches for vulnerable subjects (Eckardt et al., 2019) (Figure 6.5).

6.1.3. Consequences of Chronic Hypertension on Kidney Structure

Long-term elevation of blood pressure characterizes hypertension, an entity of extremely significant effects on renal structure and function. Specifically, chronic hypertension mechanically stresses the glomeruli and kidney vasculature, leading to changes such as glomerulosclerosis and nephrosclerosis. Such structural changes alter the normal architecture of the kidney, rendering it dysfunctional in performing its fundamental functions, such as filtration and waste elimination. Because glomerular capillaries undergo hypertrophy and ensuing apoptosis due to continuous pressure overload, the filtration surface is significantly decreased, ultimately resulting in reduced kidney function. The impact of chronic hypertension extends beyond function; it carries structural consequences, placing people at risk for chronic kidney disease (CKD) and end-stage renal disease (ESRD), so effective management and treatment in individuals with hypertension (Haidich et al., 2017) is important. The pathophysiology of kidney injury progression is best illustrated in the context of the mechanisms of various antihypertensive drugs. Certain medications, such as renin-angiotensin system inhibitors (RASI), have been discovered to cause magnificent renoprotection and are noted for their ability to oppose structural kidney damage with the coexistence of hypertension. Evidence from observational studies demonstrates that RASI use can slow the progression of kidney injury through the inhibition of glomerular hypertension and hyperfiltration, culprits that become exacerbated with long-term high blood pressure. Furthermore, RASI combinations with other antihypertensive drug classes, such as calcium channel blockers, have been studied, with multifaceted impacts on renal outcomes. This therapeutic approach highlights the importance of personalized antihypertensive treatment in preserving kidney function and integrity in hypertensive patients (Haidich et al., 2017). With diabetic nephropathy, the long-term effects of hypertension are compounded by the metabolic disturbances inherent to diabetes.

Studies have shown that elevated blood pressure exacerbates diabetic renal injury in mice through mechanisms involving the disruption of the angiotensin-converting enzyme 2 (ACE2) pathway and the upregulation of pro-fibrotic molecules, such as fibronectin. While moderate doses of certain antihypertensive medications can enhance renal injury by enhancing protective mechanisms in the kidney, the use of enormously excessive doses paradoxically may exacerbate renal damage and lead to increased impairment. This nuanced mechanism represents an exquisitely balanced state between therapeutic efficacy and injury, for which caution must be exercised in managing blood pressure in diabetic individuals to avoid adverse renal outcomes (Figure 6.6).

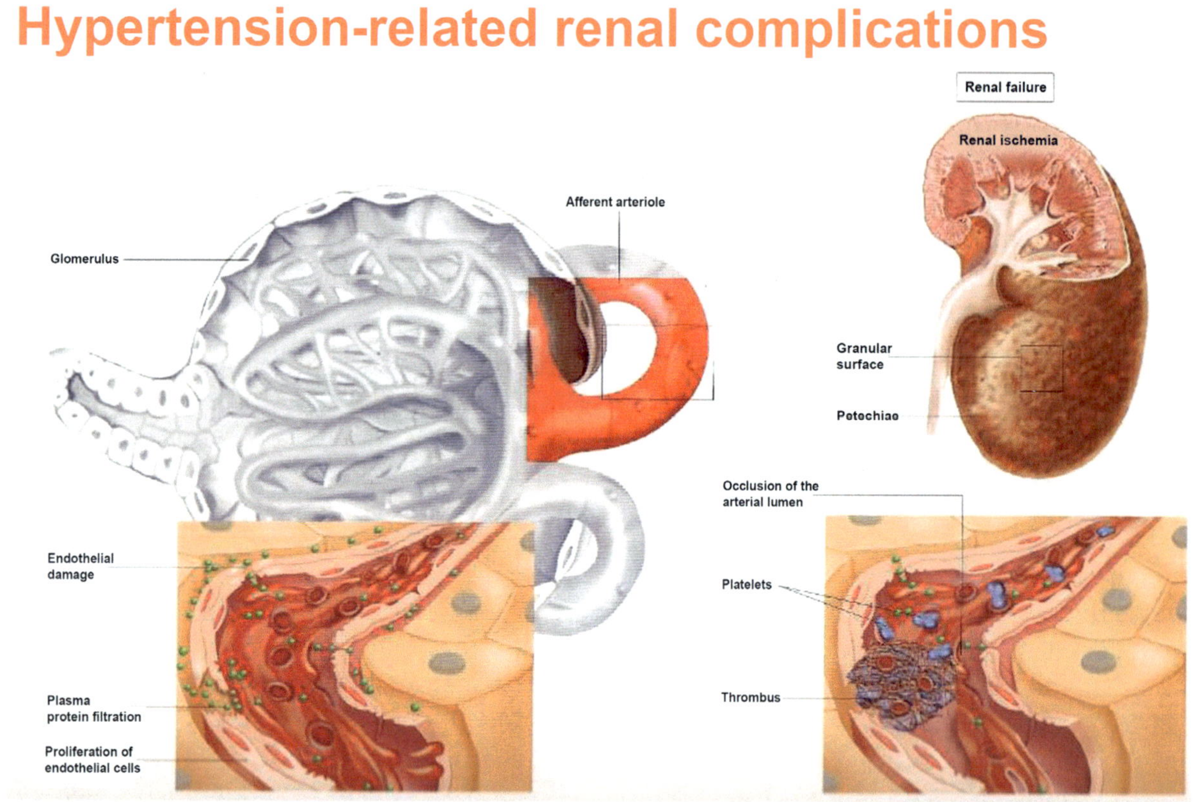

Figure 6.6. Consequences of chronic hypertension on kidney structure.

Source: https://s3.amazonaws.com/libapps/accounts/51387/images/Hypertension.jpg.

6.2. Pathophysiology of Diabetic Nephropathy

The pathophysiology of diabetic nephropathy (DN) can be complex and multi-factorial, but is largely due to the deleterious effects of chronic hyperglycemia. Exposure to chronic hyperglycemia leads to metabolic derangements with far-reaching consequences for renal structures, amongst various changes that occur, one such change is the formation of advanced glycation end products (AGEs), which trigger inflammation and fibrosis in the kidney. These alterations affect the glomerular filtration barrier, resulting in increased permeability and proteinuria, a feature of DN. Perhaps significantly, the combined interaction of hyperglycemia and hypertension increases renal damage, calling for an understanding of the subtler details of this interaction. Identifying the molecular mechanisms involved is essential for designing specific therapeutic interventions that can prevent the progression of nephropathy and preserve renal function in diabetic patients. Hypertension, strongly linked with diabetes and critical in the pathophysiology of DN, is a significant risk factor that facilitates renal deterioration. The interaction between elevated blood pressure and diabetic metabolic derangement can stimulate various mechanisms of injury to contribute to kidney damage. Of utmost significance is the stimulation of the RAAS, causing vasoconstriction, inflammation, and renal fibrosis. Evidence indicates that angiotensin II, specifically, has been known to enhance the production of profibrotic cytokines like transforming growth factor-beta (TGF-β), hence leading to glomerulosclerosis as well as tubular damage. The ensuing hemodynamic effects not only augment hypertension but also create a vicious cycle of renal damage and render it even more difficult to control patients with both these conditions. Therefore, an integrated perspective on these concurrent pathways is crucial for directing clinical interventions that treat both diabetes and hypertension. Advanced molecular research has further elucidated the pathophysiological mechanisms of DN, particularly through the mechanism of microRNAs. There is evidence that urinary microRNA profiles are modified by the progression of renal disease stages in patients with Type 1 diabetes. For instance, the levels of certain microRNAs were found to vary significantly between patients with early microalbuminuria and those with overt nephropathy, indicating their potential utility as disease stratification biomarkers. These microRNAs are involved in the modulation of critical biological pathways essential for growth factor signaling and renal fibrosis, established factors in nephropathy. By examining these microRNA profiles, researchers aim to identify new therapeutic targets with the potential to reorient disease progression and augment patient outcomes for diabetes. Identifying these correlations highlights the potential of translating molecular knowledge into clinical practice, offering promise for improved interventions in diabetic nephropathy (Eckardt et al., 2019; Krupa et al., 2013) (Figure 6.7).

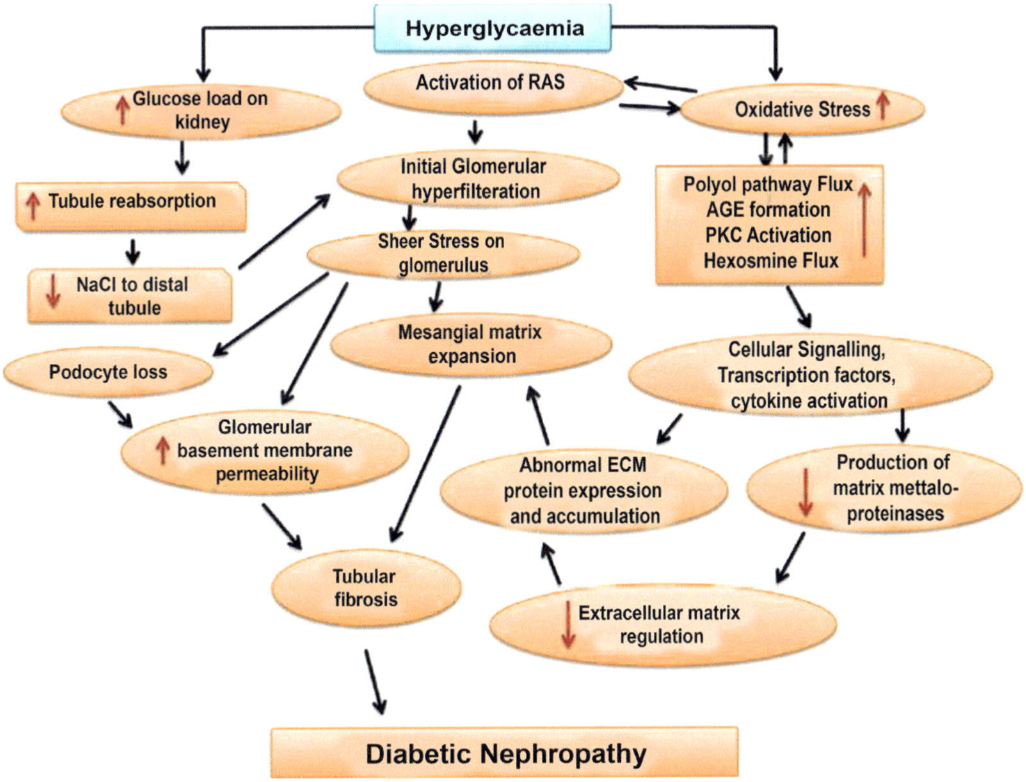

Figure 6.7. Pathophysiology of diabetic nephropathy.

Source: https://www.researchgate.net/profile/Agnieszka-Najda/publication/356748691/figure/fig3/AS:1102789392506880@1639936888247/Pathophysiology-of-Diabetic-Nephropathy-Hyperglycemia-increases-both-the-glucose-load-on.png.

6.2.1. Impact of Hyperglycemia on Kidney Tissues

The relationship between hyperglycemia and its pathologic impact on kidney tissues is a central component of the way in which hypertensive and diabetic nephropathy is conceptualized. Chronic elevation in blood glucose establishes a permissive environment for kidney damage that leans toward triggering a cascade of pathologic processes. The nephron, the functional unit of the kidney, becomes susceptible to hyperglycemic stress and thus becomes disabled in its ability to filter blood and carry out numerous homeostatic processes. Such disturbance is primarily expressed through glomerular hyperfiltration, which subsequently leads to nephron hypertrophy and subsequent renal impairment. Hyperglycemia also amplifies the formation of advanced glycation end products, leading to endothelial dysfunction and inflammation, further worsening kidney damage. Therefore, the intersection of hyperglycemia and its specific impact on renal tissues is a key solution to the pathogenesis of diabetic nephropathy and warrants significant emphasis in therapeutic strategies for managing the disease. The mechanism by which hyperglycemia impacts renal tissues is intricate and multipronged. Experimental evidence suggests that one very critical point in this process is the activation of the renin-angiotensin-aldosterone system (RAAS) during hyperglycemic conditions. This system not only regulates blood pressure but also influences renal sodium transport via multiple signaling mechanisms. Increased production of angiotensin II leads to increased sodium reabsorption, which in turn results in hypertension—a common comorbidity in diabetic patients. Increased sodium retention and ensuing hypertension can also lead to tubular damage and interstitial fibrosis of the kidney, further potentiating the impact of hyperglycemia. As described in the latest literature, the interdependent interaction between sodium transport dysregulation and hyperglycemia best characterizes the systemic effects of diabetic states on renal functions, such that specific interventions are required to decrease renal damage (Guzik et al., 2018). Added to the picture of diabetic nephropathy is the role of serum and glucocorticoid-induced kinase-1 (SGK1), which plays a central modulating role in sodium transport in the kidneys. Under a hyperglycemic state, SGK1 expression and activity are also augmented, further increasing sodium reabsorption and contributing to hypertension. Not only does this excess of SGK1 impact sodium channels utilized by nephron function, such as the epithelial sodium channel (ENaC), but it also counteracts the nephrons' ability for proper filtration and waste elimination. The interplay between SGK1 and hyperglycemia becomes pivotal in assessing the cellular changes encountered in damaged renal tissues. When dysregulated, SGK1 can contribute to the development of secondary hypertension, suggesting the need for new therapeutic strategies targeting SGK1-associated pathways for diabetic nephropathy (Bland et al., 2009). Ultimately, by controlling these mechanistic pathways, therapeutic interventions could be optimized to treat individuals suffering from both diabetes and hypertension.

6.2.2. Role of Advanced Glycation End-Products (AGEs)

The role of AGE is of increasing concern in understanding the pathophysiology of diabetic and hypertensive nephropathy. AGEs are formed through a complex process involving the reaction of reducing sugars with proteins, lipids, or nucleic acids, particularly under conditions of hyperglycemia associated with diabetes. The accumulation of AGEs not only results in structural damage to renal tissues but also activates inflammatory pathways, which accelerates microvascular complications. By causing oxidative stress, AGEs play a crucial role in endothelial dysfunction and glomerular hypertension. Their pathologic impact on the renal system highlights the need for holistic therapeutic approaches that focus on inhibiting AGE accumulation and its consequences, thereby providing a preventive intervention in diabetic nephropathy alongside hypertension. Elevated levels of AGEs have been specifically found to be directly associated with the progression of kidney disease in patients with diabetes, as evidenced by studies. In particular, AGEs have been found to play a role in glomerulosclerosis, a feature of diabetic nephropathy. Upon binding to their receptor, RAGE, they trigger a cascade of inflammatory processes and exacerbate oxidative stress, ultimately leading to kidney impairment. This pathway is particularly undesirable in that diabetic and hypertensive patients have concomitant risk factors that include endothelial dysfunction and global inflammation (Matsui et al., 2010). Thus, the finding of how AGEs modulate these conditions puts into the limelight a useful area for intervention through the reduction of AGE formation and renal health. In light of the growing incidence of diabetes globally, as documented in the literature, research into the AGE-RAGE axis may reveal new therapeutic avenues towards avoiding kidney injury (Matsui et al., 2010). Furthermore, the interconnection among AGEs, hypertension, and diabetic nephropathy highlights the unified pathophysiological processes common to the three factors, which render them challenging to treat. AGEs not only promote diabetic nephropathy but also influence the progression of hypertension via mechanisms such as arterial stiffening and vascular remodeling. Diabetic hypertension significantly increases the risk of diabetic nephropathy, thus increasing the clinical necessity of reducing AGEs and their systemic effects (Guzik et al., 2018). Investigation of the AGE-RAGE pathway may provide an entry point for new therapeutic approaches targeting cardiovascular and renal protection, as existing interventions are suboptimal. The addition of targeted therapy against AGEs may serve as an adjunct to conventional therapy, offering a multi-dimensional approach to complications arising from the double burden of diabetes and hypertension, with the final aim being to improve patient outcomes and quality of life (Figure 6.8).

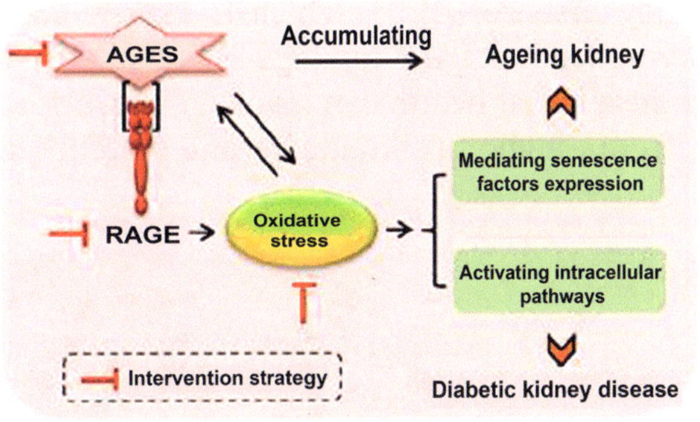

Figure 6.8. The role of advanced glycation end-products (AGEs).

Source: https://ars.els-cdn.com/content/image/1-s2.0-S0891584921003178-ga1.jpg.

6.2.3. Progression of Diabetic Nephropathy Stages

The progression of diabetic nephropathy includes the insidious deterioration of kidney function, which is traditionally categorized into five stages. Initially, patients may develop hyperfiltration when the kidneys must work harder due to elevated blood glucose levels. This first stage is not always apparent since kidney function remains within normal ranges. With long-standing diabetes, renal injury emerges, and with this emergence comes elevated urinary albumin excretion—a precursor to overt nephropathy. The development of microalbuminuria, a significant predictor of renal damage marks this stage. If left untreated, the disease will continue to advance and create macroalbuminuria. This transition highlights the importance of early detection and treatment to prevent further risks to renal function, laying the groundwork for follow-up therapies designed to sustain kidney function in the long term. As diabetic nephropathy progresses, more pronounced pathophysiologic changes occur in the renal architecture. The kidney glomeruli undergo structural modifications, such as hypertrophy and hypercellularity, which result in further reductions in glomerular filtration rate (GFR). The decrease may advance to chronic kidney disease (CKD), which is staged based on levels of GFR. Particularly when patients are moving from stage 2 to stage 3 and stage 4 CKD, careful management is called for. Strategies that promote renal health can involve the cautious delivery of medications, particularly those targeting the renin-angiotensin-aldosterone system (RAAS).

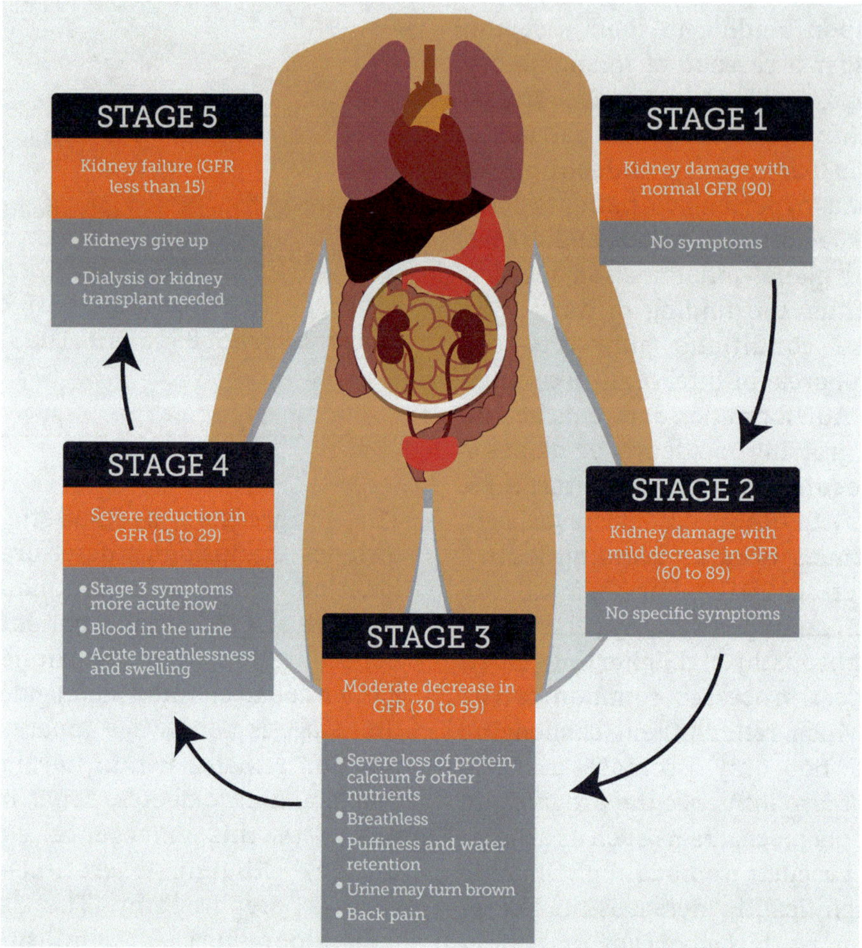

Figure 6.9. Progression of diabetic nephropathy stages.

Source: https://tambarammedicalcenter.com/wp-content/uploads/2020/11/diabetic-nephropathy.png.

These medications, such as angiotensin-converting enzyme inhibitors or angiotensin receptor blockers, have been demonstrated to decrease heart failure and risk of mortality effectively, particularly in advanced nephropathy stages, showing the importance of adequate pharmacological treatment of patients depending on their stage of CKD, as indicated by research (Johansen et al., 2018). End-stage renal disease (ESRD) is expensive, and prevention of diabetic nephropathy progression is a priority of healthcare systems worldwide. As highlighted in research, the ability to differentiate early-stage CKD with potential for progression from that without is expected to enhance clinical outcomes as well as reduce costs significantly. Early interventions, conducted in a timely manner with strict observation of the disease course, can facilitate proper management of both cardiovascular and renal diseases, resulting in favorable outcomes for patients. Conclusions made in studies lead towards the indication that the construction of an integrated model of care for diabetes patients can gain meaningful benefits, justifying the demand for careful planning efforts based on multifaceted risk factors for CKD progression. By conceptualizing CKD in primary care, healthcare systems can implement forward-thinking interventions to promote renal function, consistent with the growing body of evidence surrounding diabetic nephropathy management (Hoffmann et al., 2015) (Figure 6.9).

6.3. Risk Factors for Hypertensive Nephropathy

Hypertensive nephropathy, or renal damage from long-term high blood pressure, is more and more recognized as a significant renal complication, particularly in diabetic patients. Chronic exposure to hypertension is one of the most important risk factors since it can lead to damage of the microvasculature and glomeruli within the kidneys. This ultimately results in a gradual reduction in renal function, typically leading to end-stage renal disease if not treated. In particular, comorbid conditions accelerate the interaction between hypertension and renal damage, and obesity and hyperlipidemia are the most significant of these. Elevated body mass index (BMI) and dyslipidemia are central to the mechanisms of pathophysiology of hypertensive nephropathy and are central to prevention strategies for high-risk individuals. More recent studies also highlight the interaction between gender and the manifestation of nephropathy due to hypertension and diabetes. Findings indicate that although in general men have higher nephropathy rates than women, certain risk factors, such as obesity and hyperlipidemia, complicate this trend. Incidentally, obesity and hyperlipidemic men have a high risk of nephropathy, necessitating gender-specific predisposition-based differentiated care modalities. Besides, adherence to treatment regimens, which is typically lower in women, also plays a vital role in the development of nephropathy.

This sexual difference identifies the necessity for individualized healthcare measures that take into account biological and behavioral factors so that there is effective monitoring and intervention to prevent nephropathy onset in both sexes (Hinstersteiner et al., 2013). Finally, genetic factors also play an essential role in the risk of developing hypertensive nephropathy, particularly in specific populations. APOL1 risk alleles have been associated with kidney disease, which has indicated susceptibility among certain ethnic groups, most notably African Americans. Studies, such as those conducted by the Systolic Blood Pressure Intervention Trial (SPRINT), have shown that these genetic variables not only influence baseline renal function but are also associated with elevated urine albumin-to-creatinine ratios, an indicator of renal damage (Bild et al., 2015). Identification of these genetic predispositions underscores the necessity for continued research into targeted intervention with dual action on environmental and genetic risk factors underlying hypertensive nephropathy. The approach with both simultaneously targeted interventions represents a window towards reducing the impact of kidney disease among groups of people who are at an increased risk due to hypertension and related conditions (Figure 6.10).

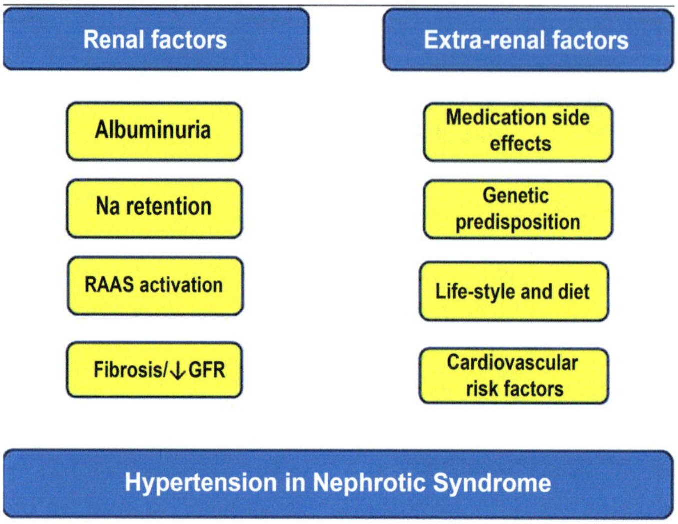

Figure 6.10. Risk factors for hypertensive nephropathy.

Source: https://www.frontiersin.org/files/Articles/456470/fped-07-00287-HTML/image_m/fped-07-00287-g001.jpg.

6.3.1. Genetic Predisposition and Family History

The relationship between family tendency and family background is critical in the elucidation of hypertensive and diabetic nephropathy. This has been repeatedly established by research to reveal that clustering of nephropathy within families indicates genetic influence as a significant contribution to the development of chronic kidney disease. Individuals with a history of end-stage renal disease (ESRD) among their families have a three- to nine-fold increased risk compared to individuals with no such familial associations. This staggering number is essential in bringing to light the intricate interface between environmental exposures and genetic predisposition in the pathogenesis of kidney diseases. Additionally, it highlights the need for early screening and treatment among affected families to avoid establishing chronic processes like diabetic nephropathy and hypertension, thereby providing healthier status in subsequent generations (Freedman et al., 2005). New evidence also suggests that genetic determinants may control the physiological processes of hypertension in individuals at risk for diabetes. There has been evidence of a considerable difference in blood pressure response to sodium consumption based on family history. Individuals who have diabetic nephropathy and whose parents have diabetes, for instance, exhibit higher systolic and diastolic blood pressure than parents without diabetic nephropathy. This salt-sensitive phenotype may serve as an intermediate marker, indicating an increased risk of subsequent nephropathy among genetically predisposed individuals. Thus, understanding these genetic and familial relationships can help clinicians devise personalized screening and treatment strategies for high-risk patients, enabling earlier interventions to curb kidney disease (Dick et al., 2017). Furthermore, localization of specific genetic loci to nephropathy provides significant information on the biology behind these conditions. Of more recent interest have been investigations identifying possible genetic markers on chromosomes for diabetic nephropathy, which may help augment our understanding of the pathophysiologic mechanisms. This study emphasizes the collaboration of multi-center consortia in gathering data on families with more than one case of diabetic nephropathy. These studies aim not only to clarify the complexities of renal pathogenesis but also to cultivate an awareness of risk factors—such as hereditary patterns—in clinical practice and public health. With full regard for genetic susceptibility, healthcare practitioners are more able to engage vulnerable populations in preventive medicine and health education, which ultimately leads to a reduction in the burden of hypertensive and diabetic nephropathy (Freedman et al., 2005) (Figure 6.11).

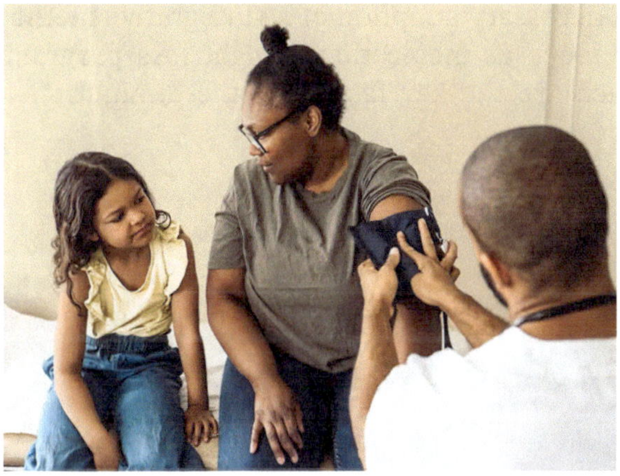

Figure 6.11. Genetic predisposition and family history for hypertensive nephropathy.

Source: https://media.post.rvohealth.io/wp-content/uploads/2022/03/mother-daughter-blood-pressure-732x549-thumbnail.jpg.

6.3.2. Lifestyle Factors: Diet and Physical Activity

Lifestyle plays a crucial role, particularly in terms of diet and physical exercise, in controlling and preventing diabetic and hypertensive nephropathy. Dietary pattern research indicates that high sodium intake and low potassium intake significantly elevate blood pressure, hence raising the risk of kidney damage in hypertensive patients. Besides, diets of processed foods are also a factor that leads to obesity, a substantial risk for diabetes and hypertension. Studies have found that the consumption of the dietary approaches to stop hypertension (DASH) diet, which emphasizes fruits, vegetables, whole grains, and low-fat milk, can significantly reduce blood pressure and overall kidney health. Such changes in nutrition not only result in more efficient control of blood pressure but also contribute to decelerating the progression of diabetic nephropathy, illustrating the contribution of nutritional treatment to clinical practice. Maintaining regular exercise is yet another important lifestyle factor that plays a crucial role in managing hypertensive and diabetic conditions. Exercise is beneficial in controlling weight, increasing sensitivity to insulin, and enhancing cardiovascular health, all of which play a significant role in blood pressure control and the prevention of diabetic nephropathy. Research has shown that both aerobic and resistance exercise can lead to substantial positive alterations in metabolic parameters, such as decreased HbA1c levels and improved blood pressure control, in diabetic patients. As patients with chronic kidney disease would usually have limited activities according to their condition, specially designed exercise regimens for moderate exercise with minimal stress are beneficial. These programs will help the patients achieve physical activity goals, improve adherence and motivation, and achieve improved outcomes to overall health in the management of nephropathy. With dietary and physical activity factors, a comprehensive method of lifestyle alteration is paramount in the avoidance of hypertensive and diabetic nephropathy complications. Correct handling must incorporate patient education on the role that lifestyle and treatment compliance play. The Joint Asia Diabetes Evaluation program also emphasizes that patients with chronic kidney disease often have poor control of risk factors, underscoring the need for an integrated approach that combines dietary management, increased physical activity, and pharmacotherapy. Establishing an enabling environment that facilitates healthy living is likely to empower patients and their families, resulting in improved health outcomes. With knowledge of disease progression and lifestyle determinants' interactions, health care professionals will be able to help their patients more in achieving their health goals and managing the adverse effects of diabetic and hypertensive nephropathy, as indicated by the findings from (Chan et al., 2016).

6.3.3. Coexisting Medical Conditions: Obesity and Hyperlipidemia

The association between hyperlipidemia and obesity is particularly significant in the context of diabetic and hypertensive nephropathy, as both are also main culprits behind the worldwide risk of cardiovascular disease and renal injury. Obesity has been defined as an increased body fat content, making the patient prone to numerous metabolic disorders like insulin resistance and dyslipidemia. Because these conditions tend to come hand in hand, their overall effect can be to aggravate hypertension and diabetes and ultimately lead to nephropathy. Moreover, the combination of obesity with lipid profile deterioration justifies the necessary adoption of an integrative method of treatment, emphasizing lifestyle modifications as much as medication. Weight loss programs have to take precedence over regular exercises, which are the key factors to the diminution of these related diseases.

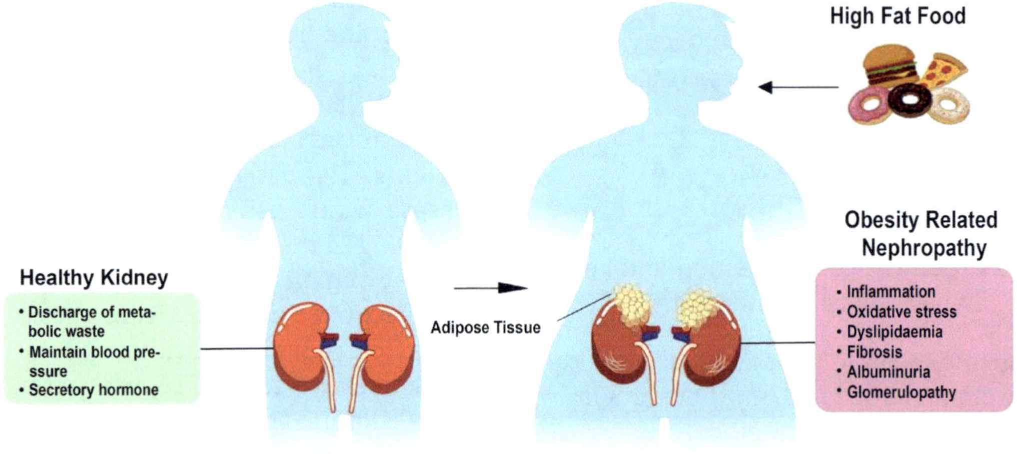

Figure 6.12. Coexisting medical conditions: obesity and hyperlipidemia in diabetic nephropathy.

Source: https://www.mdpi.com/ijms/ijms-23-00747/article_deploy/html/images/ijms-23-00747-g001.png.

The pathogenic mechanisms of these conditions illustrate the interdependent complications of their coexistence and the necessity of targeted therapeutic interventions to prevent long-term outcomes. In addition to obesity, hyperlipidemia is also a major etiologic factor in the development of diabetic and hypertensive nephropathy. Hyperlipidemia may lead to a change in lipid profile, characterized by elevated levels of low-density lipoprotein (LDL) cholesterol and triglycerides. These dyslipidemias cause endothelial dysfunction and vascular inflammation, which are key to the development of hypertension and renal damage. All individuals with this trio of obesity, hyperlipidemia, and hypertension are at increased risk of developing cardiovascular disease and chronic kidney disease. Dyslipidemia has been seen in several studies to be a common culprit for adverse outcomes in patients with diabetes, highlighting the importance of focused interventions aimed at lipid reduction. Through aggressive management of hyperlipidemia, health professionals can develop a preventive strategy that reduces the risk of hypertensive and diabetic nephropathy among vulnerable populations. The knowledge of the overlap between obesity and hyperlipidemia and their effects on hypertensive and diabetic nephropathy is significant towards embracing effective public health interventions. As national health data illustrate, age, body mass index (BMI), and ethnicity all have significance in the prevalence of these comorbidities. For instance, cohorts with higher rates of obesity and hyperlipidemia have the exact high prevalence of hypertension and diabetes (Ogunmuyiwa et al., 2023). Public health efforts must counteract these alarming trends by prioritizing education on lifestyle and early detection of metabolic disorders. Furthermore, the use of treatment regimens that act together on obesity and hyperlipidemia may enhance results and decrease the incidence of kidney complications. New approaches, such as the development of a "polypill" acting on multiple aspects of these clinical conditions, promise a multitargeted approach to significantly decrease the health impact of these related conditions (Scheen et al., 2004) (Figure 6.12).

6.4. Risk Factors for Diabetic Nephropathy

The risk determinants of diabetic nephropathy are complex, involving both modifiable and non-modifiable factors. Of most significant importance among them are glycemia and hypertension. Inadequate control of blood glucose levels manifests as advanced glycation end-products, which have the potential to cause renal injury in the long term. This is why tight glycemic control becomes crucial, as evidenced by studies that have shown the attainment of an HbA1c level of less than 7% to reduce the development of nephropathy strongly. In addition, the relationship between diabetes and hypertension cannot be overlooked; elevated blood pressure hastens renal injury in diabetic patients. Because hypertension is prevalent in diabetic patients, early management of blood pressure is essential to reduce the risk for nephropathy, particularly in patients with initial kidney disease. Therefore, interventions targeting these risk factors in the initial stages are highly significant in preventing diabetic nephropathy, leading to improved outcomes among patients. Genetic factors also play a significant role in susceptibility to diabetic nephropathy, particularly in certain populations. Genetic changes within the APOL1 gene have been identified that are associated with a higher risk of chronic kidney disease (CKD) in African Americans, a group predisposed to hypertension and diabetes as well. Specifically, the presence of APOL1 risk variants has been linked to a higher risk of lower renal function and increased urine albumin levels, both of which are markers of kidney damage. This genetic predisposition needs stricter control over diabetes and its complications in individuals carrying these variants. It is as crucial to manage environmental risk factors as it is to understand genetic ones, because then the clinician can tailor treatment to the individual's particular risk profile and thereby enhance preventive strategies against diabetic nephropathy. With respect to the psychosocial care of diabetes, compliance with treatment strategies comes across as the most crucial factor in influencing nephropathy risk. Evidence indicates that diabetic care adherence has substantial gender differences, with women reportedly having lower adherence than men. This is particularly concerning given that full adherence to drug regimens, lifestyle modification, and monitoring can strongly enhance desirable outcomes, along with preventing complications such as nephropathy. Psychological distress, as well as socio-economic problems, suffered by diabetic patients further add to the complexity of adherence, serving as barriers towards the successful management of the disease. Hence, integrating support mechanisms that address eventually, psychosocial factors become essential to improving rates of adherence, thereby reducing the possibility of diabetic nephropathy while offering an integrated system of patient care in the context of hypertensive and diabetic nephropathy (Figure 6.13).

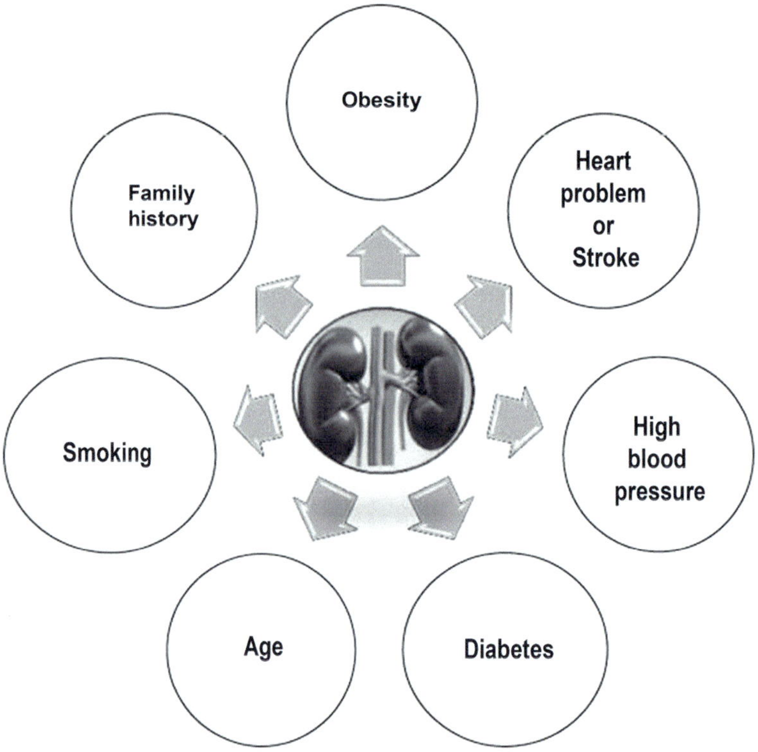

Figure 6.13. Risk factors for diabetic nephropathy.

Source: https://www.researchgate.net/publication/359691106/figure/fig1/AS:1141140996800538@1649080623755/Risk-factors-affecting-diabetic-kidney-disease.jpg.

6.4.1. Type 1 vs. Type 2 Diabetes Considerations

An understanding of the distinction between Type 1 and Type 2 diabetes is crucial in establishing their importance in nephropathy and hypertension. Type 1 diabetes, or autoimmune interference with insulin secretion in the pancreas, typically manifests during the child or adolescent period. Type 2 diabetes, which is primarily attributed to insulin resistance, is often a secondary effect of obesity and physical inactivity and tends to occur in advanced age groups. Both diabetes types have unique clinical presentations, which dictate their long-term treatment approaches. For instance, while Type 1 diabetes needs lifelong insulin therapy, Type 2 diabetes can be treated by a change in lifestyle along with drug therapy. The difference in essential pathophysiologic mechanisms between the two diabetes types warrants differential treatments, particularly when studying complications such as diabetic nephropathy, which may be caused by long-term blood glucose elevation in both types. The combination of diabetes and hypertension causes significant challenges to both Type 1 and Type 2 diabetic patients by elevating the risk of renal impairment. Hypertension also occurs most frequently with both types in association with obesity, inadequate metabolic control, and dietary habits. In Type 1 diabetes, risk for nephropathy is closely linked with duration of the disease, with more prolonged exposure being a sign of greater renal dysfunction. In Type 2 diabetes, patients usually struggle with the confluence of metabolic damage and cardiovascular risk factors, such as dyslipidemia and obesity, which can result in renal impairment. Comorbid hypertension and diabetes need effective management strategies to avert the progression of complications to end-stage renal disease. Medication compliance has recently been found to be sex-dependent, with men being more compliant with drugs for hypertension, which can potentially have essential impacts on outcome in nephropathy in all patient groups (Hinstersteiner et al., 2013). Discussing the dietary aspects in managing diabetic nephropathy brings forth landmark differences relevant to Type 1 and Type 2 diabetes. Research has highlighted the importance of dietetic intervention in retarding the evolution of nephropathy in both types, though the methods may vary. In Type 1 diabetes, glycemic control and balance of macronutrients are most important. Still, Type 2 diabetes management actually requires a concerted effort to manage weight and limit calories as a reaction to obesity. Current research suggests limiting specific food constituents, such as glycotoxins and protein-rich foods, in an attempt to combat the risk of nephropathy. The combination of micronutrients with protective effects on renal damage is another emerging field that requires further study to provide evidence-based dietary recommendations for all forms of diabetes. Understanding these nuances in diet therapy not only supports patient education but can even improve clinical outcomes in the management of diabetic nephropathy and associated hypertensive disorders (Iacobini et al., 2017) (Figure 6.14).

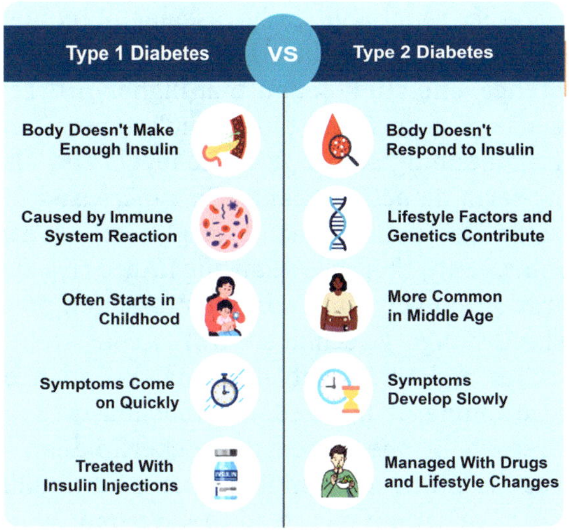

Figure 6.14. Type 1 vs. type 2 diabetes.

Source: https://images.everydayhealth.com/images/seo-graphic-content-initiative/eh--how-type-1-and-type-2-diabetes-differ-seo-graphics.png?sfvrsn=11cb28b3_3.

6.4.2. Duration of Diabetes and Glycemic Control

The duration of diabetes is also an essential factor in the pathogenesis and progression of microvascular complications, particularly nephropathy. The longer the duration of diabetes, the higher the risk of damage to the glomerular filtration apparatus, with studies proving there to be a direct association of increased diabetes duration with kidney damage. Specifically, glycemic control plays a critical role in preventing such risks, as chronic hyperglycemia provides a milieu for nephropathy. Even slight variations in glycemic indices may aggravate the progression of renal disease over time, testifying to the fact that duration of diabetes is not a straightforward temporal marker but a vital component for estimating diabetic complications. This emphasizes the need for tight glycemic control, particularly in patients with long-standing diabetes, as tight control will delay the onset and severity of nephropathy from hyperglycemia. Studies have noted that glycemic variability, rather than the mean glucose concentration, is important for predicting diabetic complications, including nephropathy. Recent systematic analyses have highlighted that the variability of HbA1c concentrations has the potential to predict renal and cardiovascular outcomes, suggesting that it is not merely the mean glucose level that matters, but also the consistency of that control from one time point to another. For instance, one study found that higher HbA1c variability is linked with an increased risk for renal disease in type 1 and type 2 diabetic patients. Consequently, clinicians would place a dual focus on maintaining stable glycemic levels and also on monitoring variability in specific terms among long-term diabetic patients. This increased focus on variability can serve as an important adjunct to standard measurements of glycemic control in assessing an individual's risk for progressive nephropathy, thereby enhancing future risk stratification and intervention. In addition, sex, diabetes duration, and glycemic control interaction provide multifaceted layers of complexity to nephropathy risk. Although glycemic control is consistently equivalent in men and women, variations in lipid profiles and treatment guideline compliance emerge as significant predictors of complications. For example, it has been established through research that risk of nephropathy is particularly increased in obese men and hyperlipidaemic women, indicating that factors outside control of glycemia influence complications. Additionally, treatment regimen adherence is found to exhibit gender variation; men tend to have improved adherence to clinical standards, thereby influencing the effectiveness of diabetic complication prevention. Therefore, comprehension of such dynamics is crucial in formulating intervention strategies that account for both the duration of diabetes and other patient-specific variables to manage and prevent diabetic nephropathy more effectively across different populations.

6.4.3. Influence of Hypertension on Diabetic Patients

Diabetes and hypertension often manifest together, subjecting the targeted individuals to an enormous health load. The combination of the two is very potent, with the prevalence of hypertension identified as twice that in diabetic patients compared to individuals who do not have the metabolic syndrome. This double occurrence enhances cardiovascular complications, which are still the leading cause of morbidity and mortality in diabetic patients. Endothelial dysfunction and inflammation of the vasculature are common factors that link these conditions, as they share similar risk factors, including obesity and dyslipidemia. The resultant high blood pressure due to hypertension complicates the already complex pathophysiology of diabetes and renders a concerning convergence of microvascular and macrovascular complications that impair renal function. It is essential to understand these associations to apply effective interventions for controlling blood pressure in diabetic patients, thereby reducing the risks of nephropathy and cardiovascular disease (Guzik et al., 2018). Hypertension affects diabetic patients more than cardiovascular issues, and it has a direct impact on renal function as well. In patients with Type 1 Diabetes, the development of hypertension is particularly harmful since hyperglycemia increases oxidative stress, leading to macro- as well as microvascular disease. It is now established that diabetic patients have a greater likelihood of developing chronic kidney disease, and hypertension accelerates its advancement. On top of this, diabetic patients' cardiac autonomic neuropathy further exacerbates the condition by deranging renal blood flow and increasing renal injury. The relationship between hypertension and compromised renal function can be a vicious cycle, as worsening renal function can lead to intractable hypertension. Therefore, detection and management of hypertension in diabetic patients is vital to preserve the kidneys and prevent the onset of nephropathy (Cappuccio et al., 2013). Management of the interaction between hypertension and diabetes calls for a combination therapeutic approach. Targeted therapies, such as aggressive insulin therapy, are beneficial for both conditions by restricting the risk of complications. The Diabetes Control and Complications Trial (DCCT) emphasizes the importance of tight glycemic control in preventing vascular complications. Additionally, newer treatments, such as glucagon-like peptide-1 (GLP-1) agonists, are on the horizon, which have the potential to improve glycemic control and also to exert vasoprotective effects.

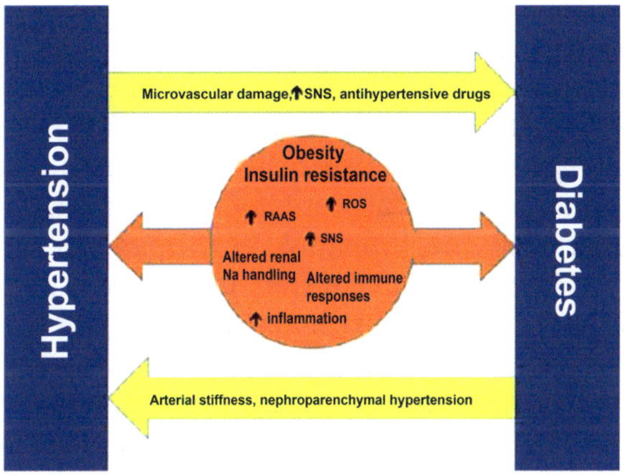

Figure 6.15. Influence of hypertension on diabetic patients.

Source: https://www.researchgate.net/profile/Rosa-Bruno/publication/283703679/figure/fig1/AS:304023967158272@1449496370445/Complex-cause-effect-relationship-between-hypertension-and-diabetes-SNS-sympathetic.png.

Such innovations reflect the need for treatment methods that are interconnected and involve both blood pressure management and metabolic control, and, in doing so, curtail the pathologic impact of hypertension in diabetic patients. The ongoing research with these therapeutic modalities holds promise for better outcomes in preventing hypertensive and diabetic nephropathy, thereby increasing the quality of life for those afflicted (Guzik et al., 2018) (Figure 6.15).

6.5. Diagnosis of Hypertensive and Diabetic Nephropathy

Diabetic and hypertensive nephropathy diagnosis is a difficult clinical presentation, and an extensive evaluation of symptoms and varied risk factors is needed. Hypertensive nephropathy is directly caused by chronic blood pressure elevation, which damages and impairs the kidneys over time. Diabetic nephropathy is primarily caused by the chronic effect of diabetes on renal structure and function. Diagnosis relies on a two-pronged strategy, comprising close observation of blood pressure, blood glucose measurement, and analysis of kidney function using serum creatinine and urine albumin-to-creatinine ratio tests. These assessments are increasingly critical since early detection of kidney impairment can trigger early intervention regimens to slow disease development and improve patient outcomes. Sex differences in the presentation and treatment of diabetic and hypertensive nephropathy complicate the diagnosis further. Previous research has indicated that nephropathy has different presentations among men and women, with the prevalence found to be higher among obese men and hyperlipidemic women. This further underscores the need for gender-sensitive approaches to clinical measurement and management. Whereas the glycemic control of women in general is as good as that of men, the incidence of nephropathy in specific subgroups diverges strongly, most significantly in the obese and hypertensive groups. By placing the diagnosis in context, considering gender differences, clinicians can more effectively define identification strategies and individualize treatment to address both the systemic and renal components of the disease, thereby optimizing guideline concordance and overall clinical outcomes. Aside from diagnostic workups initially, regular surveillance of renal function becomes essential in patients with diabetic and hypertensive nephropathy. Increased emphasis is given to the modulator roles of comorbid conditions and their effects on renal function. Overlapping disease states such as obesity and dyslipidemia, for instance, can exacerbate renal injury, as highlighted in recent studies. This common knowledge provides a sound justification for incorporating these broader cardiovascular risk factor assessments into nephrological practice. Elevated awareness of conditions like high cholesterol levels can underpin interventions such as lifestyle modification, drug therapy, and follow-up regimen. In alignment with the evidence that supports targeted medical and nutritional approaches, clinicians are urged to tailor their practice as a function of patient profile and ensure greater treatment plan and clinical guideline compliance, and one that meets the disease complexity (Hinstersteiner et al., 2013; Agabiti-Rosei et al., 2016) (Figure 6.16).

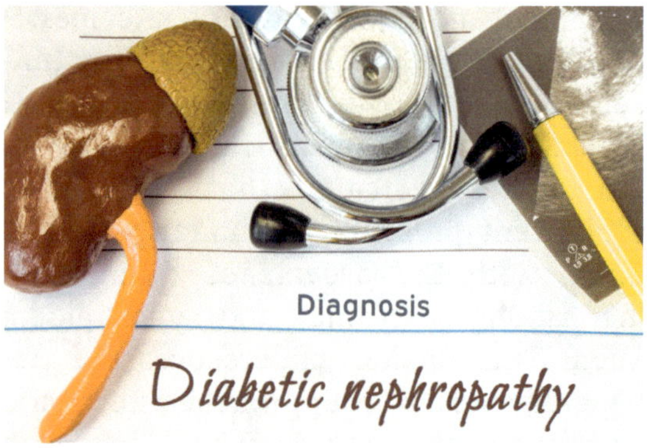

Figure 6.16. Diagnosis of hypertensive and diabetic nephropathy.

Source: https://wp02-media.cdn.ihealthspot.com/wp-content/uploads/sites/197/2019/10/iStock-908816406.jpg.

6.5.1. Clinical Symptoms and Patient History

Clinical presentations shown by hypertensive and diabetic nephropathy patients typically constitute the major predictors of the progression of the diseases. They usually include fatigue, edema, and urination changes, which can be represented as more frequent urination or more severe nocturia. These presentations are typically associated with the loss of renal function, which affects the kidneys' ability to eliminate waste. Furthermore, the worse the hypertension, the greater the risk of patients experiencing headaches and visual disturbances indicative of vascular damage within the eye's structures. Such symptoms are crucial for doctors to observe because they indicate the extent of intrarenal nephropathy and the urgency of intervention to prevent further kidney damage (Kawata et al., 2010). An extensive patient history is not necessary in assessing the clinical presentation of diabetic and hypertensive nephropathy. Yet, the patients with a previously recorded history of hypertension or diabetes are at high risk for the development of renal impairment and treatment and diagnosis are therefore more critical if done early. The duration of hyperglycemia and blood pressure control are also powerful predictors for the development of nephropathy. Family history can also determine genetic predispositions, so it is essential to monitor high-risk patients closely. Inquiring about a patient's disease history can also lead to individualized treatment regimens, which are centered on lifestyle modification and close observation of glucose and blood pressure levels, thus avoiding the onset of established renal disease (Agabiti-Rosei et al., 2016). In clinical symptom and patient history management, consideration must be given to the psychosocial issues that influence management plans. The emotional weight that conditions such as hypertension and diabetes place on patients may lead to anxiety and unpredictability of health outcomes, more so for the kidneys.

Studies have shown that worry about prognosis and coping tendencies are essential in the food behaviors of diabetic nephropathy patients (Kawata et al., 2010). If healthcare providers understand the emotional lives of their patients, they can develop a sense of communication and support that is vital in promoting treatment adherence. Improved patient outcomes are not only contingent upon physical management of symptoms but also upon concern for their psychological well-being during the course of their hypertensive and diabetic nephropathy.

6.5.2. Laboratory Tests: Urine Analysis and Blood Tests

In the diagnosis of diabetic and hypertensive nephropathy, laboratory tests such as blood work and urinalysis become valuable tools for monitoring the progression of the disease and managing treatment. Urinalysis, through proteinuria measurement, is a significant biomarker for renal injury. The identification of elevated protein content in the urine, particularly in patients with diabetes, indicates glomerular damage. Furthermore, the urine albumin-to-creatinine ratio (UACR) provides information about the extent of nephropathy. Evaluation of such parameters allows clinicians to ascertain early indicators of nephropathic alterations in patients, particularly in those groups that are genetically predisposed to kidney disease, e.g., African Americans, where APOL1 risk variants are highly associated with chronic kidney disease (Bild et al., 2015). These are complemented by blood tests, adding vital information on renal function and general health through urine analysis. The estimated glomerular filtration rate (eGFR) is derived from serum creatinine and serves as a primary measure of kidney function. For diabetic nephropathy, careful follow-up of eGFR is necessary because declining renal function indicates disease progression. Besides, blood work can measure other indicators, such as serum uric acid, which are associated with proteinuria among diabetic patients. Recent studies have brought to the forefront the association between uric acid levels and renal health. For instance, the administration of low doses of allopurinol has been shown to significantly reduce proteinuria among patients with diabetic nephropathy (Kheiri et al., 2010). Essential to comprehensive patient care, these lab tests inform prognosis and guide treatment adjustments. In aggregate, urine analysis plus blood testing is critical in effective hypertensive and diabetic nephropathy management. Through earlier detection of renal damage and ongoing assessment of disease progression, these laboratory tests optimize the clinician's ability to adjust therapy preemptively. As research continues, the understanding of specific markers and their applicability to various patient populations remains incomplete. This is a reason why repeated follow-up and customized management strategies in light of both genetic and anthropometric factors are to be followed eventually in an effort to mitigate the impact of chronic kidney disease as a result of hypertension and diabetes. Global appreciation of these laboratory results is crucial towards optimizing the outcome in chronic renal diseases (Figure 6.17).

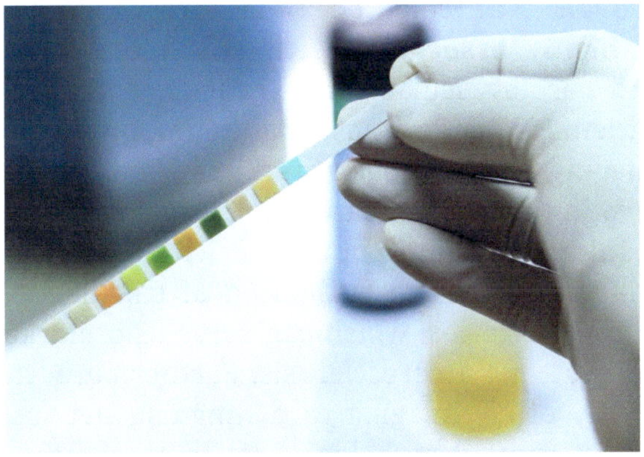

Figure 6.17. Laboratory tests.

Source: https://cdn-prod.medicalnewstoday.com/content/images/articles/319/319712/urine-sample-being-tested-with-an-indicator-strip.jpg.

6.5.3. Imaging Techniques: Ultrasound and CT Scans

The application of imaging modalities, such as ultrasound and computed tomography (CT) scans, has found a pivotal position increasingly in the diagnosis and management of hypertensive and diabetic nephropathy. Ultrasound imaging, particularly through its Doppler counterpart, provides real-time images of blood flow in the kidneys, enabling clinicians to determine renal artery stenosis and assess the kidney's structure. This is particularly meaningful since hypertensive patients are susceptible to renal injury, which in turn can lead to nephropathy. By offering a non-invasive method for studying renal structure and function, ultrasound is a vital first-line diagnostic tool that can be used to guide subsequent intervention approaches. CT scans, though, provide high-resolution imaging with the ability to delineate fine features of renal parenchyma and vascular anatomy, thus allowing identification of complications like calcification and atherosclerotic changes in renal arteries, often seen with both hypertension and diabetes. Computed tomography scans can also help in assessing renal health in diabetic patients. For instance, studies have proven that calcified renal artery plaque is highly associated with subclinical renal and cardiovascular complications in diabetic patients, again emphasizing the importance of imaging to detect such disabling conditions at a young age (Bowden et al., 2004). The high-resolution images obtained with CT scans enable a thorough evaluation of calcification in renal arteries, which can serve as a marker for systemic atherosclerosis. Furthermore, the ability of CT imaging to distinguish between different renal pathologies can help clinicians tailor management approaches. Such precision is indispensable in the management of diabetic and hypertensive nephropathy's progressive course, therefore potentially improving patient outcomes by means of efficient interventions dictated by imaging features. Moreover, integration of images from both CT scans and ultrasounds can lead to a better overall impression of kidney condition in diabetic and hypertensive nephropathy. For example, changes in renal flow can be shown with ultrasound, with associated structural changes visualized by CT imaging and related to the same flow patterns. These complementary measurements are essential, since previous studies show correlations of aortic wall motion with diseases such as diabetes and hypertension and how these impact vascular distensibility significantly (Croccia et al., 2012). Understanding such intricate relationships enables medical practitioners to make more informed risk assessments in cases of hypertension and diabetes, leading to enhanced surveillance and control measures. Ultimately, the combined strength of ultrasound and CT scans maximizes diagnostic potential while also informing preventive measures against the advancement of kidney damage in affected patients.

6.6. Treatment and Management Strategies

Effective management of diabetic and hypertensive nephropathy is a multi-component approach that places a priority on the control of hypertension and preservation of renal function. The pharmacological approaches to management are dominated by the prescription of antihypertensive drugs, which play a crucial role in preventing the cardiovascular complications associated with these conditions. The use of renin-angiotensin-aldosterone system (RAAS) blockers, such as angiotensin-converting enzyme (ACE) inhibitors and angiotensin receptor blockers (ARBs), is particularly emphasized due to their dual advantage of reducing blood pressure and protecting the kidneys. There is evidence that these drugs slow the progression of kidney disease by preventing glomerular hypertension and hyperfiltration (Barbano et al., 2016). Thus, inclusion of these drugs in therapeutic regimens is indispensable to improve outcomes in patients with diabetic and hypertensive nephropathy. Apart from pharmacologic treatment, lifestyle modification is a significant aspect of overall management regimens. blood pressure levels and improve overall well-being. Additionally, habitual exercise, weight management, and smoking cessation are among the most significant factors in reversing the multifactorial etiology of these pathologies. As high blood pressure is increasingly being recognized among young people and teenagers, as determined by recent research, healthcare practitioners must employ early detection and effective treatment methods to prevent irreversible renal injury (Agabiti-Rosei et al., 2016). These lifestyle interventions complement pharmacological therapies, providing a holistic approach that is crucial for optimizing patient outcomes. Lastly, regular monitoring of renal function and cardiovascular risk factors is essential for the ongoing management of diabetic and hypertensive nephropathy. It involves frequent measurement of serum creatinine, eGFR, and urine protein level to evaluate the efficacy of treatment programs and adjust them accordingly. Additionally, the latest trends in treating ischemic nephropathy, where optimized medical treatment is the first step, suggest that a conservative therapeutic approach to revascularization may be necessary in some cases. With increasing understanding of renal microvascular malfunction, new therapies targeting adrenergic systems and other pathways can further complement traditional strategies (Barbano et al., 2016). Such a dynamic interplay of pharmacologic, lifestyle, and monitoring interventions recognizes the significance of personalized medicine that can fulfill the challenges posed by hypertensive and diabetic nephropathy.

6.6.1. Pharmacological Interventions for Hypertension

Pharmacological interventions for hypertension play a critical role in mitigating the complications of diabetic and hypertensive nephropathy. The increasing prevalence of hypertension in adolescents and adults necessitates the application of multi-faceted treatment, particularly in its contribution to cardiovascular morbidity of long-term duration and renal damage. Various classes of antihypertensive agents, such as angiotensin-converting enzyme (ACE) inhibitors, diuretics, and calcium channel blockers, have proven successful in the management of elevated levels of blood pressure. Present guidelines lay intense stress on individualized treatment schedules, including age, comorbidities, and sex-related elements into the pharmacotherapy. Given the complex interconnection between blood pressure and renal function, blood pressure control through drug therapy not only preserves renal integrity but also reduces the risk of developing complications related to it, further substantiating the importance of aggressive management of hypertension in susceptible populations (Agabiti-Rosei et al., 2016). The interaction between diabetes and hypertension also escalates the need for effective pharmacological interventions even more. Diabetic nephropathy, a common microvascular diabetes complication, usually occurs in combination with elevated blood pressure, which makes renal impairment and cardiovascular morbidity even more problematic. Both proper glycemic control and blood pressure regulation have been found to significantly delay the development of nephropathy, emphasizing the importance of a combined therapeutic strategy. Clinical evidence further shows that certain antihypertensive medications, particularly ACE inhibitors and angiotensin receptor blockers (ARBs), have renal protective benefits, further supporting their prescription use in diabetic patients. Not only does successful blood pressure control prevent further progression of end-stage renal disease, but it also improves overall outcomes in both conditions of the patients, further supporting the call for greater awareness and intervention methods in clinical practice

(Hinstersteiner et al., 2013). Lastly, adherence to drug treatment needs to be assessed as a separate predictor of success for hypertension management among patients with diabetic nephropathy. Evidence suggests striking variations in adherence, particularly with a gender dichotomy, which may have implications for clinical outcomes in chronic disease management. For instance, nonadherence to antihypertensive treatment aimed at reducing blood pressure might result in uncontrolled blood pressure, with subsequent effects on renal status. Psychological variables, socioeconomic level, and patient education also play a significant role in adherence rates. Utilizing education interventions to address specific needs, enhancing effective provider-patient communication, and addressing special needs in high-risk populations are all key factors in achieving adherence to hypertension management programs. These measures are essential for improving the outcomes of treatment and reducing the long-term costs of diabetic and hypertensive nephropathy (Hinstersteiner et al., 2013; Agabiti-Rosei et al., 2016) (Figure 6.18).

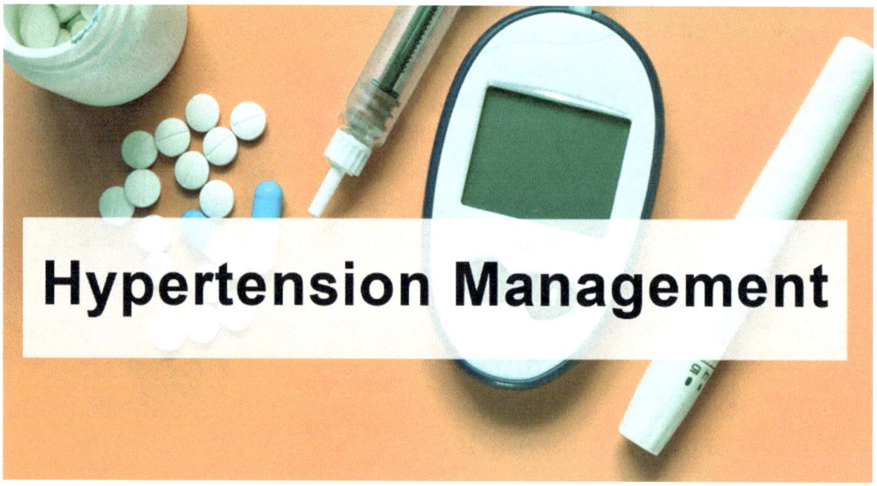

Figure 6.18. Pharmacological interventions for hypertension.

Source: https://medicaldialogues.in/h-upload/2021/08/05/158594-hypertension-management.webp.

6.6.2. Glycemic Control Strategies for Diabetes

Glycemic control is at the forefront of diabetes treatment, particularly with diabetic and hypertensive nephropathy. Pharmacologic control is not only successful but also goes hand in hand with lifestyle modifications, such as diet and exercise. Research indicates that macronutrient dietary changes, and more notably, reduced protein intake can prevent diabetic nephropathy progression by decreasing renal workload and preventing glycotoxin production, which hastens kidney damage. Moreover, these approaches also enable an all-encompassing strategy for diabetes control, not only for blood glucose but also for hypertension and dyslipidemia, two significant risk factors in DN. By combining dietary corrections with conventional therapy, the potential for positive outcomes in patients is greatly improved, demonstrating the merit of a multifaceted model of treatment for the multivariable conditions of diabetic kidney disease and its related comorbidities (Iacobini et al., 2017). In addition to nutritional management, patient education is also a significant consideration for optimal glycemic control. By way of educational programs, diabetic patients can be empowered by being given information regarding disease control, including self-blood glucose monitoring, the necessity of an adequate diet, and potential diabetic control complications. A trial evaluating the effect of intensive treatment and education regimens showed significant reductions in HbA1c and LDL cholesterol levels among participants, supporting the efficacy of patient-centered care in achieving glycemic control. This is particularly crucial in concomitant disease patients, such as those with hypertension, where successful diabetes education may help in better drug and lifestyle compliance and thus reduce the risk of developing more severe complications, such as diabetic nephropathy (Rao et al., 2015). The overlap of glycemic control strategies with nephropathy risk underscores the need for personalized therapeutic interventions. For instance, when combined with traditional glucose-lowering medications, incorporating lifestyle modifications such as increased physical activity can enhance metabolic health and increase insulin sensitivity. Research shows that structured exercise programs, aside from improving blood glucose management, also play a crucial role in lowering blood pressure, which is essential for preserving renal function. As diabetic nephropathy is typically a slow disease that is glycemic fluctuation-dependent, ongoing monitoring and compensatory action become the priority. Thus, a comprehensive and informed management plan that involves glycemic control through diet, education, and exercise makes a significant contribution to minimizing the risk of diabetic nephropathy and ultimately sustaining renal function and patients' quality of life (Iacobini et al., 2017) (Figure 6.19).

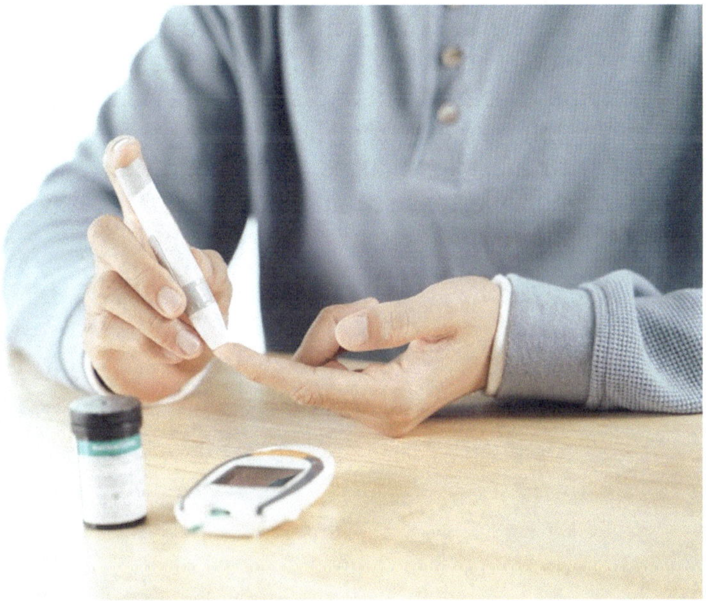

Figure 6.19. Glycemic control.

Source: https://asahealthcare.in/assets/uploads/service-48.jpg.

6.6.3. Lifestyle Modifications and Patient Education

Control of diabetic and hypertensive nephropathy is best managed with a multidisciplinary intervention, which, first and foremost, involves lifestyle modification and patient education. Patients are encouraged to adopt healthier diets, engage in regular exercise, and maintain a stable weight. Consuming a diet rich in fruits, vegetables, whole grains, and low-fat dairy products, while avoiding salt and saturated fats, has been shown to reduce blood pressure and improve glycemic control significantly. This is particularly relevant for patients like MB, whose pre-diabetic conditions, such as dyslipidemia, pose a high risk of cardiovascular complications. Furthermore, exercise not only aids in weight management but also enhances the body's physiological response to insulin, which helps to mitigate the adverse effects of diabetes and hypertension. With targeted patient education, clinicians can prepare patients to effectively incorporate these lifestyle changes into their management regimen, providing a foundation for sustained health benefits. Patient education extends beyond exercise and dietary modification to include education about the interconnection between diabetic complications and hypertension. One such example is that poorly controlled hypertension hastens the progression of diabetic nephropathy, which is essential for patient compliance. The patient must be educated about their condition and learn how to manage their own health. With such conditions as diabetic nephropathy being a significant cause of kidney failure, there is a need for awareness on prevention (MacKenzie et al., 2019). Education programs that emphasize the effects of high blood pressure and the importance of regular check-ups can stimulate patients to take proactive steps in maintaining their health. In addition, data regarding potential complications can instill a sense of urgency in adopting a new lifestyle, and patients are more likely to embrace self-care practices. Ultimately, practitioners must strive to create an enabling environment for patients as they navigate lifestyle modifications. This involves building tailored action plans taking into consideration a patient's own situation, e.g., work commitments and stress levels, of special relevance to such patients as MB with demanding professions (Abela et al., 2006). Support groups, counseling, or lifestyle coaching may be used to create additional stimulus, enabling patients to learn from and share experiences with one another. Furthermore, routine follow-up and reinforcement from healthcare professionals can help ensure patients' long-term compliance with lifestyle changes. With education and support, health practitioners can regimens for preventing hypertensive and diabetic nephropathy, thereby effectively enhancing patient outcomes and quality of life.

SUMMARY

The pathophysiological heterogeneity of hypertensive and diabetic nephropathy is indicative of an urgency for efficient diagnostic and therapeutic intervention. Considering these conditions leading to progressive renal damage, it is crucial to develop a better understanding of the underlying biomarkers that account for renal impairment. The newer methods of urinary proteomics have been found promising in identifying specific protein alterations associated with kidney disease progression. These findings suggest that urinary biomarkers are a more sensitive and specific test than traditional tests, hence improving nephrology clinical decision-making (Magalhães et al., 2016). These advancements are essential to create targeted interventions that could reverse or stabilize diabetic and hypertensive kidney injury. Microvascular health is also highlighted as a crucial determinant of the progression of diabetic nephropathy. Evidence suggests that reduced capillary density is a major initiating factor leading to kidney disruptions characteristic of metabolic syndrome (Dendorfer et al., 2012). This understanding of drugs like pioglitazone, which helps preserve the integrity of capillaries even in stable glycemic control, highlights a central mechanism of therapy. This finding is beneficial, as it teaches that microvascular integrity may be preserved beyond glucose control by molecular mechanisms. Thus, it provides the opening for pharmacologic intervention to reverse nephropathy in hypertensive and diabetic individuals with a potential reduction of end-stage renal disease burden. Ultimately, hypertensive and diabetic nephropathy is a two-edged sword that calls for multi-disciplinary effort through dynamic research and clinical innovation. The scope for utilizing developed biomarkers by urinary proteomics and maintaining microvascular architecture is a futuristic paradigm for nephrology. Combating these dual disorders requires not only an understanding of risk factors at the individual level but also an awareness of the synergistic effect on renal function. As more research unearths the complexities of these disorders, the need to close the gap between scientific knowledge and pragmatic clinical practice that can effectively treat and still prevent nephropathy's progression in vulnerable populations is more crucial than ever.

The interplay between diabetes and hypertension significantly augments the risk of developing nephropathy, and therefore, close observation and intervention protocols are required. Recent investigations highlighted the rising trend of hypertension, particularly in children and adolescents, and its chocking potential to augment renal impairment. Through establishing a more comprehensive understanding of the clinical significance of isolated systolic hypertension and of its clustering with other cardiovascular risk factors, we can better appreciate the impact of these conditions on kidney function. This data enables medical professionals to adopt an integrated approach that includes early diagnosis of high blood pressure among the young, resulting in improved clinical outcomes for patients at risk of diabetic and hypertensive nephropathy (Magalhães et al., 2016). In addition to information on the implications of hypertensions, new approaches in urinary proteomics provide a useful diagnostic tool for hypertension and diabetic nephropathy-related kidney disease. Several studies have highlighted the potential of biomarkers in urine, such as collagen breakdown products and uromodulin, for understanding underlying disease mechanisms in the future. Such biomarkers offer greater sensitivity and specificity than conventional diagnostic methods, suggesting a shift in paradigms in clinical practice. The integration of urinary proteomics into routine testing may enhance decision-making and prognostic evaluation in patients with nephropathies, ultimately leading to more personalized therapeutic management and better control of hypertensive and diabetic conditions (Magalhães et al., 2016). Lastly, hypertensive and diabetic nephropathy treatment needs a multidisciplinary strategy involving lifestyle modifications and drug therapy. Due to the complexity involved in these interrelated disorders, clinicians have a responsibility to apply evidence-based practice guidelines that integrate vast amounts of knowledge derived from both scientific research and clinical experience. Prioritization of therapy with proven interventions, including angiotensin-converting enzyme inhibitors and strict glycemic control, can substantially decrease nephropathy progression. Further, policy and public health education interventions, as well as increased screening and care among vulnerable populations such as children and adolescents, are required. These integrated strategies underscore the global collaborative effort necessary to mitigate the burden of diabetic and hypertensive nephropathy and optimize patient care outcomes (Agabiti-Rosei et al., 2016).

CLOSER LOOK

UROMODULIN

Uromodulin, or Tamm-Horsfall protein, is the most common urinary protein in normal human urine and is secreted exclusively by the thick ascending limb (TAL) epithelial cells of the loop of Henle in the kidney. It is encoded as a glycoprotein, which is secreted into the tubular lumen and undergoes extensive post-translational modification before being released into the urine. While once thought to be merely a byproduct of urine, uromodulin is now recognized as a multifunctional protein with numerous roles in kidney health, immune response regulation, and protection against urinary infections and kidney stone formation. It possesses a structure that forms high-molecular-weight polymers, enabling it to function as a capturer of pathogens and a regulator of mineral balance in the urinary tract.

Functionally, uromodulin serves several protective functions in the renal and urinary tracts. Among its significant roles is defending the urinary tract against infection by adhesively binding to uropathogenic bacteria such as *Escherichia coli* and hindering them from attaching to the urothelium. Uromodulin prevents the crystallization as well as the aggregation of calcium oxalate and other minerals, therefore averting the crystallization and aggregation of calcium oxalate and other minerals, thereby preventing kidney stone formation. Within renal tubules, it plays a crucial role in balancing salt and water absorption by controlling ion transporters and signaling pathways. Uromodulin is also immunomodulatory in function, as it can bind to and affect the function of numerous immune cells, thereby controlling local immune responses and maintaining the integrity of the renal environment.

Clinically, uromodulin is gaining broad interest as a biomarker for renal disease and function. Under normal conditions, urine uromodulin is very high in normal subjects and correlates with intact TAL function. Lower levels of urinary uromodulin have been reported to correlate with all forms of kidney disease, including acute kidney injury (AKI), chronic kidney disease (CKD), and tubulointerstitial disease, and are linked to impaired tubular function. Conversely, elevated serum concentrations of uromodulin may indicate early tubular stress or damage before changes in glomerular filtration rate are detectable. Therefore, serum and urinary uromodulin testing are being explored as potential tools for the early diagnosis of kidney disease, risk stratification, and monitoring of disease progression.

Genetically, mutations in the UMOD gene, which encodes uromodulin, are associated with a group of rare inherited kidney disorders known as autosomal dominant tubulointerstitial kidney disease (ADTKD-UMOD). The mutations result in aberrant uromodulin proteins that are misfolded and accumulate in the endoplasmic reticulum of tubular cells, leading to cellular stress, inflammation, and chronic kidney injury. Patients with ADTKD-UMOD have insidiously progressive renal failure, hyperuricemia, and early-onset gout and typically develop ESRD in mid-adulthood.

References

1. Abela, J. C. (2006). A case of hypertension. https://core.ac.uk/download/46602086.pdf (accessed on 25th June 2025).
2. Lurbe, E., Agabiti-Rosei, E., Cruickshank, J. K., Dominiczak, A., Erdine, S., Hirth, A., Invitti, C., Litwin, M., Mancia, G., Pall, D., Rascher, W., Redon, J., Schaefer, F., Seeman, T., Sinha, M., Stabouli, S., Webb, N. J., Wühl, E., & Zanchetti, A. (2016). 2016 European Society of Hypertension guidelines for the management of high blood pressure in children and adolescents. *Journal of Hypertension*, *34*(10), 1887–1920. https://doi.org/10.1097/hjh.0000000000001039Antunes, T., Briones, A. M., Burns, K., Callera, G. E., et al. (2016). Differential renal effects of candesartan at high- and ultra-high doses in diabetic mice: Potential role of ACE2/AT2R/Mas. https://core.ac.uk/download/74229872.pdf (accessed on 25th June 2025).
3. Barbano, B., Cianci, R., Coppolino, G., Di Mario, F., et al. (2016). Pharmacological effects of RAAS blockade in ischemic nephropathy. https://core.ac.uk/download/74319200.pdf (accessed on 25th June 2025).
4. Bild, D. E., Divers, J., Freedman, B. I., Hawfield, A., et al. (2015). Apolipoprotein L1 gene variants associate with prevalent kidney but not prevalent cardiovascular disease in the Systolic Blood Pressure Intervention Trial. https://core.ac.uk/download/323070317.pdf (accessed on 25th June 2025).
5. Bland, R., Hills, C. E., & Squires, P. E. (2009). SGK1 in the kidney: Disrupted sodium transport in diabetes and beyond. https://core.ac.uk/download/20442635.pdf (accessed on 25th June 2025).
6. Bowden, D. W., Carr, J. J., Dryman, B. N., Freedman, B. I., et al. (2004). Renal artery calcified plaque associations with subclinical renal and cardiovascular disease. https://core.ac.uk/download/pdf/82200764.pdf (accessed on 25th June 2025).
7. Cappuccio, F., Ceriello, A., Genovese, S., Schnell, O., et al. (2013). Type 1 diabetes and cardiovascular disease. https://core.ac.uk/download/19553374.pdf (accessed on 25th June 2025).
8. Chan, J. C., Li, X., & Luk, A. O. Y. (2016). Quality of care in patients with diabetic kidney disease in Asia: The Joint Asia Diabetes Evaluation (JADE) Registry. https://core.ac.uk/download/80961822.pdf (accessed on 25th June 2025).
9. Christensen, P. K., Clausen, P., Feldt-Rasmussen, B., Hommel, E., et al. (1999). Impaired autoregulation of the glomerular filtration rate in patients with nondiabetic nephropathies. https://core.ac.uk/download/pdf/81150428.pdf (accessed on 25th June 2025).
10. Croccia, M. (2012). Influence of cardiovascular risk factors on aortic wall motion after repair of type A aortic dissection: An ECG-gated CT study. https://core.ac.uk/download/14705456.pdf (accessed on 25th June 2025).
11. Davies, M. (2024). Abstracts of the South African Renal Congress 2024, held in Johannesburg, South Africa, 18–20 October 2024. https://core.ac.uk/download/642003950.pdf (accessed on 25th June 2025).
12. Dendorfer, A., Arany, Z., Ashoff, A., Baraka, A., Battegay, E. J., Billiet, L., Biscetti, F., et al. (2012). Pioglitazone prevents capillary rarefaction in streptozotocin-diabetic rats independently of glucose control and vascular endothelial growth factor expression. https://core.ac.uk/download/16432530.pdf (accessed on 25th June 2025).

13. Dick, B., Ferrari, P., Frey, F., Gorska, R., et al. (2017). Salt-sensitive blood pressure—An intermediate phenotype predisposing to diabetic nephropathy? https://core.ac.uk/download/85222280.pdf (accessed on 25th June 2025).

14. Eckardt, K. U., & Sievers, L. K. (2019). Molecular mechanisms of kidney injury and repair in arterial hypertension. https://core.ac.uk/download/222574030.pdf (accessed on 25th June 2025).

15. Freedman, B. I., Moossavi, S., & Satko, S. G. (2005). Genetic factors in end-stage renal disease. https://core.ac.uk/download/pdf/81117978.pdf (accessed on 25th June 2025).

16. Gorst, C., Cavalot, F., Kwok, C. S., Kontopantelis, E., Foo, R. S., Heatlie, G., Hermann, M., et al. (2015). Long-term glycemic variability and risk of adverse outcomes: A systematic review and meta-analysis. https://core.ac.uk/download/41991337.pdf (accessed on 25th June 2025).

17. Guzik, T. J., Petrie, J. R., & Touyz, R. M. (2018). Diabetes, hypertension, and cardiovascular disease: Clinical insights and vascular mechanisms. https://core.ac.uk/download/153444565.pdf (accessed on 25th June 2025).

18. Haidich, A. B., Lasaridis, A. N., Mark, P. B., Pikilidou, M., et al. (2017). Changes in kidney function in a population with essential hypertension in real life settings. https://core.ac.uk/download/82965093.pdf (accessed on 25th June 2025).

19. Heerspink, H. J. L., Mischak, H., & Pena, M. J. (2016). Proteomics for prediction of disease progression and response to therapy in diabetic kidney disease. https://core.ac.uk/download/84148392.pdf (accessed on 25th June 2025).

20. Hinstersteiner, J., Johnson, J., Kamyar, M. R., Kautzky, A., et al. (2013). Sex-specific differences in cardiovascular risk in type 1 diabetes: A cross-sectional study. https://core.ac.uk/download/9843456.pdf (accessed on 25th June 2025).

21. Hoffmann, A., Levin, A., Levin, A., Levin, A., Marengoni, A., Otero, A., Qaseem, A., et al. (2015). Early chronic kidney disease: Diagnosis, management and models of care. https://core.ac.uk/download/35435599.pdf (accessed on 25th June 2025).

22. Iacobini, C., Menini, S., Pesce, C., Pugliese, G., et al. (2017). Dietary interventions to contrast the onset and progression of diabetic nephropathy: A critical survey of new data. https://core.ac.uk/download/80314820.pdf (accessed on 25th June 2025).

23. Johansen, K. L., Ku, E., Lin, F., McCulloch, C. E., et al. (2018). Use of antihypertensive agents and association with risk of adverse outcomes in chronic kidney disease: Focus on angiotensin-converting enzyme inhibitors and angiotensin receptor blockers. https://core.ac.uk/download/323072344.pdf (accessed on 25th June 2025).

24. Kapke, D. R. (2015). Childhood type II diabetes: The risks and complications. https://core.ac.uk/download/58826199.pdf (accessed on 25th June 2025).

25. Kawata, C., Makino, H., Shikata, K., Sumiyoshi, Y., et al. (2010). Influencing factors for dietary behaviors of patients with diabetic nephropathy. https://core.ac.uk/download/12546794.pdf (accessed on 25th June 2025).

26. Kheiri, S., Momeni, A., Seirafian, S., Shahidi, S., et al. (2010). Effect of allopurinol in decreasing proteinuria in type 2 diabetic patients. https://core.ac.uk/download/143841902.pdf (accessed on 25th June 2025).

27. Krupa, A., Micera, A., Phillips, A. O., John, B., Argyropoulos, C., Lunn, D., et al. (2013). Urinary microRNA profiling in the nephropathy of type 1 diabetes. https://core.ac.uk/download/12214608.pdf (accessed on 25th June 2025).

28. MacKenzie, J. (2019). Role of anti-hypertension class drugs in the pathogenesis of diabetes mellitus complications. https://open.bu.edu/bitstream/2144/36583/7/MacKenzie_bu_0017N_14509.pdf (accessed on 25th June 2025).

29. Magalhães, P., Mischak, H., & Zürbig, P. (2016). Urinary proteomics using capillary electrophoresis coupled to mass spectrometry for diagnosis and prognosis in kidney diseases. https://core.ac.uk/download/74362547.pdf (accessed on 25th June 2025).

30. Matsui, T., & Yamagishi, S. (2010). Advanced glycation end products, oxidative stress and diabetic nephropathy. https://core.ac.uk/download/pdf/8460747.pdf (accessed on 25th June 2025).

31. Ogunmuyiwa, O. (2023). Hypertension and diabetes comorbidity: Factors that are associated with their joint occurrence. https://core.ac.uk/download/571193846.pdf (accessed on 25th June 2025).

32. Rao, L. S. (2015). Redesigning treatment strategies in type 2 diabetes by treatment intensification and patient education. https://core.ac.uk/download/33562651.pdf (accessed on 25th June 2025).

33. Scheen, A. (2004). Management of the metabolic syndrome. http://orbi.ulg.ac.be/bitstream/2268/11710/1/METABOLIC%20SYNDROME%20MANAGEMENT%202.pdf (accessed on 25th June 2025).

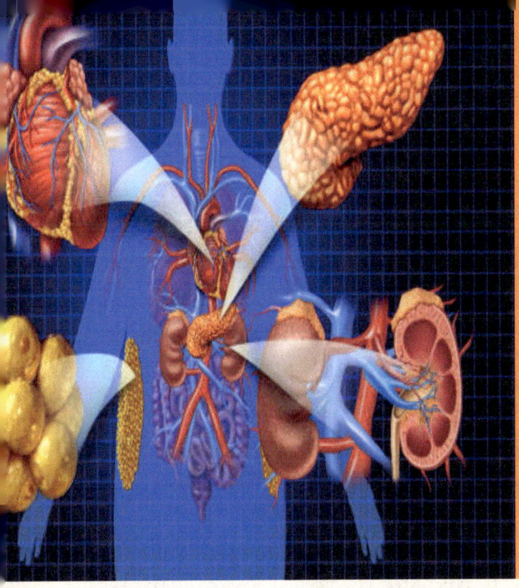

Chapter 7

RENAL INVOLVEMENT IN SYSTEMIC DISEASES

Contents

Introduction

The introduction of renal involvement in systemic diseases lays the foundation for how systemic diseases influence renal well-being. The kidneys play a crucial role in maintaining homeostasis, filtering waste products, regulating electrolyte balance, and controlling blood pressure. The effect of systemic diseases on renal function in their occurrence can lead to severe complications, including renal failure. Diseases such as systemic lupus erythematosus (SLE) show the intricate relationship between systemic disease and renal pathology. Research into SLE manifestations, particularly those involving anti-ribosomal P antibodies, underscores the importance of investigating renal implications among SLE patients. A recent study indicated that single anti-P antibodies are inversely correlated with the incidence of lupus nephritis, suggesting that some immunologic factors may contribute to differing risks for renal complications in systemic diseases (Elghali et al., 2025). The systemic nature of diseases such as periodontitis can also explain the renal involvement that ensues from chronic inflammation.

Recent research using animal models has shown that induced periodontal inflammation can have systemic effects, including alterations in renal function parameters. For instance, researchers established significant alterations in biochemical markers following the induction of periodontitis in female rats, raising concerns about the potential systemic effects of chronic inflammatory diseases on renal function. The convergence of inflammatory cascades across various systems highlights the interconnectedness between systemic inflammation and renal function. Such a convergence presents fertile ground for researching the relationship between systemic disease and renal disorders, shedding light on mechanisms that may inform clinical practice and recommendations for managing affected individuals (João et al., 2024).

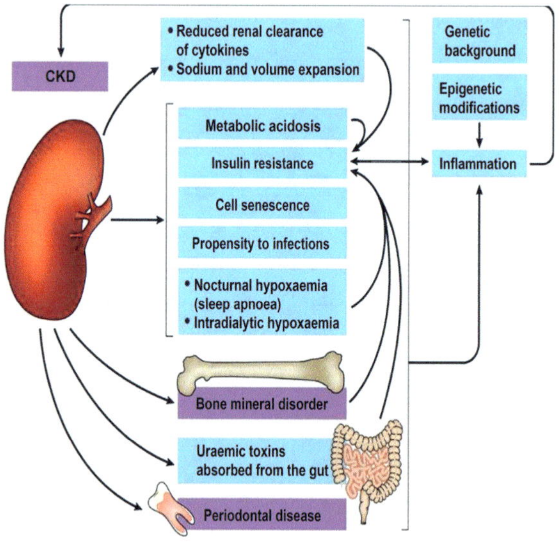

Figure 7.1. Renal involvement in systemic diseases.

Source: https://media.springernature.com/lw1200/springer-static/image/art%3A10.1038%2Fnrneph.2017.52/MediaObjects/41581_2017_Article_BFnrneph201752_Fig2_HTML.jpg.

In compiling these findings into a composite, it is crucial to consider the broader context of renal involvement in systemic diseases. Understanding the interface between systemic inflammation and renal function not only aids in the diagnosis of renal complications but also guides therapeutic interventions. By studying specific biomarkers for systemic diseases such as SLE and periodontal disease, clinicians are able to predict better the risk of renal decline in individuals affected by them. Lastly, establishing a comprehensive profile of renal involvement enables improved patient management and better outcomes in the context of systemic disease. Thus, the introduction to this essay is aimed at highlighting essential interactions between systemic disease and renal status and raising awareness of the necessity of continued research in this field to optimize care in those afflicted by these multigenerational medical issues (Figure 7.1).

Definition of Systemic Diseases

It is crucial to learn the definition of systemic diseases, as such disorders are characterized by their extensive involvement of the body, rather than being localized to a specific organ or region. Systemic diseases can affect normal homeostasis, affecting multiple organ systems, making the clinical scenario more complex. Examples are autoimmune diseases, infections, and metabolic disorders, all of which elicit complex pathophysiological reactions that can involve inflammation, deregulation of the immune response, and pathological cellular functions. The myriad manifestations of systemic illnesses make their diagnosis and control difficult since symptoms typically overlap with other illnesses. The systems biology approach to systemic disease emphasizes the interconnectedness of organs and how disturbances to one system can have cascading effects across others, frequently most severely impacting organs that are critical to fluid and electrolyte balance, as is the case with the kidneys (Ponikowski et al., 2016). The renal system is particularly susceptible to systemic disease-altered states. For instance, diabetes and hypertension are responsible for diabetic nephropathy and hypertensive renal disease, respectively, accentuating the kidneys' function as a mediator and target of systemic health. Further, systemic disorders like lupus erythematosus or vasculitis have renal involvement as a concomitant, either as glomerulonephritis or renal failure. These renal complications highlight the significance of diagnosing kidney injury at an early point in the course of systemic diseases to avert long-term morbidity. Most importantly, renal pathologies in conjunction with systemic diseases tend to complicate existing health conditions, thereby leading to a more extensive spectrum of organ dysfunction and system failure, stressing the severity of interdisciplinary management (Singer et al., 2016).

The characterization of systemic diseases, therefore, must encompass their multidimensional interactions among numerous body systems, particularly in relation to renal implications. Because systemic diseases have the potential to alter renal physiology and induce states such as chronic kidney disease or acute renal failure, there is a need for an integrated care approach to patient treatment that involves both systemic and organ-specific factors. Continuing advances in therapy and monitoring of systemic disease can maximize outcomes, particularly in terms of renal status. With a greater understanding of systemic pathologies, the introduction of additional knowledge will be essential in developing integrated management regimens that can address both the systemic features of these diseases and their direct effects on the kidney. It is by the appreciation of the multi-factorial mechanisms through which systemic diseases affect the renal system that one can enhance patient management and prognosis in clinical practice (Ponikowski et al., 2016).

Overview of Renal Involvement

The kidneys play a crucial role in the overall health of the body, and their involvement in systemic disease can often reveal the intricacy of the illness. Kidney impairment can result from numerous systemic diseases, including autoimmune diseases, infection, and metabolic disease. For instance, in systemic lupus erythematosus (SLE), the kidneys can be directly affected, leading to lupus nephritis, a serious complication. This serious complication can produce significant morbidity if not adequately controlled. The interplay between renal disease and disease activity is atypical, with the renal function altering both as a marker and a precipitant of the systemic symptoms. Increased disease activity has been associated with renal complications, and this underlines the necessity of regular monitoring and intervention to minimize long-term damage and improve patient outcomes. An appreciation of renal involvement in systemic disease is, thus, crucial for successful disease management. The role of vitamin D comes to the forefront in the context of systemic diseases, particularly those involving the kidneys. In fact, it is evidenced that vitamin D deficiency contributes to the pathogenesis of diseases like SLE, for which vitamin D has been associated with disease activity and renal manifestations. Low levels of serum vitamin D have been associated with an increased frequency of disease flare-ups and renal manifestations among SLE patients, supporting the potential that vitamin D may serve not only as a biomarker but also as a therapeutic target. Given the inverse relationship between vitamin D status and both renal function and fatigability in these patients, it should become routine to monitor vitamin D status in SLE management. Although controversy exists concerning effect and causation, treatment of vitamin D deficiency is imperative, and systemic disease requires multi-modal management, including proper assessment and supplementation policy to ensure optimal renal function and overall patient well-being (Navarro-Trivio, 2020). Another significant example of renal engagement is cardiorenal syndrome type 5 (CRS-5), where cardiac and renal failure are concurrent expressions of an associated systemic process. This model emphasizes the systemic origin of disease processes, whereby renal impairment may arise from or worsen cardiac disease. The pathophysiology of CRS-5 is multifactorial, involving numerous biochemical and hemodynamic changes that occur in response to both cardiac and renal stressors. As an example, sepsis is employed as a model to study CRS-5 in order to elucidate how inflammatory mediators can have deleterious effects on organ systems. Understanding such mechanisms is crucial for establishing effective therapeutic interventions, as early diagnosis and appropriate regimen management can significantly alter the clinical course for those afflicted with the complication. The systemic involvement of both the heart and kidneys underscores the need for an integrated strategy in patient monitoring and treatment in the context of systemic illness, thereby highlighting the interdependence of body systems in disease presentation and progression (Mehta et al., 2013).

Importance of Understanding Renal Implications

Careful familiarity with renal implications is necessary in the context of systemic disease because these conditions often come with renal involvement that may have a devastating effect on the overall outcome of patients. The kidneys have the task of maintaining homeostasis, regulating fluid balance, electrolyte composition, and eliminating waste products. Therefore, when systemic conditions such as autoimmune diseases or infections such as COVID-19 impose their action on the renal function, it could lead to serious complications such as acute kidney injury, hypertension, and chronic kidney disease. For instance, studies have reported that viral infections exert a profound impact on renal pathology, characterized by acute tubular necrosis and inflammation processes in the kidneys, as well as systemic symptoms, thereby complicating management plans and prognoses (Oprinca et al., 2024). In this regard, the identification of renal implications becomes crucial for clinicians to develop effective therapeutic plans based on renal health in the overall management of systemic diseases. Moreover, the relationship between systemic diseases and renal implications tends to form a series of complications that may further escalate existing health conditions. Such conditions as scleromyxedema pictorially illustrate such interrelations; the systemic manifestations, such as muscle weakness and dysphagia, imply underlying pathologies that may even include renal failure. Awareness of such an association may enhance diagnostic sensitivity and prompt effective management, ultimately leading to improved patient outcomes and quality of life. Additionally, renal impairment may affect drug pharmacokinetics, necessitating individualized dosage adjustments. With the complexity of such cases and their presentations on multiple levels, identifying renal implications assists healthcare workers in distinguishing between primary kidney pathologies and secondary ones secondary to systemic diseases, thereby facilitating better therapeutic targeting (Mohareb et al., 2022). Finally, a cognizant knowledge of renal implications encompasses not only the assessment of renal function but also the multidisciplinary management of patients. Collaborative efforts among nephrologists, rheumatologists, and primary care physicians become essential when managing patients with systemic diseases involving the kidneys. Through interprofessional communication, the healthcare team can create comprehensive treatment plans that encompass potential renal complications associated with systemic diseases. For example, a patient suffering from systemic sclerosis needs tests that include renal screening for any earliest signs of renal involvement because timely intervention can avoid severe implications. Such embedding of knowledge about renal implications, therefore, constitutes a necessary step toward improving healthcare quality in the context of systemic diseases with the motive of better patient outcomes as well as disease management at large (Figure 7.2).

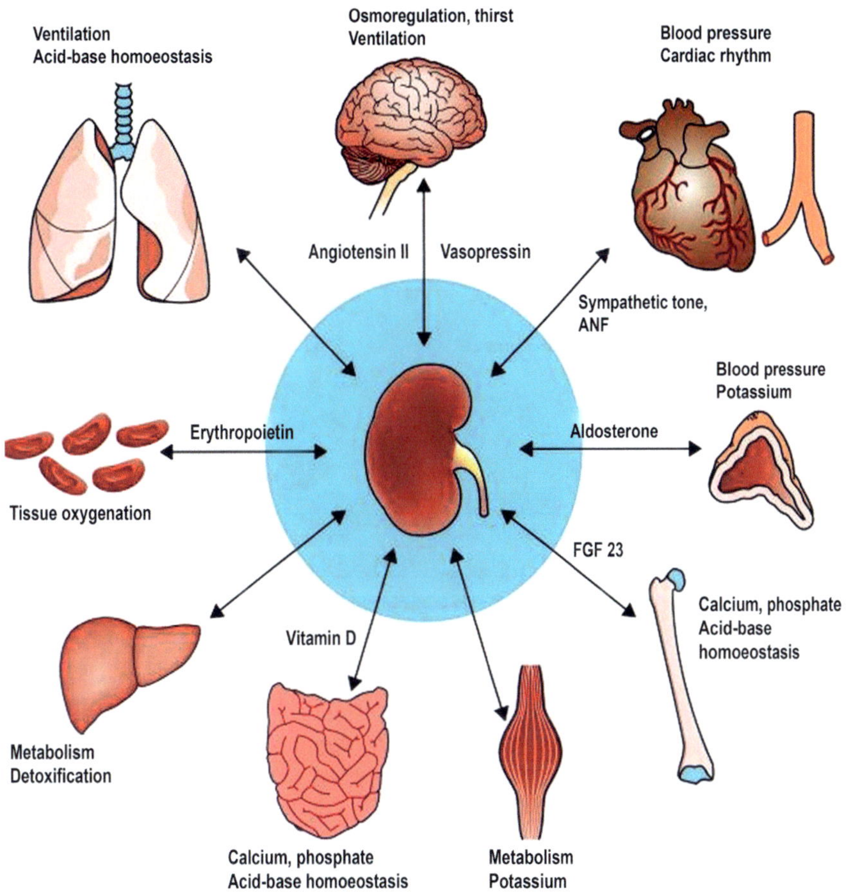

Figure 7.2. Importance of understanding renal implications.

Source: https://ars.els-cdn.com/content/image/1-s2.0-S0140673613604390-gr2.jpg.

7.1. Pathophysiology of Renal Involvement

The pathophysiology of renal disease in systemic disease is multifactorial, most commonly involving intricate interplay among renal tissue response and immune dysregulation. A good example is systemic lupus erythematosus (SLE) with glomerulonephritis (GN) being a leading cause of morbidity and mortality. In SLE, the inappropriate activation of the innate and adaptive immune system leads to the production of autoantibodies that deposit in the glomeruli, ultimately resulting in inflammation and renal damage. B lymphocyte contribution is particularly notable, as these cells have been shown to produce not only autoantibodies but also pro-inflammatory cytokines that increase renal injury. The ongoing pathological processes damage the normal renal function, manifesting as proteinuria and hypertension, and complicating the management of the overall disease in infected patients. Furthermore, the renal effects of SARS-CoV-2 infection reflect the intimate interdependence between systemic inflammation and renal pathophysiology. COVID-19 has been a poly-syndromic illness, where acute kidney injury (AKI) is a frequent complication in hospitalized patients. Both the elevation of inflammatory markers and the direct viral effects on renal cells cause damage to kidney tissues.

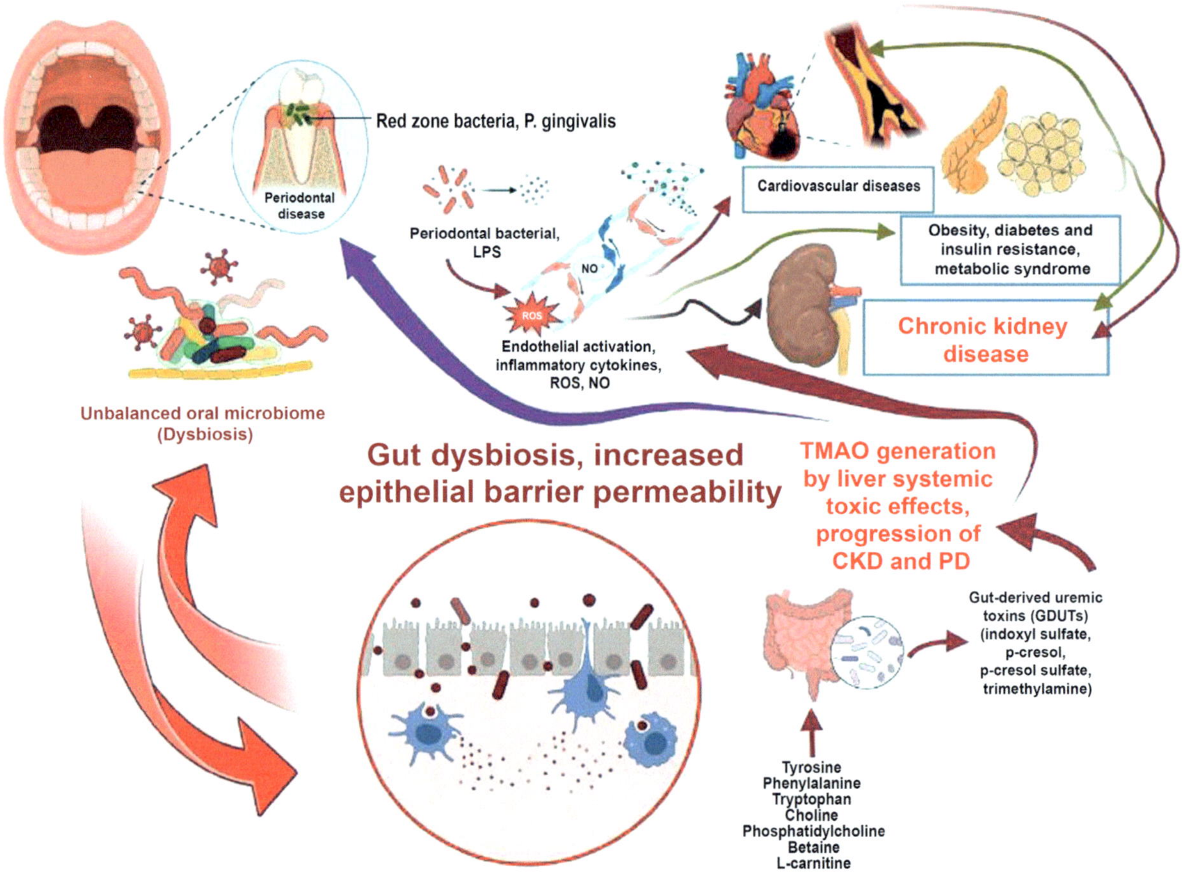

Figure 7.3. Pathophysiology of renal involvement in systemic diseases.

Source: https://pub.mdpi-res.com/biomedicines/biomedicines-11-03033/article_deploy/html/images/biomedicines-11-03033-g002.png?1699776803.

The severity of COVID-19 is immense, with almost 85% of survivors having extrapulmonary complications, including renal ones. This highlights the need for prompt clarification of the mechanisms of renal injury during systemic infections, as they may have long-term consequences for kidney function and patient outcomes (Marzoog, 2023). Lastly, inflammatory cytokines are essential in mediating renal injury in systemic conditions like SLE and COVID-19. For instance, the role of interleukin-40 (IL-40) in the pathogenesis of lupus nephritis has emerged as a critical aspect through recent research. The cytokine is reported to have altered levels among active GN patients, thereby piquing interest in its application as a biomarker of renal involvement in SLE. Elevated IL-40 in renal biopsy specimens entails its participation in immune-mediated renal architectural breakdown. Understanding such cytokines and pathways will help guide the development of therapies aimed at minimizing renal complications of systemic disease (Rizzo et al., 2022). Ultimately, targeted treatment aimed at the underlying pathophysiologic mechanisms may lead to improved outcomes in patients and more effective management of renal manifestations of systemic disease (Figure 7.3).

7.1.1. Mechanisms of Kidney Damage

An understanding of the pathogenesis of renal injury is crucial for clarifying the complex interaction between systemic disease and renal disease. Damage to the glomerulus is one such mechanism wherein podocyte function is altered and glomerular permeability is increased. Diabetes mellitus is just one instance of factors that cause hyperglycemia and lead to a cascade of biochemical reactions, ultimately resulting in the production of advanced glycation end products (AGEs). Such substances not only increase inflammation but also cause fibrosis of renal tissues, which adversely affects glomerular filtration rates in the long term. In addition, hypertensive states impose mechanical stress on renal vasculature, which causes nephrosclerosis and further exacerbates kidney damage. All of these successive insults ultimately result in the pathogenesis of chronic kidney disease (CKD), underscoring the relevance of early therapy for systemic diseases to avoid renal consequences. Another significant nephrotoxicity mechanism occurs through inflammatory and immune-mediated damage, which is well evident in infections and autoimmune conditions. As an example, acute kidney injury (AKI) may result from systemic diseases such as COVID-19, where the virus was reported to infect renal tissue to produce acute tubular damage and glomerulonephritis. The systemic inflammatory response to such infections can trigger a cascade of immune mediators that not only result in direct damage to renal cells but also induce secondary complications, such as inflammation of the vasculature. In COVID-19, inflammatory cytokines play a key role in contributing to renal injury, causing tubular cell damage and loss of renal function. The interaction between the inflammatory and kidney injury pathways underscores the need to investigate therapeutics that are targetable to affect these pathways, presenting a therapeutic option for the preservation of renal function in systemic diseases like COVID-19 (Litvinov et al., 2020). Additionally, cellular senescence within the kidneys is a critical pathway that can result in kidney injury, particularly in the context of aging and chronic disease. Research indicates that senescent cells induce a senescence-associated secretory phenotype (SASP), which amplifies inflammation and fibrosis in renal tissues, leading to functional deterioration. Mitochondrial damage and impairment of the DNA damage repair mechanism have been identified as the reasons for the acceleration of renal senescence, thereby impairing renal cell regenerative capacity. As senescent cells accumulate, they produce a pro-inflammatory cytokine environment, ultimately leading to a microenvironment that is detrimental to renal function. The search for pharmacologic strategies, such as senolytics, to target specifically senescent cells within the kidneys offers therapeutic strategy to combat renal damage and improve outcomes in patients with chronic kidney disease (Franzin et al., 2021).

7.1.2. Role of Inflammation in Systemic Diseases

The role of inflammation in systemic illness has garnered considerable attention, as it is both an etiology and a response to tissue injury in most disease processes. Two-way association is best demonstrated by illnesses like ANCA-associated vasculitis (AAV), where systemic inflammation is observed to result in severe renal impairment. ANCA positivity has been linked to necrotizing inflammation of blood vessels, ultimately leading to renal impairment if left untreated. Moreover, recent findings highlight the interaction between the complement pathway and inflammation in AAV, suggesting that overactivation of the alternative complement pathway further leads to renal TMA, a marker of advanced interaction between inflammatory biomarkers and kidney damage. As renal involvement in systemic diseases progresses, identifying such inflammatory mediators becomes crucial in the development of targeted therapies that address both systemic and renal manifestations of these conditions (Gentile et al., 2023).

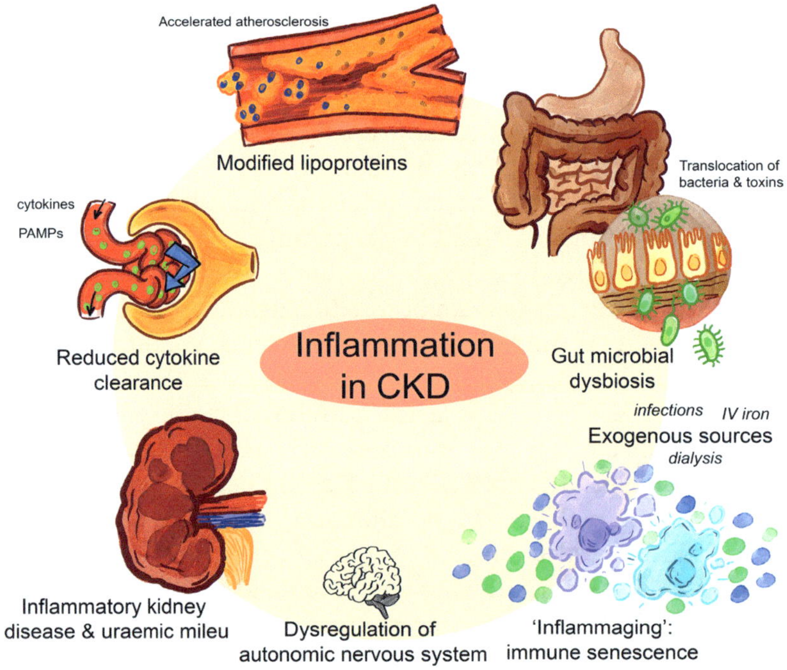

Figure 7.4. Renal role of inflammation in systemic diseases.

Source: https://www.ahajournals.org/cms/10.1161/STROKEAHA.124.047070/asset/fb6a32c5-7c03-4c78-92e3-749c6038534c/assets/graphic/strokeaha.124.047070.fig01.jpg.

Inflammations extend beyond AAV to various systemic diseases, including diabetes, which significantly contributes to renal complications. In diabetic kidney disease (DKD), low-grade inflammation and oxidative stress are central to its pathogenesis, and hence, renal status becomes difficult to control clinically. The interaction between local and systemic inflammation with respect to DKD is key because it can happen through a variety of metabolic derangements leading to renal fibrosis and ultimately end-stage renal disease. Specifically, the gut-kidney axis has also been of particular interest because it contributes to modulating inflammation in DKD. Metabolites produced by the gut microbiota control the systemic immune response, illustrating how inflammation can be induced by both intrinsic and extrinsic factors, making clinical outcomes even more challenging to predict. Elucidating this interplay between inflammation and renal function in systemic disease is essential to trigger effective treatment strategies (Cheng et al., 2022). Further, understanding the inflammatory contribution to systemic diseases necessitates an awareness of the therapeutic targets by which renal disease can be alleviated. Current research is testing the potential of anti-inflammatory medications to modulate disease trajectories and improve renal outcomes in systemic diseases. For instance, butyrate, a short-chain fatty acid produced by gut microbiota, is effective in preventing diabetic complications through its anti-inflammatory action, including histone deacetylase inhibition. This highlights not only the involvement of inflammation in disease pathogenesis but also the therapeutic choices that modulate these inflammatory processes in an effort to preserve renal function. As our understanding matures, research must continue to untangle the complex interactions between renal and inflammatory status in systemic disease, until treatment modalities emerge that might induce better patient outcomes in more than one affected system (Figure 7.4).

7.1.3. Impact of Systemic Circulation on Renal Function

The intricate relationship between systemic circulation and renal function is significant in understanding the ways in which systemic disease may influence renal health. Several physiological factors, including blood pressure and vascular integrity, are significant predictors of renal perfusion and its resultant function. When systemic circulation is compromised, either by hypertension or by vascular disease, the kidneys will be insufficiently perfused with blood and thus develop renal ischemia and consequent dysfunction. For example, systemic sclerosis is accompanied by vascular derangement that may directly compromise renal perfusion, manifested as elevated serum creatinine values and proteinuria in systemic sclerosis patients. It has been shown through research that patients with systemic sclerosis experience more critical renal impairment compared to those with rheumatoid arthritis, where systemic disease renal function should be monitored vigilantly (Božić et al., 2023). In addition, the impact of systemic circulation extends not only to direct hemodynamic changes but also to the action of drugs used in managing systemic conditions. Tumor necrosis factor (TNF) inhibitors, which are commonly used in chronic inflammatory diseases, have been related to instances of drug-induced vasculitis that may significantly impact renal function. Because such treatments aim at enhancing signs of systemic inflammation, they will incidentally trigger complications such as renal involvement or even the need for dialysis. What complicates the management of such a case is balancing the therapeutic impact against the potential caustic impact, thereby necessitating ongoing monitoring of renal parameters, such as serum creatinine and proteinuria (Przygocka et al., 2023). The dual function of systemic circulation as both a regulator and a potential disruptor of renal function highlights the interactive balance between the kidneys and systemic disease. In renal involvement in systemic disease, there is a need for an integrated understanding of pathophysiologic interactions between renal function and systemic circulation. Renal function can serve as a measure of the systemic severity of the disease, given that renal impairment will always follow deteriorating disease manifestations. Such an agreement only underscores the necessity of detecting and treating renal abnormalities in systemic patients at an early stage. Clinicians should perform routine renal screening, including urine analysis and imaging investigations, to adequately evaluate renal status. These measures can prevent further complications and enhance patient quality of life by facilitating early interventions, promoting a multidisciplinary approach that encompasses nephrology and systemic disease management. By understanding the intricate relationship between systemic circulation and kidney function, healthcare professionals are better equipped to address the complexities presented by patients with systemic diseases (Božić et al., 2023) (Figure 7.5).

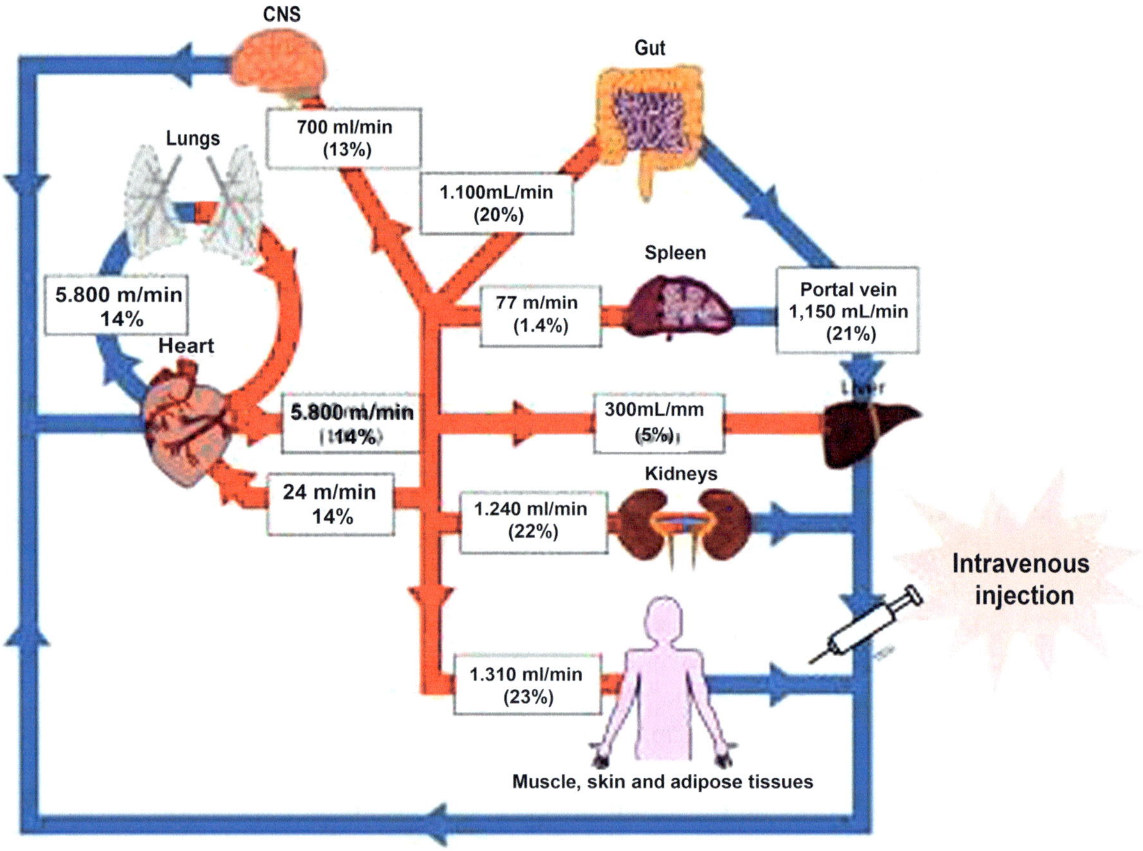

Figure 7.5. Impact of systemic circulation on renal function.

Source: https://ars.els-cdn.com/content/image/1-s2.0-S0168365911009527-gr1.jpg.

7.2. Common Systemic Diseases Affecting the Kidneys

The kidneys are vital organs responsible for maintaining fluid balance, electrolyte balance, and excreting waste. They are usually the site of systemic diseases that compromise their structural integrity and functional performance. Autoimmune conditions such as lupus erythematosus and IgA vasculitis can result in widespread renal involvement in the form of glomerulonephritis. Particularly,

IgA vasculitis, which is prevalent in the pediatric age group, presents with systemic features such as skin rashes, gastrointestinal involvement, and arthralgias. The association of gastrointestinal pathology with renal pathology in these patients demarcates the multifactorial etiology of systemic kidney diseases. In fact, research shows that gastrointestinal-symptomatic children are at risk for renal complications and thus, systemic and kidney disease could potentially share similar mechanisms in causing disease (Kili et al., 2025). Coming to infectious diseases, COVID-19 has emerged as a significant threat to the kidneys since it is systemic.

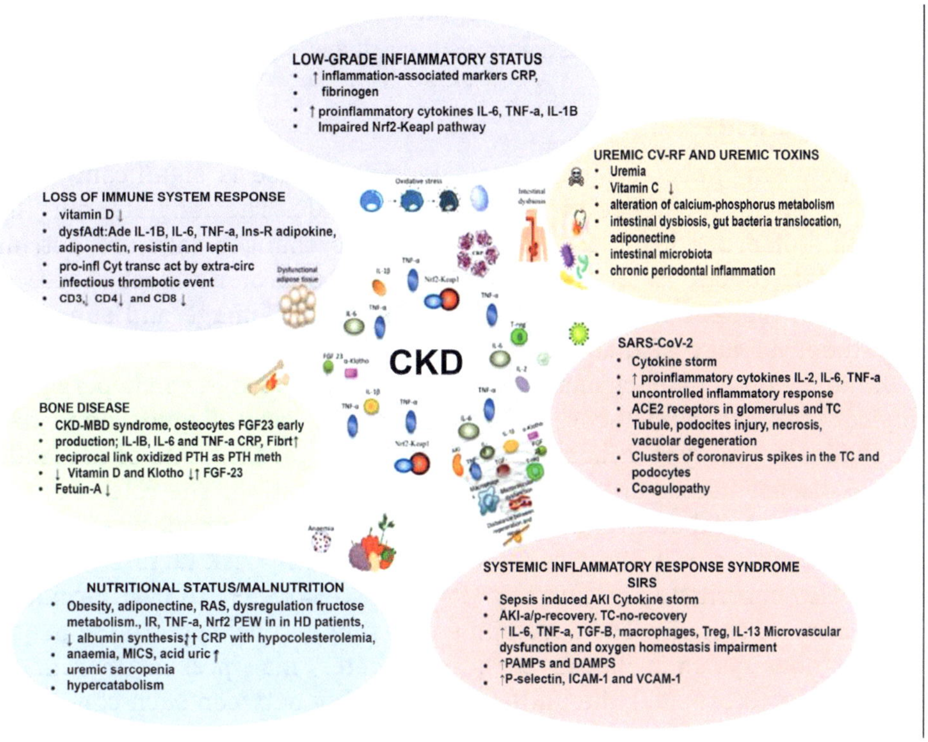

Figure 7.6. Systemic diseases affecting the kidneys.

Source: https://www.mdpi.com/life/life-11-00419/article_deploy/html/images/life-11-00419-g001.png.

The COVID-19 virus has been shown to target kidney cells by attaching through the angiotensin-converting enzyme 2 (ACE2) receptor, which is richly expressed in renal tissue. Various renal injuries have been described in asymptomatic patients without prior kidney disease, indicating the capacity of the virus in producing acute kidney injury. Clinical manifestations may include renal dysfunction, characterized by increased serum creatinine levels and altered urine output. Interestingly, hypertension, diabetes, and obesity are comorbidities that have a tremendous impact on worsening the extent of renal complications resulting from COVID-19 infection. From these results, it is evident that the influence of systemic illnesses on renal function tends to extend beyond the immediate effects of the disease itself, as the interaction with existing health conditions has a multiplier effect on kidney-related difficulties (Santos et al., 2024). Other than autoimmune and infectious diseases, systemic conditions such as hypertension and diabetes mellitus are the principal causes of renal impairment. Long-standing hypertension causes nephrosclerosis, a process of impeding renal blood flow that eventually results in kidney failure. Diabetes, however, may cause nephropathy, defined by the occurrence of microalbuminuria and progressing to end-stage renal disease if not controlled well. These conditions underscore the importance of early treatment and management strategies that consider both systemic health and renal function. With the rise of diabetes and hypertension globally, understanding their mechanisms and kidney impacts is central to public health programs aimed at reducing renal morbidity. Collectively, the interaction between these systemic diseases and kidney status underscores the rationale for integrated approaches to patient care, encompassing both treatment and prevention of downstream kidney disease (Figure 7.6).

7.2.1. Diabetes Mellitus

The relationship between Diabetes Mellitus and kidney disease is significant, particularly with the continuous rise in the incidence of diabetes worldwide. The long-standing hyperglycemia associated with this disorder leads to several metabolic changes that are detrimental to the renal organs and their functions. Untreated diabetes has one of its most severe complications in the development of diabetic nephropathy with glomerular damage and subsequent CKD. The multifactorial pathophysiology of diabetic renal disease includes increased oxidative stress and inflammation within the renal parenchyma, further propagated by long-term hyperglycemia exposure. These pathological processes underscore the importance of early diagnosis and treatment since over 40% of individuals with type 2 diabetes will eventually get CKD, one of the leading etiologies of end-stage renal disease necessitating dialysis or transplantation. The role of hypertension as a concurrent risk factor for diabetic renal disease cannot be underemphasized. Data indicate that factors such as hypertension and diabetes mellitus are not only risk factors for the development of renal cysts but also contribute significantly ($P=0.000$, $OR=2.969$) to cyst formation in patients undergoing renal ultrasonography. The development of simple renal cysts in the majority of female patients illustrates how systemic illness, such as diabetes, may present in renal pathology. In addition, it is necessary to consider the underlying interplay between such conditions and indeed how proper management of blood pressure among diabetic patients may be able to reduce the risk of renal exacerbation. This two-way relationship underscores the need for multimodal care strategies that address both cardiovascular and metabolic control to improve patient outcomes. In considering the potential of treatments for diabetic nephropathy, it becomes increasingly crucial to emphasize newer therapies that have the potential to alter the disease course. Recent clinical studies have explored the use of mineralocorticoid receptor antagonists like finerenone, which have proven to restrict the progressive nature of diabetic kidney disease. The findings of trials like FIGARO-DKD and FIDELIO-DKD draw attention to the pivotal role that these drugs can play in improving renal outcomes by targeting the oxidative and inflammatory pathways triggered by hyperglycemia. These modalities of treatment have been successful, not just in slowing down the deterioration of kidney function but also in lowering cardiovascular morbidities in diabetic patients. As chronic kidney disease is becoming more and more a prevalent complication of Diabetes Mellitus, further research into the biochemical events involved and refinement of the modes of treatment is essential for enhancing the quality of life of those afflicted (Figure 7.7).

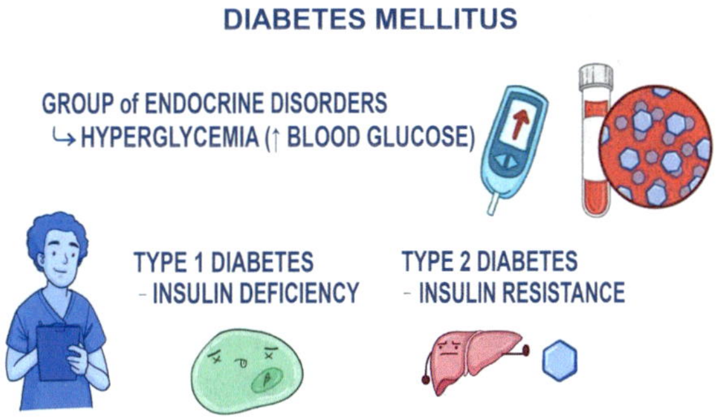

Figure 7.7. Diabetes mellitus.

Source: https://www.osmosis.org/_next/image?url=https%3A%2F%2Fd16qt3wv6xm098.cloudfront.net%2FrYDmLEhXTIa31kql5T6ImjTiQeesycwM%2F_.jpg&w=3840&q=75.

7.2.2. Hypertension

Hypertension is a frequent disorder with grave consequences for renal function, particularly in patients with diseases affecting the whole body, such as systemic sclerosis (SSc). As blood pressure increases, the risk of developing renal involvement grows, and thus, hypertension is a critical point in deciding on the overall prognosis of patients. In SSc, there has been a high prevalence of renal crisis documented within studies compared to European-derived populations, and also a marked 7% prevalence in African American patients—highlighting the variability in presentation of disease between populations (Boin et al., 2017). This association helps to emphasize the necessity for very tight blood pressure monitoring in systemic disease patients and the role of hypertension as an antecedent to renal failure. The pathophysiological mechanisms of hypertension in systemic disease generally involve endothelial dysfunction and microvascular injury, most pronounced in SSc. Elevated serum uric acid (UA) is a key marker of both inflammation and vascular stiffness, providing useful information regarding the severity of these conditions. Research has identified a powerful positive relationship between serum UA and creatinine and pulmonary artery pressure in SSc patients, suggesting more generalized syndromic significance of these common laboratory findings (Amoroso et al., 2016). Thus, practitioners must understand the intricate interplay between hypertension, renal function, and systemic disease activity so that they can institute effective treatments to address the multifaceted dimensions of patient welfare. Furthermore, the interaction between hypertension and renal disease in systemic disorders underscores the urgent need for multidisciplinary treatment approaches. Proper management of high blood pressure leads to improved renal outcomes, especially in patients with evidence of vascular damage. Blood pressure control interventions not only decrease the immediate damage due to hypertension but also slow renal disease in these patients. By acknowledging hypertension as a multidimensional issue embedded in systemic pathology, healthcare professionals can more effectively work with treatment protocols while increasing the quality of life for patients and minimizing the risk of devastating complications associated with renal insufficiency and systemic disease as a whole (Figure 7.8).

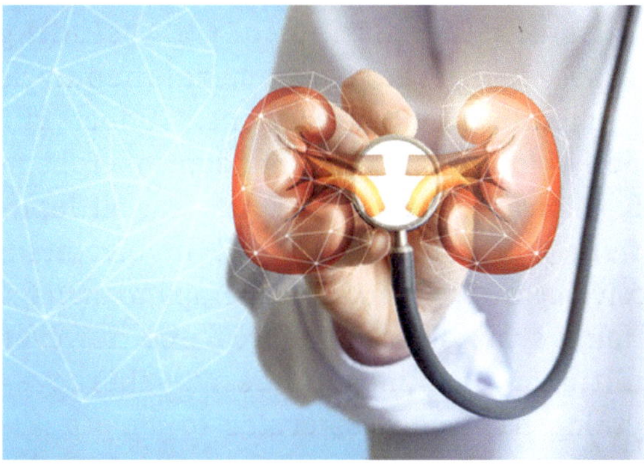

Figure 7.8. Hypertension and kidney health.

Source: https://metrohospitals.com/wp-content/uploads/2024/02/hypertension-and-kidney.jpg.

7.2.3. Systemic Lupus Erythematosus

Systemic lupus erythematosus (SLE) is a prototype of a systemic autoimmune disease with variable presentation and potential for extensive renal involvement. Renal injury in SLE, also known as lupus nephritis, affects a considerable percentage of patients and is capable of producing severe morbidity. SLE is more complex since it involves two or more organ systems, and the pathophysiology, therefore, needs to be understood holistically to treat it optimally. Recent studies have shown that environmental triggers, such as viral infections, may be a decisive component in the initiation of SLE. Furthermore, post-COVID-19 phenomena have highlighted the potential relationship between viral infections, such as Epstein-Barr virus, and the initiation of autoimmune diseases, including SLE, underscoring the multifactorial etiology of these diseases (Clive et al., 2024). The implication of this relationship is the recognition of triggers for efficient management and the avoidance of renal complications. Lupus nephritis is associated with a range of pathological changes that can significantly compromise renal function, underscoring the importance of stringent clinical observation.

Histologic distinctions, including diffuse proliferative glomerulonephritis and membranous alterations, reflect the underlying immune dysregulation inherent in SLE. Clinical guidelines require that all lupus patients, regardless of renal involvement, receive hydroxychloroquine therapy to manage systemic symptoms and reduce flares. However, traditional immunosuppressive therapy—anything from corticosteroids to agents like cyclophosphamide and mycophenolate mofetil—are usually employed in the management of more severe manifestations of lupus nephritis (Athanassiou et al., 2023). These treatments are effective, though they have side effects that need serious consideration and patient education regarding the risk-benefit ratio. In the last few years, the identification of biologic agents has revolutionized SLE treatment, particularly among patients with significant renal activity. Targeting specific immunologic mechanisms, such as B-cell function, has been encouraging in improving patient outcomes. Medications such as belimumab and rituximab have emerged as valuable additions to the therapeutic arsenal, particularly when conventional immunosuppressants cannot provide adequate disease flare control or are burdened with intolerable side effects (Athanassiou et al., 2023).

The evolving treatment paradigm of SLE reflects a more advanced approach aimed at enhancing patient quality of life, while also minimizing renal damage. With increasing research focusing on the role of personalized medicine in treatment protocols, understanding the impact of renal complications in SLE remains crucial for optimal treatment and patient outcomes (Figure 7.9).

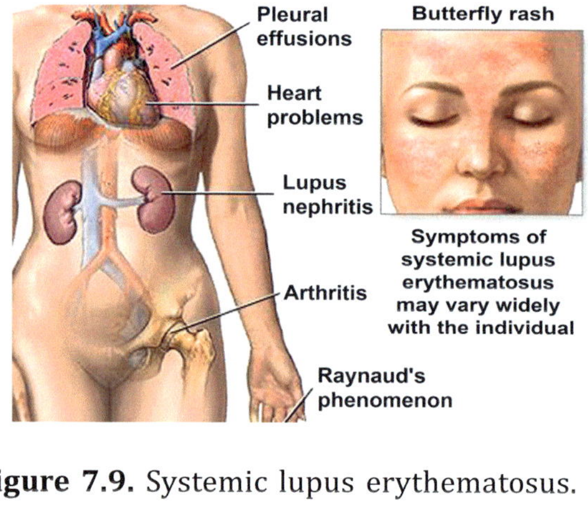

Figure 7.9. Systemic lupus erythematosus.

Source: https://medlineplus.gov/ency/images/ency/fullsize/17134.jpg.

7.3. Clinical Manifestations of Renal Involvement

Renal involvement is a significant clinical presentation in most systemic diseases that complicate the pathogenesis of these diseases. A case in point is systemic lupus erythematosus (SLE), whose many manifestations range from renal injury to be harmful to patient prognosis. Studies have demonstrated variable renal manifestations in SLE that can range from mild proteinuria to fixed renal failure, emphasizing kidney involvement in autoimmune disease. Late-onset SLE patients, compared to early-onset individuals, have reduced frequencies of renal symptoms but still present with issues that can hinder renal function and overall morbidity. It is essential to recognize these differences to individualize treatment protocols for patients, as early intervention can prevent irreparable kidney damage and provide a clearer direction for managing the systemic manifestations of the disease effectively (Gokcen et al., 2024). In cases of spondyloarthritis (SpA) with renal involvement, there is an additional dimension of systemic disease burden. SpA patients can manifest a range of renal complications, including proteinuria, hematuria, and nephrotic syndrome.

In a retrospective study of SpA patients, 7.4% were found to have renal abnormalities, indicating the importance of renal monitoring in these patients. The multifactorial etiologies of renal impairment in SpA, such as secondary renal amyloidosis and IgA nephropathy, reflect the complex relationship between systemic inflammation and kidney function. Moreover, diagnosis usually occurs years after the initial diagnosis of SpA, which is reflective of a subclinical course of renal symptoms to include in patient treatment (Bouden et al., 2023). Recognition of clinical manifestations of renal involvement in systemic diseases is crucial for improving patient management. Early recognition of renal impairment can lead to a more effective therapeutic strategy, averting the potential effects of chronic renal insufficiency. Both SLE and SpA demonstrate the absolute necessity for an interdisciplinary approach to monitor renal function as well as systemic disease activity, since renal pathology can be a sign of underlying disease activity. Clinicians should be vigilant in evaluating renal health, with regular laboratory tests and urinalysis constituting the standard. Proactive monitoring through such measures can enable early intervention and improve the quality of life for patients with systemic illnesses involving the kidneys, ultimately ensuring comprehensive care and management of their overall well-being (Bouden et al., 2023; Gokcen et al., 2024) (Figure 7.10).

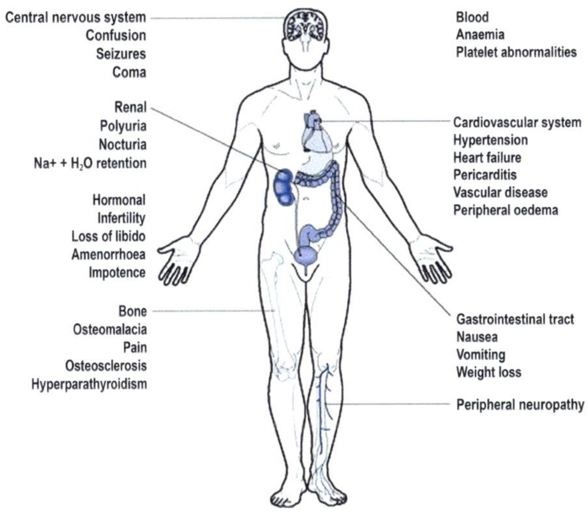

Figure 7.10. Clinical manifestations of renal involvement in various systemic diseases.

Source: https://basicmedicalkey.com/wp-content/uploads/2016/06/B9780702042935000312_f18-06-9780702042935.jpg.

7.3.1. Symptoms of Kidney Dysfunction

It is essential to recognize the signs of kidney impairment, particularly in systemic diseases where renal involvement can impact overall well-being. Typical presentations of kidney disease include manifestations such as fatigue, edema, and alterations in urine output. Fatigue resulting from the buildup of waste products in the bloodstream, commonly referred to as uremia, can be experienced by patients. Moreover, fluid overload may lead to evident edema in the legs and eyelids. The frequency of the urine may also be abnormal, either too frequent or too infrequent, and may indicate compromised kidney function. These manifestations illustrate the kidney's role in maintaining homeostasis and highlight the importance of careful evaluation in patients with renal involvement and systemic diseases. In disorders such as systemic lupus erythematosus (SLE), renal manifestations can become more severe and complex. Up to 50% of SLE patients present with evidence of renal disease, and the disease can evolve into severe conditions such as lupus nephritis, characterized by inflammatory damage to the renal tissues. The typical presentation is hematuria, proteinuria, and hypertension, which over time can progressively lead to impairment of kidney function. Presence of high inflammatory markers and other laboratory abnormalities typically trails these signs, necessitating a potential diagnosis of lupus nephritis. The relationship between systemic disease and renal function underscores the importance of vigilant monitoring and management to prevent deleterious consequences, including cardiovascular disease and end-stage renal disease, as reported by Abasse (2024). Also, kidney failure may extend beyond its physiological representation to affect neurological status, particularly in systemic disorders like SLE. Involvement of the central nervous system can manifest through various neurological symptoms, including confusion, seizures, or mood alterations. Research has established CNS processes to be prevalent in SLE patients (21% to 95% experiencing some degree of involvement in CNS), underscoring the interlinked relationship between renal function and neurological status. Such symptoms may be due to secondary complications, including infections or renal cause-based hypertension, that result in such crises as stroke or cerebrovascular accident. Thus, the interdependent relationship between renal impairment and neurologic manifestations highlights the absolute need for complete assessment and explicit interventions among patients suffering from systemic disease, as identified through studies of SLE patients (Kim et al., 2024) (Figure 7.11).

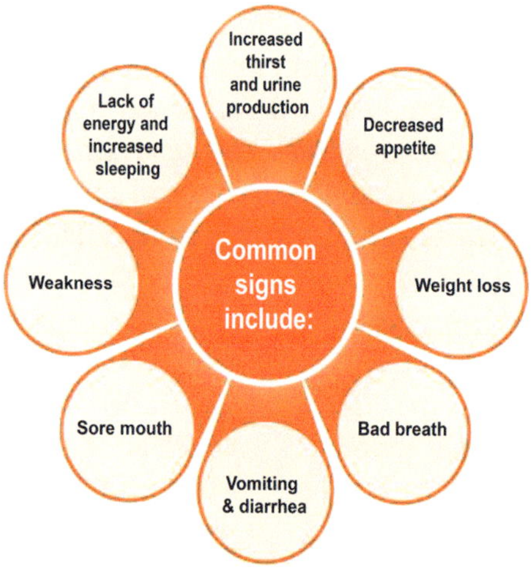

Figure 7.11. Symptoms of kidney dysfunction.

Source: https://www.medicaidhospital.com/wp-content/uploads/2016/05/kidney-disease-common-signs_400_en.jpg.

7.3.2. Laboratory Findings in Systemic Diseases

The study of laboratory findings is of utmost significance in diagnosing and understanding renal involvement in systemic illnesses. Systemic lupus erythematosus (SLE), for instance, is complicated by its complexity, which frequently leads to significant renal consequences, including lupus nephritis. Advances in urinary peptidomic technology have enabled researchers to study the potential utilization of urinary biomarkers that are able to label renal involvement in SLE patients specifically. In a recent study, researchers analyzed urine samples by capillary electrophoresis coupled with mass spectrometry to develop a biomarker panel that discriminates between SLE and healthy controls. Such advances underscore the importance of laboratory findings as physicians work to enhance patient risk stratification with the ultimate goal of more effective drug treatment regimens (Braun et al., 2007). Another significant area of laboratory diagnosis for systemic diseases is the assessment of cryoglobulinemia, which occurs in both cutaneous vasculitis and glomerulonephritis. This is a serious complication, per se, secondary to infections such as hepatitis C, with life-threatening implications for the patient, potentially leading to end-stage renal failure. Laboratory findings that reveal the existence of cryoglobulins are crucial in the diagnosis and proper management of this serious complication. Furthermore, novel antiviral therapy holds promise for causal treatment, thereby preventing the renal sequelae of such systemic diseases. Laboratory findings play a role here that is much greater than diagnosis; they are a critical component in guiding therapeutic interventions and facilitating improved patient care by informing treatment of the primary systemic disease (Braun et al., 2007). Furthermore, the integration of advanced laboratory techniques has revolutionized the landscape of renal disease diagnosis associated with systemic conditions. Identification of biomarkers through new techniques not only aids in early detection but also enables monitoring of disease progression and responsiveness to treatment. The identification of specific urinary peptides specific to various systemic diseases, such as SLE, serves to indicate a paradigm shift towards individualized medicine. These laboratory test modality advances are necessary because they provide clinicians with valuable information regarding the biochemical pathways of systemic diseases, making therapeutic interventions more precise and improving the overall management of renal complications associated with these diseases (Burkly et al., 2018) (Figure 7.12).

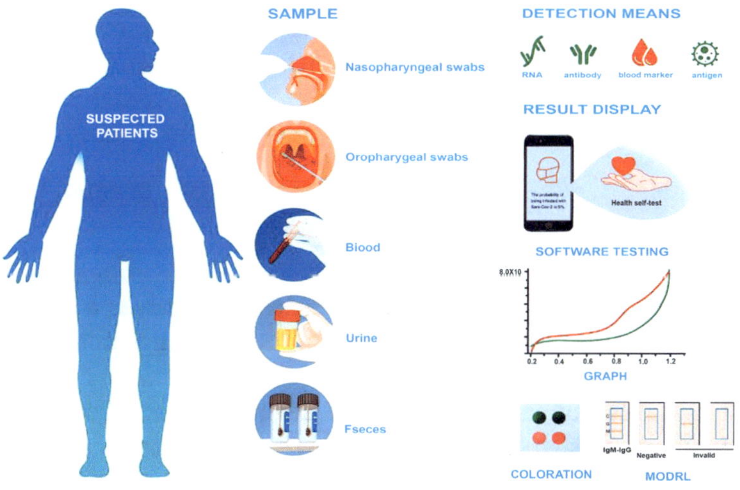

Figure 7.12. Laboratory findings in systemic diseases.

Source: https://media.springernature.com/full/springer-static/image/art%3A10.1038%2Fs41392-021-00731-z/MediaObjects/41392_2021_731_Fig1_HTML.png.

7.3.3. Imaging Techniques for Renal Assessment

Assessment of renal involvement in systemic disease necessitates the use of an extensive array of sophisticated imaging modalities. These imaging modalities help clarify renal anatomy, function, and disease, thereby enhancing diagnostic accuracy and treatment planning. Ultrasound remains a necessary first-line imaging modality due to its non-invasive nature and ability to image renal anatomy in real-time. It is helpful for identifying obstructions, cysts, and masses. Furthermore, Doppler ultrasound can assess renal blood flow, providing valuable information about vascular compromise secondary to systemic diseases. Although ultrasound is helpful for diagnostic purposes, its inability to accurately evaluate parenchymal disease necessitates the use of adjunctive imaging modalities, particularly in instances where the underlying pathology is not immediately apparent. Computed tomography (CT) and magnetic resonance imaging (MRI) are more advanced techniques of renal assessment and are employed to the maximum in assessing complex cases. CT is commonly employed for its fine resolution and economic efficiency, making it the optimal choice for diagnosing renal masses, stones, and trauma. Moreover, CT angiography provides visualization of the renal vasculature, which is essential in cases of renal artery stenosis. MRI has an advantage when radiation exposure is a concern or when contrast media cannot be avoided. Imaging modalities, such as non-contrast MRI, can highlight vascular and vasogenic alterations in the kidneys, which are particularly beneficial in assessing systemic conditions, such as ANCA-associated vasculitis (Lubas et al., 2022). Therefore, the integration of CT and MRI into renal imaging represents a comprehensive approach for diagnosing renal impairment in systemic illnesses. In addition to conventional imaging, advanced modalities such as PET have been valuable in evaluating renal involvement with systemic illness. PET scans not only show images of renal anatomy but also quantify metabolic activity, allowing clinicians to differentiate between inflammatory processes that are not evident on CT or MRI. This is particularly valuable in autoimmune disease where acute shifts in renal metabolism correlate with disease activity. Furthermore, the inclusion of PET with CT (PET/CT) offers enhanced localization of disease activity, benefiting from the use of anatomical landmarks, which is especially useful in directing therapeutic interventions. The increasing role of quantitative imaging techniques, such as dynamic contrast-enhanced MRI, which is capable of quantifying renal perfusion and function, further justifies the use of a multidisciplinary approach to renal imaging. Lastly, the selection of the appropriate imaging modality is essential for optimizing outcomes in renal involvement due to systemic diseases, enabling the detection and treatment of early disease.

7.4. Diagnostic Approaches

Accurate diagnosis of renal involvement in systemic illnesses involves a multidisciplinary process that includes clinical examination, laboratory studies, and imaging modalities. Clinicians initiate the diagnostic process by eliciting an accurate history of the patient and conducting a physical exam, which in most instances unearths signs such as hematuria, proteinuria, or hypertension. Such presentations may arouse suspicion of intrinsic renal impairment in systemic disease such as vasculitis. Subsequently, laboratory tests, including blood tests and urinalysis, yield critical data on kidney function and detect biomarkers of kidney damage. For instance, elevated serum creatinine levels and the presence of specific antibodies may indicate conditions such as ANCA-associated vasculitis. The synthesis of these findings is required since it assists in the resolution of differential diagnoses and the direction of further investigation aimed at elucidating the specific renal involvement in systemic disease, ultimately determining an efficacious management strategy. Imaging techniques play a central role in the diagnostic arsenal for evaluating renal involvement in systemic diseases. Kidney ultrasound is often the initial imaging modality used due to its non-invasive nature and ability to assess kidney size, configuration, and the presence of masses or obstruction. More advanced modalities, such as CT and MRI, are more adept at providing precise information regarding renal vasculature and abnormal structures that may be related to systemic illnesses. For example, CT angiography can identify vascular lesions that are associated with vasculitides, thus informing appropriate treatment options.

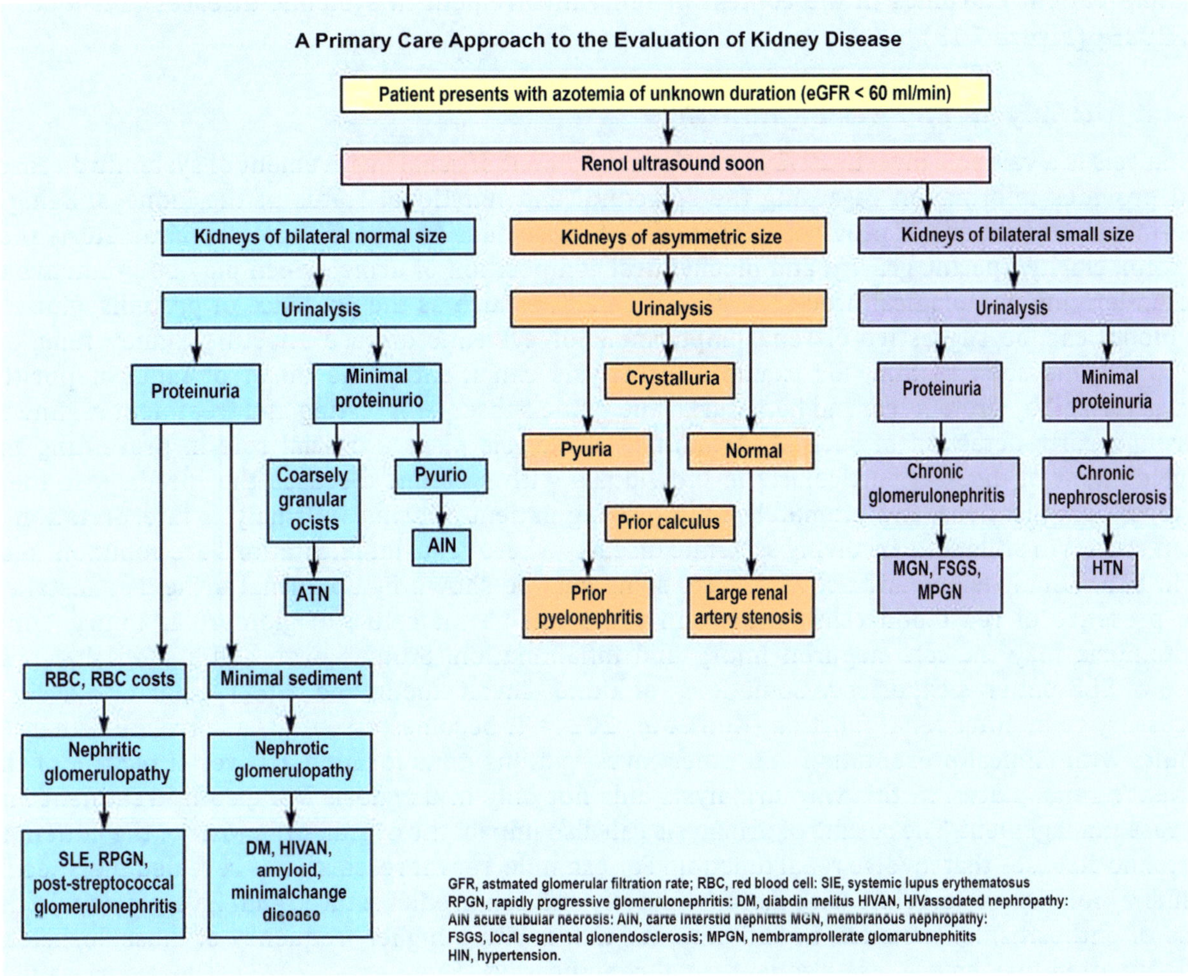

Figure 7.13. Diagnostic approaches of renal involvement in systemic diseases.

Source: https://s3.amazonaws.com/HMP/c360/imported/transfer/Table_Care_of_kidneyDisease.jpg.

The use of imaging in combination with other diagnostic modalities enhances a detailed understanding of the renal space, allowing clinicians to arrive at a more accurate diagnosis and initiate timely interventions tailored to the individual patient presentation (Zerhoudi et al., 2025). In essence, renal biopsy remains the definitive means of proving renal involvement in systemic disease. Direct visualization of renal tissue during the procedure reveals histopathologic patterns that can significantly influence treatment decisions. In vasculitis, for instance, it identifies lesions that are indistinguishable from necrotizing crescentic glomerulonephritis, a condition that requires emergent and aggressive therapy. The utility of renal biopsies as a diagnostic tool is further enhanced by the addition of ancillary studies, such as immunofluorescence and electron microscopy, which provide a detailed description of the underlying immunopathological processes. With changing treatment paradigms, particularly the use of new biologic agents, accurate histological diagnosis has become central to personalizing therapy. Finally, a robust diagnostic procedure, comprising clinical, laboratory, imaging, and histopathological examinations, is fundamental to achieving optimal patient outcomes in the context of renal involvement in systemic diseases (Zerhoudi et al., 2025) (Figure 7.13).

7.4.1. Urinalysis and Its Significance

Urinalysis is a valuable investigative aid in the assessment of renal involvement of systemic diseases and provides information regarding the structural and functional status of the kidneys. Being a non-invasive technique, it provides clinicians with the means to examine various parameters, such as color, clarity, specific gravity, and biochemical composition of urine, which may be predictive of the underlying pathological process. Pathologic results, such as the presence of proteins, glucose, or blood, can be suggestive of renal impairment or systemic disease affecting kidney function. In conditions such as SLE, for example, urinalysis can identify the onset of lupus nephritis, characterized by proteinuria and hematuria, and guide subsequent testing and treatment regimens. Through early detection of such abnormalities, urinalysis plays a crucial role in preventing the development of disease, particularly in individuals with systemic diseases that predispose them to renal complications, and ultimately, in improving patient outcomes. Urinalysis interpretation is most crucial in situations involving systemic disease, where renal manifestations are common, such as in SLE. Renal lesions and active disease signs may be shown by abnormal urine. For instance, the presence of red blood cells or casts in urine can be indicative of glomerular injury, while proteinuria may indicate nephron injury and inflammation. Studies have highlighted that over 50% of SLE patients experience some form of kidney involvement, and thus regular urinalysis is necessary to monitor renal function (Kim et al., 2024). It becomes essential to correlate urinalysis results with clinical presentation and other investigations, thus forming an overall picture of the patient's renal status. In this way, urinalysis aids not only in diagnosis but also in treatment and disease management. The results of urinalysis can also impact the overall prognosis of the patient in systemic diseases that involve renal function. For example, recent research has revealed thatspecific urinary biomarkers correlate with disease severity and can predict future renal involvement. In the case of enthesitis, for instance, in SLE patients, those with a higher frequency of musculoskeletal inflammation may have a less frequent renal complication (Fagni et al., 2023). These correlations facilitate easier adjustments by medical practitioners to tailor treatment interventions and anticipate potential complications. Regular urinalysis, therefore, forms a critical part of managing systemic diseases as a valuable predictor of renal health and the overall systemic effect of these conditions. Such detailed characterization allows clinicians to act preventively and adjust treatment protocols effectively, enhancing the overall management of the patient in the complex syndrome of systemic diseases.

7.4.2. Blood Tests for Renal Function

The evaluation of renal function through blood testing is a crucial component of assessing renal involvement in systemic diseases. Serum creatinine, blood urea nitrogen (BUN), and electrolyte panel tests are all blood laboratory tests that provide helpful information about renal health and systemic function. Serum creatinine is often used to estimate the glomerular filtration rate (GFR), a crucial factor in determining kidney function. Higher serum creatinine concentrations may indicate renal dysfunction, in most cases justifying an investigation of potential systemic diseases that could cause renal impairment. BUN concentration also reflects the kidneys' ability to clear waste products from the blood, providing a measure of renal function in systemic diseases. Collectively, these blood tests are essential for the early diagnosis and treatment of renal manifestations of many systemic illnesses and ultimately decide on optimal clinical interventions and improved patient outcomes. In patients with systemic diseases such as diabetes and hypertension, monitoring renal function by blood tests becomes particularly important. Systemic illnesses can have a significant impact on kidney function and develop into chronic kidney disease (CKD) if left untreated. Among the most important blood tests, the complete metabolic panel (CMP) allows practitioners to monitor eGFR and proteinuria, both of which are important markers of renal function. An abnormal amount of protein can be a marker of glomerular damage, and a declining eGFR can be a sign of worsening renal condition. Through early blood testing in patients with pre-existing conditions, the premature development of end-stage renal disease is avoided. Second, performing the tests promptly to create treatment plans also helps appropriate management of the systemic disease as well as renal complications that may arise, capturing the integrated nature of renal and systemic health. Blood test findings analysis in relation to renal function not only aids in the diagnosis of kidney disease but also serves as a critical prognostic factor in the event of systemic diseases. For instance, elevated creatinine and BUN can represent acute kidney injury secondary to systemic disease such as sepsis or dehydration. Monitoring these variables can help clinicians distinguish between renal pathologies and other complications in states of systemic disease. The incorporation of longitudinal data from laboratory tests can also be helpful in forecasting disease trajectory and designing treatment regimens on an individual basis. Because systemic disorders are likely to have multifaceted effects on renal health, investigating these parameters through blood studies provides a comprehensive understanding of a patient's overall condition, enabling the development of protective management strategies that can improve both renal and systemic conditions. Bringing blood study data into clinical practice would allow practitioners to more effectively handle renal involvement in systemic disease (Figure 7.14).

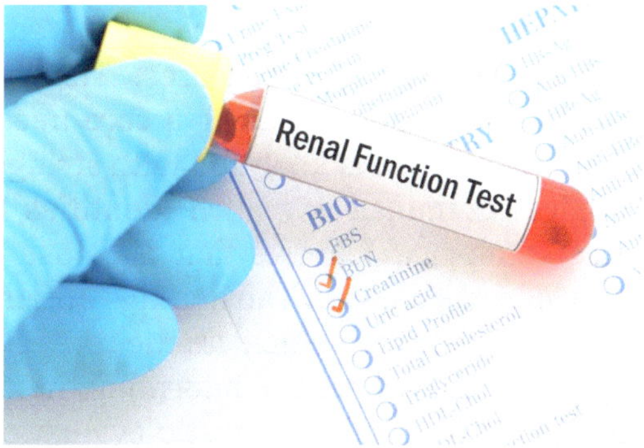

Figure 7.14. Blood tests for renal function.

Source: https://blog-revamp.s3.ap-south-1.amazonaws.com/wp-content/uploads/2023/08/13005555/image2-22-1024x683-1-1.jpg.

7.4.3. Biopsy Indications and Procedures

The most fundamental indication for renal biopsy lies in the need for a definitive diagnosis in those with an ambiguous clinical presentation or deranged laboratory results. The technique is particularly valuable in patients with nephrotic syndrome or acute kidney injury manifestations, where nonspecific findings mask the underlying pathology. Because systemic disease frequently presents with renal involvement, early biopsy can help distinguish between primary renal disease and secondary presentation due to systemic disease. In addition, accurate diagnosis is essential to initiate appropriate regimens of treatment since the treatment varies substantially between disorders such as lupus nephritis and focal segmental glomerulosclerosis. The ability of renal biopsy to identify the etiology of renal dysfunction positions it as an effective diagnostic aid in the clinical management of systemic diseases affecting the kidney. Technical maneuvers for renal biopsy comprise patient selection, imaging guidance, and histopathologic interpretation. Performed commonly percutaneously, renal biopsies most often use ultrasound or CT scan for precise placement of the needle and circumvent complications such as bleeding and injury to nearby structures. Tissue is obtained most frequently using a core needle, which once removed is analyzed with stringent histological examination, which identifies the crucial pathological features that diagnose the majority of renal disease. The findings obtained from such analyses can elucidate the role of the kidney in systemic illnesses, informing therapy recommendations and prognostic evaluations. Except for the potential dangers associated with the procedure itself, such as complications, the value of acquiring important diagnostic information makes renal biopsy an essential component of renal pathology treatment in systemic illnesses, as evidenced by various retrospective analyses of renal biopsy indications and outcomes (Teixeira et al., 2014). Familiarity with the epidemiological patterns of renal biopsy indications contributes to our understanding of renal disease in various populations. Accounts of the frequency of specific indications, such as nephrotic syndrome and acute kidney injury, are essential information about patterns of renal disease. For instance, the Madeira Islands investigation, spanning over two decades of native kidney biopsies, identified nephrotic syndrome as the most common indication for biopsy, accounting for over one-third of all cases (Teixeira et al., 2014). Besides, the study also provided a demographic report wherein gender demonstrated a strong correlation with primary pathological diagnoses. The data not only aid clinical practice but also identify burgeoning trends in renal disease that correlate with systemic conditions. Continued monitoring of these indicators can be a helpful guide in shaping healthcare policy for renal involvement in systemic diseases (Figure 7.15).

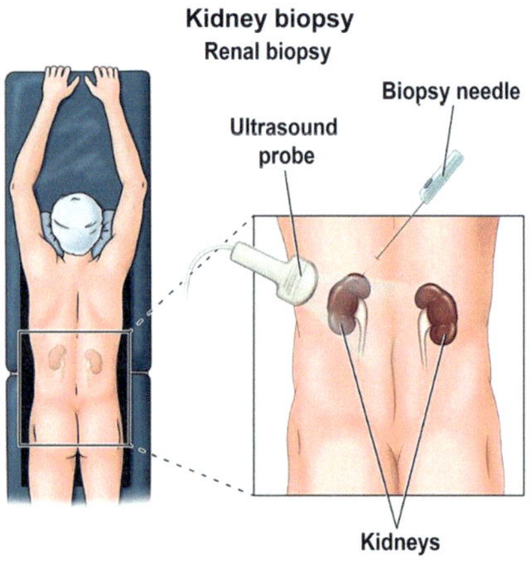

Figure 7.15. The indication for renal biopsy.

Source: https://my.clevelandclinic.org/-/scassets/images/org/health/articles/kidney-biopsy.

7.5. Treatment Strategies

Effective therapeutic strategies for renal presentations of systemic diseases, particularly SLE, are based on early diagnosis and focused treatment. The most important tool in formulating an appropriate treatment regimen is the kidney biopsy, which provides valuable histopathological data necessary to differentiate lupus nephritis (LN) from other types of renal diseases. Kidney biopsies have been suggested even in patients with low-grade proteinuria, as, despite minimal proteinuria values, more severe forms of LN may be present (Karlsson et al., 2023). Early diagnosis of LN can facilitate early treatment with immunosuppressive drugs, significantly improving patient outcomes. This underscores the necessity for an integrated strategy, whereby clinicians accord priority to suspected renal complications in patients with biopsy operations, therefore facilitating on-time modifications in the therapy plan based on the proper degree of renal involvement. In addition to immunosuppressive therapy, dyslipidemia control has been a significant element in therapy regimens for SLE patients presenting renal complications. Research indicates a strong correlation between renal damage and dyslipidemia in SLE, characterized by elevated triglycerides and low-density lipoprotein (Huang et al., 2023). This kind of association suggests that dyslipidemia is not only a comorbidity but may be a contributing factor to renal damage. It can be treated by managing lipid disorders through lifestyle modifications and pharmacological therapy, thereby reducing the disease burden and improving renal function. By incorporating lipid-lowering measures into the treatment plan of SLE patients, clinicians can address one additional aspect of systemic engagement, thereby refining the therapeutic paradigm for renal well-being in these subjects. Additionally, the use of glucocorticoids in the management of SLE, particularly about renal participation, requires careful attention. Even though glucocorticoids remain a cornerstone in the management of acute exacerbations of LN, their association with severe dyslipidemia is a matter of concern from a clinical perspective (Huang et al., 2023). Supraphysiological glucocorticoid use has been associated with exacerbation of lipid derangements, which itself can contribute to cardiovascular risk and renal dysfunction. Thus, clinicians are caught between balancing the benefits of glucocorticoid therapy and risks. Individualized management plans, incorporating regular monitoring of renal function and lipid profiles, are critical to maximizing patient care. Dealing with these complex areas of SLE management can enable clinicians to significantly enhance the treatment effectiveness and quality of life for patients with systemic lupus erythematosus (SLE) and renal disease (Figure 7.16).

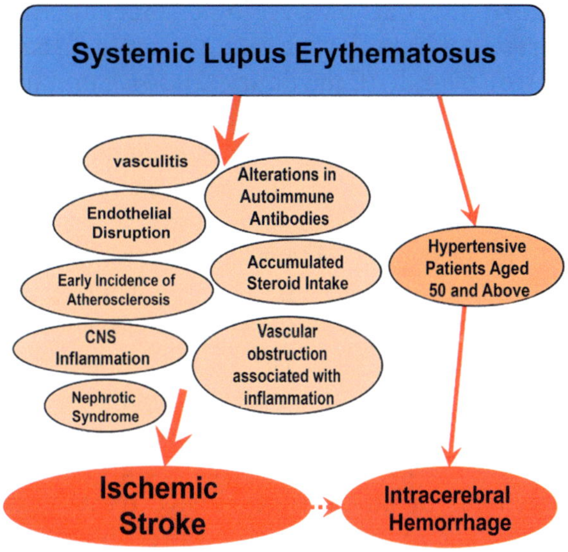

Figure 7.16. Systemic lupus erythematosus (SLE)

Source: https://www.mdpi.com/medicines/medicines-11-00015/article_deploy/html/images/medicines-11-00015-g001.png.

7.5.1. Management of Underlying Systemic Disease

Treatment of underlying systemic conditions significantly contributes to the management of renal disease, as various conditions can have a profound impact on renal function. Lupus and vasculitides are diseases with renal manifestations that can make the overall prognosis of the patient poorer. Systemic lupus erythematosus (SLE), for instance, can be associated with lupus nephritis, affecting up to 60% of patients during the course of their illness. Early diagnosis and early therapy are vital to prevent irreversible damage to the kidneys. Renal biopsies are supported through clinical pathways if patients have proteinuria beyond certain thresholds or renal function shows evidence of worsened renal health. This type of comprehensive evaluation enables individualized treatment approaches, utilizing immunosuppressive drugs that target the specific underlying pathophysiologic mechanisms, thereby improving renal and systemic disease control overall (Chowdhury, 2024). Similarly, in the management of vasculitides and the underlying systemic disease to minimize renal disease involves a team of experts. Renal vasculitis is an inflammation of blood vessels that can lead to secondary kidney complications, such as rapidly progressive glomerulonephritis. Since renal disease can occur in granulomatosis with polyangiitis and other conditions, appropriate management begins by guaranteeing proper diagnosis using clinical evaluation and renal biopsy. The histopathological features guide the choice of immunosuppressive treatments, including glucocorticoids and biologics targeted at the specific underlying vasculitic subtype. Notably, the management plan must incorporate regular monitoring of renal function and laboratory values to minimize toxicity and improve treatment adherence. Such an integrated approach is essential to optimize patient outcomes and reduce long-term risk of chronic kidney disease (Chowdhury, 2024). In addition to pharmacological treatment, the management of comorbidities and the promotion of lifestyle modifications are integral to the management of primary systemic diseases with renal involvement. Systemic patients typically have conditions that result in renal impairment, such as hypertension and diabetes. Therefore, regularly monitoring blood pressure, blood glucose, and lipids is essential for preserving kidney function. Educational interventions that stimulate medication compliance and promote diet modifications can significantly contribute to enhancing renal and overall well-being. Furthermore, engaging patients in self-management plans enhances compliance and enables them to actively manage their health. Ultimately, a holistic system integrating pharmacological, monitoring, and lifestyle strategies offers complete and efficient management of systemic disease patients with compromised kidney function (Issayeva et al., 2023).

7.5.2. Renal-Specific Therapies

The exploration of renal-targeted treatments for systemic illnesses is crucial in maximizing patient outcomes, for instance, in SLE. SLE is particularly notorious for inducing catastrophic renal injury in the form of LN. New evidence suggests that urinary peptidomic biomarkers may also serve as novel markers of early-onset disease, thereby reinforcing patient risk stratification and informing therapy. In a more recent study, a panel of 65 urinary peptides was characterized, which precisely differentiated SLE patients from healthy controls with 83% sensitivity and 73% specificity (Burkly et al., 2018). These results demonstrate the promise that non-invasive diagnostic tools hold for the development of renal-specific therapies that are sensitive to early pathologic alterations, enabling more efficient and timely treatment of renal involvement in systemic diseases. Furthermore, the advent of targeted therapies has revolutionized the management of renal complications associated with systemic diseases. Corticosteroids and immunosuppressants have played a crucial role in preventing renal inflammation and halting the progression to irreversible disease. The evolution of biologic agents, such as monoclonal antibodies targeting specific pathways or groups of pathways implicated in the immunologic mechanisms of renal injury, has provided new therapeutic options. These therapies aim not only to manage symptoms but also to address disease processes, thus enhancing the efficacy of treatment protocols specifically targeting the kidney. Heterogeneity of such therapy is especially beneficial in circumstances where the usual therapies are bound to fail; e.g., biologics may represent an option for patients with severe side effects from traditional immunosuppressives (Brém et al., 2020). This individualized approach is the hallmark of renal treatment in the realm of systemic disease, expanding the range of patient care.

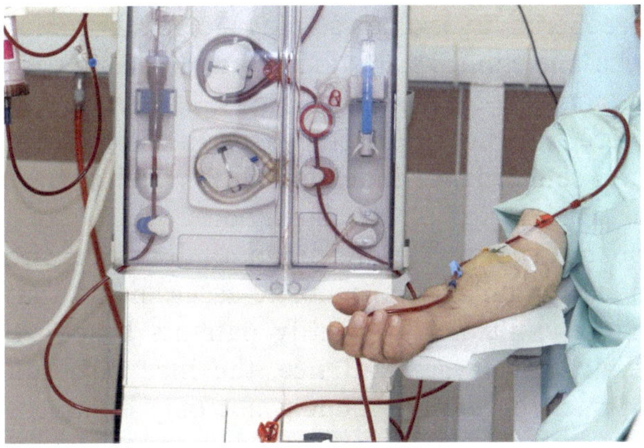

Figure 7.17. Renal-specific therapies.

Source: https://cdn-prod.medicalnewstoday.com/content/images/articles/152/152902/dialysis-can-carry-out-the-function-of-the-kidneys.jpg.

The role of pharmacogenomics in renal-specific medication cannot be overstated, either, as it holds promise for individualizing treatment protocols based on a patient's genetic profile. With the potential for differential drug responses, awareness of the genetic determinants of drug metabolism and efficacy can optimize therapy in cases of renal involvement in systemic disease. With ongoing research further revealing the complexities of drug interaction and metabolism, clinicians can now individualize treatment protocols for managing such situations optimally. For instance, detection of patients at risk for nephrotoxicity enables clinicians to modify dosing or select alternative therapies, thereby eliminating risks from conventional treatment regimens. The incorporation of pharmacogenomic data ensures a more sophisticated and patient-centered management of renal-specific therapies, ultimately maximizing the treatment of systemic diseases that compromise renal function (Figure 7.17).

7.5.3. Role of Lifestyle Modifications

Lifestyle modifications are also crucial in the treatment of renal involvement in systemic disease, acting not only as prophylactic measures but also as therapy. Risk factors for renal complications secondary to systemic diseases such as diabetes and hypertension can be mitigated by patients through healthier lifestyles. For instance, maintaining a balanced diet and a healthy weight can reduce the stress placed on the kidneys to allow them to function optimally. The body is also helped through dietary changes such as limiting sodium intake and restricted protein consumption, which help manage blood pressure and control proteinuria, diseases that usually are elevated in chronic kidney disease patients. The facilitation of such adaptations underscores the significance of comprehensive patient education on lifestyle adaptations as part of comprehensive renal care; such adaptations hence significantly influence patient outcomes during systemic diseases (Visseren et al., 2021). Exercise is another vital component of lifestyle adaptations that can dramatically affect kidney health. Daily exercise not only supports a healthy weight but also enhances cardiovascular well-being, which is critically essential for patients with systemic diseases whose renal function is compromised. Research has demonstrated that higher activity levels may lead to better blood pressure control, reduced insulin resistance, and improved overall quality of life, all of which contribute to decreased risk of renal decline. Also, specific exercise regimens according to the patient's abilities can be helpful in managing present conditions such as diabetes and obesity, thus further protecting kidney functions. Therefore, promotion of an active lifestyle becomes even more essential in clinical practice directed towards the maintenance of renal health, particularly in patients with established systemic diseases (Arthur et al., 2018). Beyond diet changes and physical training, the psychological aspect of well-being must never be overlooked in life change planning. Systemic illnesses are often accompanied by emotional upset, and this can negatively affect overall well-being and treatment compliance. Stress management tactics, such as mindfulness, cognitive behavioral therapy, and support groups, can lead to improved coping skills, thereby ensuring healthier lifestyle choices. Patients who engage in stress-reducing behaviors are likely to comply with dietary recommendations and exercise regimens. Therefore, the integration of mental health care into physical health interventions promotes a holistic approach to managing renal involvement in systemic disease. Such an approach is critical because it empowers patients, enhances their quality of life, and ultimately leads to improved health outcomes (Visseren et al., 2021).

7.6. Prognosis and Outcomes

The prognosis of renal involvement secondary to systemic disease varies significantly in severity and in underlying condition. In systemic sclerosis (SSc), for instance, renal complications are often manifested as asymptomatic reductions in glomerular filtration rate (GFR), increased renal arterial resistance, and more severe manifestations, such as scleroderma renal crisis (SRC). One SSc patient study indicated that while most patients had stable renal function for five years, some 4.9% developed SRC, which often necessitated dialysis. This highlights the requirement of ongoing monitoring, as the development of intrarenal arterial stiffness has a negative correlation with GFR. Therefore, effective management interventions must include intermittent clinical evaluation and imaging techniques to anticipate and manage renal involvement before widespread damage, which thereby affects patient outcomes and quality of life (Barbano et al., 2018). In the case of nephrectomy for nonmetastatic kidney cancer, prognosis can be significantly enhanced by the application of preoperative predictive models. A trial that considered 1,889 patients who underwent resection identified significant preoperative variables, such as age, gender, tumor size, and clinical stage, that were correlated with recurrence-free survival rates. The variables were utilized to develop a prognostic model of a concordance index of 0.747, which is high as a predictor of the likelihood of recurrence post-surgery. The findings underscore the need for tailored prognostic assessments that allow clinicians to stratify patients based on their unique risks. Hence, the incorporation of such predictive models not only enhances patient empowerment through evidence-based decision-making but also optimizes clinical outcomes through individualized follow-up therapy and interventions (Soyupak et al., 2012). The overall prognosis of patients with renal involvement due to systemic diseases cannot but be improved upon by early detection and management. Both in systemic sclerosis and kidney cancer, the identification of risk factors is also instrumental for patient outcomes. While SSc patients can have stable renal function for several years, patients with renal crisis can experience severe complications that necessitate aggressive treatments, making their treatment more complicated. Similarly, high-risk patients who are identified for nephrectomy at an earlier stage can stimulate the use of targeted surveillance strategies, refining them with forward-thinking interventions. Thus, the complexity of managing renal involvement in systemic diseases underscores the necessity of multidisciplinary expertise, prioritizing more severe appraisals and personalized treatment protocols to enhance prognostic outcomes and patient well-being.

7.6.1. Factors Influencing Renal Prognosis

Understanding the determinants of renal prognosis in patients with systemic disease provides valuable insights into disease management and patient outcomes. An important factor influencing renal prognosis is the quality and extent of organ involvement in systemic disease such as systemic sclerosis (SSc). Renal complications, particularly scleroderma renal crisis, are found to be closely linked with lower survival rates. In a multicenter French series, other complicating factors for renal involvement and prognosis are age at diagnosis, functional capacity at baseline, and pulmonary hypertension. Older age and diffuse cutaneous SSc, in particular, are associated with significantly higher risks of adverse outcomes, implying that the extent of skin involvement could be related to the evolution of renal impairment. Finally, early recognition of such essential factors can help in individualizing monitoring and intervention strategies to retard renal decline and improve overall prognosis in the setting of systemic illness (Varga et al., 2020). In the setting of viral infection, current research emphasizes the impact of SARS-CoV-2 on renal prognosis, especially in individuals with a history of cardiovascular and renal disease. The virus acts upon angiotensin-converting enzyme 2 (ACE2) receptors, which are ubiquitously present in the kidneys, leading to both acute kidney injury and chronic renal impairment. Systemic vasculopathy due to COVID-19 can worsen the existing renal pathology and illustrate the mutual nature of the interaction between kidney function and systemic inflammatory reactions. In addition, the manifestation of inflammatory cells that accumulate and extreme endothelial dysfunction, as observed at the time of postmortem examination in infected individuals, suggests that vascular integrity plays a critical role in renal prognosis. Hence, familiarity with viral pathophysiology related to renal function is required for formulating preventive modalities and therapeutic interventions, particularly in vulnerable patient populations with an increased burden of renal impairment (Varga et al., 2020). The interaction of environmental factors and genetic susceptibilities also plays a significant role in determining renal outcomes in systemic diseases. Autoantibody disease profiles for conditions such as SSc are also important prognostic indicators, with specific autoantibodies correlating with varying amounts of organ involvement, including renal. For instance, patients who are anti-Scl70 antibody-positive have a worse disease course with increased renal-associated morbidity. Additionally, extrinsic factors such as hypertension, obesity, and lifestyle choices can augment threats to renal deterioration in diverse patient populations. Such multifaceted effects necessitate an integrated therapeutic approach that encompasses genetic markers and modifiable risk factors in clinical assessment. By refining prognostic models to include such factors, healthcare providers can optimize patient management plans, ultimately leading to improved prognosis through evidence-based, focused interventions to preserve renal function in systemic disease settings (Pokeerbux et al., 2019).

7.6.2. Long-Term Effects of Systemic Diseases on Kidney Health

In assessing the long-term effects of systemic conditions on kidney health, diabetes nephropathy and hypertension are both important factors that lead to renal damage. Diabetic nephropathy is a chronic disorder caused by prolonged hyperglycemia, which leads to glomerular hypertension and hyperfiltration and eventually results in renal damage. Subsequently, this microvascular complication results in increased proteinuria and reduced glomerular filtration rates, ultimately leading to end-stage renal disease (ESRD) in the majority of patients. Interestingly, the prevalence of diabetic nephropathy in diabetic individuals may range between 20% and over 40%, reflecting a significant kidney disease burden. Hypertension, also typically coexistent with diabetes, exacerbates renal damage through direct mechanisms such as increased intraglomerular pressure and endothelial dysfunction, further adding to the decline in kidney function over a period of time (Visseren et al., 2021). Moreover, systemic autoimmune diseases such as systemic lupus erythematosus (SLE) have a severe impact on renal function, leading to a condition known as lupus nephritis. This involves the complication caused by the deposition of immune complexes in the kidney, which evokes inflammatory responses and damages renal tissue. Chronic lupus nephritis results in scarring and permanent damage, ultimately leading to CKD. Clinical evidence indicates that approximately 50% of SLE patients will develop some form of renal involvement during their lives, so early assessment and treatment are essential. Long-term management strategies that focus on both systemic inflammation and renal protection are essential for minimizing the adverse effects of lupus nephritis, including an elevated risk of cardiovascular diseases (Steven et al., 2021). Furthermore, the interface between chronic systemic diseases, like heart failure and COPD, and renal function cannot be prevented. These conditions are more likely to precipitate a multifactorial reduction in renal function through mechanisms such as renal hypoperfusion secondary to decreased cardiac output, or via the effects of systemic inflammation and oxidative stress. Patients with heart failure, for instance, usually present with deteriorating renal function due to hemodynamic instability, which leads to a syndrome known as cardiorenal syndrome. This syndrome can generate a vicious cycle, with renal impairment exacerbating the signs of heart failure and vice versa. The long-term effects of systemic disease on renal function necessitate comprehensive and multidisciplinary treatment, including regular monitoring of renal function and the application of proactive measures to prevent progressive renal deterioration (Visseren et al., 2021) (Figure 7.18).

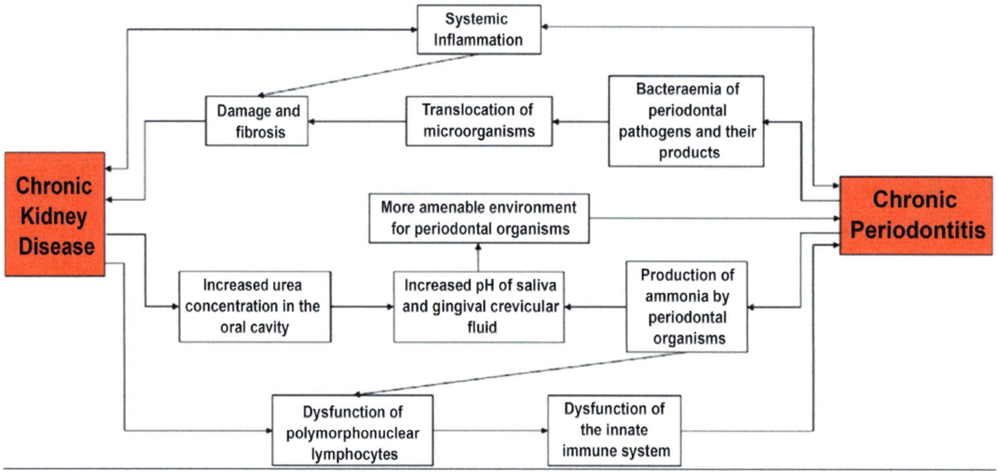

Figure 7.18. Long-term effects of systemic diseases on kidney health.

Source: https://www.researchgate.net/profile/Chris-Van-Der-Gast/publication/339209322/figure/fig3/AS:1032318248550411@1623135258540/Possible-interactions-between-the-systemic-effects-of-CKD-and-CP.png.

7.6.3. Importance of Early Intervention

The significance of early treatment in managing renal involvement in systemic disease cannot be overstated. Conditions such as SLE have a propensity to reveal renal complications that may initially not have clinical manifestations. The insidious course of LN may result in extensive renal injury before diagnosis because patients may have few indications of renal dysfunction despite background pathological changes. Early recognition through meticulous surveillance of the laboratory values, such as antinuclear antibodies and complements, is essential to the early initiation of treatment and prevention of irreversible damage. Such a case, for instance, with immediate therapy following abnormal laboratory findings, exemplifies improved renal results and serves as a reminder to the practitioner of the necessity for greater clinical acuity. Treatment of renal involvement is also becoming increasingly multidisciplinary. Early intervention often requires collaboration among nephrologists, rheumatologists, and primary care physicians to provide comprehensive patient care. Such collective effort is most beneficial in the early initiation of therapeutic interventions that can delay the advancement of renal disease. Therapy with immunosuppressive drugs, such as corticosteroids, in SLE patients with renal manifestations can stabilize both renal function and patient clinical outcomes. The case of a patient with silent LN, who presented with minimal symptoms but ultimately required a renal biopsy, is exemplary of the requirement for active clinical engagement. Through the creation of an interdisciplinary network, clinical teams are better positioned to expedite diagnosis and treatment, thereby enhancing patient quality of life and alleviating the burden of chronic renal injury (Elfar et al., 2024). Furthermore, early intervention of renal disease will have significant effects on the prognosis of long-term health in patients with systemic illnesses. Studies indicate that when patients receive early intervention for renal complications of illnesses like SLE, they experience better disease activity monitoring, resulting in lower morbidity and improved survival. For example, a patient who demonstrated acute neurological worsening, as in specific case reports, benefited from aggressive immunosuppressive therapy initiated early following diagnosis. Not only did the treatment correct renal inflammatory disorders, but it also prevented severe neurological damage, underscoring the importance of early intervention (Elfar et al., 2024). Ultimately, early detection, interdisciplinarity, and timely intervention collectively create an effective model for managing renal involvement in systemic diseases, ensuring optimal patient outcomes and long-term health sustainability.

SUMMARY

The intricate relationship between renal disease and systemic disease mirrors the sophistication of autoimmune pathophysiology, particularly in SLE. The findings imply that certain biomarkers, namely anti-P antibodies, are powerful predictors of individual clinical manifestations and renal injury. Isolated anti-P antibody patients possessed a distinct profile with reduced frequencies of renal and articular involvement compared to other antibody profiles. This directs towards a potential for stratifying patient risk based on serological markers, which may guide therapeutic interventions and monitoring approaches. Through such correlations, health professionals can better tailor treatments, thereby enhancing overall patient care for those suffering from systemic diseases with renal complications (Elghali et al., 2025). Advances in high-tech genomic tools have also elucidated pathophysiological mechanisms of renal complications in systemic diseases. The discovery of genes like ELF1, linked with disease activity and kidney damage in SLE, represents a significant step towards the elucidation of the molecular basis of such disorders. In particular, ELF1's differential expression in relation to various disease manifestations, urinary protein excretion, and complement activation suggests its potential as a biomarker for renal complications. By combining genetic data with clinical presentations, researchers can develop more precise diagnostic criteria and targeted treatments. Not only does this enhance our knowledge of disease pathogenesis but it also aligns with the trend of personalized medicine in the field of autoimmune disorders (Zhang et al., 2024). On a broader scale, the convergence of renal involvement with systemic disease is an indication of the necessity of a multi-dimensional diagnostic and treatment strategy. Continued research into biomarkers and genetics holds the potential to improve outcomes for patients with these complex diseases. Comparison of clinical findings associated with specific antibody profiles and the groundbreaking interrogation of genomic data hold the key to future developments that could revolutionize the way nephrology and rheumatology are treated. As the science progresses, the potential to enhance renal complications in systemic diseases becomes increasingly tangible, with assured better health outcomes among populations afflicted by such disorders. Prioritizing renal assessment in systemic conditions can provide avenues to more patient-centered care, indicating the importance of multidisciplinary care in chronic disease (Elghali et al., 2025).

The interaction between systemic diseases and renal participation highlights the character of kidney pathology in various settings. Autoimmune diseases, as a case in point, share the potential to manifest with renal implications, mirroring the tendency for the kidneys to both be a target and an actor in systemic immune activity. Sjögren's syndrome and immunoglobulin G4-related diseases are both good examples; both diseases result in inflammatory alterations that impair renal function. The impact of such autoimmune illnesses extends beyond symptomatic implications, leading to chronic renal disease if not controlled, thus underlining the significance of proper comprehension and early treatment in patients presenting systemically with autoimmune diseases (Vincentiis et al., 2017). Acute kidney injury (AKI) is also a significant concern of renal involvement in systemic diseases, typically arising from a multitude of underlying causes, including systemic infection, surgery, and pre-existing disease. The global trend toward surgery has been followed by a rising incidence of AKI, emphasizing the integration of surgical practice and kidney function. AKI is challenging in that it jeopardizes not just renal function but patient mortality and quality of life as well. Current pharmacological therapy is primarily aimed at symptom relief rather than preventing permanent injury. Therefore, it is essential to know the molecular mechanisms involved in AKI to develop targeted therapy that can treat the condition more efficiently and restrict its systemic implications (Human et al., 2015). Additionally, being aware of the molecular mechanisms that lead to renal failure in systemic diseases facilitates the development of more effective treatment strategies. Stimulation of pathways such as the renin-angiotensin-aldosterone system (RAAS) reflects a common thread among specific renal pathologies. The complex interactions between many cascades of signaling, including but not limited to those with tumor necrosis factor alpha (TNF) and transforming growth factor beta (TGF), are involved in the pathogenesis and exacerbation of renal injury. Perhaps most striking, however, is the unexpected contribution of the glutamatergic axis, historically associated with neural function, to the multifactorial nature of renal injury. Through explanation of these complex interactions, researchers to identify potential pharmacological targets, paving the way for new therapies that can prevent renal injury in patients with systemic disease (Human et al., 2015).

CLOSER LOOK

CARDIORENAL SYNDROME TYPE 5

Cardiorenal Syndrome (CRS) type 5 is a complex and multifactorial clinical syndrome in which an intrinsic systemic disorder causes cardiac and renal impairment simultaneously. Unlike with other types of CRS, where primary disease in one organ (either the kidney or heart) leads to secondary dysfunction of the different organ, type 5 involves acute or chronic systemic diseases like sepsis, systemic lupus erythematosus (SLE), diabetes mellitus, or amyloidosis that impact both the cardiovascular and renal systems at the same time. This simultaneous organ damage reflects the interconnected pathophysiology between the kidneys and heart and demonstrates how systemic inflammation, immune dysregulation, and hemodynamic instability can drive multi-organ injury. In type 5 CRS, damage to both organs is not sequential but concurrent, resulting from shared pathological mechanisms such as cytokine storm, oxidative stress, microvascular derangement, and pathological neurohormonal activation.

Sepsis is the most common and clinically significant etiology of type 5 cardiorenal syndrome. During sepsis, widespread inflammatory activation leads to vasodilation, capillary leakage, and hypotension, resulting in tissue hypoperfusion and cellular injury in the myocardium and renal parenchyma. The inflammatory mediators such as tumor necrosis factor-alpha (TNF-α), interleukins (IL-1, IL-6), and nitric oxide are held accountable for cardiac depression (septic cardiomyopathy) and acute kidney injury (AKI). In addition, mitochondrial impairment and apoptosis of cardiac myocytes and renal tubular cells are also causative of organ failure. Deposition of immune complexes and complement activation, with the involvement of other systemic illnesses such as SLE or systemic vasculitides, can lead to glomerulonephritis and myocarditis together. Endothelial dysfunction, atherosclerosis, and advanced glycation end-products resulting from chronic hyperglycemia in diabetes cause diabetic nephropathy as well as cardiomyopathy. Diagnosis of CRS type 5 requires a high index of suspicion and systems-based approach, considering the global systemic process rather than isolated organ dysfunction. Clinical evaluation includes determining the etiologic systemic disease and quantifying the degree of renal and cardiac dysfunction through laboratory and imaging studies. Biomarkers such as serum creatinine, estimated glomerular filtration rate (eGFR), troponins, B-type natriuretic peptide (BNP), and inflammatory markers (e.g., CRP, procalcitonin) aid in diagnosis and monitoring. Imaging techniques, such as echocardiography and renal ultrasonography, provide additional information about the structural and functional status. Early diagnosis is essential because the coexistence of both heart and kidney dysfunction has a far poorer prognosis, higher rates of morbidity and mortality, and longer hospital stays.

Management of CRS type 5 is particularly challenging because therapeutic methods must simultaneously address both renal and cardiac dysfunctions and target the underlying systemic cause. Fluid resuscitation, vasopressor therapy, and rapid and aggressive treatment of the infection are critical in sepsis-induced type 5 CRS. Fluid management should be, however, strictly controlled to avoid worsening pulmonary edema or kidney injury. In autoimmune or metabolic disease, immunosuppression, glycemic control, and organ-protective measures are paramount. Supportive therapy in severe forms can involve renal replacement therapy and inotropic support. Coordination of nephrologists, cardiologists, and intensivists is of paramount importance for optimal patient outcomes.

References

1. Gigante, A., Barbano, B., Barilaro, G., Quarta, S., Gasperini, M. L., Di Mario, F., Romaniello, A., Amoroso, A., Cianci, R., & Rosato, E. (2016). Serum uric acid as a marker of microvascular damage in systemic sclerosis patients. *Microvascular Research, 106*, 39–43. https://doi.org/10.1016/j.mvr.2016.03.007Athanassiou, P., & Athanassiou, L. (2023). Current treatment approach, emerging therapies and new horizons in systemic lupus erythematosus. *Life, 13.* https://www.semanticscholar.org/paper/7dfcb2a414fa3b7c93feda0cf5e08fc9878130f9 (accessed on 25th June 2025).
2. Barbano, B., Cianci, R., Gasperini, M. L., Gigante, A., et al. (2018). Prognostic factors of renal involvement in systemic sclerosis. https://core.ac.uk/download/159268972.pdf (accessed on 25th June 2025).
3. Boin, F., Carns, M., Chung, L., Criswell, L. A., et al. (2017). Clinical and serological features of systemic sclerosis in a multicenter African American cohort: Analysis of the genome research in African American scleroderma patient's clinical database. https://core.ac.uk/download/323074312.pdf (accessed on 25th June 2025).
4. Bouden, S., Ben Messaoud, M., Saidane, O., Rouached, L., Ben Tekaya, A., Mahmoud, I., Tekaya, R., et al. (2023). AB1062 Renal involvement in spondylarthritis. *Annals of the Rheumatic Diseases.* https://www.semanticscholar.org/paper/8fa43658533d61c5ad6ace14f848572e79865001 (accessed on 25th June 2025).
5. Božić Majstorović, L., & Ovcina, I. (2023). AB0884 The importance of renal impairment in systemic sclerosis. *Annals of the Rheumatic Diseases.* https://www.semanticscholar.org/paper/cec4afa842ae46e96d5f4d8ba3559e2652768c15 (accessed on 25th June 2025).
6. Braun, G. S., Horster, S., Ihrler, S., Schmid, H., et al. (2007). Cryoglobulinemic vasculitis: Classification and clinical and therapeutic aspects. https://core.ac.uk/download/12175185.pdf (accessed on 25th June 2025).
7. Brém, E., Koyfman, A., & Long, B. J. (2020). Oncologic emergencies: Immune-based cancer therapies and complications. https://core.ac.uk/download/305124082.pdf (accessed on 25th June 2025).
8. Burkly, L. C., Mischak, H., Mullen, W., Pejchinovski, M., et al. (2018). Urine peptidome biomarkers for diagnosis of patients with systemic lupus erythematosus. https://core.ac.uk/download/82958552.pdf (accessed on 25th June 2025).
9. Burnett, A. L., Nehra, A., Breau, R. H., Culkin, D. J., Faraday, M. M., Hakim, L., Heidelbaugh, J. J., et al. (2018). Erectile dysfunction: AUA guideline. *The Journal of Urology, 200*, 633–641. https://doi.org/10.1016/j.juro.2018.05.004 (accessed on 25th June 2025).
10. Campbell, S. C., Uzzo, R. G., Allaf, M. E., Bass, E. B., Cadeddu, J. A., Chang, A., Clark, P. E., et al. (2017). Renal mass and localized renal cancer: AUA guideline. *The Journal of Urology, 198*, 520–529. https://doi.org/10.1016/j.juro.2017.04.100 (accessed on 25th June 2025).
11. Campbell, S. C., Uzzo, R. G., Karam, J. A., Chang, S. S., Clark, P. E., & Souter, L. (2021). Renal mass and localized renal cancer: Evaluation, management, and follow-up: AUA guideline: Part II. *The Journal of Urology, 206*, 209–218. https://doi.org/10.1097/ju.0000000000001912 (accessed on 25th June 2025).

12. Cheng, X., Zhou, T., He, Y., Xie, Y., Xu, Y., & Huang, W. (2022). The role and mechanism of butyrate in the prevention and treatment of diabetic kidney disease. *Frontiers in Microbiology, 13.* https://www.semanticscholar.org/paper/7c37034466219f7eaf649841a86b45c71f1549d9 (accessed on 25th June 2025).

13. Chowdhury, M. N. (2024). Renal involvement in vasculitis: An evidence-based approach. *Bangladesh Journal of Medicine.* https://www.semanticscholar.org/paper/378895141d0a1057ff7a7e34919dd2fb54ca5eef (accessed on 25th June 2025).

14. De Vincentiis, M., De Virgilio, A., Fusconi, M., Gallo, A., et al. (2017). Sialendoscopic management of autoimmune sialadenitis: A review of literature. https://core.ac.uk/download/98339930.pdf (accessed on 25th June 2025).

15. El Abasse, Z. (2024). Peculiarity of systemic lupus erythematosus with cardiac involvement in case report and literature review. *Clinical Cardiology and Cardiovascular Interventions.* https://www.semanticscholar.org/paper/c1a844db383b416eb3f245757151de2eceb7a85b (accessed on 25th June 2025).

16. Elfar, E., Baldwin, C., Sukhija, G., Thoroughgood, J., Rabee, H., Rutherford, A., Mahto, A., et al. (2024). OA19 Acute confusion, reduced conscious levels and stroke in systemic lupus erythematosus resulting from cerebral vasculitis. *Rheumatology Advances in Practice, 8.* https://www.semanticscholar.org/paper/aba98ac6746c2c453d38196c50cae444caa174ab (accessed on 25th June 2025).

17. Elghali, M., Yosr, B., Syrine, D., Mahbouba, J., Nabil, S., & Sonia, H. (2025). Isolated anti-ribosomal P antibodies are associated with reduced risk of renal and articular involvement in systemic lupus erythematosus patients. An observational study from one center. *Rheumatologic, 63,* 27–34. https://www.semanticscholar.org/paper/3d94d1b2e20ee949da5e22db8578331c49aa3be6 (accessed on 25th June 2025).

18. Estarreja, J., Pimenta, A. C., Botelho, J., Vilares, A., Mendes, J., Rocha, J., Pinto, R., et al. (2024). Blood count, endocrine, immunologic, renal, and hepatic markers in a case-control animal study of induced periodontitis in female rodents. *Frontiers in Physiology, 15.* https://www.semanticscholar.org/paper/23925b6e9a829b921a6c0baea495d062bf3c50ab (accessed on 25th June 2025).

19. Fagni, A., Bettiol, A., Silvestri, E., Fedi, R., Palermo, A., Urban, M. L., Mazzotta, R., et al. (2023). AB0667 Characterizing ultrasound-proven enthesitis in systemic lupus erythematosus: Prevalence and identification of disease subset with less frequent renal involvement. *Annals of the Rheumatic Diseases.* https://www.semanticscholar.org/paper/dcaee6a9e0319e9d717d8463a381635c0be410bb (accessed on 25th June 2025).

20. Franzin, R., Stasi, A., Ranieri, E., Netti, G., Cantaluppi, V., Gesualdo, L., Stallone, G., et al. (2021). Targeting premature renal aging: From molecular mechanisms of cellular senescence to Seno lytic trials. *Frontiers in Pharmacology, 12.* https://www.semanticscholar.org/paper/1f4c32c50589919a5dadb417364c9aa398681f13 (accessed on 25th June 2025).

21. Gentile, M., Maggiore, U., Manenti, L., Fenaroli, P., Delsante, M., Fiaccadori, E., & Rossi, G. M. (2023). #2533 Prognostic significance of arteriolar C4d positivity as a marker of microangiopathy in ANCA-associated vasculitis. *Nephrology Dialysis Transplantation.* https://www.semanticscholar.org/paper/516756ba1962a9816c58971d3f26d21cc3beaeb3 (accessed on 25th June 2025).

22. Gokcen, N., & Çefle, A. (2024). Clinical features of late-onset systemic lupus erythematosus. *Anti-Aging Eastern Europe.* https://www.semanticscholar.org/paper/3e98e5922007c4ea360b0aa54fd1af7e6a9597ad (accessed on 25th June 2025).

23. Hasan, M. (2023). Silent lupus nephritis: Unmasking the subtle burden of renal involvement in systemic lupus erythematosus–A case report. *Community Based Medical Journal.* https://www.semanticscholar.org/paper/940aef2f2b6624072d55a7c62b91dd9c936c92b8 (accessed on 25th June 2025).

24. Huang, S., Zhang, Z., Cui, Y., Yao, G., Ma, X., & Zhang, H. (2023). Dyslipidemia is associated with inflammation and organ involvement in systemic lupus erythematosus. *Clinical Rheumatology, 42*, 1565–1572. https://www.semanticscholar.org/paper/3e73051cde53d84ce65f5528c167ed545d097d09 (accessed on 25th June 2025).

25. Human, C., & Husi, H. (2015). Molecular determinants of acute kidney injury. https://core.ac.uk/download/46559950.pdf (accessed on 25th June 2025).

26. Issayeva, E., Aseeva, N., Nikishina, A., Mesnyankina, A., Solovyev, S., Issayeva, S., Saparbayeva, M., et al. (2023). AB0622 Lupus nephritis: Is the kidney biopsy currently necessary in the management of lupus nephritis? *Annals of the Rheumatic Diseases.* https://www.semanticscholar.org/paper/937520d3571eaa7a65235be3e1a058474a27e1f4 (accessed on 25th June 2025).

27. Kamal, S., Jehangir, R., Yaqoob, M., Tariq, H., Quddos, H., Ullah, B., & Ullah, R. (2025). Early detection of renal cyst on ultrasonography and their associated risk factors. *Insights–Journal of Health and Rehabilitation.* https://www.semanticscholar.org/paper/4d907a56e4786b4710fb5d15f553c79fbd665393 (accessed on 25th June 2025).

28. Karlsson, L., Zickert, A., Svenungsson, E., Schmidt-Mende, J., Faustini, F., & Gunnarsson, I. (2023). Urinary aberrations in systemic lupus erythematosus not always indicative of lupus nephritis: A cross-sectional cohort study. *Clinical Rheumatology, 42*, 2981–2986. https://www.semanticscholar.org/paper/4573af2a04ff21eab9d7a12d45c69473edc4ca11 (accessed on 25th June 2025).

29. Kim, J. H., Shin, J. I., Kim, J. H., & Lee, K. (2024). A rare case of childhood-onset systemic lupus erythematosus associated end-stage renal disease with cerebral abscess and hemorrhage. *Childhood Kidney Diseases.* https://www.semanticscholar.org/paper/1a197916db5a7c66b3e5838399be81e9b74f3af0 (accessed on 25th June 2025).

30. Kitsiou, A. L. P., Caforio, A., Porta-Sanchez, A., Vahanian, A., Iung, B., Carrera, C., Szymanski, C., et al. (2013). ESC core curriculum for the general cardiologist (2013). https://core.ac.uk/download/55756305.pdf (accessed on 25th June 2025).

31. Litvinov, S., Savin, A. V., Kukhtina, A. A., & Sitovskaya, D. A. (2020). Clinical and morphological parallels of lung and kidney damage in COVID-19. *Nephrology (Saint-Petersburg).* https://www.semanticscholar.org/paper/dc65ac4adc5587b8b4023b6d81f4fbd61d5e3edf (accessed on 25th June 2025).

32. Lubas, J., Staszewski, A., Maliborski, M., Mosakowska, M., Spłocharski, G., Bilbin-Bukowska, A., Wołoszyńska, I., et al. (2022). Vascular and vasogenic manifestations of systemic ANCA-associated vasculitis with renal involvement in non-contrast brain MRI in patients with acute disease onset. *Journal of Clinical Medicine, 11.* https://www.semanticscholar.org/paper/7af69de6939a1ebb934959ef21986b74d185d9d6 (accessed on 25th June 2025).

33. Marzoog, B. A. (2023). Pathophysiology of cardiac cell injury in post-COVID-19 syndrome. *New Emirates Medical Journal.* https://www.semanticscholar.org/paper/4a24e9c3ced02e781b2de4fbe27b9488e202df37 (accessed on 25th June 2025).

34. Mehta, R., Rabb, H., Shaw, A., Singbartl, K., Ronco, C., McCullough, P., & Kellum, J. (2013). Cardiorenal syndrome type 5: Clinical presentation, pathophysiology and management strategies from the eleventh consensus conference of the Acute Dialysis Quality Initiative (ADQI). *Contributions to Nephrology, 182*, 174–194. https://www.semanticscholar.org/paper/542a9e3d8d05d21407dad0f0f9e955bd65306a81 (accessed on 25th June 2025).

35. Mohareb, M., Ugwoke, A., & Gendi, N. (2022). OA14 A case of scleromyxedema with muscle involvement including myotonia and dysphagia. *Rheumatology Advances in Practice, 6.* https://www.semanticscholar.org/paper/04d5289b4de3ac125e4479f0c9ff5ddab8bf7626 (accessed on 25th June 2025).

36. Navarro-Trivio, F. J. (2020). Vitamin D level and its influence on systemic lupus erythematosus: An overview. *Volume 5*, 1–3. https://www.semanticscholar.org/paper/46fc21c8eb2a1a047204770f670b15f2e57f7185 (accessed on 25th June 2025).

37. Oprinca, C., Mohor, A., Bereanu, L. A., Oprinca-Muja, Lilioara-Alexandra, Bogdan-Duică, I., Fleacă, S., Hașegan, A., et al. (2024). Detection of SARS-CoV-2 viral genome and viral nucleocapsid in various organs and systems. *International Journal of Molecular Sciences, 25.* https://www.semanticscholar.org/paper/56a30d76225e613705bc52cdf9a371c341a66665 (accessed on 25th June 2025).

38. Petrea Cliveți, C. L., Ciortea, D., Miulescu, M., Candussi, I. L., Chirilă, S., Verga (Răuță), G. I., Bergheș, S. E., et al. (2024). A new case of pediatric systemic lupus erythematosus with onset after SARS-CoV-2 and Epstein-Barr infection—A case report and literature review. *Current Issues in Molecular Biology, 46*, 8642–8657. https://www.semanticscholar.org/paper/937d267466688007a8eeb506e0608b6c4bff6e90 (accessed on 25th June 2025).

39. Pokeerbux, M. R., Giovannelli, J., Dauchet, L., Mouthon, L., Agard, C., Lega, J.-C., Allanore, Y., et al. (2019). Survival and prognosis factors in systemic sclerosis: Data of a French multicenter cohort, systematic review, and meta-analysis of the literature. *Arthritis Research & Therapy, 21.* https://doi.org/10.1186/s13075-019-1867-1 (accessed on 25th June 2025).

40. Ponikowski, P., Voors, A. A., Anker, S. D., Bueno, H., Cleland, J. G. F., Coats, A. J. S., Falk, V., et al. (2016). 2016 ESC Guidelines for the diagnosis and treatment of acute and chronic heart failure. *European Heart Journal, 37*, 2129–2200. https://doi.org/10.1093/eurheartj/ehw128 (accessed on 25th June 2025).

41. Przygocka, A., Berti, G. M., Campus, A., Tondolo, F., Vischini, G., Fabbrizio, B., La Manna, G., et al. (2023). Rituximab as possible therapy in TNF inhibitor-induced IgA vasculitis with severe renal involvement. *BMC Nephrology, 24.* https://www.semanticscholar.org/paper/21e192785ce99f8a9f6b5e073e78567251ddbe0d (accessed on 25th June 2025).

42. Rizzo, L., La Barbera, M., Lo Pizzo, L., Mohammadnezhad, V. L., Lentini, D., Donzella, F., Ciccia, F., et al. (2022). POS0101 Potential involvement of IL-40 and IL-40 producing cells in systemic lupus erythematosus and lupus-associated nephritis. *Annals of the Rheumatic Diseases.* https://www.semanticscholar.org/paper/a152429cec75753b181ec89246a4931172911d34 (accessed on 25th June 2025).

43. Sağlam, M. K., Yıldırım, S., Ergüven, M., & Sungur, M. A. (2025). Gastrointestinal features of pediatric IgA vasculitis and their association with renal complications: An observational study. *European Journal of Pediatrics, 184.* https://www.semanticscholar.org/paper/f258c0ed0047f8f9834d6121973dc9586b66454b (accessed on 25th June 2025).

44. Santos, T. M. M., de Souza, A. D., Sá, A. C. M., Moreira, J. L., Batista, L. C., Amorim, M. C., Moreira, M. R., et al. (2024). Renal histopathological lesions associated with SARS-CoV-2 infection in patients with no history of kidney disease: A systematic review. *Journal of Advances in Medicine and Medical Research.* https://www.semanticscholar.org/paper/8099782a119b750bc0e6b895cd81f9e631a16f9c (accessed on 25th June 2025).

45. Severino, R. S. (2024). Medical use of finererone in patients with diabetes mellitus and chronic kidney disease. *Journal of Diabetes, Metabolic Disorders & Control.* https://www.semanticscholar.org/paper/971171ea52c8b7500ca87df6a260408fab5df230 (accessed on 25th June 2025).

46. Singer, M., Deutschman, C. S., Seymour, C. W., Shankar-Hari, M., Annane, D., Bauer, M., Bellomo, R., et al. (2016). The Third International Consensus Definitions for Sepsis and Septic Shock (Sepsis-3). *JAMA, 315,* 801–801. https://doi.org/10.1001/jama.2016.0287 (accessed on 25th June 2025).

47. Soyupak, C., Gogus, C., Karabulut, E., Ozen, H., Turkeri, L., Yaycioglu, O., et al. (2012). Patients with kidney cancer. https://core.ac.uk/download/227071316.pdf (accessed on 25th June 2025).

48. Teixeira, A. A., Araújo, J., Brinca, A., Carvalho, F., et al. (2014). Doença renal na Região Autónoma da Madeira: Experiência de vinte e sete anos de biópsias de rim nativo. https://core.ac.uk/download/71739053.pdf (accessed on 25th June 2025).

49. Varga, Z., Flammer, A. J., Steiger, P., Haberecker, M., Andermatt, R., Zinkernagel, A. S., Mehra, M. R., et al. (2020). Endothelial cell infection and endotheliitis in COVID-19. *The Lancet, 395,* 1417–1418. https://doi.org/10.1016/s0140-6736(20)30937-5 (accessed on 25th June 2025).

50. Visseren, F. L. J., Mach, F., Smulders, Y. M., Carballo, D., Koskinas, K. C., Bäck, M., Bénétos, A., et al. (2021). 2021 ESC Guidelines on cardiovascular disease prevention in clinical practice. *European Heart Journal, 42,* 3227–3337. https://doi.org/10.1093/eurheartj/ehab484 (accessed on 25th June 2025).

51. Zerhoudi, R., Bourzeg, K., Eljazouli, H., Elmasrioui, J., Yahya, A., Ztati, M., Eljamili, M., et al. (2025). Beyond the kidneys: Cardiac involvement in ANCA vasculitis. *Cardiology and Angiology: An International Journal.* https://www.semanticscholar.org/paper/f6d800eb83a3e6201dceec26094554c4d6e2ef7d (accessed on 25th June 2025).

52. Zhang, Y., Cai, M., Huang, X., Zhang, L., Wen, L., Zhu, Z., Gao, J., et al. (2024). ELF1 serves as a potential biomarker for the disease activity and renal involvement in systemic lupus erythematosus. *Scientific Reports, 14.* https://www.semanticscholar.org/paper/73df1cb74e1a786077f1e7ce70490e9ee9a0a0e9 (accessed on 25th June 2025).

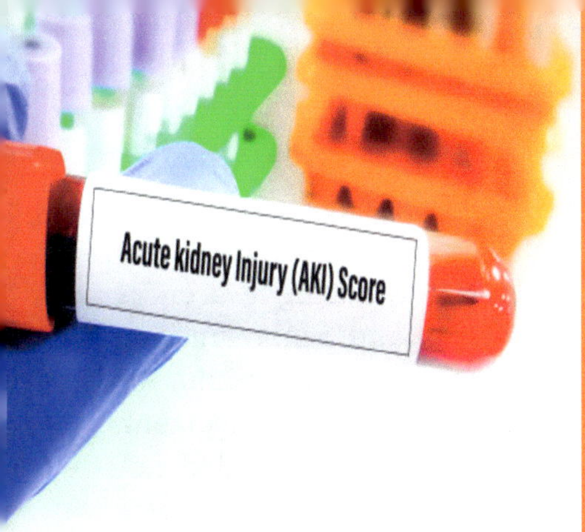

Chapter 8
ACUTE KIDNEY INJURY (AKI)

Contents

Introduction

Acute kidney injury (AKI) is a significant clinical entity representing an acute reduction in renal function, occurring from hours to days. Not only does it disrupt the kidney's function to stabilize electrolytes and regulate acid-base balance, but it also potentially causes irreversible damage if left unchecked. The causes of AKI are varied, ranging from underlying medical problems such as diabetes and hypertension to acute causes including trauma and operations. Notably, the high incidence of surgeries globally has resulted in a concerning growth in AKI cases, thereby aggravating concerns regarding mortality rates and healthcare spending. Current interventions for the management of AKI are symptomatic in character with no efficient curative treatment, and reflect an increasing necessity to explore and expand research in this significant area of nephrology (Human et al., 2015). Understanding the molecular processes that control AKI is essential to elucidating its intricate pathophysiology. The disease initiates a cascade of several signaling pathways leading to cell damage and dysfunction.

For instance, the renin-angiotensin-aldosterone system (RAAS) is a key player that triggers downstream processes like immune responses via the NF-κB pathway. Other key pathways, including those of tumor necrosis factor-alpha (TNF) and transforming growth factor-beta (TGF), are implicated in the pathological development of AKI. Moreover, recent data provide evidence of the involvement of the glutamatergic axis—a pathway traditionally implicated in neurological processes—in the process of renal injury. Therefore, a highly differentiated understanding of these molecular interactions is necessary for the development of targeted pharmacologic therapy with the goal of diminishing the effect of AKI and preventing long-term kidney damage (Human et al., 2015).

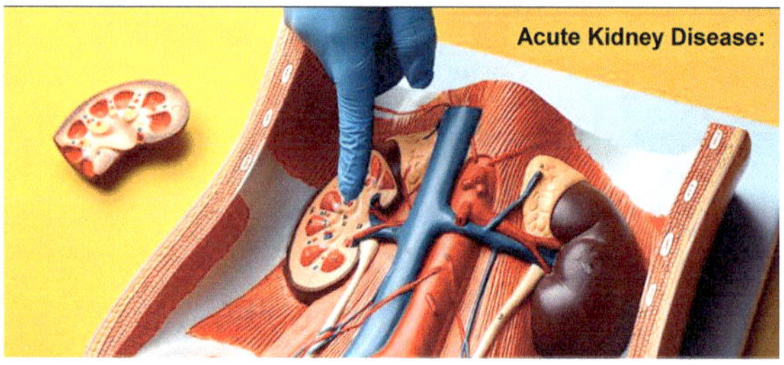

Figure 8.1. Understanding acute kidney injury (AKI).

Source: https://images.nirmalsuperspecialityhospital.com/Understan_23_07_2024_11_07_34.png.

Of particular concern is the development of pregnancy-associated acute kidney injury (PRAKI), which accentuates the unique issue confronting some groups. Even though the incidence of PRAKI has decreased with better obstetric care and legal reforms in reproductive health among developed countries, the condition remains a priority in the majority of developing nations. The maternal and fetal complications that are generally associated with it are incredibly severe, and they also cause increased rates of morbidity and mortality. Hypertension-related disorders, obstetric hemorrhage, sepsis, and acute fatty liver of pregnancy are some of the causes of PRAKI. Therefore, raising awareness about these risk factors and renal function adaptations in pregnancy is paramount for the early detection and adequate management. These elements must be comprehended not only to reduce maternal and fetal risks but also to improve overall obstetric outcomes in such populations (Figure 8.1).

Definition of Acute Kidney Injury

Acute kidney injury (AKI) is a critical clinical syndrome with acute loss of renal function, with significant prognostic implications for patient outcome. Briefly described, AKI is an acute reduction in renal function that occurs over a short duration and could present as decreased glomerular filtration rate (GFR) resulting in the accumulation of waste products in the circulation. The clinical syndrome is characterized by a heterogeneous etiology that encompasses prerenal, intrinsic, and postrenal etiologies. The identification of AKI is of utmost importance given its prevalence in the health care setting, where it may arise rapidly, particularly in people who are at risk, such as surgery patients or those with a history of existing medical conditions. Formal AKI definitions have been revised, with the 2012 kidney disease: Improving global outcomes providing structured guidance that enhances our understanding of the condition and reminds us of the need for early action to prevent renal damage (Kellum et al., 2013). Clinically, the Acute Kidney Injury Network (AKIN) criteria are central to the diagnosis and staging of AKI, and also in providing a standardized treatment approach. According to these definitions, AKI is characterized by an abrupt increase in serum creatinine, a rise of 0.3 mg/dL or greater within 48 hours, or a relative increase of greater than 50% from the baseline value. Or else, oliguria, defined as a urine output of less than 0.5 mL/kg per hour for six hours or more, can be employed as a diagnostic criterion. These conditions bring into focus the necessity of early diagnosis as well as careful monitoring of renal function, particularly among patients who are hospitalized and potentially at risk of AKI. Precision in the definition of AKI not only contributes to clinical diagnosis but also brings into focus the necessity of timely preventative treatment and intervention to avoid complications of AKI (Malhotra et al., 2015). Additionally, knowledge of the etiology and pathophysiology of AKI is crucial for developing effective treatment modalities. AKI can be caused by multiple factors, such as dehydration, nephrotoxins, and acute glomerulonephritis, each requiring specific interventions. AKI requires a multidisciplinary approach to be treated effectively, involving the correction of inciting causes, avoidance of additional renal injury, and careful surveillance of renal function. Evidence-based practice recommendations require monitoring of fluid balance, normalization of blood pressure, and avoidance of nephrotoxic medications, emphasizing the need for an active strategy in susceptible patients. By and large, AKI remains a vital issue for modern medicine, with ongoing research and clinical guideline development being required to enhance outcomes in affected patients and reduce the morbidity of this preventable disease (Kellum et al., 2013).

Importance of Understanding AKI

AKI is a severe clinical problem, and understanding its etiology, pathophysiology, and impact on patient outcomes is essential. The importance of understanding AKI extends beyond clinical care itself; it is pivotal in creating a framework for effective prevention and intervention programs. AKI frequently precedes more advanced disease states like CKD and ESRD, placing significant healthcare burdens and impacting the quality of life for these patients. A comprehensive understanding of AKI can guide healthcare providers in identifying risk factors, enabling them to recognize at-risk groups early. Such awareness is crucial, as it allows for timely intervention that can prevent the course of renal damage and minimize the risk of injurious long-term sequelae, thereby improving patient care and the efficiency of the health system. Furthermore, the relationship between acute kidney injury and postoperative morbidity indicates the need for extensive education and awareness in clinical practice. In particular, postoperative acute kidney injury (PO-AKI) is common in patients who undergo major surgeries and has dangerous consequences for their health pathways. Older age and comorbidities during admission may increase susceptibility to PO-AKI, and therefore, healthcare professionals have to spot high-risk patients early before surgery. Grasping the clinical parameters that characterize AKI, most significantly through KDIGO classification, enables practitioners to obtain the tools needed to observe kidney function and apply preventative measures closely. Managing AKI in a surgical setting not only reinforces the importance of thorough preoperative evaluation but also fosters the development of personalized care strategies that prioritize kidney health, thereby improving overall patient outcomes (Bihorac et al., 2021). Ultimately, a general understanding of acute kidney injury directs research and health policy, informing advances in therapeutic practice and resource allocation. Investment in AKI research can yield more accurate diagnostic tools and therapies, allowing for tailored interventions to individual patients. Health systems that encourage awareness of AKI can implement targeted practitioner and patient education, thereby increasing knowledge about risk factors and management. As illustrated within the health setting, prevention of CKD can yield substantial economic impacts; hence, education on AKI can become a catalyst for more integrated CKD prevention programs designed to avoid CKD advancing to ESRD (Hoffmann et al., 2015). By conceptualizing AKI as a central component of renal disease within primary care, healthcare systems can facilitate improved patient pathways, ultimately leading to better cardiovascular and renal outcomes within the population (Figure 8.2).

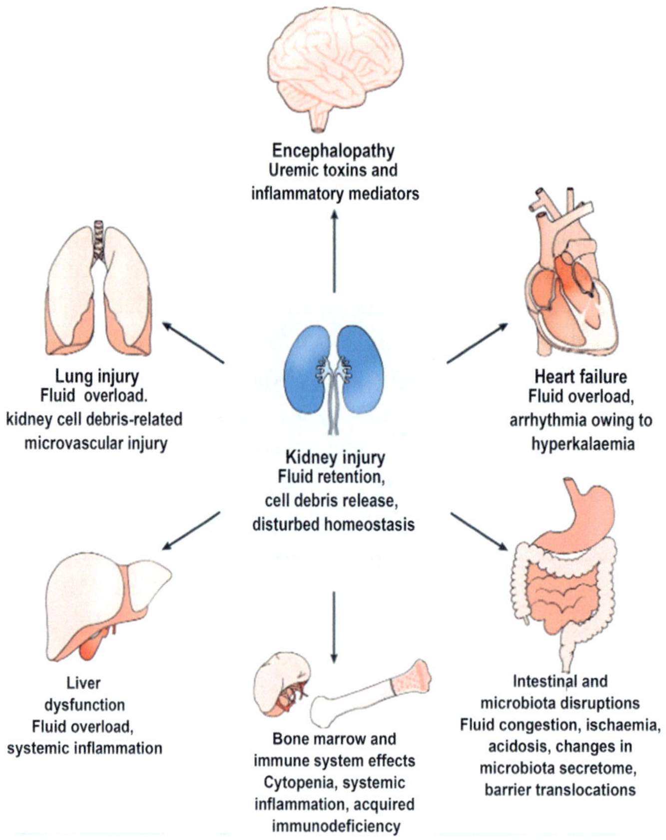

Figure 8.2. Understanding AKI.

Source: https://media.springernature.com/lw1200/springer-static/image/art%3A10.1038%2Fs41572-021-00284-z/MediaObjects/41572_2021_284_Fig3_HTML.png.

8.1. Causes of Acute Kidney Injury

The multifactorial pathophysiology of acute kidney injury (AKI) is primarily attributed to the unique interaction of a variety of intrinsic and extrinsic determinants. Perhaps the most frequent cause is prerenal azotemia, which results from decreased renal perfusion due to hypovolemia, heart failure, or systemic vasodilation. Decreased renal blood flow is particularly prevalent in the elderly, who, with advancing age, undergo increased physiological changes that render them increasingly vulnerable to renal damage. In this population, comorbid conditions like diabetes or hypertension further complicate them towards renal dysfunction and hence AKI during hospital stay or critical illness. Furthermore, AKI often develops from iatrogenic causes, in which medical interventions unintentionally accelerate the deterioration of renal function. With more hospitals and intensive care units acknowledging the significance of AKI prevention, awareness of these causes becomes a necessity for effective management and intervention strategies, particularly for vulnerable populations (Calvaruso et al., 2020). Drug-induced nephrotoxicity is another significant cause of AKI and an inherent problem in inpatients and outpatients. 20–60% of hospital inpatients are said to experience AKI secondary to drugs, and the most common causative drugs are antimicrobials. While vital in the treatment of infections, some antibiotics are capable of inducing various forms of renal injury, ranging from acute tubular necrosis to interstitial nephritis.

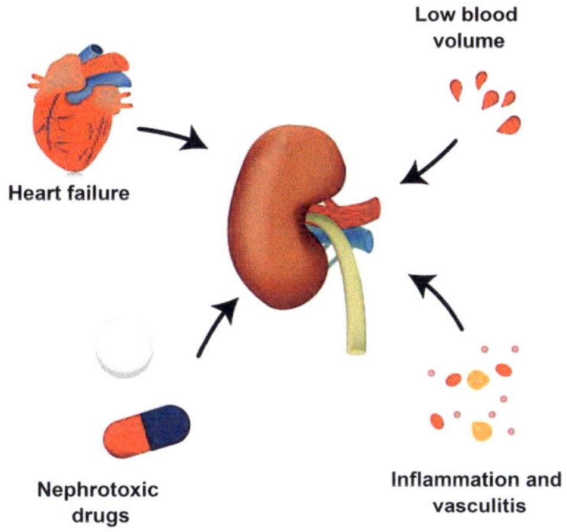

Figure 8.3. Causes of acute kidney injury.

Source: https://wp04-media.cdn.ihealthspot.com/wp-content/uploads/sites/464/2024/08/Acute-Kidney-Injury-1.jpg.

The risk of nephrotoxicity is higher with coexistent renal disease or with the concomitant use of two or more nephrotoxic agents. Understanding the pathogenic processes of such harmful effects allows for more informed clinical decisions and the introduction of preventive measures to mitigate risk. For clinicians, recognizing the characteristics of antimicrobial-induced nephrotoxicity enables early intervention, ultimately reducing the incidence of AKI and its associated morbidity (Abishek et al., 2023). Induction of AKI can also be induced by many systemic diseases, indicating the intricate relationship between renal function and overall physiological status. For instance, sepsis and septic shock can lead to kidney damage through hemodynamic instability, inflammation, and the release of nephrotoxic mediators. Under these conditions, a cascade of pathophysiological responses occurs, compromising renal perfusion and function. The aged with multiple comorbidities are most susceptible to sepsis attacks and raise the risk for developing AKI. Besides, other systemic diseases such as liver failure or cardiovascular instability may further compromise renal function, making AKI a multi-factorial syndrome. Hence, in developing prevention and management protocols to prevent the incidence of AKI and improve patient outcomes, an in-depth understanding of these systematic etiologies becomes relevant (Calvaruso et al., 2020) (Figure 8.3).

8.1.1. Pre-Renal Causes

The occurrence of AKI is typically triggered by pre-renal causes that disrupt the delicate balance between renal perfusion. The conditions are normally brought about by situations that compromise blood flow to the kidneys and therefore their ability to excrete waste. Hypovolemia is a very prevalent pre-renal cause and can result from many situations, including excessive loss of fluid due to severe dehydration, hemorrhage, or sequestration of fluids in burns. A decreased effective circulating blood volume leads to diminished renal perfusion, thereby jeopardizing the glomerular filtration rate (GFR). A patient with severe volume depletion, for instance, typically has an elevated serum creatinine, indicating the kidneys' response to compromised perfusion. Understanding these mechanisms is critical in managing susceptible patients and in the early interventions to ensure blood volume and kidney function are preserved. But yet another significant pre-renal cause of AKI is cardiac failure, which impairs the heart's function to pump blood properly, and therefore decreases renal perfusion.

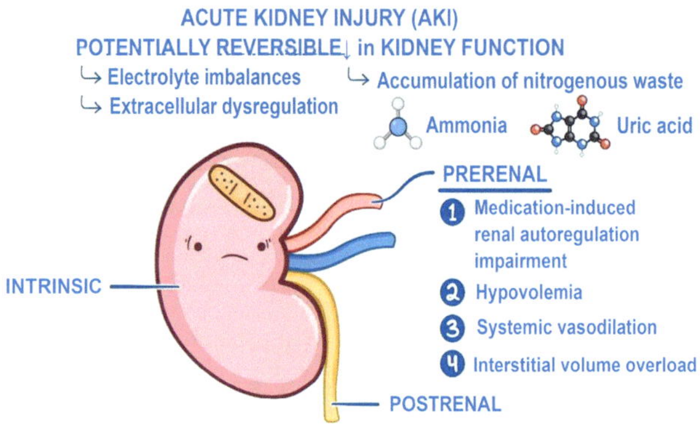

Figure 8.4. Pre-renal acute kidney injury.

Source: https://d16qt3wv6xm098.cloudfront.net/9X_1YbqmQmWK6v9oR193lj44RmqxNT7S/_.jpg.

Myocardial infarction or congestive heart failure can significantly lower the quantity of blood being sent to the kidneys, causing relative hypoperfusion. Under such conditions, the kidneys can react actively by activating the renin-angiotensin-aldosterone system (RAAS), with the goal of retaining water and sodium to maintain circulating blood volume. Chronic cardiac insufficiency can nevertheless increase the hazard of renal ischemia, resulting in tubular injury and subsequent kidney injury. As observed in recent clinical experience, maximizing cardiac function in patients with renal impairment can significantly improve outcomes. Therefore, an understanding of the interaction between renal function and cardiac status is crucial for delivering effective patient care. In addition to hypovolemia and cardiac disease, drug-related alterations in renal blood flow can also be pre-renal causes of AKI. Non-steroidal anti-inflammatory drugs (NSAIDs), for example, can inhibit the synthesis of prostaglandins, which cause vasoconstriction of the afferent arterioles and impaired glomerular perfusion. Additionally, drugs that modify renal hemodynamics, including angiotensin-converting enzyme inhibitors, can be risky in some patients, especially volume-depleted ones. The interaction of pharmacologic agents with pre-renal phenomena further complicates the clinical scenario. Therefore, a comprehensive understanding of these pre-renal mechanisms enables healthcare professionals to identify vulnerable patients and tailor treatment modalities accordingly. Identification of these factors is crucial when adhering to the Kidney Disease: Improving Global Outcomes guidelines for AKI prevention and management (Kellum et al., 2013; Human et al., 2015) (Figure 8.4).

8.1.2. Intrinsic Renal Causes

Of the many etiologies of AKI, intrinsic renal etiologies are very important due to their direct impact on renal parenchyma. Etiologies of ATN, acute interstitial nephritis, and glomerulonephritis have different pathophysiologic mechanisms. ATN, most often due to ischemia or nephrotoxins, disrupts the delicate structure and function of the renal tubules, initiating a chain of cellular injury and inflammation. Conversely, acute interstitial nephritis, most commonly caused by allergic reactions to drugs or infections, damages the renal interstitial tissue and thereby impairs nephron function. Furthermore, diseases such as glomerulonephritis include autoimmunity that causes direct injury to the glomeruli, reducing filtration capacity. It is essential to understand these intrinsic renal etiologies of AKI to design specific therapeutic strategies and enhance outcomes for patients. The connection between intrinsic renal etiology and organ function implications is of great clinical importance. AKI has been found to have systemic effects in addition to affecting renal function, potentially altering liver metabolism and other organ systems after insult.

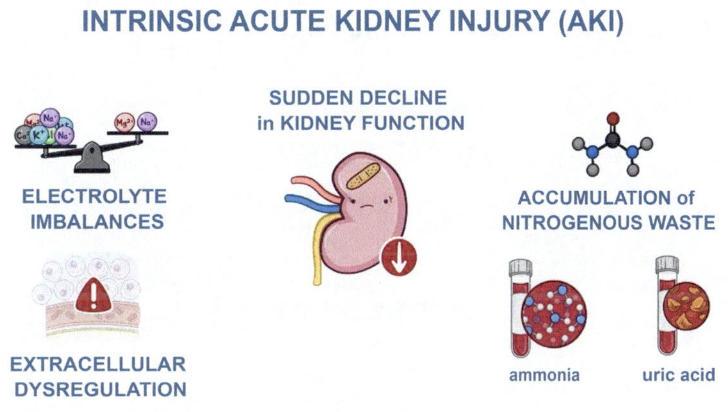

Figure 8.5. Intrinsic acute kidney injury.

Source: https://d16qt3wv6xm098.cloudfront.net/6pphYWScSqu9oC-Y1uZrQXJWTxmPy2-O/_.jpg.

The drug metabolism of CKD patients, for instance, has been changed due to reduced hepatic cytochrome P450 activity, compounded by AKI. This renders dosing with drugs more complex because pharmacologic responses may significantly vary from individual to individual, particularly in those with intrinsic renal impairment. The need for individualized dosing regimens based on kidney function underscores the complex interplay between renal impairment and overall health, a testament to the fact that intrinsic renal etiologies must be diagnosed in both acute treatment and chronic care regimens in AKI. Understanding of ischemia and reperfusion injury (IRI) is another added layer of complexity in the intrinsic causes of renal injury. IRI occurs as a result of transitory ischemic events, which are often encountered in procedures like a kidney transplant, when the blood supply is momentarily obstructed. This impact not only produces acute kidney injury but also influences chronic graft survival with the potential to influence late outcomes through mechanisms such as interstitial fibrosis and tubular atrophy. Emerging research has identified some of the molecular pathways of IRI, providing promising avenues for intervention. The modulation of these pathways may be useful in developing new therapeutic opportunities for reducing the deleterious effects of IRIs, ultimately improving patient prognosis. Thus, knowledge of the intricate pathways of intrinsic renal causes enriches the discussion on AKI and highlights avenues to enhance therapeutic advances (Figure 8.5).

8.1.3. Post-Renal Causes

In the context of AKI, post-renal etiologies predominantly arise from obstructions in the urinary tract. These obstructions occur at various levels, including the ureters, bladder, and urethra, but are more likely to significantly block the passage of urine and thus lead to a decline in kidney function. Common etiologies of post-renal AKI include kidney stones, malignancies, prostate hypertrophy in males, and urethral stricture. Identification of such causes is of utmost significance, as early intervention can often reverse AKI progression. For instance, removal of an obstructing stone or relief of bladder outlet obstruction will normalize renal function, emphasizing the necessity of a comprehensive diagnostic workup in suspected post-renal etiologies. Further, the presence of post-renal causes underscores the importance of careful monitoring in specific patient populations, particularly those with underlying urological conditions.

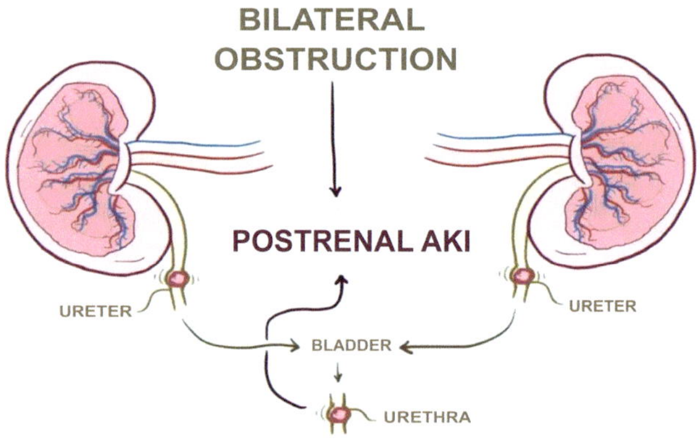

Figure 8.6. Post-renal causes of acute kidney injury.

Source: https://www.osmosis.org/_next/image?url=https%3A%2F%2Fd16qt3wv6xm098.cloudfront.net%2Fl8k1bSSXRDaXvBJ_ecSGFvTrTo6SVhRr%2F_.jpg&w=3840&q=75.

For instance, patients who are to undergo extensive spinal surgery or significant abdominal and pelvic surgery may be at risk for urinary retention or obstruction as a consequence of anatomical changes. The clinical presentation of post-renal AKI is subtle. It can be characterized by an increase in serum creatinine with preserved urine output in the initial phase, thus rendering it difficult to diagnose. Clinicians must therefore maintain a heightened index of suspicion, particularly for those patients presenting with symptoms of obstruction or urinary tract obstruction. Appropriate management interventions, such as imaging assessment and catheterization of the bladder, are imperative in addressing the inherent etiologies, with an emphasis on securing timely intervention to avert unnecessary kidney damage. Further, if one does not treat post-renal causes, the long-term implications are extensive, resulting in precipitous declines in kidney function and high morbidity rates. Studies indicate that among those patients suffering from post-renal AKI, who do not receive timely intervention, can have prolonged hospital stays and a higher risk of complications in the form of infection or the need for dialysis (Hooda et al., 2022). Furthermore, long-term effects of post-renal AKI cannot be overlooked, as there is evidence to show it correlates with the faster deterioration of chronic kidney disease (CKD) in patients suffering from it (Anderson et al., 2020). Understanding the interconnectedness of post-renal etiologies and ultimate kidney health underscores the need for comprehensive care strategies that treat not only short-term treatment but also the prevention of potential kidney complications in the future. This expanded perspective is necessary to achieve improved patient outcomes within the framework of AKI and its diverse etiologies (Figure 8.6).

8.2. Risk Factors for AKI

AKI is increasingly recognized as a severe complication in many clinical contexts, contingent to a large extent on many risk factors. Age is the most significant factor among them, as older patients are more likely to have comorbid conditions that may compromise their kidney function. A reduced glomerular filtration rate is not unusual in this subgroup, for example, and therefore they are more susceptible to the effects of acute insults during surgery or hospitalization.

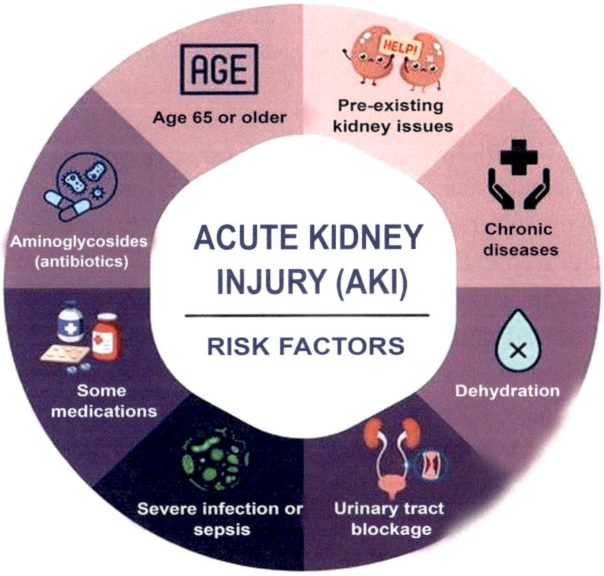

Figure 8.7. Risk factors for AKI.

Source: https://scontent.fdel11-1.fna.fbcdn.net/v/t39.30808-6/485887945_1005980281629719_4213628303930740090_n.jpg?stp=dst-jpg_p526x296_tt6&_nc_cat=100&ccb=1-7&_nc_sid=127cfc&_nc_ohc=IBLsP4xebxAQ7kNvwF-7P3C&_nc_oc=AdmxW0ajidDCQ6Pf09w0uNrBvPEFqK7UrdrmbZOZC4iW6G3FvXpQ4W2gIOhmgX-FPjZzsQ6lto2weyUa7ZbkpiKj&_nc_zt=23&_nc_ht=scontent.fdel11-1.fna&_nc_gid=NDuzii-HXDQyFZZl9N97_Q&oh=00_AfPsT0bBVY6pI7GEqfI7qGAgbaFznY5ucX7i0F4R8rmnqQ&oe=68584E81.

The literature suggests that comorbid conditions such as diabetes, heart failure, and hypertension contribute to the vulnerability further, and thus, the risk of AKI development is higher. It is, therefore, vital to acknowledge the contribution of comorbidities as well as age so that at-risk patients can be identified and measures can be taken for the prevention of AKI development. Additionally, some interventions and patient care measures may increase or decrease AKI risks. One specific concern has been diuretic administration, which has been linked to a risk for AKI, especially when aggressively given to patients who are at risk for renal failure. In cardiac surgery, variables such as intraoperative transfusion volume with packed red blood cells and cross-clamp times for the aorta have been shown to have an association with oliguric AKI requiring RRT (Perez-Valdivieso et al., 2009). Awareness of these modifiable factors can lead to improved surgical results and fewer instances of AKI through careful planning and intentional intervention among surgical patients at risk. Lastly, the impact of pre-operative renal impairment cannot be exaggerated in the context of AKI. Surgical patients with compromised renal function are at a heightened risk for acute worsening, which is more likely to result in an intensification of chronic kidney disease after surgery (Baptista et al., 2012). As an instance, evidence indicates that patients needing RRT after AKI are subject to very high rates of mortality and increased durations of stay in the hospital, highlighting the need for intervention in renal health before surgery. Identification of patients with established renal disease before performing high-risk surgery is essential in minimizing the risk of AKI and maximizing the quality of life and prognosis of the patient. This preventive approach can significantly reduce the adverse outcomes associated with acute renal damage (Figure 8.7).

8.2.1. Age and Gender

The association of age with AKI occurrence has drawn considerable attention in medical research, particularly against the backdrop of increasing global health concerns. Evidence has repeatedly established that older age groups are predisposed to AKI, predominantly due to the physiological decline of renal function with age. With advancing age, the kidneys undergo physiological changes that can affect glomerular filtration rates and toxin removal, making them more susceptible to disease states that lead to AKI. Add to this the comorbid conditions that are prevalent in older patients, such as diabetes and hypertension, that amplify the vulnerability, particularly when an acute insult is superimposed, such as in COVID-19. As observed in recent studies, the likelihood of developing AKI increases exponentially with advancing age, a role for which preventive measures and vigilance of renal function in older patients receiving acute care interventions are particularly pertinent (Cheruiyot et al., 2023). Gender also plays a role in the scenario for acute kidney injury, with differing risk factors and variable outcomes in males and females. Epidemiologic data suggest that men, on average, are more vulnerable to AKI, possibly as a product of behavioral as well as biological factors. Men, for example, have greater rates of incidence of specific comorbidities, such as cardiovascular disease and hypertension, which are significant risk factors for AKI. Lifestyle factors, such as diet and alcohol consumption, may be gender-specific and influence renal function. The impact of gender can be further augmented by variations in the clinical course and prognosis of AKI. Women have been reported in some studies to have improved survival following AKI, but their long-term renal function could be compromised. Awareness of such gender differences is essential for applying gender-sensitive strategies in the prevention and management of AKI (Bottle et al., 2014). The dynamic between gender, age, and risk for acute kidney injury emphasizes the complexities of patient care in populations with considerable variation. Medical providers must consider both age and gender when they evaluate patients for AKI since these two elements have significant effects on both occurrence and clinical outcomes.

The realization that older individuals, particularly men, are at higher risk can steer targeted screening and trigger intervention, which is essential to improve patient prognosis. On the contrary, the realization that young women are likely to exhibit varied AKI patterns can inform personalized treatment approaches. The intersection of these demographic elements underscores the importance of patient integration and individualization in addressing AKI effectively, ultimately leading to improved health outcomes among vulnerable populations with acute renal complications (Bottle et al., 2014; Cheruiyot et al., 2023).

8.2.2. Pre-Existing Health Conditions

Most pertinent is the interface between initial health conditions and AKI development, whereby these conditions might predispose individuals to renal injury. Specifically, diabetes mellitus and hypertension have been shown to compromise long-term renal function in such a way that the kidneys become susceptible to acute injury. In patients with diabetes, for instance, vascular disease can lead to kidney ischemia, which subsequently predisposes them to AKI during acute stress such as dehydration or sepsis. Moreover, suppose patients with chronic renal impairment are subjected to acute stressors. In that case, the cumulative injury leads to sharp decreases in kidney function, turning a chronic process into an acutely lethal event. A deep understanding of the interaction between pre-existing conditions and acute kidney disorders is at the core of efficient prevention and management. Pre-existing conditions not only increase the risk for AKI but also play a significant role in defining the clinical evolution of affected patients. As an example, in cases of liver transplantation, pre-existing renal insufficiency has been linearly related to the progression to new-onset CKD. Such. This. Relationship highlights the complex interaction between chronic illness and acute renal insults because patients transitioning from stable chronic to their acute presentation may be at risk.

The multifactorial origin of AKI following transplant is particularly evident where pre-existing disease influences intra-operative events, such as ischemia-reperfusion injury, that can augment kidney injury. Understanding how these interconnected processes are carried out is crucial for managing and long-term care of at-risk patients with both AKI and CKD, thereby improving overall patient outcomes. Furthermore, the transition from acute kidney injury to chronic kidney disease underscores the importance of early detection and intervention strategies. AKD's recognition, which bridges the gap between CKD and AKI, shows how timely and correct intervention of current conditions can alter the dynamics of emerging kidney disease. Identification of risk factors and monitoring, for example, patients with the Model for End-stage Liver Disease score, become imperative to prevent AKI in the course of management of acute illness. Adequate management strategies that address both chronic inciting health conditions and acute attacks can substantially improve patient survival rates and reduce long-term complications. By targeting the multifactorial processes driving AKI in patients with significant pre-existing conditions, healthcare practitioners can conceptualize interventions that ensure renal protection and optimize overall patient quality of life (Evison et al., 2016; Dewitte et al., 2017) (Figure 8.8).

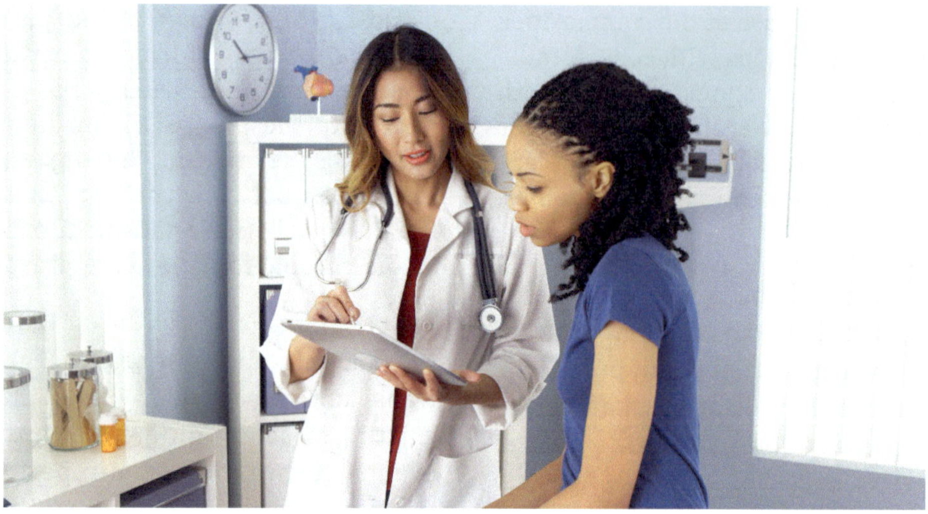

Figure 8.8. Pre-existing medical conditions.

Source: https://external-content.duckduckgo.com/iu/?u=https%3A%2F%2Fblog.withfaye.com%2Fwp-content%2Fuploads%2F2023%2F11%2Fpre_exsisitng_conditions_3.jpeg&f=1&nofb=1&ipt=81c019a3c4742a20c69ded006e9b8c8f8cf77b355eff427dd203c9f7d510d179.

8.2.3. Medications and Environmental Factors

The drug-AKI interaction is a significant area of research, particularly in light of the increased prevalence of this disorder in susceptible populations. Certain drugs, such as NSAIDs and antibiotics, have been recognized as nephrotoxic agents that can cause AKI in susceptible patients. The kidneys play a significant role in drug metabolism and excretion, and impaired renal function leads to altered pharmacokinetics, causing drug concentrations that are toxic and risk-increasing injury. Moreover, acute patients commonly receive more than one medication simultaneously, which enhances the potential for drug interactions leading to AKI. Knowledge of the pharmacologic profiles and interactions of these agents is essential for clinicians seeking to decrease risk and implement appropriate monitoring measures for patients at risk for renal injury. Environmental factors also play a crucial role in the etiology and development of AKI, underscoring the need for an integrative approach to patient care. For instance, living in contaminated areas has been associated with increased occurrences of diseases related to the kidneys, which suggests that environmental toxins can exacerbate preexisting renal vulnerability. In addition, water levels of hydration also rely on environmental conditions such as temperature and access to clean water, which have a central role in guaranteeing optimum function of the kidneys. In the elderly population, these determinants play a more significant role, as older individuals usually have physiological alterations that compromise their kidneys' ability to clear drugs and maintain homeostasis. Hence, it is paramount to target environmental determinants to prevent AKI as well as in treatment strategies to combat AKI, particularly in vulnerable populations. The overlap between drugs and environmental determinants is a rich tapestry that can influence AKI dramatically. Elderly patients, who are usually comorbid and polypharmacologically, are at increased risk considering that they are exposed to adverse environmental conditions or nephrotoxic drugs. Taking into consideration news on elderly patients acknowledges that considering a high proportion of them use five or more drugs, it raises the danger of toxic effects, including renal injury (Tirrell et al., 2016). Identification of environmental stressors, such as dehydration in adverse climatic conditions, further complicates the challenge of AKI management among these patients. With the objective of creating effective intervention frameworks, integrating medication management with an understanding of environmental health factors is imperative in framing overall care strategies aimed at reducing the incidence and severity of acute kidney injury among susceptible groups.

8.3. Symptoms and Diagnosis

AKI is characterized by a combination of signs and symptoms, which are often vague and thus difficult to diagnose. The most obvious symptom is typically decreased urine output, but it can also be accompanied by fatigue, nausea, and lower extremity edema resulting from fluid retention. Changes in mental status arise when toxins become accumulated in the blood. Because the symptoms may overlap with those of other illnesses, such as congestive heart failure or diabetes, healthcare professionals need to exercise a careful eye for the entire clinical presentation of the patient. For instance, the diabetic patient might come with signs of nausea and vomiting alongside decreased urination that necessitates additional examination to make a conclusive diagnosis of AKI and its cause, because several other concurrent health conditions could easily mislead the clinical relevance of these signs. AKI diagnostic findings are focused primarily on changes in serum creatinine and urine output. The Kidney Disease: Improving Global Outcomes (KDIGO) guidelines establish specific thresholds for these parameters that initiate an AKI diagnosis, traditionally categorized into three stages. A rise in serum creatinine by 0.3 mg/dL over 48 hours or a reduction in urine output to below 0.5 mL/kg/h for six hours is typical of AKI. It is critical that practitioners perform a thorough investigation, such as laboratory research, that can reveal electrolyte imbalance or metabolic acidosis.

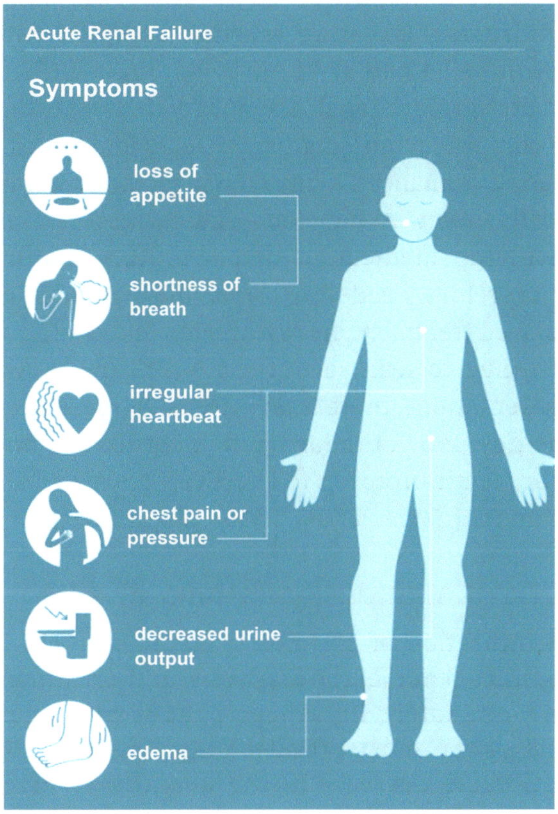

Figure 8.9. Symptoms and diagnosis for AKI.

Source: https://www.verywellhealth.com/thmb/hbfKjTYzh6J1q2H4ASwzFTkB7A4=/1500x0/filters:no_upscale():max_bytes(150000):strip_icc()/acute-renal-failure-symptoms-5ae1f536ff1b780036287ecb.png.

As seen from recent experience, such as in a case involving a patient with hyperglycemia, early detection is essential to manage potential complications due to AKI. Through proper guidelines, health professionals can better manage the intricacies of AKI diagnosis and effectively handle its immediate effects (Juan et al., 2025). Due to the multifactorial etiology of AKI, identification of comorbidities linked to AKI and their role in renal impairment becomes crucial for successful management. As has been evident from recent research, acute conditions like drug reactions and metabolic crises can have a profound impact on aggravating AKI. Some syndromes, i.e., drug reaction complex with eosinophilia and systemic symptoms (DRESS), create an additional diagnostic challenge due to complex symptomatology. Delay in diagnosis leads to enhanced kidney damage and systemic involvement. A judicious clinical assessment involving medication and symptom history is therefore needed to avoid misdiagnosis or delayed treatment. As researchers and clinicians continue to learn about the spectrum of AKI presentations, there is an increasing realization to develop standardized diagnostic and therapeutic protocols to effectively treat affected patients (Cortes et al., 2024) (Figure 8.9).

8.3.1. Common Symptoms of AKI

Identification of common symptoms in AKI is significant for early diagnosis and treatment and ultimately influences patient outcomes. One of the most prevalent signs is an easily noticeable decrease in the quantity of urine produced, also known as oliguria, which can manifest as either less frequent urination or a drastic reduction in urine volume. This symptom indicates impaired kidney function and suggests potential accumulation of waste products in the blood, potentially leading to subsequent complications if left untreated. The patient may also present with fluid overload, resulting in unanticipated swelling, particularly in the lower limbs, ankles, and face. These signs reflect the kidneys' role in maintaining fluid and electrolyte balance impaired in AKI. Therefore, the practitioners must be vigilant in monitoring these symptoms to enable early interventions that can counteract the progression of kidney injury (Human et al., 2015). In addition to oliguria, patients with AKI typically present with a range of systemic symptoms that are indicative of intrinsic metabolic derangement. Of these, weakness and fatigue are normally seen, and they are due to the accumulation of toxins secondary to defective kidney function. This can lead to a generalized decline in physical function and quality of life, also contributing to the clinical presentation. Nausea, vomiting, and loss of appetite may also be present as a result of the body's efforts to eliminate waste products that are not being efficiently filtered out by the kidneys. These GI symptoms lead to an imbalance of metabolism that further deteriorates the patient's condition and contributes to their feeling of malaise. Consequently, a clear understanding of common symptoms is necessary for incorporating supportive measures into AKI management (Human et al., 2015). Another critical element of AKI symptomatology is the potential alteration in the patient's mental status that may be observed in more severe cases. Confusion, disorientation, and somnolence may result from the accumulation of uremic toxins and electrolyte imbalances that affect cerebral function. In addition, patients may have persistent headaches that may be a sign of hypertension or other metabolic disorders resulting from kidney malfunction. Complications may develop as the AKI progresses, such as metabolic acidosis or electrolyte imbalance, further justification for early detection of such signs. This multidimensional symptomatology necessitates a cautious examination by healthcare professionals to ensure timely interventions that respond to both the renal and systemic impacts of acute kidney injury (Human et al., 2015).

8.3.2. Diagnostic Tests and Procedures

The etiology of AKI is substantially reliant on a synergy of traditional and novel diagnostic procedures and tests. Traditionally, serum creatinine has been the universal criterion for AKI diagnosis; however, serum creatinine may not be significantly elevated until advanced renal insufficiency, potentially leading to delayed therapy. To address this deficiency, researchers have investigated novel biomarkers that can indicate kidney injury earlier. For instance, research has established that the uNGAL and the uNGAL-to-urinary creatinine ratio (UNCR) measurement can identify AKI sooner than serum creatinine. In one study, a 7-fold elevation in UNCR indicated AKI at an average of eight days, which contrasts with a significant increase in serum creatinine recorded at sixteen days (Cowgill et al., 2016). The urgent need for more timely diagnostic strategies underscores the necessity of translating these advanced biomarkers into daily practice. Additionally, integration of molecular and genetic testing into AKI diagnostic recommendations offers substantial promise. Advances achieved in the field of personalized medicine enabled the identification of several biomarkers that correlate with renal pathology. Methods such as genomics and proteomics have been developed, providing insights into donor and recipient kidney health beyond standard parameters. For example, some SNPs related to the complement system might predict baseline risks for allograft injury before transplantation, and this might be pivotal in the management of AKI in renal transplant patients. Additionally, multi-gene expression panels can predict graft acceptance in patients after transplant and thus provide valuable information for effective monitoring of immunosuppression (Khatri et al., 2011). Such emerging techniques represent a shift to more patient-specific, subtle approaches in the diagnosis and management of AKI. Overall, the new development in tests and procedures now demands evolution in clinical practice. The multifactorial etiology of AKI necessitates a multidirectional diagnostic strategy that extends beyond the usual serum markers. Clearly, the integration of biomarkers like uNGAL, in conjunction with extensive molecular profiling, can enhance the early recognition and management of AKI. Such advancements in diagnostic methods, aside from possibly improving patient outcomes, have the ability to make renal health easier to manage. With more research underway to uncover the mechanisms of kidney damage, it is essential for medical professionals to stay updated on advances so that they can incorporate them into clinical practice effectively, enabling early intervention and optimal patient care for AKI cases (Figure 8.10).

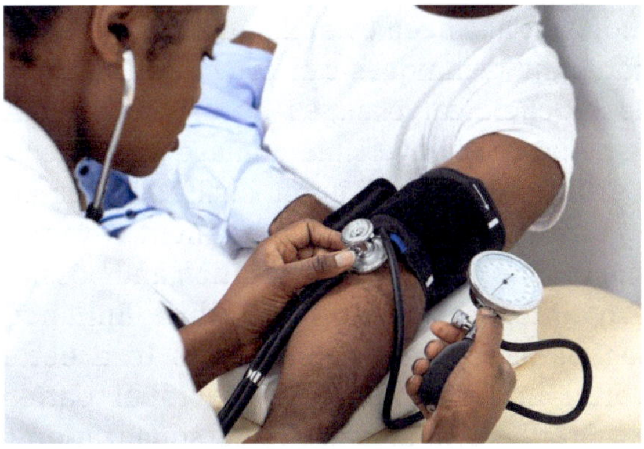

Figure 8.10. Diagnostic tests and procedures for AKI.

Source: https://kcuk.cdn.ngo/media/images/AKI_-_blood_pressure.width-700.jpg.

8.3.3. Importance of Early Detection

The significance of early detection of AKI in managing it cannot be overstated, particularly when considering its multifactorial etiology and the pathophysiologic intricacies of AKI. Early detection of AKI plays a critical role in preventing its acceleration to severe renal injury, leading to irreversible kidney failure along with increased morbidity. The diversity of AKI causes, from trauma and surgery to intrinsic disease, underscores the need for healthcare providers to roll out stringent screening strategies with alacrity. According to Gwinner et al. (2016), timely intervention might be key to preventing electrolyte imbalance and renal necrosis. Early recognition enables targeted treatment approaches that stabilize renal function and significantly improve patient outcomes, resulting in a better quality of life and reduced costs to the healthcare system. The addition of new diagnostic modalities is necessary for the early detection of AKI. Traditional markers of renal injury, such as serum creatinine and urine output, are too insensitive for early detection. New methods, including proteomic analysis of urine and blood, hold promise for new frontiers in the diagnosis of non-invasive AKI and its etiology. Based on a critical appraisal of multiple studies, it has been established that these new proteomic techniques can provide insight into the biochemical changes occurring in renal tissue before irreversible damage (Gwinner et al., 2016). Expansion upon such advances is a key turning point in AKI management, with real-time monitoring of renal condition and possible early intervention now possible. Enhanced diagnostic capability contributes to a better overall understanding of individual patient risk profiles and aids in the personalization of treatment approaches. Besides, the effects of delayed diagnosis not only extend to patient health but also extend deeper into larger healthcare systems due to increased morbidity and costs associated with late-stage kidney disease. As suggested by Human et al. (2015), a growing incidence of AKI has been associated with growing volumes of surgery, indicating the need for active prevention to avert harm. The application of systematic protocols to the early detection of AKI can reduce the incidence of adverse outcomes, thus shortening hospital stays and decreasing healthcare expenditures. In the process, awareness of the importance of early recognition in AKI serves not only to enhance the treatment of individual patients but also to alleviate the financial strain on healthcare systems. By placing a high value on early intervention, we can change the pattern of AKI management from prevention to cure, ultimately enhancing both clinical outcomes and public health (Figure 8.11).

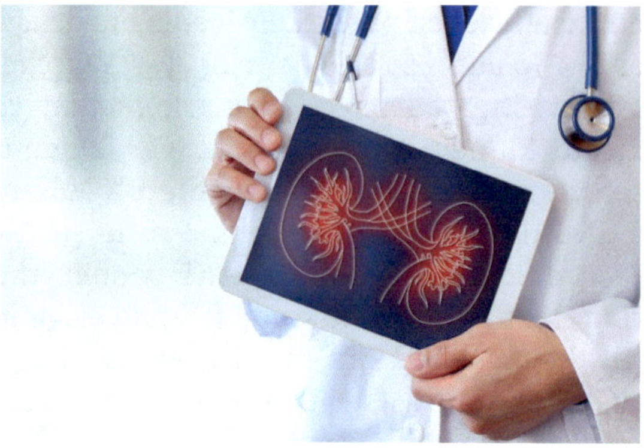

Figure 8.11. The importance of early detection in kidney disease.

Source: https://www.durhamnephrology.com/wp-content/uploads/2023/09/image2-1024x683.jpg.

8.4. Pathophysiology of AKI

The pathophysiology of AKI is complex, involving a broad range of biochemical and cellular changes that disrupt normal renal physiology. Initially evoked by ischemia or nephrotoxins, AKI is characterized by a sudden decrease in the glomerular filtration rate (GFR), leading to the accumulation of waste in the circulation. This loss can be due to intrinsic, prerenal, or postrenal causes, of which intrinsic causes often lead to direct damage to the renal parenchyma. Notably, ischemia-reperfusion injury is also a significant contributor, as reperfusion after an ischemic insult can exacerbate tissue damage through oxidative injury and inflammatory activation. Thus, disrupted cellular homeostasis results in cell necrosis and apoptosis, which causes an overall decline in renal function, making it difficult for the patient's outcome and management. Analysis of cellular mechanisms of AKI reveals intricate layers of dysregulated lipid metabolism, which have increasingly been recognized as primary causal determinants. , where the cytotoxic action of excess lipid accumulation takes a central role in AKI pathogenesis, is a key phenomenon. Lipid accumulation can initiate mitochondrial dysfunction, leading to a loss of energy and an increase in oxidative stress in renal cells. Afolarin et al. (2024) introduces the new idea of "immunometabolic" lipotoxicity, where abnormal lipid signaling intersects with immune mechanisms to intensify kidney injury. Such an intersection refers to a broad field of metabolic disturbances that can enhance AKI, which calls for therapeutic options. Therapy for lipotoxicity not only provides a way to limit injury but also illuminates the pathophysiologic roles of metabolic dysregulation in AKI formation. Further, enhanced understanding of ischemia and reperfusion injury (IRI) has elucidated specific molecular mechanisms involved in AKI pathophysiology. Not only is IRI pertinent to AKI in various clinical situations, such as transplantation, but it also illustrates the long-term impact of acute events. Underlying mechanisms of IRI include an inflammatory cascade of pathways, oxidative stress, and dysregulation of cell signaling, which act synergistically to cause post-injury complications such as fibrosis and chronic graft dysfunction in transplant recipients. Berger et al. (2020) provide insights into these intricate mechanisms and suggest new therapeutic modalities against the involved pathways of IRI. By understanding these molecular mechanisms, researchers aim to maximize graft survival and minimize renal injury, thereby enhancing the management of patients with AKI (Figure 8.12).

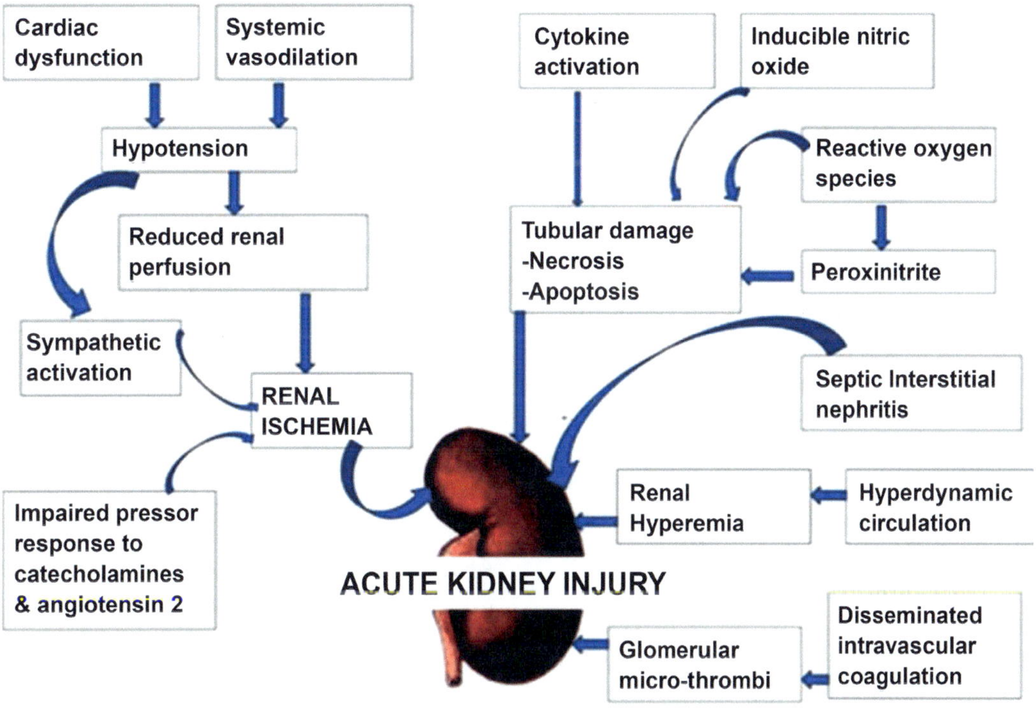

Figure 8.12. Pathophysiology of acute kidney injury.

Source: https://www.researchgate.net/publication/368759160/figure/fig2/AS:11431281122235527@1677241396538/Pathophysiology-of-Acute-Kidney-Injury-33.png.

8.4.1. Mechanisms of Kidney Injury

It is essential to understand the processes of kidney injury to treat AKI, a disease that presents significant clinical dilemmas. Ischemia-reperfusion injury is one of the dominant mechanisms, a process that frequently occurs in surgery, such as liver transplantation. The original kidney cell injury due to insufficient blood supply may be exacerbated later during reperfusion of the blood, leading to a cascade of cell damage. Post-reperfusion syndrome (PRS) has the potential to influence outcomes in patients significantly. As seen in Evison et al. (2016), underlying conditions such as an increased Model for End-stage Liver Disease score or baseline renal dysfunction exacerbate such complications, demonstrating the interaction between renal function and surgical outcome. Identifying the mechanism by which these initial ischemic events lead to long-standing renal complications offers therapeutic data that may reduce the prevalence of AKI in vulnerable populations. Another key area of AKIs pathophysiology is that of oxidative stress. This mechanism holds particular relevance to populations with an aging demographic who present a risk factor for increased susceptibility to injury. As discussed by Bonventre et al. (2014), the aging kidney undergoes hemodynamic alterations and increased oxidative stress, rendering the organ vulnerable to acute insults. The accumulation of reactive oxygen species may exceed the antioxidant defenses, leading to cellular damage, apoptosis, and dysrepair. Increased inflammation and decreased autophagic processes secondary to aging further exacerbate this oxidative environment, thereby amplifying vulnerability to AKI. Exploring how senescence affects these mechanisms may reveal potential targets for preventing or minimizing AKI, particularly in elderly patients or those with underlying comorbidities that can further strain renal function. Ultimately, inflammation is a crucial mediator of AKI pathogenesis and progression. Upon injury, the kidneys initiate inflammatory responses that, although initially helpful, can lead to further renal parenchymal damage if left uncontrolled. The invasion of immune cells and the release of pro-inflammatory cytokines have the potential to initiate a cycle of injury enhancement through fibrosis, resulting from chronic inflammation, which ultimately leads to chronic kidney disease. The interaction of inflammatory mechanisms and AKI suggests the possibility of developing anti-inflammatory therapy as a treatment regimen. As both Evison et al. (2016) and Bonventre et al. (2014) observe, the interacting complexity of ischemia, oxidative stress, and inflammation, each in combination, reveals the multifactorial nature of kidney injury in AKI. Clarification of these interacting processes is crucial for improving management regimens, ultimately leading to better patient outcomes following acute renal insults.

8.4.2. Impact on Kidney Function

The impact of AKI on renal function is profound, and it has serious consequences on the patient's survival and health outcomes. Most recent research indicates that the prevalence of AKI, particularly when it manifests as sudden rises in serum creatinine, is not only confined to the hospital environment but also in the primary care setup. A study pointed out that patients with rising creatinine levels tend to have increased mortality, with unadjusted 30-day survival rates of as low as 82.3% for those with severe AKI versus 99.9% in those with no AKI. This stark contrast emphasizes the need for early detection and prevention strategies, as it is possible that, promptly, the disastrous consequences associated with deteriorating renal function in various health facilities can be prevented, thus significantly contributing to holistic patient care and management strategies (Bottle et al., 2014). Other than primary healthcare facilities, the long-term effects of AKI on renal function are particularly alarming in CKD patients. A pertinent clinical trial, DAPA-CKD, showed that patients with CKD who have severe albuminuria are at risk for sudden deteriorations in kidney function, with doubling serum creatinine levels being a key endpoint. The deterioration was significantly less in those receiving dapagliflozin, transmitting a hopeful therapeutic pathway to stem kidney function decline. Perhaps most importantly, the trial demonstrated that the timing of AKI-associated serious adverse events was not significantly different between placebo and treatment, suggesting that anticipatory risk factor management will be a vital determinant in the preservation of kidney function in at-risk groups (Cherney et al., 2021). Preventive measures and evidence-based treatment recommendations are central to managing the complexities of AKI and its effects on kidney function. The recognition of AKI as a multifaceted condition necessitates an interdisciplinary approach to effectively address its etiology and management. From optimizing fluid management to employing nephroprotective strategies, healthcare providers are encouraged to adhere to inclusive guidelines that reduce the incidence of AKI. Furthermore, integrating patient education into therapy protocols will enable individuals to recognize previous indicators of kidney dysfunction and seek early intervention from healthcare workers. By doing so, it is possible to maximize patient outcomes and prevent the long-term impact of AKI on kidney function. Ultimately, a multidimensional view of AKI can lead to an improved quality of life for affected individuals and reduce the burden on healthcare systems as a whole (Figure 8.13).

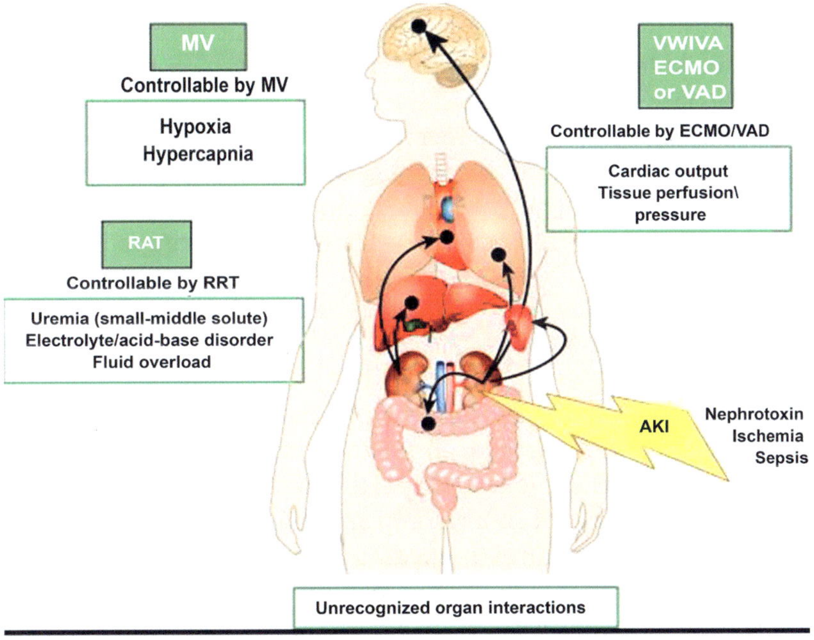

Figure 8.13. The impact of acute kidney injury (AKI) on kidney function.

Source: https://www.kidneyinternational-online.org/cms/10.1016/j.kint.2015.11.019/asset/583c12ed-c77c-456e-9554-6d4a68c14ade/main.assets/gr1.jpg.

8.4.3. Consequences of Prolonged AKI

Complications of extended AKI extend far beyond the loss of renal function and carry significant implications for overall health and quality of life. Of significance among the serious consequences is augmented morbidity as a result of extended AKI, which then goes on to lead to a more challenging hospital course. Studies have proven that patients who develop AKI have longer lengths of stay and higher healthcare costs compared to those without this complication. Furthermore, the incidence of adverse events, such as infections and cardiovascular events, increases exponentially in AKI patients, particularly in vulnerable subgroups, including the elderly and those with pre-existing comorbidities. The pathophysiologic stress that other organ systems are exposed to from chronic renal dysfunction drives these complications and suggests that the implications of AKI could be multifactorial and highly interwoven with the overall clinical context of the inpatient (Hosohata et al., 2018). Prolonged AKI is also linked with disturbed drug metabolism and elimination, making patient management even more complicated. Kidneys are vital organs in the clearance of numerous pharmacologic agents, and acute renal injury may produce marked changes in drug clearance processes. Changes in hepatic drug metabolism occur in patients with AKI. Still, growing concern is now regarding the appropriateness of standard dosing recommendations that have been conventionally extrapolated from patients with chronic kidney disease (CKD). Specifically, fluctuations in enzyme activities, e.g., cytochrome P450 (CYP) enzymes, can lead to drug accumulation and increased risks of toxicity in AKI patients. Therefore, individualized therapy is recommended here, where vigilant monitoring of the drug's effect and logical adjustment of the dosage become essential in these patients (Abosaif et al., 2014). Long-term outcomes of chronic AKI are significant, as it is associated with a higher risk of progression to chronic kidney disease and end-stage renal disease. Evidences show that a single episode of AKI can put patients at risk for subsequent renal insult and its development to chronic impairment of kidney function. Moreover, patients with a history of severe AKI may continue to be at higher risk for cardiovascular disease and other systemic complications well after the initial hospital discharge. It is thus increasingly necessary to have in mind not only acute treatment but also sound approaches to monitoring and minimizing long-term risk after an AKI event. Hence, it is crucial to understand the far-reaching effects of chronic AKI to further patient outcomes and guide appropriate preventive measures in at-risk groups (Hosohata et al., 2018).

8.5. Treatment Options

The treatment of AKI largely depends on the etiology and severity of the condition. The initial management thus involves identifying and eliminating reversible causes of renal impairment, such as dehydration or nephrotoxic agents. Supportive management is vital since it can restore kidney function and prevent additional injury. In prerenal etiology, fluid resuscitation may be the answer, but obstructive aetiology requires immediate relief of the urinary tract obstruction. The earlier the diagnosis and treatment, the better the patient's outcome, emphasizing the importance of regular observation and laboratory tests in high-risk patients for developing AKI. Once the initial treatment is underway, renal replacement therapy (RRT) is then typically opted for by medical practitioners as a choice for the patient with a severe compromise of the kidneys. The two principal modalities of RRT are intermittent renal replacement therapy (IRRT) and continuous renal replacement therapy (CRRT). New evidence suggests that CRRT may have advantages over IRRT in the critically ill patient, particularly about fluid balance and hemodynamic stability. In terms of cost-effectiveness in comparison, CRRT has evidenced a slightly better gain in quality-adjusted life years (QALYs), although it is more costly initially. 1000 patient analysis indicates that while the initial expense of CRRT is greater, the extended cost can be lower due to reduced dialysis-dependence-related hospitalizations, making CRRT a better option in severe AKI cases

(Bagshaw et al., 2014; Bagshaw et al., 2017). Apart from dialysis methods, drug interventions can also potentially aid in the management of AKI. The prudent use of nephroprotective drugs such as N-acetylcysteine and fenoldopam has emerged as a strategy for minimizing kidney damage, though their efficacy is controversial among specialists. Further, dietary changes such as protein restriction may help manage metabolic abnormalities associated with AKI. With our growing understanding of AKI, novel treatment modalities, such as stem cell therapy and biomarker-guided therapy, are being investigated, with the promise of improved outcomes. AKI treatment overall must include a multifaceted approach aimed at early intervention, ongoing monitoring, and possibly new therapies to optimize recovery and prevent long-term complications (Figure 8.14).

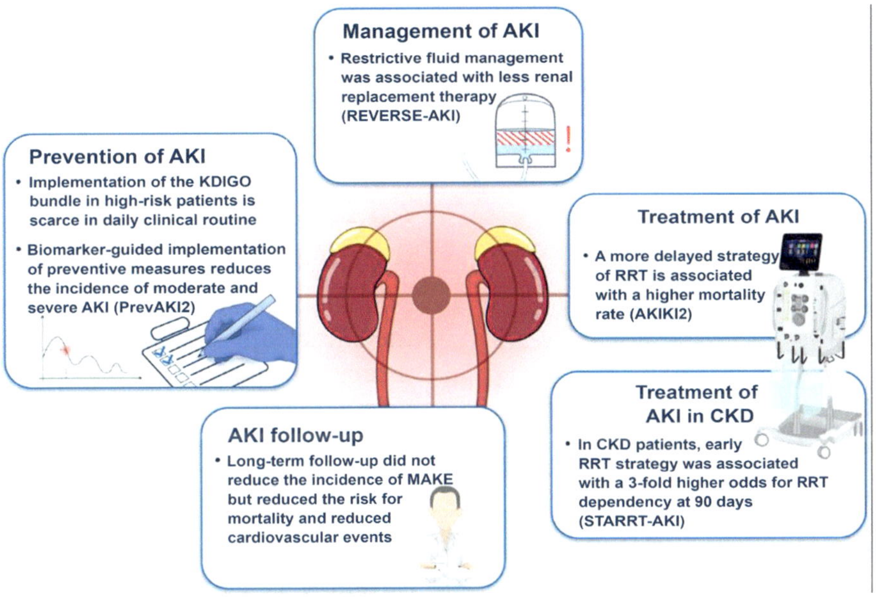

Figure 8.14. The treatment options for acute kidney injury (AKI).

Source: https://media.springernature.com/lw1200/springer-static/image/art%3A10.1007%2Fs00134-023-07061-4/MediaObjects/134_2023_7061_Fig1_HTML.png.

8.5.1. Medical Management

The clinical management of AKI demands a complete understanding of its pathophysiology as well as the concomitant risk factors that cause kidney dysfunction. Its detection is also critical, considering that it has been recognized as a common precursor to chronic kidney disease and has significant implications regarding the mortality and morbidity of patients. The Kidney Disease: Improving Global Outcomes (KDIGO) guidelines are an integral resource in AKI management, providing a standardized approach to the definition, evaluation, and management of this condition. Key points of these recommendations are the importance of its early detection and risk stratification, which can direct therapeutic intervention in an attempt to minimize the course of renal damage and improve patient outcomes, in keeping with best practices of critical care medicine and nephrology (Kellum et al., 2013). Physicians also need to be able to distinguish between its various stages and causes so that they can efficiently manage AKI. The KDIGO guideline clearly defines and stratifies AKI based on the sudden decline in kidney function, typically within a week. This differentiation enables clinicians to individualize interventions that may include volume expansion, drug regimen modification, and close monitoring of electrolyte status. It is also essential to adopt a patient-specific approach, considering comorbid conditions that may exacerbate kidney injury or hinder recovery. Because AKI and CKD are now recognized as a continuum of processes, detection of AKD has also been proposed in patients who experience ongoing pathophysiologic processes following AKI, highlighting the need for personalized treatment approaches responsive to the continuum of renal well-being (Dewitte et al., 2017).

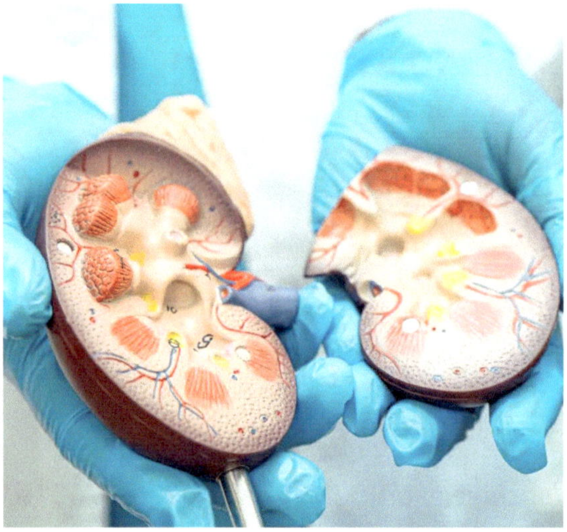

Figure 8.15. The medical management of acute kidney injury (AKI).

Source: https://medwayhospitals.b-cdn.net/wp-content/uploads/2024/07/Acute-Kidney-Injury-AKI.webp.

In the clinical setting, non-dialytic management approaches are a crucial component of treating AKI. These strategies focus on preserving kidney function through pharmacological and supportive measures. Careful consideration of factors such as volume status, electrolyte balance, and avoidance of nephrotoxicity is at the heart of optimizing AKI outcomes. Moreover, integration of interdisciplinary care can enhance AKI treatment by unifying nephrologists with primary care providers to deliver evidence-based interventions early in the development of kidney injury. By employing the data provided by the KDIGO guidelines and ongoing clinical investigations, practitioners can further customize their approach to treating AKI to not only recover renal function as rapidly as possible but also avoid long-term complications associated with kidney injury (Kellum et al., 2013) (Figure 8.15).

8.5.2. Dialysis and Renal Replacement Therapy

The management of AKI often necessitates the initiation of dialysis and RRT as critical interventions. From these interventions, homeostasis in patients whose kidney function has been severely impaired can be reestablished to ensure that toxic substances and excess fluids that the failing kidneys are unable to remove effectively are eliminated. Advances in RRT technologies have expanded the range of alternatives available to healthcare professionals, making it increasingly important to have individualized treatment regimens. For instance, advancements in continuous renal replacement therapy (CRRT) devices enable the early treatment of critically ill patients, aligning with the evolving understanding of the dynamic process of fluid balance and solute removal, as emphasized in the consensus report on nomenclature harmonization in extracorporeal blood purification therapies (Bagshaw et al., 2016). Modalities of dialysis, such as hemodialysis and peritoneal dialysis, differ in their treatment approaches for AKI. Hemodialysis involves the use of a dialyzer to filter outside the body, while peritoneal dialysis utilizes the peritoneal cavity as a membrane for removing solute and fluid. The efficacy of both treatments is dependent on varied factors like patient parameters, clinical presentation, and severity of renal failure. The employment of an effective dialysis treatment can directly influence patient outcomes and recovery patterns, and thus the significance of well-informed clinical decision-making. Additionally, the Kidney Disease: Improving Global Outcomes standards emphasize the need for ongoing assessment of renal function during the progression of RRT to modify treatment regimens accordingly, based on the complications presented by AKI (Kellum et al., 2013). As continuous development occurs in the extension of RRT practice, its recognition in treating multi-organ dysfunction syndromes has further enhanced its significance within critical care units.

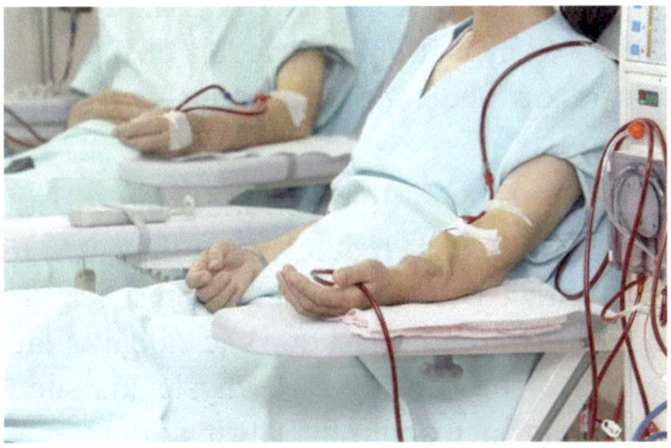

Figure 8.16. Renal replacement therapy.

Source: https://www.news-medical.net/image-handler/picture/patient%20monitored%20by%20electronic%20sphygmomanometer%20during%20dialysis%20session-Picsfive_thumb.jpg.

Extracorporeal therapies, such as therapeutic plasma exchange and liver support, are becoming essential components of multi-modal treatment regimens in patients developing AKI in the context of other severe conditions. Continuous technological advancement and protocol refinement will inevitably redefine the landscape of renal replacement therapy, making it more efficient and safer. Tackling the intricate issues encompassed by RRT not only facilitates improved survival rates but also prevents long-term sequelae encompassed by traumatic kidney damage. In this regard, the inclusion of multidisciplinary expertise remains at the core of improving care standards in tackling AKI with dialysis and renal replacement technologies (Bagshaw et al., 2016) (Figure 8.16).

8.5.3. Supportive Care and Monitoring

The management of AKI involves ongoing supportive care and close monitoring to maximize patient benefits. Supportive care is involved in a range of interventions aimed at preserving renal function and preventing ongoing injury. This may include optimizing hemodynamics through fluid adjustments, maintaining electrolyte balance, and providing sufficient nutrition. Because the pathophysiology of AKI is multifactorial, healthcare workers must be proactive in closely monitoring renal parameters, such as urine output and serum creatinine. This monitoring is a valuable tool in the detection of renal function decline and in making early interventions to prevent AKI complications. Ultimately, a concerted strategy of supportive care and regular monitoring can have a significant impact on trajectories of recovery, highlighting the value of an integrated approach to the care of this potentially life-altering complication. In addition to general supportive care, the inclusion of biomarker advances has promise for enhancing the monitoring of AKI. Traditional markers, such as serum creatinine, preferentially signal renal injury once significant impairment has occurred, triggering the search for more sensitive substitutes. Increasing evidence suggests that urinary biomarkers may serve as predictors to their onset in AKI, with interventions begun earlier. Urinary sodium concentration and fractional excretion of potassium, for instance, have been proposed as dynamic indicators of renal microcirculatory stress and GFR reduction. The inclusion of such innovative monitoring strategies may provide clinicians with insightful information regarding changes in renal function, enabling timely adjustments to management and improving patient outcomes. With progress in the subject area, health systems must adopt evidence-based methods by incorporating new tools into conventional AKI care practices. Training also plays a critical role in delivering effective monitoring and supportive care to AKI patients. Health care professionals must be capable of recognizing evidence of renal impairment and be aware of the ramifications of various treatment modalities. This knowledge is not only crucial for making informed clinical decisions but also for effective patient and family communication regarding the nature of the disease and the necessity of ongoing monitoring. Case-based learning can be particularly beneficial, providing tangible examples that illustrate the need for timely interventions in AKI management. The development of continued education and sensitization on the part of healthcare providers can contribute to better overall quality of care in patients who present with AKI, ultimately leading to better long-term outcomes and prevention of progression to chronic kidney disease, as highlighted within the literature (Kovačević et al., 2024; Maciel, 2024).

8.6. Prevention Strategies

Effective prevention of AKI entails a holistic strategy that includes the early identification of risk factors, optimized management of intrinsic conditions, and close monitoring of high-risk populations. It is among the most critical things to identify those patients with pre-existing states such as diabetes and hypertension, which predispose them to renal damage. The Cardio-Renal Syndrome Consensus Conference underscored the need for an appreciation of the interdependence of heart and kidney health, with the implication that acute or chronic dysfunction of one organ can significantly impact the other (Ahmed et al., 2010).

The use of systematic screening protocols will facilitate the detection of those at risk so that early intervention can take place, which may prevent the progression of kidney injury. Furthermore, hydration is also a key preventive step, especially when contrast agents are involved in imaging. Research has established that intravenous hydration before and following procedure can substantially reduce the incidence of contrast-induced AKI. However, there is some controversy regarding the efficacy of various hydration regimens, highlighting the need for patient-specific strategies that depend on individual patient states (Hoste et al., 2019). In addition to hydration, restriction of the use of nephrotoxic medications in intensive therapies is pivotal.

By meticulous evaluation and even alteration of drug regimens, medical practitioners can significantly curtail the risk of AKI in susceptible patients. In the end, education and enlightenment account for preventing AKI. Physicians should be well-informed about the latest guidelines and evidence-based recommendations so that they can effectively advise patients on preventive measures. Engaging patients in the learning process regarding their own disease state and influencing variables that could impact kidney function encourages active prevention. Educating the general populace through public programs carried out within the community will ensure greater awareness of the risks contributed by undiagnosed diseases and facilitate lifestyle changes that are kidney-friendly. Lastly, a concerted effort among support systems, healthcare staff, and patients will empower vulnerable populations, lower the rates of AKI, and contribute to better overall health outcomes (Figure 8.17).

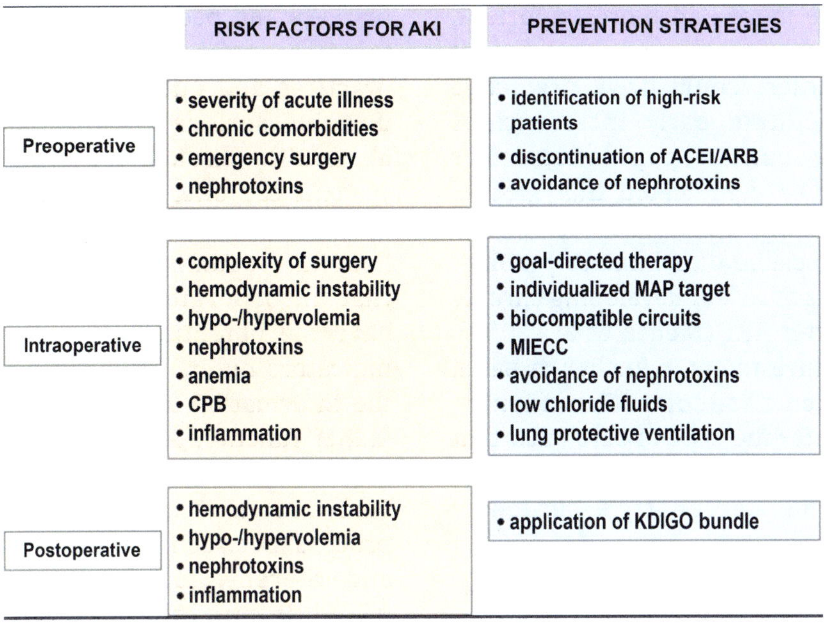

Figure 8.17. Prevention of acute kidney injury.

Source: https://media.springernature.com/lw685/springer-static/image/chp%3A10.1007%2F978-3-030-93433-0_18/MediaObjects/524014_1_En_18_Fig1_HTML.png.

8.6.1. Identifying High-Risk Patients

Identification of high-risk patients is an integral part of effective treatment for Acute Kidney Injury (AKI), as prompt intervention can significantly improve patient outcomes. Recent studies emphasize the utility of combining clinical characteristics with new biomarkers for the prediction of long-term kidney disease risk after AKI. Research involving 723 patients with AKI admitted to the hospital revealed that using machine learning techniques to evaluate 75 potential predictors accurately predicted individuals at risk for making significant adverse kidney events (MAKEs) within three years. The study identified primary factors, such as albuminuria and soluble TNF receptor-1, as robust predictors, indicating the potential of these tools in enhancing AKI patient treatment plans (Menez et al., 2024). By focusing interventions on high-risk individuals, healthcare providers can maximize follow-up care to decrease the incidence of advanced renal complications ultimately. Pre-existing conditions, such as intravenous iodinated contrast exposure during radiographic procedures, may augment the risk for AKI development. In particular, CKD before the procedure is a commonly accepted risk factor with increased risk for AKI in these patients. One recent retrospective study proved the efficacy of the Abbott iSTAT creatinine assay in identifying patients at medium to high risk of developing AKI after contrast exposure. Employing laboratory-based eGFR as the gold standard, the study established that the iSTAT assay accurately stratified patients based on their eGFR levels, enabling clinicians to take appropriate measures before administering contrast (Hawkins, 2024). In this way, clinicians can actively promote to protect vulnerable populations and tailor preventive measures to mitigate the risk of AKI. The integration of new diagnostic technologies with clinical practice yields a significant advancement in identifying high-risk patients, which is crucial for minimizing the complications of AKI. With the growing prevalence of AKI, efficient screening strategies become more and more important. Combining traditional clinical assessment with new biomarkers could drive predictive function and facilitate early interventions among selective patient populations. For instance, studies have indicated that models merging clinical assessments and biomarkers can achieve appreciable discriminatory ability to identify persons at risk of developing chronic kidney disease after AKI (Menez et al., 2024). Consequently, an investment in further research and the implementation of such screening techniques will alter the type of care such that high-risk individuals are adequately surveilled and cared for, and the country's burden of kidney disease is reduced.

8.6.2. Implementing Protocols in Healthcare Settings

Effective implementation of protocols in health facilities is critical in AKI management, a severe complication that is common among critically ill patients. The development of brief, evidence-based protocols helps healthcare workers identify risk factors and implement effective prevention strategies. For instance, a recent study demonstrated that AKI prevalence among intensive care unit patients was 49.2%, which highlights the necessity of targeted interventions among high-risk populations, such as older adults with hypertension and sepsis (Ahmed et al., 2025). Through systematic implementation of protocols, clinicians can coordinate the delivery of care to become more effective, leading to better early detection, timely intervention, and potentially optimized patient outcomes. The development of well-defined procedures is not only vital in minimizing the dangers associated with AKI but also in creating a proactive healthcare environment where patients' safety and quality of care rank foremost. Incorporating technological advancements into healthcare procedures can significantly enhance the management of AKI. Telehealth programs, with a focus on lay health workers and peer support systems, have been found to improve patient self-management practices and outcomes in other comparable domains, such as vascular illness (Kennedy et al., 2013). Through these models, healthcare systems can offer ongoing support to patients at risk for AKI, with early intervention and hospital readmission prevention. Protocols that incorporate technological integration have the potential to monitor critical health indicators online, enabling patients to receive the information and tools required to sustain kidney function. Adoption of such technologies requires thorough planning for training medical staff and ensuring a smooth communication process between different support systems, and thereby, technology becomes a good friend in the quest to prevent AKI from progressing. Proper utilization of protocols in the management of acute kidney injury also includes building interdisciplinary collaboration within healthcare teams. By fostering open communication among nephrologists, nurses, and other healthcare professionals, an integrated approach to managing AKI can be developed. Interdisciplinary teamwork is highly essential because several elements are involved in the etiology of AKI, necessitating input from numerous medical specialties to provide effective treatment and preventive measures. Regular joint team sessions, combined with educational activities, can facilitate a unified strategy for patient management, enabling the rapid adjustment of protocols as new evidence emerges. As evidence continues to elucidate the role of variables such as age, hypertension, and sepsis in AKI development, being able to adjust with a flexible yet uniform protocol structure will be key to maximizing outcomes in high-risk populations (Ahmed et al., 2025).

8.6.3. Patient Education and Awareness

Patient education and awareness are imperative in the management of AKI. Effective patient education empowers patients with information about their condition, helps them recognize early warning signs, and encourages active participation in their treatment regimens. Through gaining a comprehensive understanding of their health status, patients can make informed decisions about lifestyle modifications, medication, and follow-up care. Besides, educational programs may facilitate the early identification of risk factors of AKI, which would initiate preventive actions to curtail its prevalence. Under the coordination of healthcare providers in developing and implementing customized educational programs, the emphasis on patient-specific demands comes to the forefront, complementing broad-based health programs to increase outcomes as well as reduce hospitalization. Moreover, the provision of information by healthcare providers cannot be overstated. Interprofessional teams of nephrologists, nurses, dietitians, and pharmacists can collaborate to develop a robust education platform that addresses the multifaceted problems of AKI. Optimal utilization of each profession's strengths, patient education can be maximized not only to tackle the medical aspects of AKI but also nutritional advice and lifestyle changes. For instance, patients who receive information regarding dietary modifications have shown improved compliance with nutritional restrictions, which are advocated for by improved dietary monitoring, and this can significantly aid in the health and recovery of the kidneys. Shared decision-making initiatives further enhance activation in patients, as patients feel encouraged to participate proactively in their care process, resulting in better health outcomes despite the challenges posed by AKI (Awdishu et al., 2019). AKI awareness is not confined to the clinical setting and overflows into community programming and public health activities. Recognizing that AKI disproportionately affects disadvantaged populations, targeted educational initiatives can encourage heightened awareness of risk factors and preventive practices. For instance, community health programs that focus on the importance of hydration, regular health screenings, and the management of chronic diseases reduce the occurrence of AKI. In addition, research indicates the need for prevention and care coordination policy, particularly for conditions with abundant evidence but minimal policy implementation, such as patient self-management and palliative care (Morton et al., 2015). By integrating patient education and awareness into these broader public health interventions, stakeholders can collectively contribute to alleviating the AKI burden and improving health equity within heterogeneous populations (Figure 8.18).

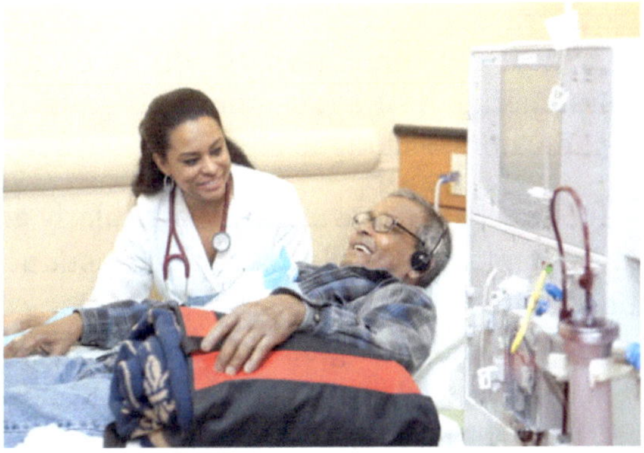

Figure 8.18. Patient education and awareness for acute kidney injury (AKI).

Source: https://www.kidney.org/sites/default/files/aki_to_dialysis.png.

SUMMARY

AKI is a multifaceted clinical syndrome that extends beyond the scope of kidney dysfunction to involve other organ systems. The interaction between AKI and extra-renal complications underlines the need for a complete understanding of its pathophysiology and ramifications. As research continues to unveil the extended effects of AKI on systemic health, clinicians are prompted to adopt an integrated approach in addressing the implicated patients. This involves not only addressing the kidney injury but also monitoring and responding to the potential cascade of other organ dysfunctions that may arise as a result of AKI. Recognition of these inter-relationships is pivotal in optimizing patient outcomes, underscoring the critical value of prompt and effective intervention. AKI management also involves meticulous drug dosing and potential drug interactions, especially in critically ill patients. Patients with chronic kidney disease are found to cluster in a therapeutic margin of efficacy when medications are prescribed. Dosing tables derived from populations with chronic kidney disease would lead to under- or over-dosing of AKI patients due to the confounding factors that are specific to this condition. Importantly, new findings suggest that AKI can interfere with hepatic cytochrome P450 (CYP) function, making the pharmacokinetics of many drugs employed in clinical settings complex. Hence, following individualized drug prescribing regimens becomes necessary, particularly for more acutely ill patients, to limit side effects and encourage AKI recovery (Abosaif et al., 2014). Last but not least, the complexity in treating AKI underscores the need for ongoing research and education in the medical field. Even though current guidelines represent a minimal model for the treatment of AKI, the ever-changing nature of clinical information confirms the need for personalized treatment modalities. More research into genetic factors controlling CYP expression and drug regimens' responses among patients can enhance outcomes and point to best practices. Additionally, interprofessional collaboration among nephrologists, pharmacists, and critical care practitioners will be crucial in advancing treatment strategies. With a growing understanding of AKI, it can be envisioned that efforts will be made to strive for improved patient care indicators, leading to significant strides in the care of this severe condition (Black et al., 2015).

It is worth recognizing AKI, particularly given its multifactorial nature and heterogeneous causes of development. The illness can arise suddenly based on intrinsic renal disease, for example, in patients with COVID-19, where complications develop due to thrombotic events, virus-induced tubular cell injury, and even glomerulonephritis. Hypovolemia, multi-organ failure, and rhabdomyolysis represent other extrinsic reasons for AKI development. Importantly, of note is the observation that mortality risk increases in tandem with AKI events, demonstrating the need for clinical vigilance. Early identification and prevention of risk factors throughout treatment are crucial, as well as the implementation of appropriate renal-specific monitoring protocols to assist in the elimination of AKI-related complications. These prevention strategies are crucial in enhancing patient outcomes, underscoring the correlation between early diagnosis and optimal management practices in acute care settings (Selby et al., 2020). This clinical setting is also marred by the discouraging reports on AKI, especially among vulnerable groups like neonates in NICUs. Studies have shown that up to 30% of neonates admitted to NICUs are diagnosed with AKI, which has increased mortality rates and possible sequelae into CKD. Although the level is alarming, under-recognition of AKI persists, particularly when serum creatinine levels are the only criterion used. A retrospective study of at-risk neonates highlighted the matter, where follow-up testing for the diagnosis of early CKD was inadequate. Few AKI-positive patients were properly consulted by nephrology, and AKI was noted adequately in discharge summaries, generating gigantic long-term management issues. Long-term monitoring and follow-up measures must be initiated to ensure these high-risk patients are appropriately managed and future renal complications are minimized (Roy et al., 2020). The implications of AKI are multidimensional in nature and thus necessitate a comprehensive understanding of its clinical implications, particularly in terms of early detection and management. Given the fact that AKI presents through multiple syndromes ranging from fluid overload to electrolyte imbalance, early intervention is of utmost importance. In COVID-19 patients suffering from AKI, for instance, careful fluid management becomes a therapeutic intervention to prevent further renal damage. Furthermore, with the new evidence of neonatal renal damage following AKI, follow-up care that involves specialized and focused monitoring of kidney function and associated health status is imperative. A concerted effort through healthcare teams can facilitate the provision of long-term assessments for optimal recovery and protection against long-term complications in high-risk patients. Thus, the integration of evidence-based care into AKI care guidelines is expected to yield improved outcomes and enhance the quality of treatment offered to the affected population (Roy et al., 2020; Selby et al., 2020).

CLOSER LOOK

URINARY NEUTROPHIL GELATINASE-ASSOCIATED LIPOCALIN (NGAL)

Urinary NGAL, also known as lipocalin-2, is a new and highly promising biomarker for the early detection of AKI. NGAL, a 25-kDa protein, is part of the lipocalin superfamily that is constitutively expressed at low levels in most tissues under basal conditions, including the kidney, liver, lung, and gastrointestinal tract. Its levels are significantly increased upon tissue injury, infection, or inflammation. In the setting of renal pathology, NGAL is rapidly induced and secreted by damaged tubular epithelial cells of the nephron, most notably in the distal nephron and collecting ducts, often within a few hours following injury, making it a considerably more immediate marker of renal injury than traditional markers like serum creatinine. Due to its rapid increase and ease of detection in urine, urinary NGAL has emerged as a valuable tool for detecting subclinical AKI before the onset of overt symptoms or laboratory abnormalities.

The clinical advantages of NGAL are its timing and sensitivity. Traditional markers for renal injury, like serum creatinine, are indirect and delayed measures of renal function; they may take 24–48 hours to increase after there is severe nephron injury. Urinary NGAL, on the other hand, can rise 2–6 hours after renal injury, allowing doctors to diagnose and treat AKI sooner. It holds great importance in settings such as cardiac surgery, sepsis, contrast-induced nephropathy, and critical illness, where early detection of kidney stress or injury would play a pivotal role in enhancing patient outcomes. Urinary NGAL is particularly useful in intensive care and emergency settings, where it can be employed to risk-stratify patients, direct therapy, and reduce the progression of chronic kidney disease or the need for dialysis.

At a molecular basis, NGAL is a transporting protein of iron and participates in innate immunity by inhibiting bacterial growth through iron sequestration. Its urinary elevation in AKI is not only a reflection of increased synthesis by injured tubular cells but also a result of decreased reabsorption and increased filtration by injured glomeruli. Outside of AKI, elevated urinary levels of NGAL have also been reported in chronic kidney disease (CKD) and glomerulonephritis, as well as in other inflammatory urinary tract diseases. Interpretation would require being context-specific because non-renal conditions such as systemic infections, tumors, and inflammatory illnesses also increase NGAL.

NGAL testing is typically performed using immunoassays, and either urine or plasma can be employed; however, NGAL in the urine is a more reliable marker of tubular injury to the kidney. In recent years, commercial point-of-care NGAL assays have become more widely available, making them more convenient to use in the clinic. NGAL, for all its advantages, is not yet used in every clinic because there is still some heterogeneity in the assay methods, it is not free of cost, and there has to be more standardization of diagnostic values.

References

1. Abishek, A., & Venkateswaramurthy, N. (2023). A review on antibiotics induced nephrotoxicity. *International Journal of Basic & Clinical Pharmacology*, *12*(4), 600–606. https://doi.org/10.18203/2319-2003.ijbcp20231899Abosaif, M., Andres-Hernando, C., Andres-Hernando, C., Philips, B., Boucher, J., Bougle, A., Brown, S., et al. (2014). Xenobiotic metabolism: The effect of acute kidney injury on non-renal drug clearance and hepatic drug metabolism. https://core.ac.uk/download/19937736.pdf (accessed on 25th June 2025).
2. Ahmed, A., Maisel, A., Alberti, M., Palazzuoli, A., Mebazaa, A., Ammann, P., Ammann, P., et al. (2010). Cardio-renal syndromes: Report from the consensus conference of the Acute Dialysis Quality Initiative. https://core.ac.uk/download/pdf/8389436.pdf (accessed on 25th June 2025).
3. Ahmed, M. S., Harun-Ur-Rashid, M., Alam, H., Moral, S., et al. (2025). Risk factors and prevalence of acute kidney injury among intensive care unit patients: A comprehensive study in a tertiary care setting. https://core.ac.uk/download/655504092.pdf (accessed on 25th June 2025).
4. Ambrosy, A. P., Antohi, E. L., Butler, J., Chioncel, O., et al. (2018). Improving post discharge outcomes in acute heart failure. https://core.ac.uk/download/228066233.pdf (accessed on 25th June 2025).
5. Andant, T., Anderson, K., Andersson, C., Badawy, A., Balwani, M., Bissell, M., Bissell, D., et al. (2019). Acute hepatic porphyria's: Review and recent progress. https://core.ac.uk/download/323074395.pdf (accessed on 25th June 2025).
6. Anderson, A. H., Appel, L. J., Chen, J., Feldman, H. I., et al. (2020). Research-based versus clinical serum creatinine measurements and the association of acute kidney injury with subsequent kidney function: Findings from the Chronic Renal Insufficiency Cohort study. https://core.ac.uk/download/323063254.pdf (accessed on 25th June 2025).
7. Awdishu, L., Moore, T., Morrison, M., Trzebinska, E., et al. (2019). A primer on quality assurance and performance improvement for interprofessional chronic kidney disease care: A path to Joint Commission certification. https://core.ac.uk/download/323064308.pdf (accessed on 25th June 2025).
8. Bagshaw, S. M., Balducci, A., Baldwin, I., Barbarigo, L., et al. (2016). Nomenclature for renal replacement therapy and blood purification techniques in critically ill patients: Practical applications. https://core.ac.uk/download/153365476.pdf (accessed on 25th June 2025).
9. Bagshaw, S. M., Bellomo, R., Ethgen, O., Kellum, J. A., et al. (2014). Economics of dialysis dependence following renal replacement therapy for critically ill acute kidney injury patients. https://core.ac.uk/download/77160386.pdf (accessed on 25th June 2025).
10. Bagshaw, S. M., Bellomo, R., Ethgen, O., Kellum, J. A., et al. (2017). Economics of dialysis dependence following renal replacement therapy for critically ill acute kidney injury patients. https://core.ac.uk/download/85217361.pdf (accessed on 25th June 2025).
11. Baptista, A., Barroso, E., Ferreira, A. C., Monteiro, M. C., et al. (2012). Orthotopic liver transplantation in familial amyloidotic polyneuropathy is associated with long-term progression of renal disease. https://core.ac.uk/download/71736710.pdf (accessed on 25th June 2025).

12. Berger, S. P., Leuvenink, H. G. D., Nieuwenhuijs-Moeke, G. J., Pischke, S. E., et al. (2020). Ischemia and reperfusion injury in kidney transplantation: Relevant mechanisms in injury and repair. https://core.ac.uk/download/288817401.pdf (accessed on 25th June 2025).
13. Bihorac, A., Bihorac, A., Bonavia, A., Chronopoulos, A., Frisch, A., Hollinger, A., Linkermann, A., et al. (2021). Postoperative acute kidney injury in adult non-cardiac surgery: Joint consensus report of the Acute Disease Quality Initiative and Perioperative Quality Initiative. https://core.ac.uk/download/457642644.pdf (accessed on 25th June 2025).
14. Black, C., Fluck, N., Marks, A., Mitchell, M., et al. (2015). Long-term prognosis after acute kidney injury (AKI)–What is the role of baseline kidney function and recovery? A systematic review. https://core.ac.uk/download/29151088.pdf (accessed on 25th June 2025).
15. Bonventre, J. V., Parrish, A. R., & Wang, X. (2014). The aging kidney: Increased susceptibility to nephrotoxicity. https://core.ac.uk/download/28951924.pdf (accessed on 25th June 2025).
16. Bottle, A., Lassnigg, A., Wonnacott, A., Levey, A. S., Talabani, B., Farmer, C. K. T., Hsu, C. Y., et al. (2014). Do acute elevations of serum creatinine in primary care engender an increased mortality risk? https://core.ac.uk/download/30711854.pdf (accessed on 25th June 2025).
17. Calvaruso, M., Castellano, G., Franzin, R., Gesualdo, L., et al. (2020). Molecular mechanisms of AKI in the elderly: From animal models to therapeutic intervention. https://core.ac.uk/download/541253459.pdf (accessed on 25th June 2025).
18. Cherney, D. Z. I., Chertow, G. M., Correa-Rotter, R., DAPA-CKD Trial Committees and Investigators, et al. (2021). A pre-specified analysis of the Dapagliflozin and Prevention of Adverse Outcomes in Chronic Kidney Disease (DAPA-CKD) randomized controlled trial on the incidence of abrupt declines in kidney function. https://core.ac.uk/download/480392438.pdf (accessed on 25th June 2025).
19. Cheruiyot, S. (2023). Risk factors and outcomes of acute kidney injury among COVID-19 patients at a tertiary hospital in Kenya. https://core.ac.uk/download/597995915.pdf (accessed on 25th June 2025).
20. Chinudomwong, P., & Siribamrungwong, M. (2016). Relation between acute kidney injury and pregnancy-related factors. https://core.ac.uk/download/pdf/82590811.pdf (accessed on 25th June 2025).
21. Cortes, M., Cho, K. W., Chowdhury, N. M., Mays, J. N., & Shin, C. H. (2024). Amoxicillin-induced drug reaction with eosinophilia and systemic symptoms (DRESS) syndrome with acute onset of diffuse rash and acute kidney injury (AKI). *Cureus, 16*. https://www.semanticscholar.org/paper/bed8fcc217af740a2671547d68b090c8b1ea6c83 (accessed on 25th June 2025).
22. Cowgill, L. D., Kanakubo, K., Kowalkowski, K. L., LeRoy, B. E., et al. (2016). Urinary neutrophil gelatinase-associated lipocalin as a marker for identification of acute kidney injury and recovery in dogs with gentamicin-induced nephrotoxicity. https://core.ac.uk/download/323068609.pdf (accessed on 25th June 2025).
23. Dewitte, A., Ishani, A., Ishani, A., Morden, A., Pai, A. B., Schneider, A. G., Lewington, A. J., et al. (2017). Acute kidney disease and renal recovery: Consensus report of the Acute Disease Quality Initiative (ADQI) 16 Workgroup. https://core.ac.uk/download/84041861.pdf (accessed on 25th June 2025).

24. Evison, F., Ferguson, J., Gunson, B., Mitterhofer, A. P., et al. (2016). Acute kidney injury and post-reperfusion syndrome in liver transplantation. https://core.ac.uk/download/74320327.pdf (accessed on 25th June 2025).

25. Gonzalez, J. P., Vendrame, F., Gempel, S., Roach, K. E., Kirk-Sanchez, N., & Wong, M. (2025). Using metabolic parameters to inform emergency care referral in a patient with a hyperglycemic induced acute kidney injury: A case report. *Physiotherapy Theory and Practice*. https://www.semanticscholar.org/paper/784600620c41817035e13ac05a4e9cc1698abac3 (accessed on 25th June 2025).

26. Gwinner, W., Husi, H., Marx, D., Metzger, J., et al. (2016). Proteomics for rejection diagnosis in renal transplant patients: Where are we now? https://core.ac.uk/download/46559952.pdf (accessed on 25th June 2025).

27. Hawkins, R. (2024). A-332 identifying at-risk patients pre-IV contrast administration via POCT creatinine measurement. *Clinical Chemistry*. https://www.semanticscholar.org/paper/f3c6f251a37c029872fb285e9e0342555dc110dd (accessed on 25th June 2025).

28. Hoffmann, A., Levin, A., Levin, A., Levin, A., Marengoni, A., Otero, A., Qaseem, A., et al. (2015). Early chronic kidney disease: Diagnosis, management and models of care. https://core.ac.uk/download/35435599.pdf (accessed on 25th June 2025).

29. Hooda, F. (2022). Prevalence & factors associated with acute kidney injury in patients undergoing percutaneous coronary intervention at a tertiary healthcare facility in Tanzania. https://core.ac.uk/download/597995949.pdf (accessed on 25th June 2025).

30. Hosohata, K., Inada, A., Iwanaga, K., Oyama, T., et al. (2018). Acute kidney injury (AKI). https://core.ac.uk/download/322438077.pdf (accessed on 25th June 2025).

31. Hoste, E. A. J., & Vandenberghe, W. (2019). Contrast-associated acute kidney injury: Does it really exist, and if so, what to do about it? https://core.ac.uk/download/225020701.pdf (accessed on 25th June 2025).

32. Human, C., & Husi, H. (2015). Molecular determinants of acute kidney injury. https://core.ac.uk/download/46559950.pdf (accessed on 25th June 2025).

33. Kellum, J. A., & Lameire, N. (2013). Contrast-induced acute kidney injury and renal support for acute kidney injury: A KDIGO summary (part 2). https://core.ac.uk/download/55800526.pdf (accessed on 25th June 2025).

34. Kellum, J. A., & Lameire, N. (2013). Diagnosis, evaluation, and management of acute kidney injury: A KDIGO summary (part 1). https://core.ac.uk/download/55846642.pdf (accessed on 25th June 2025).

35. Kennedy, A., American Diabetes Association, Turner, B., Blickem, C., Brownson, C., Dennis, C., Murray, C., et al. (2013). Telephone-based self-management support by 'lay health workers' and 'peer support workers' to prevent and manage vascular diseases: A systematic review and meta-analysis. https://core.ac.uk/download/42478287.pdf (accessed on 25th June 2025).

36. Khatri, P., Roedder, S., Sarwal, M. M., Vitalone, M. J., et al. (2011). Biomarkers in solid organ transplantation: Establishing personalized transplantation medicine. https://core.ac.uk/download/323074810.pdf (accessed on 25th June 2025).

37. Kovačević, S., Mitović, N., Brkić, P., Ivanov, M., Životić, M., Miloradovic, Z., & Nesović Ostojić,

J. (2024). Hyperbaric oxygenation: Can it be a novel supportive method in acute kidney injury? Data obtained from experimental studies. *Cells, 13.* https://www.semanticscholar.org/paper/a274766c5433d0e8c5cff30423cd97dcda98ea8d (accessed on 25th June 2025).

38. Maciel, T. (2024). Optimizing postoperative acute kidney injury monitoring using a urine biochemical approach—Time to bring more dynamism to serum creatinine evaluation! *Indian Journal of Critical Care Medicine: Peer-reviewed, Official Publication of Indian Society of Critical Care Medicine, 28*, 729–733. https://www.semanticscholar.org/paper/718b620ed36def4ed643dfaf7d0453d34ddb7c46 (accessed on 25th June 2025).

39. Malhotra, K. (2015). Dialysis in the acute setting. https://core.ac.uk/download/159354553.pdf (accessed on 25th June 2025).

40. Menez, S., Kerr, K. F., Cheng, S., Hu, D., Thiessen-Philbrook, H., Moledina, D., Mansour, S. G., et al. (2024). Biomarker panels for predicting progression of kidney disease in acute kidney injury survivors. *Clinical Journal of the American Society of Nephrology, 20*, 337–345. https://www.semanticscholar.org/paper/a6474e39fdbc16dbd63585a823db302ef161e86f (accessed on 25th June 2025).

41. Morton, S., & Dunn, W. (2015). Addressing the health needs of an aging America: New opportunities for evidence-based policy solutions. https://core.ac.uk/download/75783019.pdf (accessed on 25th June 2025).

42. Otunla, A. A., Davies, A. H., Shalhoub, J., & Shanmugarajah, K. (2024). Lipotoxicity and immunometabolism in ischemic acute kidney injury: Current perspectives and future directions. https://core.ac.uk/download/604365208.pdf (accessed on 25th June 2025).

43. Perez-Valdivieso, J. R., Bes-Rastrollo, M., Vives, M., Garcia-Fernandez, N., & Monedero, P. (2009). Cardiac-surgery associated acute kidney injury requiring renal replacement therapy: A Spanish retrospective case-cohort study. https://core.ac.uk/download/83572934.pdf (accessed on 25th June 2025).

44. Roy, J. P., Goldstein, S., & Schuh, M. P. (2020). Under-recognition of neonatal acute kidney injury and lack of follow-up. *American Journal of Perinatology*. https://www.semanticscholar.org/paper/f1dc7b45abe04cb17c4b75c0b459be724f4f31ce (accessed on 25th June 2025).

45. Selby, N. M., Forni, L. G., Laing, C. M., Horne, K. L., Evans, R. D. R., Lucas, B. J., & Fluck, R. J. (2020). COVID-19 and acute kidney injury in hospital: Summary of NICE guidelines. *BMJ, 369*. https://www.semanticscholar.org/paper/445fd8c60ee633405c1b9a77534b42b4437a15ff (accessed on 25th June 2025).

46. Tirrell, G. (2016). The emergency department evaluation and outcomes of elderly fallers. https://open.bu.edu/bitstream/2144/15371/1/Tirrell_bu_0017N_10816.pdf (accessed on 25th June 2025).

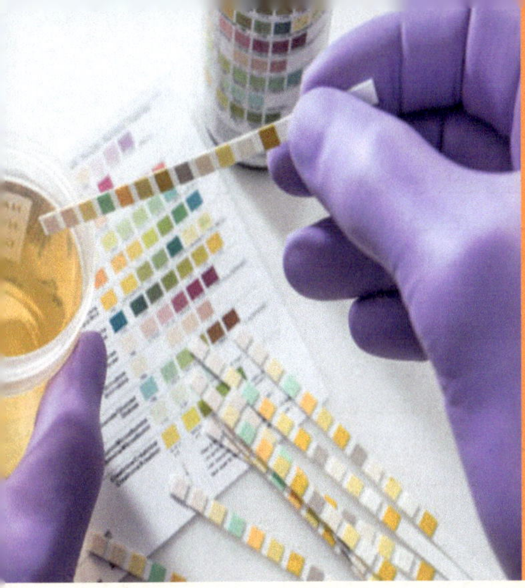

Chapter 9

CHRONIC KIDNEY DISEASE (CKD)

Contents

Introduction

Chronic kidney disease (CKD) is a significant public health issue globally due to its increasing prevalence and associated morbidity and mortality. Defined as progressive impairment of kidney function with time, CKD can progress to end-stage renal disease (ESRD), requiring dialysis or transplantation. CKD affects millions of individuals, but often remains unrecognized until advanced stages due to the lack of early symptoms or these being confused with other conditions. The main risk factors for CKD include diabetes, hypertension, and a family history of kidney disease, underlining the need for higher awareness and frequent screening of the at-risk population. Understanding the pathophysiology, risk factors, and complications of CKD is fundamental to the development of strategies for effective prevention and management that can improve patient outcomes and reduce the burden of care for this long-term condition. Literature highlights the intricate relationship between cardiovascular disease and CKD, noting that patients with CKD are at a significantly higher risk for cardiovascular morbidity and mortality. Recent findings suggest that atherosclerosis markers such as carbamylated albumin (C-Alb) are potential prognostic indicators in patients with CKD. As inflammation and atherosclerosis are closely linked in the pathology of cardiovascular disease, understanding them may facilitate earlier interventions and optimize the overall management of the patient (Daschner et al., 2024). The cardiovascular disease burden for patients with CKD would potentially further complicate their clinical management, such that a holistic approach would be required, considering renal as well as cardiovascular wellbeing. Therefore, co-management of the two related conditions is crucial for enhancing the quality of life and survival in CKD patients. Additionally, statistics indicate that children are also suffering from cystic kidney disease variations, like pediatric cystic kidney disease (CyKD), which develops into CKD in adulthood. Studies have revealed that CyKD patients have varying symptoms and complications, from recurrent urinary tract infections to hypertension (Grli et al., 2024). This would imply an immediate need for early detection and constant monitoring of infected children to reduce the long-term consequences of CKD. As the pathogenesis of CKD is better elucidated, it increasingly seems that pediatric and adult cases must be addressed with individualized therapy according to the unique needs of each group. Exploring genetic markers and disease progression in both populations may ultimately enhance prognostic utility and treatment response in chronic kidney disease overall (Figure 9.1).

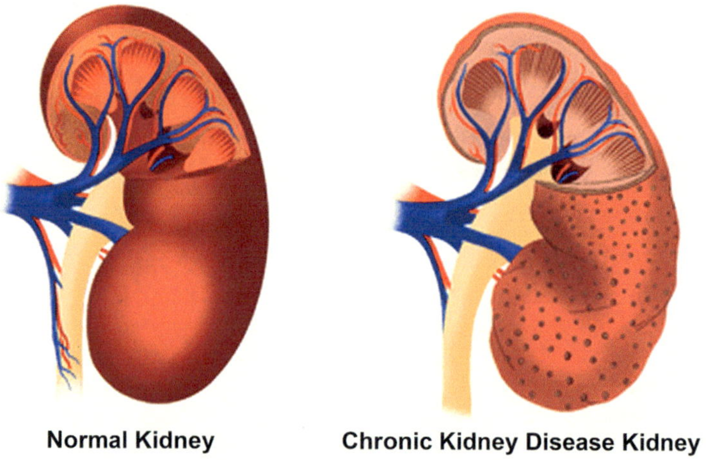

Figure 9.1. Chronic kidney disease (CKD).

Source: https://www.verywellhealth.com/thmb/mw2fcDjx_CEefzd397D3Knw1h_w=/400x250/filters:no_upscale():max_bytes(150000):strip_icc()/VWH_UremiaCauses-notext-7a60f1b2873c4b66917ddf975c052d0d.png.

Definition of Chronic Kidney Disease

CKD is a chronic disease characterized by a gradual reduction in kidney function over several months to years. CKD is responsible for filtering waste products and excess water from the blood and plays a critical role in maintaining homeostasis within the body. CKD is traditionally classified into five stages based on the glomerular filtration rate (GFR), a measure of kidney function. Stages range from mild kidney impairment (Stage 1) to final-stage renal disease (Stage 5), necessitating dialysis or renal transplant. Early detection of CKD is crucial, as timely treatment slows the course of the disease, improving patient outcomes and quality of life. Awareness of the etiologic causes—such as diabetes and hypertension—is also crucial because these are principal causal factors in the pathogenesis and aggravation of CKD. One of the most pressing CKD-related issues is that of comorbidities, specifically iron deficiency (ID) and hyperkalemia (HK). Iron deficiency occurs very frequently in patients with CKD. It is associated with many poor outcomes, like reduced quality of life, as well as increased rates of hospitalization. As stated in recent literature, monitoring iron status through indicators such as serum ferritin and transferrin saturation is crucial for the effective management of these patients (Rohr et al., 2023). Hyperkalemia is also a sinister risk in CKD, with the risk of arrhythmias and death, particularly when renin–angiotensin–aldosterone system inhibitor therapy is withheld once the potassium levels are elevated (Costa et al., 2023). Therefore, clinicians must regularly observe and treat these complications to provide the maximum possible care for CKD. All clinicians, patients, and researchers must be aware of the complex definition of CKD. CKD is not only the result of an acute cause but most often a combination of chronic systemic illnesses that contribute to its effect. With the progression of CKD, the kidneys' inability to regulate electrolytes, fluid status, and waste excretion initiates a cascade of metabolic aberrations. Such patients are therefore at risk of cardiovascular disease events, anemia, and disorders of bone mineral, all of which illustrate the interconnectedness of renal well-being and general health. The importance of early detection and management is supported by evidence that patients with well-monitored CKD can be healthier and decrease complications. Therefore, a comprehensive understanding of CKD, its definition, stages, risk factors, and treatment is crucial in meeting the challenges caused by this debilitating disease.

Importance of Understanding CKD

CKD not only endangers immediate health but also causes long-term complications that can significantly decrease a patient's quality of life. CKD must be understood since it affects various body systems, including reproductive system function, with severe hormonal disturbances leading to menstrual disorders in females. Research shows that the majority of female patients present with amenorrhea, oligomenorrhea, or menometrorrhagia, further adding to their complicated overall health care. Pinpointing the trends and prevalence of these disruptions will be important in developing interventions that address both physical health and psychosocial well-being among CKD patients. A focus on reproductive health assessment in CKD management can enable healthcare providers to enhance patient outcomes, ensuring that females receive holistic care that addresses their individual health concerns relevant to kidney disease (Ullah et al., 2025). Knowledge of CKD influences the entire arena of associated comorbidities, such as anemia, which often accompanies the condition. CKD anemia arises from several causes, including diminished erythropoietin production and a chronic inflammatory response, leading to extreme tiredness, decreased functional capacity, and a generally compromised quality of life. The development of novel therapeutic agents, like Vadadustat, represents a significant shift in treatment for anemia in this group. Vadadustat replicates the body's natural response to low oxygen levels, promoting more stable erythropoietin production than traditional erythropoiesis-stimulating agents (ESAs) that have been censured for associated risks. Hence, understanding the intricacy of CKD, such as its link with anemia and potential treatment options, is essential to improve the patient's care and chance of better management (Gul et al., 2025). Furthermore, an overall picture of CKD encompasses its socioeconomic burden. CKD patients have a heavy burden of healthcare costs, lost productivity, and related issues of access to receiving appropriate medical care. These constitute a pattern of health inequalities aggravated by inadequate information and knowledge of kidney disease among the general population. Educating patients will help break these harmful cycles, empowering them to take charge of their well-being and access early medical attention. Educational interventions and outreach campaigns for both patients and healthcare providers can raise awareness of CKD, enhance early detection, and enhance treatment plan adherence. By so doing, society can confront the total burden of CKD, improve health care for victims, and restrict future healthcare expenses (Figure 9.2).

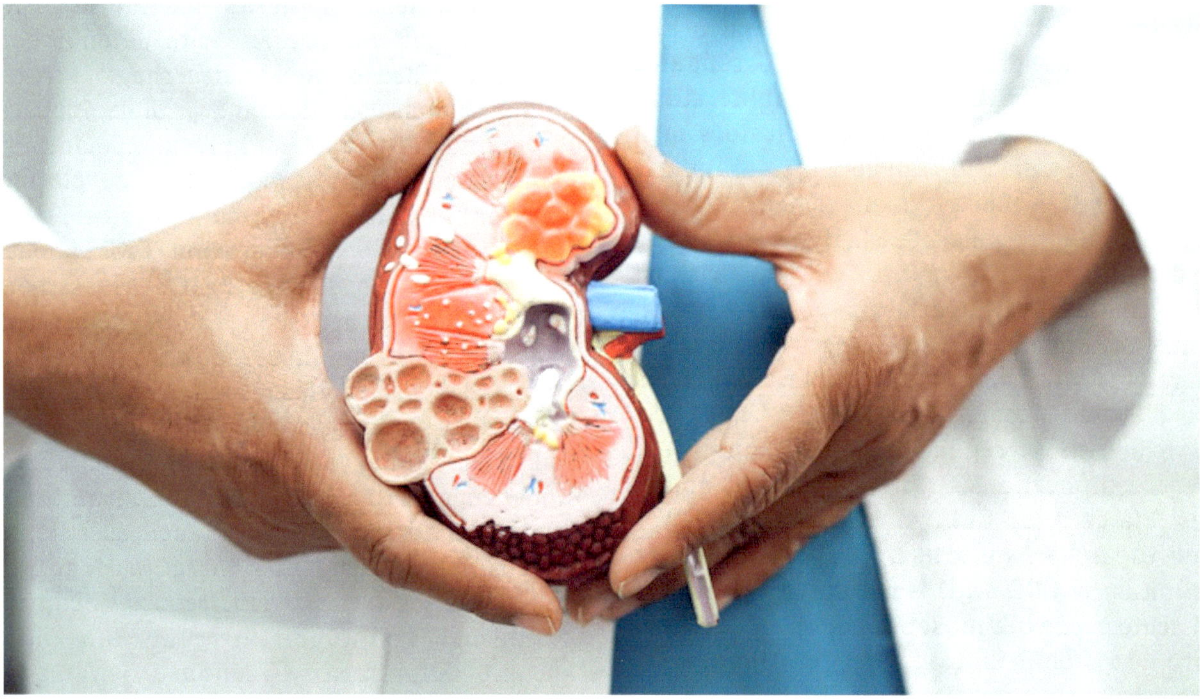

Figure 9.2. Understanding chronic kidney disease and importance of early prevention.

Source: https://images.moneycontrol.com/static-mcnews/2024/05/20240513112134_kidney.png ?impolicy=website&width=770&height=431.

9.1. Causes of Chronic Kidney Disease

Chronic kidney disease (CKD) can be caused by numerous underlying reasons, most of which are systemic diseases. The most significant cause is diabetes mellitus, which accounts for a considerable percentage of CKD cases in adults. The pathophysiologic action of hyperglycemia leads to nephropathy, as the kidneys' filtration units are destroyed. The ultimate effect is compromised kidney function. Beyond diabetes, hypertension is a second primary risk factor in CKD; inadequately controlled, it can lead to long-term damage to renal vasculature. Notably, both hypertension and diabetes not only cause CKD but also accelerate cardiovascular morbidity and mortality, contributing to the public health burden of kidney disease as reported by various supporting studies (Ahmed et al., 2018). Management of modifiable risk factors is also crucial in preventing the development and progression of CKD. Contributing further to the CKD crisis is the burden of glomerular diseases, which also cause a considerable fraction of the disease prevalence. For instance, nephrotic syndrome, which is a syndrome of proteinuria beyond what is expected for glomerular injury, predominantly occurs in children and has a substantial potential for the later development of CKD (Muryawan et al., 2015). The pathogenic mechanisms are usually immune-mediated inflammation or systemic disease, for example, lupus. They alter kidney function and structure dynamically, leading to progressive renal damage. The linkage of glomerular disease with CKD highlights the need for early diagnosis and intervention, particularly in children who can live with chronic disease states for extended durations. Identification and intervention of such underlying pathological states can decrease the incidence of CKDs and improve overall health outcomes. Lastly, lifestyle and environmental determinants are the major contributors to the risk of CKD. Obesity, for instance, is now a strong risk factor because it has been associated with numerous comorbidities such as type 2 diabetes and hypertension. In addition, excessive alcohol consumption and cigarette smoking are toxic to the kidneys either directly or indirectly by worsening underlying disease. There are also socioeconomic determinants of the occurrence of CKDs, with lower income levels limiting access to healthcare and increasing the likelihood of having unexpressed risk factors. Preventive interventions aimed at improving eating habits, motivating practice of exercise, and preventing risky lifestyles are able to challenge these risks and, as an ultimate consequence, slow down the burden of CKD among the population. The interplay of these diverse causes points to the necessity of multifaceted public health programs dedicated to kidney health promotion (Figure 9.3).

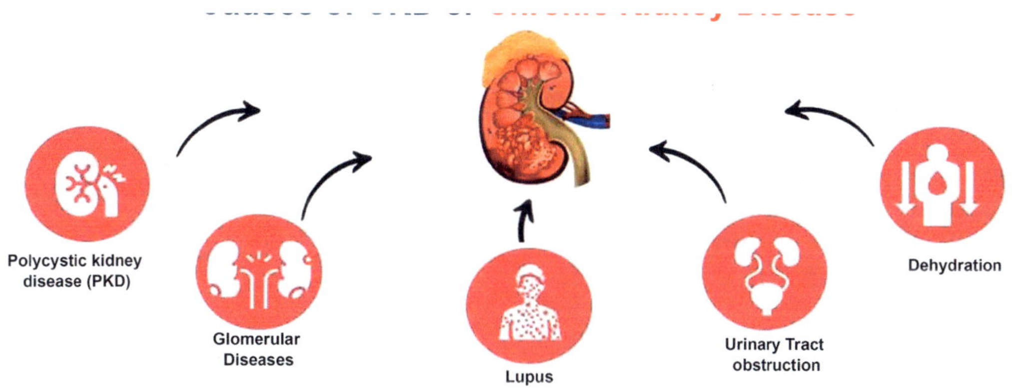

Figure 9.3. Causes of chronic kidney disease.

Source: https://www.ganeshdiagnostic.com/admin/assets/images/product section/Causes%20of%20CKD%20or%20Chronic%20Kidney%20Disease_1702038386.webp.

9.1.1. Diabetes Mellitus

The relation between CKD and Diabetes Mellitus is multifarious and interactive. Diabetes mellitus, particularly type 2, is one of the leading causes of CKD all over the world, through the key primary mechanisms of hyperglycemia and insulin resistance. Hyperglycemia causes glomerular hyperfiltration, ultimately resulting in glomerulosclerosis—a key element in diabetic nephropathy development. Additionally, diabetes exacerbates the inflammatory response in renal tissues and increases oxidative stress, thereby accelerating kidney damage. This highlights the significance of early diagnosis and aggressive management of diabetes to counteract its impact on kidney function, as many patients with CKD may be undiagnosed until advanced stages. The intertwined nature of the two diseases underscores the importance of comprehensive healthcare interventions that closely track and manage both diabetes and CKD. Moreover, physiopathologic interaction between CKD and diabetes creates a self-sustaining feedback loop that makes treatment harder and worsens patient prognosis. With decreasing renal function, the ability to clear glucose and insulin from the body also decreases, leading to worsening hyperglycemia and increased insulin resistance. This deterioration necessitates careful reconsideration of diabetic control in patients with CKD, particularly on the pharmacologic armamentarium at hand. Some anti-diabetic agents like metformin are traditionally contraindicated in advanced CKD due to the danger of lactic acidosis. In contrast, others, such as sodium-glucose cotransporter-2 (SGLT2) inhibitors, have been found to exhibit renal protective effects. Therefore, it is crucial to understand how diabetes medication affects blood glucose levels and kidney function in order to provide optimal care for patients susceptible to both conditions, which highlights the need for therapeutic intervention advancements (Robin et al., 2023). Preventive strategies are of the utmost importance for addressing the interrelated complexities of diabetes and CKD. Public health interventions aimed at reducing cases of diabetes, such as promoting healthier lifestyle habits—i.e., improved diet quality, physical activity, and smoking cessation—are essential. Lifestyle changes have proven beneficial not only in the prevention of the onset of diabetes but also in the management of its complications, such as CKD. The need for early screening and monitoring of renal function in diabetic patients cannot be overstressed; health awareness and education campaigns must encourage regular investigations to identify changes in kidney function. Furthermore, emerging evidence suggests that combining treatments against the respective pathogenic processes of diabetes and CKD may offer new opportunities for improving patient outcomes and reducing the overall burden of these chronic diseases (Owolabi et al., 2025) (Figure 9.4).

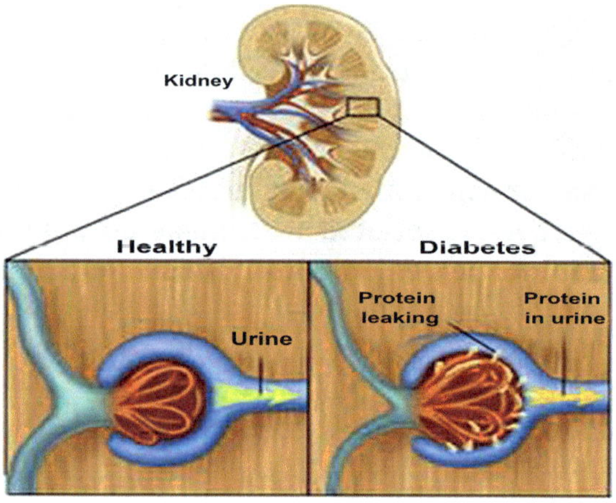

Figure 9.4. Diabetes and chronic kidney disease.

Source: https://lh6.googleusercontent.com/proxy/ImYF_BNq9YXk4aewo6N4-ySQGPppUqserxJdfODT__YxEE5lTTRzFqcQOIbSmJpq-mgdgWnhIsAN00V1qqwUTXxQxoKjeOWSYHxc9Z_-ec9f5CilVRMRbNNxs1s5TLU7I4ZEx8DSkd1sH1Z2O_uD62GDU5llkyU.

9.1.2. Hypertension

Hypertension has been referred to as the silent killer since it is often asymptomatic, yet its impact on CKD is immense and profound. The relationship between hypertension and CKD is bidirectional; high blood pressure both leads to the development of kidney disease and exacerbates existing CKD. When the kidneys lose function, they may lose the ability to maintain blood pressure, adding to hypertension. In fact, studies have shown that adequate control of blood pressure is vital in slowing the progression of CKD, which emphasizes the significance of early identification and intervention strategies in treating patients with hypertension and risk of kidney damage (Marrone et al., 2025).

Hence, there is a need to recognize the complex interaction between these diseases in developing comprehensive treatment strategies that take into account both blood pressure control and kidney status. While the worldwide burden of CKD continues to rise, especially in the developing world, hypertension as a causative agent cannot be overlooked. A very high correlation between the severe stages of hypertension and the development of CKD has been observed by recent studies, as has been observed in studies conducted in settings such as Indonesia. For instance, data pointed towards a strong correlation between stage 2 hypertension and CKD, with patients showing distinct differences in body mass index (BMI) and blood pressure by gender (Octivani et al., 2025). This suggests the need for culturally sensitive clinical management techniques. By recognizing the specific physiological and lifestyle determinants that impact hypertension and CKD across different groups, healthcare systems can enhance treatment adherence and improve patient outcomes. Thus, hypertension control is not only significant on a case-by-case patient basis but also a requirement for population-based public health action aimed at reducing the burden of CKD. Hypertension prevention and control are significant not only in terms of individual patient disease but also in minimizing the socioeconomic impact of CKD. Treatments for hypertension, such as lifestyle intervention—dietary modification and increased physical activity—were shown to significantly reduce the development of CKD (Marrone et al., 2025). Furthermore, integrating plant-based dietary approaches into hypertension management could potentially yield twin benefits: enhancing cardiovascular health and, perhaps, slowing the progression of CKD. With increasingly globalized dietary trends moving toward plant-based diets, practitioners need to place special emphasis on these guidelines, especially for those at risk of developing both hypertension and CKD. Systemic preventive interventions, such as blood pressure management and dietary education, not only improve the well-being of patients but also, as a consequence, decrease healthcare expenditure due to CKD, thereby providing a more sustainable health outcome against these collectively interdependent chronic diseases (Figure 9.5).

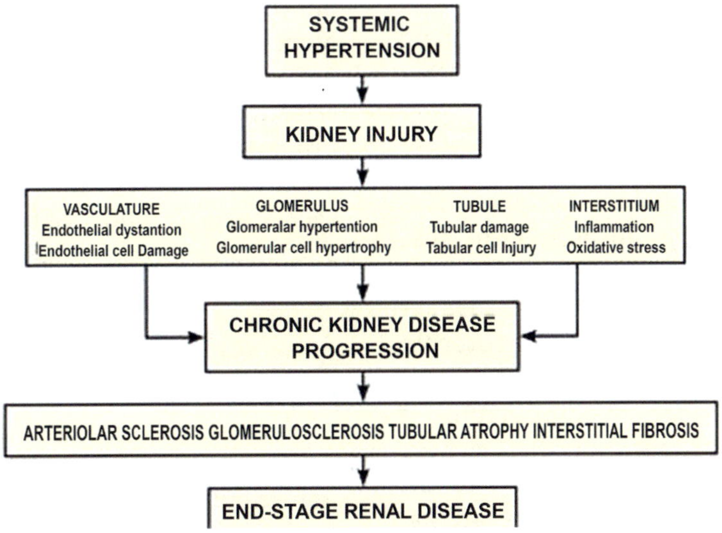

Figure 9.5. Hypertension and chronic kidney disease.

Source: https://mdatl.com/wp-content/uploads/2021/04/fig1-1-2.jpg.

9.1.3. Genetic Factors

The molecular genetics of CKD has been increasingly gaining attention as researchers try to identify the complexities involved in this multifaceted condition. Several genetic factors are implicated in susceptibility and disease progression of CKD, and some populations are found to be more susceptible based on inherited traits. Most importantly, the identification of specific genetic polymorphisms has played a pivotal role in elucidating the biological pathways leading to renal injury. These discoveries not only allow for an appreciation of CKD on a fundamental level but also aid in risk stratification within heterogeneous populations. This heterogeneity serves as a reminder of the necessity of further effort being directed towards ethnic and geographical differences, particularly in developing countries where CKD occurs in unique epidemiological patterns, as emphasized by ongoing studies such as the Indian Chronic Kidney Disease (ICKD) study (Yadav et al., 2017). In addition to traditional genetic factors, epigenetic alterations are now being considered in the CKD discussion. Epigenetic alterations can affect gene expression without altering the underlying DNA sequence and may be influenced by environmental factors and lifestyle. Epigenetic alterations may have an important role to play in CKD pathophysiology as recent research has highlighted, creating a dynamic interaction between heritable risk and environmental forces. Insights into these epigenetic mechanisms may enable the discovery of novel biomarkers that predict disease progression and inform therapeutic protocols. Moreover, the viability of epigenotype-based diagnostics presents exciting opportunities for personalized treatment of CKD, where therapeutic interventions are tailored to the patient's genetic and epigenetic susceptibility (Ekström et al., 2017). The translation of genetic and epigenetic research into the clinic has the potential to make a significant impact on CKD outcomes. With such advancements through initiatives such as the ICKD study, it is possible to have enhanced risk factor identification, which in turn can offer targeted interventions that slow down the progression of the disease. This approach recognizes that CKD is not just a consequence of environmental exposures but a complex interaction of genetic predisposition influenced by environmental and lifestyle factors. Therefore, understanding the genetic contributions to CKD can lead to more effective prevention and therapeutic programs. Lastly, building and sustaining this intersection of clinical practice and genetics is critical to addressing the growing CKD burden worldwide, and thus driving progress in both patient outcomes and scientific knowledge, an imperative (Yadav et al., 2017).

9.2. Symptoms and Diagnosis

The presentations of CKD will be subtle and insidious, with early detection being challenging. The presentation at the early stages will be fatigue, weakness, and minor fluctuations in blood pressure, which can easily be brushed off as a result of other diseases or lifestyle conditions. The symptoms will become more pronounced in advanced disease stages, typically manifested by edema of the ankles and feet secondary to fluid overload, changes in urine output, and chronic nausea. These presentations can have a significant impact on a patient's quality of life, illustrating the importance of early detection. Moreover, it is not until late stages that most patients with CKD are informed of their diagnosis; one study has shown that up to fifty-four percent of individuals did not know about their diagnosis, indicating a severe lack of patient education that needs to be addressed (Ellis et al., 2016). Diagnosis of CKD typically involves a synergy of clinical assessment, laboratory evaluation, and imaging. Initial testing may begin with patient history and physical, with a focus on risk factors such as diabetes, hypertension, and family history of kidney disease. Serial laboratory studies, such as measurement of serum creatinine and urinalysis, to estimate the glomerular filtration rate (GFR) and serve as the primary measure of renal function. The ability of the kidneys to filter out waste comes down with advancing CKD, and accurate staging of the disease from stage 1 to stage 5 is necessary to determine the proper treatment modalities. Last but not least, the role of a multidisciplinary team comprising nephrologists, dietitians, and primary care providers is crucial in diagnosing and managing CKD effectively. In addition, the emotional effect of CKD diagnosis cannot be underestimated, since most patients develop depression and anxiety when they are informed of their diagnosis. The ensuing emotional response can also make treatment adherence and self-management activities more challenging. Education plays a significant role in overcoming such challenges, whereby patients' higher knowledge levels about CKD have been associated with better patient outcomes. A study shows that increasing patient knowledge about their condition can enable them to become actively involved in management plans, potentially slowing the progression of the disease (Ellis et al., 2016). In healthcare workers' attempts to increase CKD awareness and education, prompt detection of symptoms and facilitating effective interventions will ultimately lead to improved patient outcomes and quality of life (Figure 9.6).

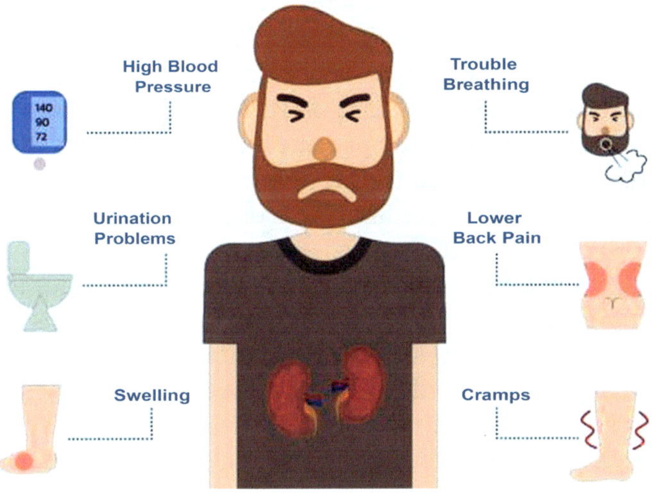

Figure 9.6. The symptoms of chronic kidney disease (CKD).

Source: https://sa1s3optim.patientpop.com/assets/images/provider/photos/2682657.jpeg.

9.2.1. Common Symptoms of CKD

CKD is also stealthy in its onset, producing a range of nonspecific symptoms that can have a significant impact on a patient's lifestyle. In some cases, the initial presentation of CKD may be characterized by fatigue, which results from the cumulative effects of multiple factors, including anemia and the accumulation of toxins in the blood that a healthy kidney would normally remove. They may also manifest with an overall feeling of malaise, and they also become lethargic, a condition that leads to decreased activity. It is also crucial for physicians to detect this early presentation because it typically leads to further investigation of the kidneys and eventually to an early diagnosis and treatment that halts disease progression. Edema, or swelling, particularly in the lower limbs, ankles, and feet, is another common symptom found with CKD. This edema occurs due to the fact that the kidneys become less effective in fluid balance as they become less capable of excreting excess water and sodium. As the condition of fluid buildup progresses, puffy eyes or swollen extremities may be mistaken for exhaustion or aging. In addition, abnormalities of urine volume, i.e., either polyuria (increased urination) or oliguria (decreased urination), are frequently associated with CKD. The altered urinary patterns may also be important indicators of worsening kidney function, making it extremely crucial for individuals with risk factors to take special care regarding their hydration levels and urinary patterns. Apart from this, the systemic presentation of CKD can occur through gastrointestinal upset in the form of nausea, vomiting, and anorexia. As the body retains toxins in the bloodstream, patients often become food-averse, resulting in nutritional disorders and involuntary weight loss. This exacerbates the fatigue and malaise already experienced with the disease. Additionally, skin changes, including dryness, pruritus, and development of rashes, are often met, most commonly as a result of an imbalance in mineral metabolism, such as secondary hyperparathyroidism. Physicians must be aware of these different manifestations of CKD not only because they compromise patient health but also because they are essential markers for effective management interventions to maximize patient outcomes.

9.2.2. Diagnostic Tests and Procedures

The diagnosis of CKD is highly based on performing many diagnostic tests and procedures, which serve to identify kidney function pathology. Traditional methods, such as laboratory tests that measure serum creatinine and glomerular filtration rate (GFR), remain pivotal in evaluating kidney function; however, the tests are insufficient to provide a clear indication of the development of CKDs. As hinted at by the increasing prevalence of CKD, which is projected to exceed 2 million patients undergoing dialysis by 2030, the medical community is under extreme pressure to enhance diagnostic accuracy, as well as early detection techniques. Advanced technologies, such as biomarkers and imaging modalities, are also employed; however, these are nonspecific for all stages of the condition. With improved diagnostic capacity, health practitioners can initiate early treatments, potentially slowing the progression of CKDs and medical complications (Ghafar et al., 2025). Following initial screening, doctors must consider more advanced diagnostic technologies that leverage technology to boost CKD surveillance. The integration of machine learning (ML) algorithms in diagnosis has gained momentum, as it has the potential to transform the dynamics of patient care. The new applications of AI algorithms, as outlined in recent studies, demonstrate the increasing accuracy of CKD diagnoses. For instance, ML algorithms such as Gaussian Naïve Bayes, gradient boosting, and decision trees have been shown to have promising predictive capability, all with accuracies of over 98% in controlled settings. The model hybrid methods, especially employing random forest classifiers as meta-classifiers, are promising for enhancing CKD diagnosis. These advancements depict the ever-evolving nature of how health care workers conduct CKD screening, highlighting the urgency and importance of fully embracing the use of technology in clinical practices (Khalid et al., 2023). The combined worth of such diagnosis technology is not only crucial for the identification of CKD but also fundamental to the effective control of its development. Diagnostic screening tests serve as pivotal entry points for monitoring subsequent therapeutic decisions and patient management strategies, ultimately leading to improved clinical outcomes. As the global burden of CKD rises, it cannot be overstated that coming up with valid, affordable, and cost-effective diagnostic processes is a priority. Confirmation of these machine learning algorithms across different populations in subsequent research must be a priority to enable their application. By addressing existing issues like data quality and algorithmic optimization, researchers can further enhance the validity of these diagnostic tests. Ultimately, an integrated strategy that combines both existing and emerging diagnostic technologies may offer the most promise for effectively mitigating the CKD epidemic (Ghafar et al., 2025) (Figure 9.7).

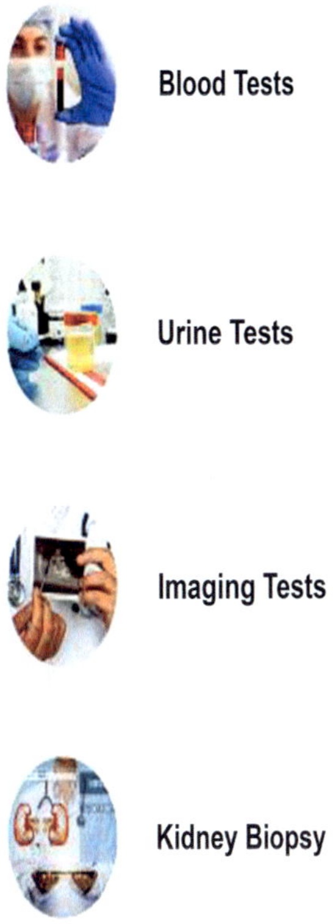

Figure 9.7. The diagnosis of chronic kidney disease (CKD).

Source: https://images.drlogy.com/assets/uploads/img/admin/health_blog/editor-img/chronic_kidney_disease_diagnosis_-_drlogy.webp.

9.2.3. Staging of Chronic Kidney Disease

Detection of the stage of CKD is necessary to manage and intervene effectively. Staging is primarily based on the estimated glomerular filtration rate (eGFR), which assesses kidney function and enables clinicians to understand the extent of kidney damage. The CKD stages are divided as follows: Stage 1 is characterized by a normal eGFR of 90 mL/min or greater, with or without the presence of structural or functional abnormalities. Stages 2 through 4 outline progressively declining kidney function, with Stage 2 being a mild reduction of eGFR (60-89 mL/min), Stage 3 subdivided into sub-stages A (45-59 mL/min) and B (30-44 mL/min), and Stage 4 being a severe decline (15-29 mL/min). Stage 5, end-stage renal disease, occurs when eGFR drops below 15 mL/min, which requires dialysis or transplantation to be performed for the patient to survive. CKD stages classification not only enhances disease comprehension but also provides a treatment strategy and prognosis for patients. For instance, patients presenting with earlier stages will be favorably responsive to therapies that will retard the disease progression, including lifestyle modification and pharmacologic therapy. On the other hand, those presenting in advanced stages tend to have more difficult management problems, which may include triggering renal replacement therapy. It is also essential to follow up on other parameters such as proteinuria, blood pressure, and electrolytes, which have a significant impact on outcomes of the patient. The variation in response to treatment among individuals highlights the necessity of tailoring care plans to the individual stage and the underlying etiology of CKD. Individualized approach is essential in treating the multi-factorial nature of CKD, particularly in high-risk populations. The addition of other diagnostic techniques and biomarkers may further delineate CKD staging and treatment. Recent evidence suggests that novel markers, such as Cystatin C and urinary biomarkers, can contribute to adding prognostic value beyond traditional measures, including serum creatinine values. With concomitant diseases, such as malignancies, assessment is complicated because some oncologic treatments may induce acute kidney injury (AKI), making CKD staging more difficult (Benoit et al., 2016). Further evidence is also presented in that variability in the determination of the creatinine level significantly affects patients' prognosis with sepsis and subsequent AKI (Dhondt et al., 2015). This shifting situation highlights the need for ongoing research and the development of more precise techniques in the diagnosis and classification of CKD, with the ultimate goal of enhancing patient management and outcomes (Figure 9.8).

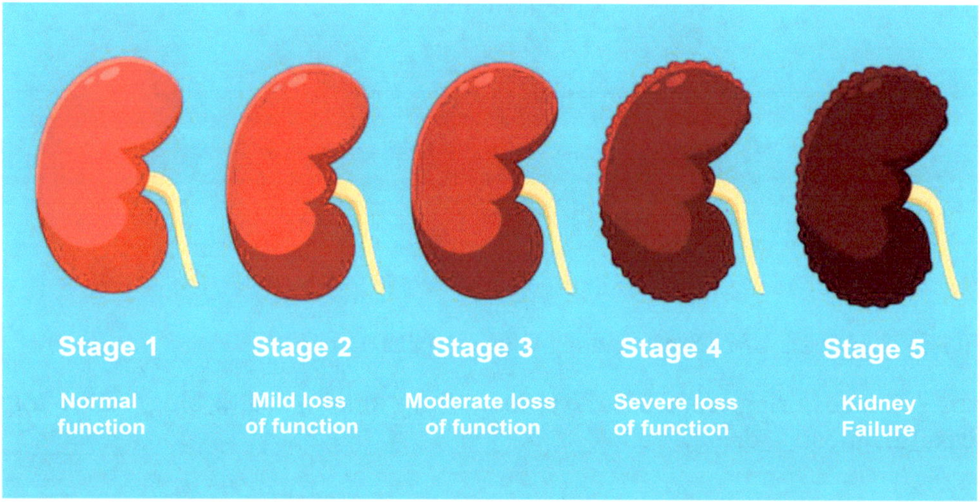

Figure 9.8. Staging of chronic kidney disease.

Source: https://gracelaboratory.com/wp-content/uploads/2024/11/The_5_Stages_of_Chronic_Kidney_Disease_HN3600_Cover_Sized-1-1024x577-1200x675.png.

9.3. Risk Factors

CKD risk factors are complex and multiplex and are often associated with each other, making the determination of their significance regarding disease progression necessary. Diabetes mellitus and hypertension are among the most significant of these and are responsible for a substantial proportion of CKD. Nephropathy arises from diabetes through hyperglycemia-mediated changes in glomerular function, while hypertension exacerbates kidney damage through chronic vascular injury. Research indicates that individuals with a history of such conditions are most vulnerable, which supports the need for early screening and active management strategies. Moreover, as noted by the National Kidney Foundation Kidney Disease Outcomes Quality Initiative (NKF-KDOQI), an understanding of how such chronic conditions interact and lead to compromised glomerular filtration rates can inform specific interventions to avoid progression to end-stage renal disease (Astor et al., 2011). Age is also a critical risk factor for CKD, with the elderly demonstrating higher disease incidence due to structural and functional alterations of the kidneys. Aging inevitably leads to a reduction in renal reserve and the loss of compensatory mechanisms, thereby predisposing individuals to kidney insults.

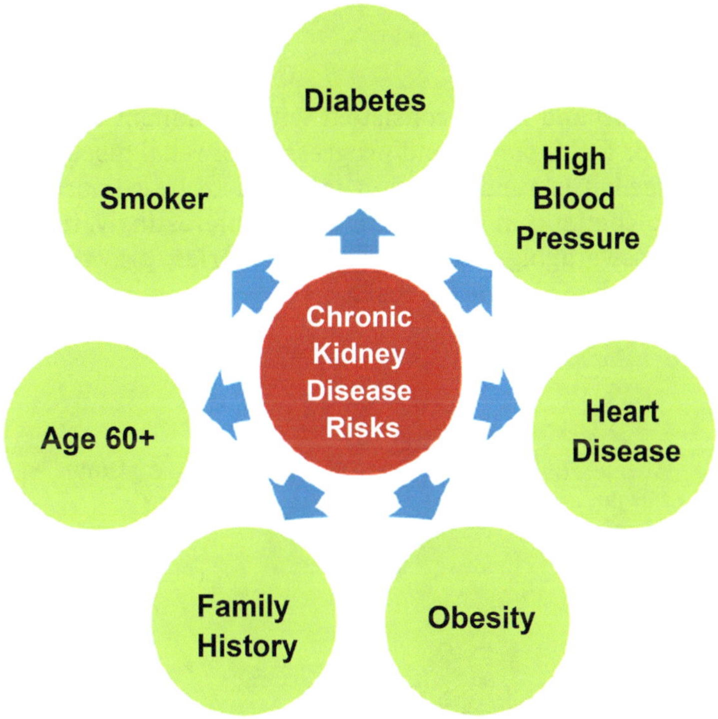

Figure 9.9. The risk factors associated with chronic kidney disease (CKD).

Source: https://www.holstonmedicalgroup.com/wp-content/themes/hmg1/assets/images/photo-kidney-risk.png.

Complicating matters, most older patients have multiple comorbid conditions, such as cardiovascular disease or metabolic syndrome, that enhance their risk. The impact of age on renal function is compounded by a chronic inflammatory illness commonly found in the aging population, which has the potential to accelerate the rate of renal function decline. Additionally, studies indicate a high level of association of age with vulnerability to acute kidney injury after surgical procedures like orthotopic liver transplantation, and this can lead to chronic renal issues (Baptista et al., 2012). Identifying such dynamics highlights the need to develop specific prevention and management measures for older populations. Lifestyle factors such as obesity, cigarette smoking, and dietary habits are also significant predictors of risk for CKD. Obesity causes the onset of diabetes and hypertension, which creates a vicious cycle that significantly increases the risk of renal damage. Cigarette smoking, which has long been recognized for its adverse effect on the vasculature, can exacerbate existing kidney disease as well as accelerate CKD progression. Additionally, a poor diet with excessive sodium, inadequate potassium intake, and suboptimal nutrient utilization can negatively impact kidney function. With such a complex interplay of risk factors, population health interventions through lifestyle modification become an absolute necessity in reducing CKD prevalence. Appropriate education about wellbeing, dietetics, and exercise can help individuals make improved lifestyle choices that ultimately minimize the burden of kidney disease on society. Here, awareness of risk factors and management remains of prime concern for healthy outcomes in high-risk patients for CKD (Figure 9.9).

9.3.1. Age and Gender

The relationship between CKD and age is consistent with prominent epidemiologic trends, as age itself is a primary risk factor for the onset and progression of renal disease. As individuals become elderly, the physiologic decline in renal function is added to by comorbidities such as diabetes and hypertension that are common in older individuals. Interestingly, it has been found through research that with progressive aging into older age categories, prevalence and severity of CKD increase, which results in higher healthcare costs.

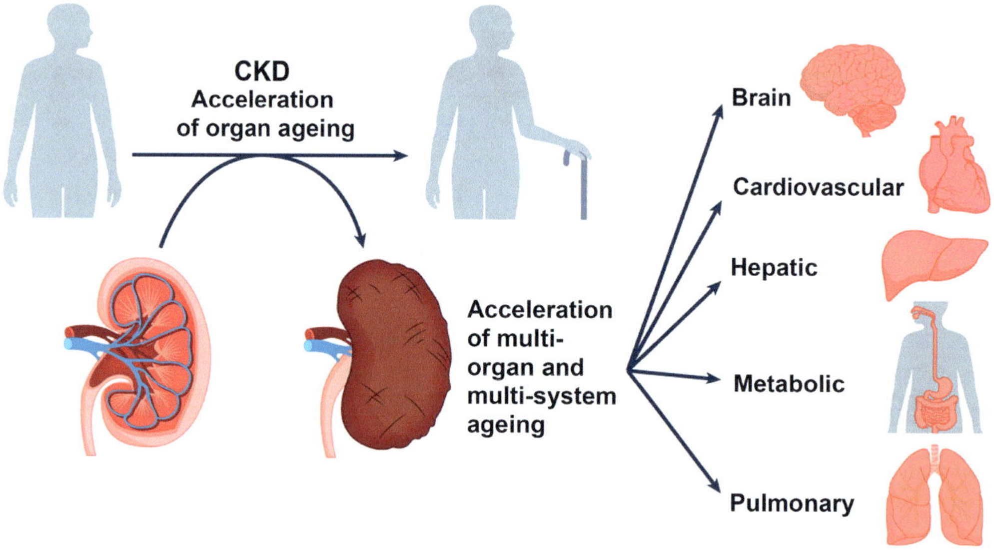

Figure 9.10. Chronic kidney disease promotes ageing in a multiorgan disease network.

Source: https://media.springernature.com/full/springer-static/image/art%3A10.1038%2Fs41581-023-00729-6/MediaObjects/41581_2023_729_Fig1_HTML.png.

Further evidence for age-related reductions in glomerular filtration rate (GFR) reveals that older patients experience more rapid loss of renal function, thereby placing them in a high-risk category based on compromised physiological reserve, which further complicates management strategies for CKD. Apart from age, gender also plays a key role in the prevalence and impact of CKD. Data indicate that women overall have a lower prevalence of CKD compared with men , but when diagnosed, they will have more severe disease. The gender difference may be due to differences in biological and sociocultural factors, including hormonal influences and sex-specific exposure to risk factors. Interestingly, women and minority patients have been shown to possess a high degree of knowledge gaps regarding dietary sodium restrictions, which are critical in CKD management. Published literature reveals that women have lower odds of identifying precise sodium intake limits, mirroring broader knowledge barriers that likely affect their compliance with dietary guidelines, calling for tailored educational interventions to ensure effective CKD management (Anderson et al., 2015).

In addition, the interaction of age and sex in CKD is similarly extended to cardiovascular risk, which is an inherent consideration given that patients with CKD are at higher risk for cardiovascular events. Data indicate that increments in the coronary artery calcification score are directly related to declining renal function, demonstrating that older patients with CKD may be disproportionately at risk due to cardiac disease. Specifically, mildly to moderately affected CKD in middle-aged patients has significantly increased CAC scores compared to healthier individuals, thereby placing them at risk for ischemic heart disease (Budoff et al., 2011). Such a coincidence of age and gender is an indication of the multifaceted nature of managing CKD, which calls for multifaceted interventions that take patient demographics into consideration to improve outcomes and reduce the particular vulnerabilities encountered by different population cohorts (Figure 9.10).

9.3.2. Lifestyle Choices

The prevalence of CKD has been linked to numerous habits of life that have the potential to influence kidney function significantly. Dietary habits, physical exercise, and the use of drugs have come to be seen as critical components in the progression and development of CKD. In developed countries, an increase in the prevalence of CKD is primarily linked to chronic degenerative non-communicable diseases (CDNCDs) such as diabetes and hypertension, which are most often caused by unfavorable lifestyle habits. In particular, non-optimal dietary habits, characterized by high salt and saturated fat intake, are responsible for increased body weight and elevated blood pressure, which in turn further increase the loss of kidney function. Detailed knowledge of such lifestyle factors is of the highest significance, as they not only affect the individual's particular health outcomes but also raise broader public health concerns that necessitate aggressive intervention strategies for controlling CKD prevalence (Marrone et al., 2025). In the management of CKD, the adoption of specific dietary habits has been shown to have a beneficial effect on disease control. Recent research points to the efficacy of vegetable-based diets in decelerating and inhibiting CKD progression. Through the implementation of mostly vegetable-based diets, one can reduce his or her consumption of damaging substances that are usually components of animal proteins while enhancing his or her nutritional and antioxidant intake. These eating patterns, such as the Mediterranean Diet and Low Protein Diet with a plant food dominance, have been associated with improved kidney function and overall health outcomes in CKD patients. Furthermore, these diets are ecologically sustainable by mitigating greenhouse gas emissions from animal agriculture, exemplifying a symbiotic convergence between ecological stewardship and health (Marrone et al., 2025). As health systems get more overwhelmed, implementing such changes in diet can bring tremendous health benefits while alleviating some cost pressures. For CKD, a whole-system lifestyle approach includes not only eating healthier, but also incorporating physical activity and stress management. Regular exercise enhances cardiovascular health, promotes weight management, and improves psychological well-being, all of which are essential for individuals at risk for CKD or those with the disease itself. In addition, traditional practices like Swasthavritta in Ayurvedic medicine stress conforming to daily routines to seasonal change in the interest of equilibrium and prevention of disease. This paradigm of preventive health targets lifestyle modification for enhancing the quality of life and could prove essential to the treatment of non-communicable disorders like CKD. By fostering a proactive approach to well-being through deliberate lifestyle choices, individuals can optimize health benefits and significantly reduce the economic burden of CKD on the healthcare system.

9.3.3. Family History

Family history plays a critical role in the management and understanding of CKD. Genetic susceptibility is a significant determinant of a patient's risk of developing CKD, as specific genetic markers make the individual susceptible to the disease. Family histories indicate that patients with a family history of kidney disease have a higher risk of having a similar issue, which implies a hereditary component related to CKD. This hereditary connection highlights the importance of obtaining meticulous family histories in clinical assessment to identify at-risk populations. Further, familiarity with family history facilitates tailoring of prevention and early intervention, such as lifestyle modification or screenings, for those with a genetic susceptibility to CKD. Thus, it emphasizes active health management among those with a history of kidney disease in the family because they are bound to experience higher risks owing to environmental or life determinants that tend to augment their genetic risk. In contemporary medicine, family history collection and interpretation have come to be emphasized within risk stratification for CKD. As genetic research unravels the etiology of CKD, family patterns then become central to individualized care planning. The relationship between CKD and family history can be determined through studies demonstrating a correlation between lifestyle, diet, and environmental influences and genetic susceptibility. For instance, the impact of salt overindulgence on renal function in scenarios where patients possess familial risk factors illustrates the interplay between intrinsic genetics and extrinsic behavior in CKD pathogenesis. This established correlation between family history and CKD susceptibility encourages patients and clinicians alike to engage in global health conversations, which results in recognition of prevention strategies tailored to those with hereditary predisposition toward kidney disease. Hence, a detailed assessment of family history is worth its weight in gold when planning healthy intervention strategies. The role of family history in genetic reasons is not the only factor, but also environmental and behavioral factors that contribute to the development of CKD. Conditions like diabetes and hypertension, prevalent in most families, add another layer to the risk of chronic kidney disease. Family dynamics often shape lifestyle choices that affect health, such as exercise and diet, making both genetic and behavioral risk factors inseparable. Family interventions that focus on health behaviors are likely to optimize clinical management of CKD. Research has shown that families involved in aggregate health-promoting strategies, including sodium intake reduction via diet or physical activity improvement, can decrease their aggregate risk for CKD substantially. Therefore, family history knowledge not only aids in recognizing genetic risk but can also be utilized for the formation of nurturing environments to provide improved health outcomes. This comprehensive use of family history ultimately leads to its central role in chronic kidney disease management and prevention (Figure 9.11).

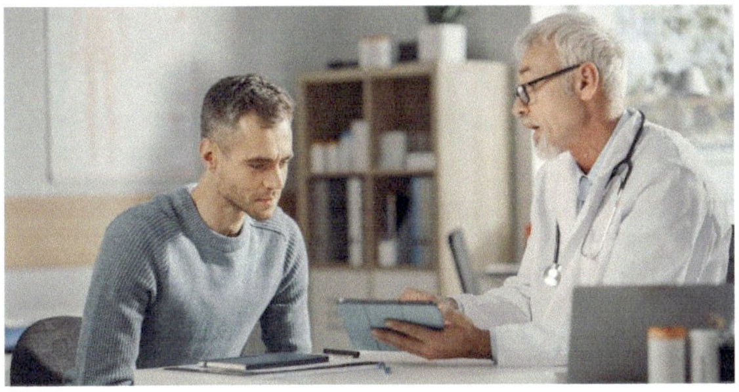

Figure 9.11. Family history in the chronic kidney disease (CKD).

Source: https://mumcdnstorage.blob.core.windows.net/dwnews/2022/12/asthma-referral-uptake_800x400.jpg.

9.4. Complications Associated with CKD

The complications of CKD are multifaceted in nature, and cardiovascular disease has been the most prevalent among them. CKD patients have a prothrombotic state with a related risk of hemorrhage, thereby leading to increased morbidity and mortality.

The combination of endothelial dysfunction and CKD coagulopathy makes CKD patients vulnerable to thrombotic complications, which can further contribute to cardiac complications. Interestingly, the increased rates of hospitalization in this group are inexorably connected with cardiovascular comorbidities. The increasing incidence of such complications highlights the importance of tailored clinical assessments to mitigate risks and enhance patient outcomes. Therefore, understanding the molecular mechanisms of these hemostatic changes is crucial in formulating effective treatment modalities for controlling cardiovascular risk in CKD patients (Saeed et al., 2024). Another significant complication of CKD that requires attention is the risk of infectious diseases, particularly influenza. Patients with chronic kidney and liver disease are particularly vulnerable to severe influenza infection, further undermining their compromised health status. According to a recent study, it appears that the dangerous trend of low influenza vaccination rates among CKD patients exists, even though these patients are at higher risk for developing severe complications. Evidence suggests that a small percentage of this population is interested in receiving the vaccine, indicating low awareness and a lack of risk perception. Favorable correlations with past vaccination experience and willingness to be vaccinated suggest that education and outreach would be an efficient intervention to improve coverage. By addressing the frequently raised concerns about vaccine safety and efficacy, healthcare providers can promote higher levels of immunization among this high-risk group, resulting in an overall improvement in outcomes (Eder et al., 2021). Anemia is also a severe complication of CKD, resulting from decreased erythropoietin production and aberrations of iron regulation. Anemia not only coexists with fatigue and compromised quality of life but also aggravates cardiovascular risk, adding another dimension to the clinical presentation of CKD patients. The condition is a sign of the delicate balance of renal function, systemic inflammation, and nutrition that may be disrupted in CKD patients. Correction of anemia in these patients is vital, typically requiring interventions such as erythropoiesis-stimulating agents or iron supplementation. Furthermore, understanding the complexities of anemia management in CKD highlights the need for integrated treatment strategies that address the root pathologies and the full spectrum of complications associated with chronic kidney disease. Effective anemia management is thus pivotal to enhancing the quality of life and reducing overall morbidity for CKD patients (Figure 9.12).

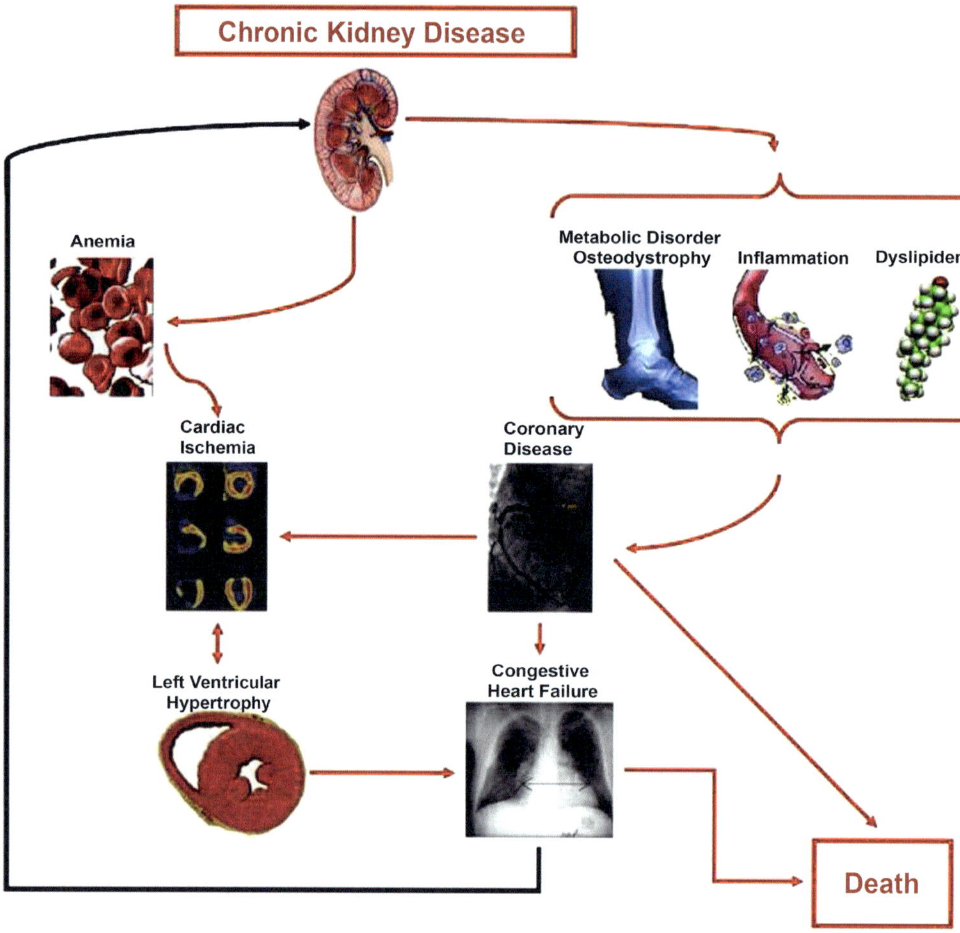

Figure 9.12. Complications Associated with CKD.

Source: https://www.primarycare.theclinics.com/cms/10.1016/j.pop.2008.01.008/asset/b7de6cd1-c9d7-4896-9b0d-114e174f302f/main.assets/gr1_lrg.jpg.

9.4.1. Cardiovascular Disease (CVD)

The intricate relationship between CKD and CVD reflects a significant health problem, given the fact that these two diseases frequently co-occur and amplify patient morbidity as well as mortality. CKD progresses through a series of physiological changes, including hypertension and dyslipidemia, which are the primary etiologies of CVD. With impairment of kidney function, vascular resistance increases due to the loss of blood pressure control, which in turn leads to resultant hypertension. Additionally, dysregulation of metabolic processes in CKD can lead to elevated levels of LDL cholesterol, thereby increasing the risk of atherosclerosis and its cardiovascular complications. Practitioners thus need to understand these interplay mechanisms so that sound management strategies that address the CVD implications of CKD patients and their disease outcomes can be designed. Interventions targeting the cardiovascular risk factors in patients with CKD hold significant potential for maximizing patient prognosis. Pharmacological measures, such as the use of renin-angiotensin system blockers, have been shown to decrease hypertension and show renal protection, thereby lowering the risk of CVD. Additionally, novel therapeutic advances in diabetes, particularly glucagon-like peptide-1 receptor agonists (GLP-1RA), have been observed to improve glycemic control with no increase in the risk of hypoglycemia. The administration of GLP-1RA not only controls diabetes but also potentially enhances cardiovascular and renal benefits in patients with diabetic kidney disease. Clinical trials are ongoing to determine these associations, so clinicians must consider overall treatment approaches that treat both CKD and its resulting cardiovascular disease states, ultimately benefiting the patient. The multifactorial condition of CKD also has a complex interaction of inflammatory and hormonal factors involved in CVD.

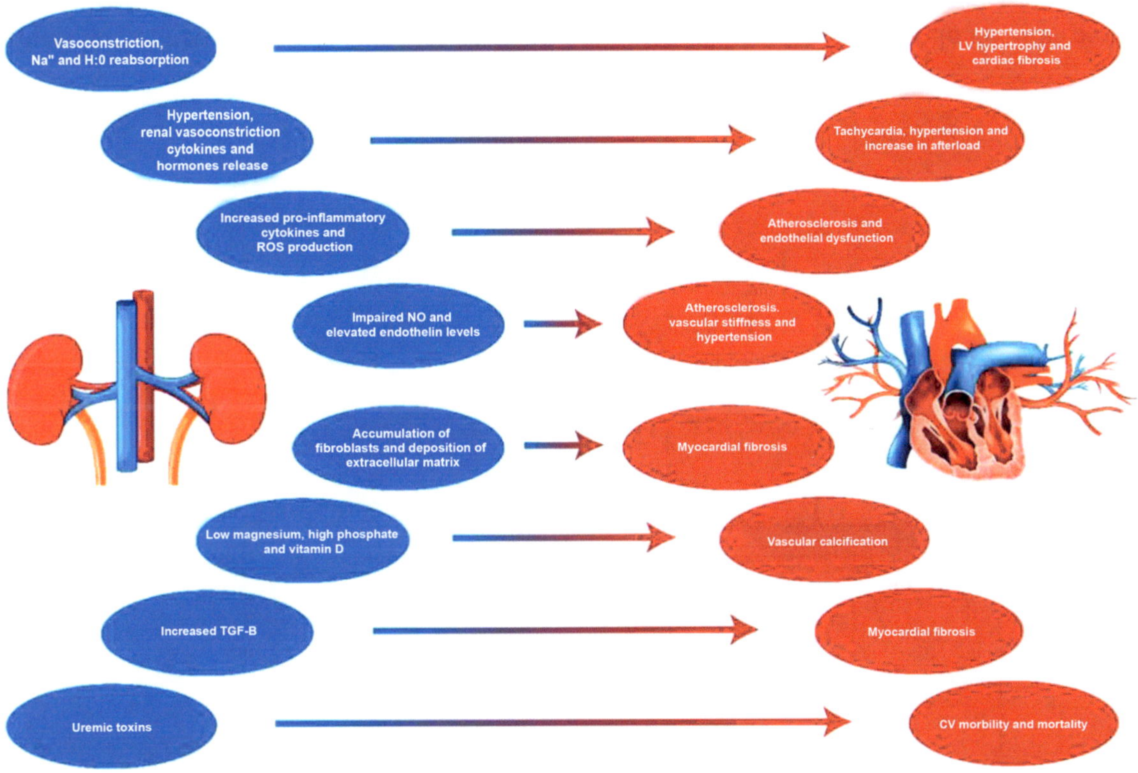

Figure 9.13. Exploring cardiovascular complications in chronic kidney disease.

Source: https://www.mdpi.com/biomolecules/biomolecules-14-01393/article_deploy/html/images/biomolecules-14-01393-g001.png.

Elevated proinflammatory cytokines, such as interleukin-1 and interleukin-6, may play a crucial role in exacerbating kidney and cardiovascular complications, and are areas that warrant further investigation in targeted therapy. Additionally, metabolic abnormalities, including increased abnormal adipocytokine levels and vitamin D deficiency, continue to promote the inflammatory process and potentially increase the risk of CVD. Given the existing data on the relationship between CKD and a range of undesirable cardiovascular events, a coordinated approach that considers dietary management, exercise, and new pharmacological modalities must be undertaken. By identifying and demarcating these concurrent risk factors, physicians can plan improved, tailored interventions in the prevention of cardiovascular disease in patients with CKD to reduce mortality and enhance the quality of life in this high-risk population (Figure 9.13).

9.4.2. Anemia

Anemia is a prevalent and severe complication in individuals with CKD, with grave implications for their overall health and welfare. Anemia arises primarily due to the kidney's failure to synthesize erythropoietin (EPO), a hormone required for red cell production. The decrease in EPO levels and lack of available iron for hemoglobin production typically leads to a state of anemia with lower hemoglobin levels. Organization. The World Health Organization has described anemia as a hemoglobin value less than 13 g/dL in men and less than 12 g/dL in women, but in CKD, the threshold may be open to reconsideration to include consideration of the particular physiological changes that are occurring.

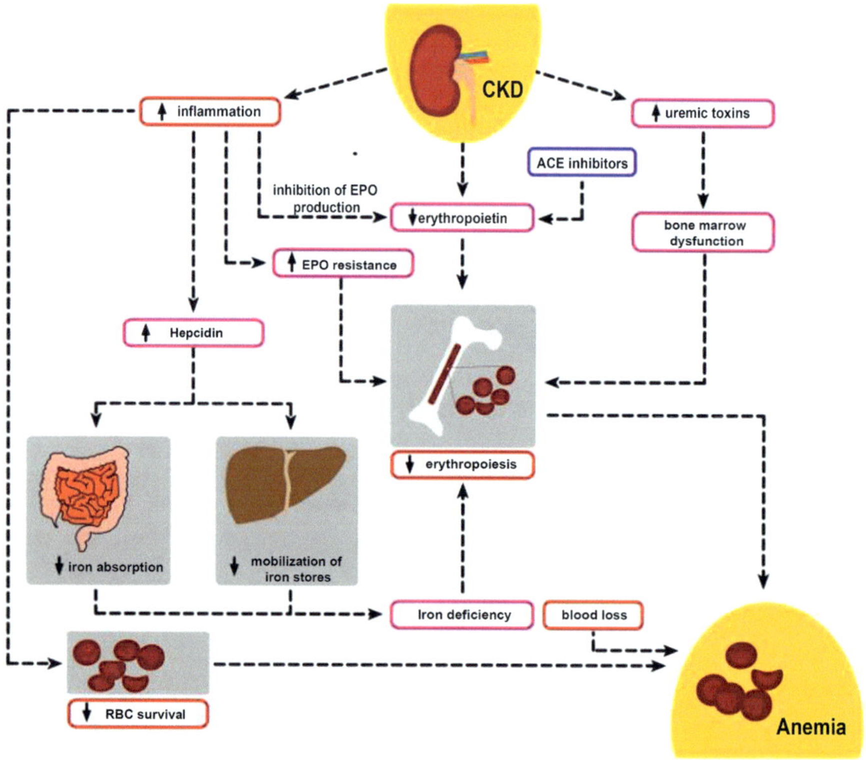

Figure 9.14. Anemia of chronic kidney disease.

Source: https://pub.mdpi-res.com/biomedicines/biomedicines-12-01191/article_deploy/html/images/biomedicines-12-01191-g001.png?1716804850.

The resulting anemia can exacerbate symptoms of fatigue and decrease the capacity to exercise, thus affecting the health-related quality of life in CKD patients immensely. Anemia treatment in CKD is complicated, with a delicate balance among multiple treatment strategies to meet individual patient needs. Erythropoiesis-stimulating agent therapy is widely used in managing such anemia, particularly in those cases where treatment is non-curative. New recommendations suggest that when hemoglobin levels drop below 10 g/dL, ESAs can be administered to stimulate erythropoiesis and increase hemoglobin levels, thereby alleviating anemia symptoms. It has been proven in research that co-administration of iron supplements with ESAs will improve hematopoietic response, with a greater increase in the level of hemoglobin and a decrease in red blood cell transfusions. This interaction highlights the importance of an integrated therapy regimen that addresses both erythropoiesis and iron deficiency, which are commonly found in the CKD population (Bohlius et al., 2019). The inclusion of new therapies, such as Auryxia® (ferric citrate), proves the progress in managing anemia of CKD. Auryxia stands out not only as a dual-purpose phosphate binder and an iron replacement therapy but also because, to a certain extent, it can improve clinical parameters in CKD patients. By managing phosphate levels well and simultaneously plugging the iron deficiency gap, Auryxia has shown promise in lowering the incidence of fibroblast growth factor 23 (FGF23), which is a risk factor for cardiovascular morbidity in CKD patients. This twin benefit can ultimately translate to improved cardiovascular well-being and overall health in patients with CKD-associated anemia, addressing a key aspect of patient therapy. With more data becoming known about the long-term effects of these therapies, anemia management in CKD will continue evolving, ensuring improved patient outcomes (Bino et al., 2019) (Figure 9.14).

9.4.3. Bone Disease

The interplay between CKD and bone disease is complex and multifaceted, primarily resulting from secondary alterations in mineral metabolism that occur with progressive CKD. As renal function deteriorates, the kidney's capacity for phosphate excretion is lost progressively, leading to hyperphosphatemia, which is a common complication in advanced CKD. This hyperphosphatemia can cause secondary hyperparathyroidism and aggravate bone density loss, creating a condition known as renal osteodystrophy. This bone disease presents as alterations in bone strength and quality, accompanied by an increased risk of fractures. The intricate interplay between vitamin D metabolism and parathyroid hormone (PTH) only serves to exacerbate the condition, as renal insufficiency disrupts vitamin D activation, which is crucial for optimal bone integrity. The current treatment methods emphasize the importance of appropriate management of mineral and bone disorder (MBD) to obtain optimal results in patients with CKD. Treatment includes the use of phosphate binders that decrease phosphate absorption from the diet, thus regulating hyperphosphatemia. One of the new treatments is sucroferric oxyhydroxide (PA21), which is a noncalcium phosphate binder that has proven effectiveness in reducing serum phosphate with reasonable safety. Clinical trials indicate that PA21 not only lowers phosphate levels considerably but also positively regulates PTH levels without interfering with vitamin D treatment, ultimately offering a dual benefit in the management of MBD in patients with CKD (Griveas et al., 2019). Regular monitoring and strict adherence to the treatment schedule are necessary to promote the overall metabolic status of patients with CKD-related bone disease. Long-term management of bone disease in the context of CKD involves continuous monitoring of treatment safety and efficacy to prevent potential side effects. Although treatment like PA21 has been shown to reduce phosphorus levels effectively, the risk for osteonecrosis and other complications of hyperparathyroidism must be monitored well in the clinic. Lifestyle modifications such as diet and exercise must also be addressed as a significant element to optimize bone health. Though pharmacologic treatment still remains the predominant mode of treatment, patient education regarding physical activity and nutrition can be used as an adjunctive measure to reduce the risk of fractures further and improve the overall quality of life. Finally, a multidisciplinary approach that incorporates medical management with lifestyle modification may be the most effective system for reversing the effects of CKD on bone disease, thereby leading to enhanced patient health and survival (Ha et al., 2025) (Figure 9.15).

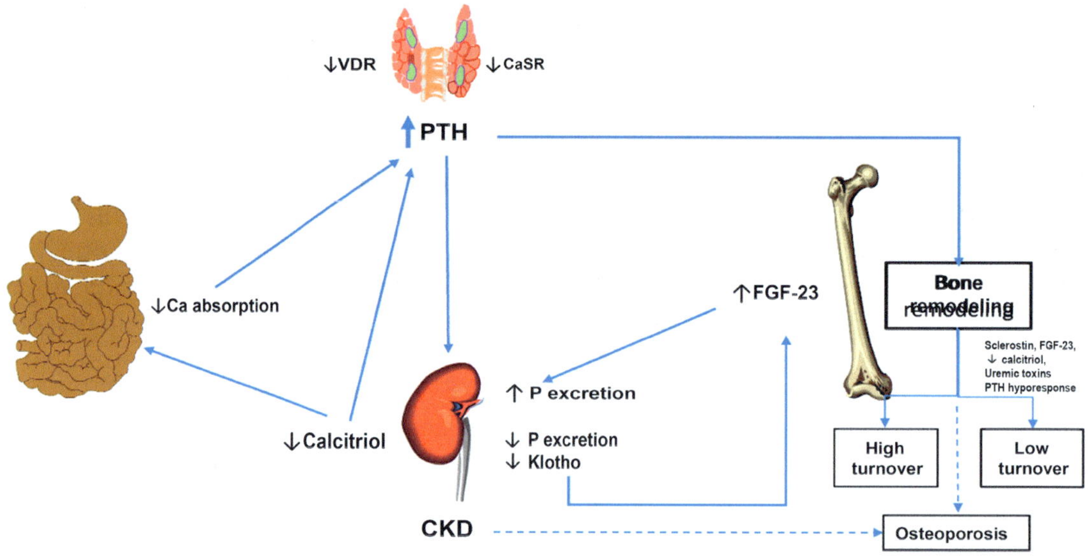

Figure 9.15. Bone disease in chronic kidney disease.

Source: https://www.mdpi.com/nutrients/nutrients-15-00167/article_deploy/html/images/nutrients-15-00167-g002.png.

9.5. Treatment Options

The management of CKD entails a comprehensive approach that hinders the progression of the disease and alleviates complications. A massive thrust is given to pharmacologic therapy in the form of the use of ACE inhibitors and Angiotensin II Receptor Blockers (ARBs). These medications have been shown to provide renal protection through the reduction of proteinuria and blood pressure, both of which are typical markers of renal injury. Emerging therapies, such as sodium-glucose co-transporter 2 (SGLT2) inhibitors, have also proven useful in CKD retardation and cardiovascular risk reduction. Patients are closely monitored for kidney function and any changes in pharmacotherapy, highlighting the importance of personalized therapy plans tailored to each patient's health condition and treatment response. In addition to pharmacotherapeutic interventions, lifestyle modification is of critical value in CKD management. The patient should maintain a diet that is kidney-friendly, with a low intake of sodium, potassium, and phosphorus, and proper hydration. Exercise is also encouraged as it can contribute to weight control and better cardiovascular outcomes. Furthermore, adequate management of comorbid conditions, particularly diabetes and hypertension, is a priority. It incorporates patient education and self-management strategies that enable patients to take an active role as care partners in their care process. CKD management can be significantly enhanced by focusing on both pharmacologic and lifestyle concerns, which eventually result in improved outcomes among patients (Amann et al., 2018). As the CKD progresses to End-Stage Kidney Disease (ESKD), treatment options become more challenging, often necessitating renal replacement therapy in the form of dialysis or kidney transplantation. Dialysis supplies artificial renal replacement by removing waste products and excess fluid from the body. While this therapy is essential for sustaining life, it has its own set of complications and lifestyle changes that impact the quality of life in patients. Kidney transplantation, on the other hand, assures a possible cure with functional recovery of the kidney but is based on organ availability and suitable donor-recipient compatibility. Additionally, clinical research studies for new therapies and interventions, including gene-based therapies, also provide promise for the future. In general, the scenario of treating CKD and ESKD is dynamic, necessitating further research and innovation for improved patient care (Amann et al., 2018) (Figure 9.16).

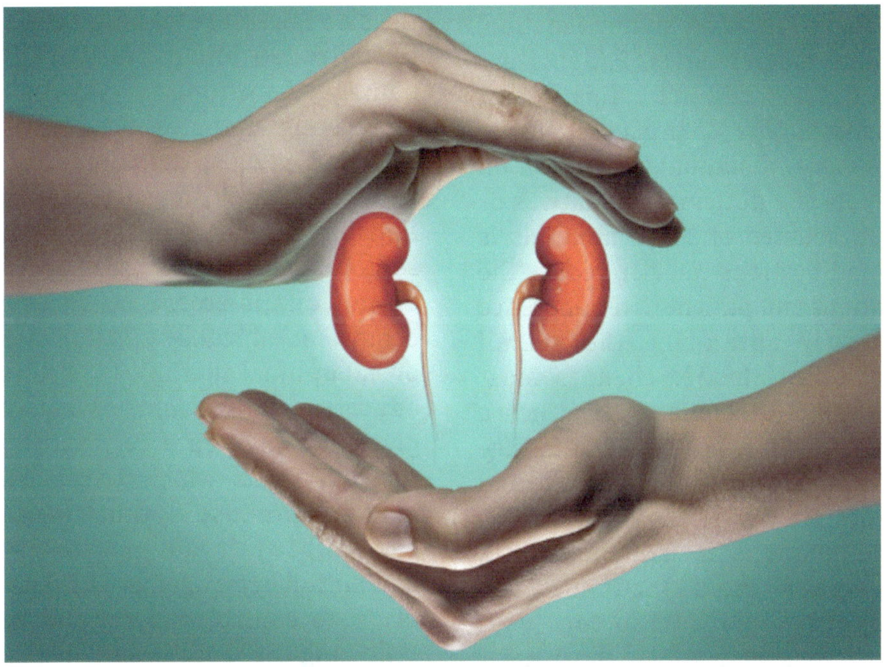

Figure 9.16. The management of chronic kidney disease (CKD).

Source: https://medicine.unimelb.edu.au/__data/assets/image/0006/4961220/varieties/medium.png.

9.5.1. Lifestyle Modifications

Lifestyle modifications are an integral part of the treatment of CKD, with significant influence on disease evolution and general health outcomes. The most critical strategy may be through dietary modifications, including strict adherence to a renal-specific diet that is low in sodium, limited in protein, and controlled in potassium. This type of diet not only decreases the burden on the kidneys but also helps to manage comorbidities such as hypertension and diabetes, which are prevalent in CKD patients. Physical exercise is another cornerstone of lifestyle modification, whereby frequent moderate exercise can enhance cardiovascular function, improve insulin sensitivity, and contribute to weight management—ideal factors that lower the risk of CKD. By adopting these dietary and physical activity changes, patients can significantly slow the worsening of kidney damage, making an active contribution to CKD management and enhancing their quality of life. In CKD, fluid management is also imperative, particularly as kidney function declines. Fluid consumption is generally difficult in patients, leading to edema and hypertension if not well managed. Healthcare practitioners advise individualized fluid management protocols based on the patient's existing kidney function, fluid balance, and comorbidities. Patients are also advised to develop mindful eating habits, avoiding excessive intake of processed foods high in phosphorus and sodium. Education on reading food labels and noticing alternatives or so-called hidden sources of these minerals is critical. These modifications can also reduce the risk of complications and patient non-adherence to therapy, thereby optimizing the overall management of CKD. Lifestyle changes must be supported by interdisciplinary healthcare interventions in order to become voluntary long-term habits. Additionally, psychosocial and behavioral factors are key to the effectiveness of lifestyle modifications in managing CKD. Counseling or group therapy support can enhance the capacity of patients to cope with lifestyle changes better, especially in the context of the predominantly intimidating experience of having CKD diagnosis. As an adjunct to teaching efforts, health professionals should help patients develop self-monitoring habits, such as regular weighing, compliance with a diet, and blood pressure monitoring. These habits instill responsibility and empower patients throughout their care. Total lifestyle modifications, such as these psychological factors, all contribute to the prevention of CKD complications, significantly reducing the morbidity and mortality rates within this population. The combined dedication of patients and healthcare staff to these changes underscores the significance of lifestyle modifications in the management of total chronic kidney disease (Alfieri et al., 2025; Mohamad, 2024).

9.5.2. Medications

CKD is often treated with a multidrug regimen tailored to the patient's individual needs. Medications play a significant role in controlling the various complications of CKD, such as hypertension, diabetes, and electrolyte disturbances. Antihypertensive medication is also commonly required in patients to maintain the blood pressure within a target range because uncontrolled blood pressure increases renal damage. Additionally, diabetic patients with underlying diabetes may also need control of blood glucose with medications that can be safely administered to patients with renal function. The drug regimen is essential in that some of these drugs will need to be adjusted or not administered at all in patients with compromised kidney function to prevent toxicity or suboptimal therapy. Medication compliance education for patients is equally significant, given the high rate of patients not knowing their diagnosis, which reflects a deficiency that may compromise optimal management (Ellis et al., 2016). In addition to antihypertensive and antidiabetic agents, CKD patients are given drugs to control mineral and bone disorders, reflecting the multifaceted interaction between kidney health and bone metabolism. Drugs like phosphate binders and vitamin D analogs are frequently used to manage conditions such as hyperphosphatemia, which is a common finding in CKD owing to the poor renal excretion of phosphate. Mineral metabolism abnormalities have the potential to cause significant consequences, including cardiovascular disease, which makes the management of these imbalances even more critical. Therefore, healthcare practitioners must regularly monitor lab results and adjust medication dosages accordingly. Effective communication between healthcare providers helps maximize the effectiveness of care, ensuring that the drug regimen is directly related to the evolving patient condition and overall wellness (Awdishu et al., 2019). As CKD stages progress, the drug regimens of the patients can become more complex, and therefore, close monitoring and titration are necessary. Opening channels of communication between the healthcare team and patients is one method of encouraging adherence, as well as enabling patients to express concerns about their medications. Patient involvement in the discussion of treatment plans enhances both comprehension and the adoption of self-management behaviors, ultimately improving health outcomes. The necessity for constant education about CKD cannot be overstated, considering that most patients possess inadequate knowledge about their condition as well as its management. Effective patient education measures are crucial to developing awareness and encouraging proactive involvement in their care plans. Through the synchronization of effective medication management with intensive education, the potential for improved health outcomes in CKD patients can be significantly enhanced (Ellis et al., 2016) (Figure 9.17).

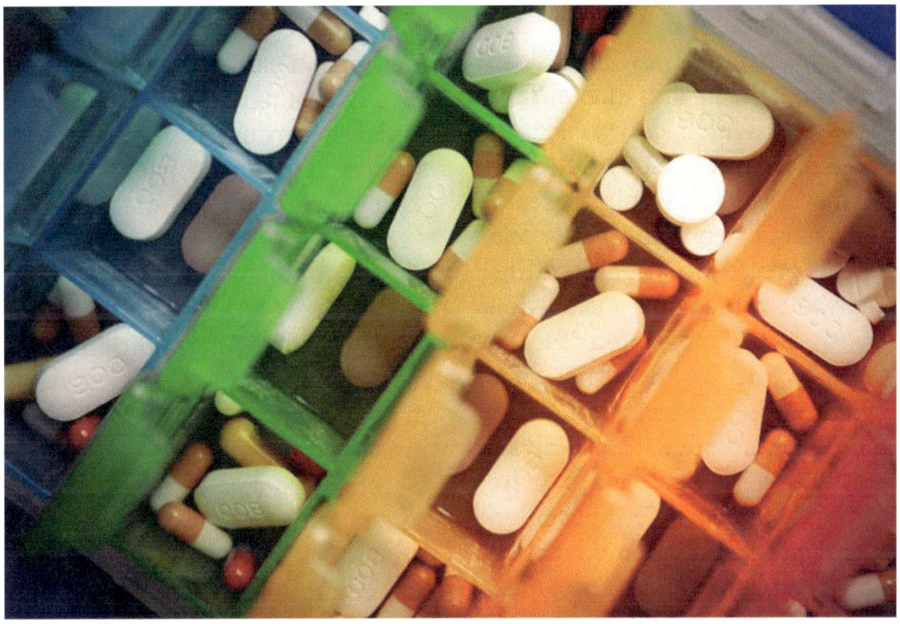

Figure 9.17. Medicines for chronic kidney disease (CKD).

Source: https://kcuk.cdn.ngo/media/images/medication_-_medicines_for_CKD_-_colourful_pil.width-700.jpg.

9.5.3. Dialysis and Transplantation

The management of CKD typically ends up involving renal replacement therapies, which are predominantly dialysis and transplantation. Dialysis is a life-sustaining approach for patients whose kidneys are no longer efficient in clearing waste products from the blood. There are two principal forms of dialysis: hemodialysis and peritoneal dialysis. Both have inherent pros and cons, from the logistics of treatment sessions to their impact on patients' everyday lives. Of importance, the selection of a particular dialysis modality is determined by patient-specific considerations, including comorbidities present, lifestyle factors, and clinical markers. The ultimate goal is always the same: to alleviate symptoms, maintain metabolic homeostasis, and ultimately optimize patient quality of life until a more definitive therapy, such as transplantation, becomes an option. Transplantation is largely the most ideal treatment for patients with end-stage renal disease (ESRD) who have exhausted all other forms of therapy, including dialysis. A successful kidney transplant not only enhances the quality of life but also significantly decreases cardiovascular risks, which are highly elevated in CKD patients. Renal transplant recipients have superior benefits, particularly with the avoidance of long-term complications of dialysis. Yet, as much benefit is conferred by transplantation, new issues are raised. Recipients must deal with the pitfalls of immunosuppression, which carry risks of graft rejection and increased susceptibility to infection. Furthermore, cardiovascular disease continues to be a primary cause of morbidity and mortality among this group of patients, calling for continuing cardiovascular risk evaluation and management after transplantation (Jardine et al., 2014). Interprofessional care also plays a crucial role in enhancing the quality of life for patients undergoing dialysis and those receiving or recovering from transplantation. A well-managed CKD based on an interprofessional model has demonstrated remarkable improvement in clinical outcomes. For instance, a recent article highlighted that patients benefited from an organized system of care through interaction among nephrologists, nurses, dietitians, and social workers (Awdishu et al., 2019). Such collaboration not only enables seamless patient referral to transplantation but also facilitates aggressive monitoring and management of health values, such as blood pressure and cardiovascular disease risk factors. As healthcare's future unfolds, uptake of systematic interprofessional practices will be pivotal in the identification of patients who may benefit from early referral to transplantation, thereby optimizing patient outcomes and satisfaction in long-term CKD care.

9.6. Prevention Strategies

Prevention of CKD plays a crucial role in minimizing disease incidence and morbidity. Timely intervention to slow the course of the disease is made possible by early detection, which is the key to prevention. Regular screening for risk factors, such as hypertension, diabetes, and obesity, can help identify high-risk patients (Ahmed et al., 2010). Patient education is also an essential component of this, with attention to lifestyle modification such as diet, exercise, and the importance of medication compliance. Furthermore, general care must include regular evaluation of kidney function through serum creatinine and urine studies to identify any emergent signs of kidney injury. Such proactive measures can significantly decrease the health care burden of CKD, while simultaneously improving patient outcomes by allowing early therapeutic intervention. In addition to interventions at the individual level, community-level interventions also hold promise for preventing CKD. Public health interventions to raise awareness of CKD's risk factors can prompt better lifestyle choices and consideration of the importance of regular visits to healthcare providers. For instance, health fairs and community workshops, as group activities, can promote key information regarding the role of balanced eating and exercise (Arnold et al., 2018). Collaborations with local healthcare professionals can facilitate screenings and the distribution of educational materials to underprivileged communities, thereby addressing care gaps. Through establishing a culture for preventive health behaviors, communities are able to take the forefront in reducing CKD prevalence and thus help lead healthier populations and lower healthcare costs. New studies on the biological and environmental determinants of kidney function may introduce novel prevention models. Studies examining the mechanisms by which certain species are resistant to kidney disease provide valuable insights that can be applied to human health (Arnold et al., 2018). For instance, knowledge about the protective factors observed in animals like the naked mole rat or a hibernating bear can be utilized to create new treatments and prevention strategies for CKD. Such collaborative work between nephrologists and experts from other fields has the potential to enhance awareness of both susceptibility and protective mechanisms related to kidney health. Such coordinated efforts underscore the value of integrating information from different scientific fields and ultimately establishing successful prevention strategies and therapeutic interventions against CKD. Increased research activities and knowledge transfer can help healthcare professionals better handle the complexities of chronic kidney disease (Figure 9.18).

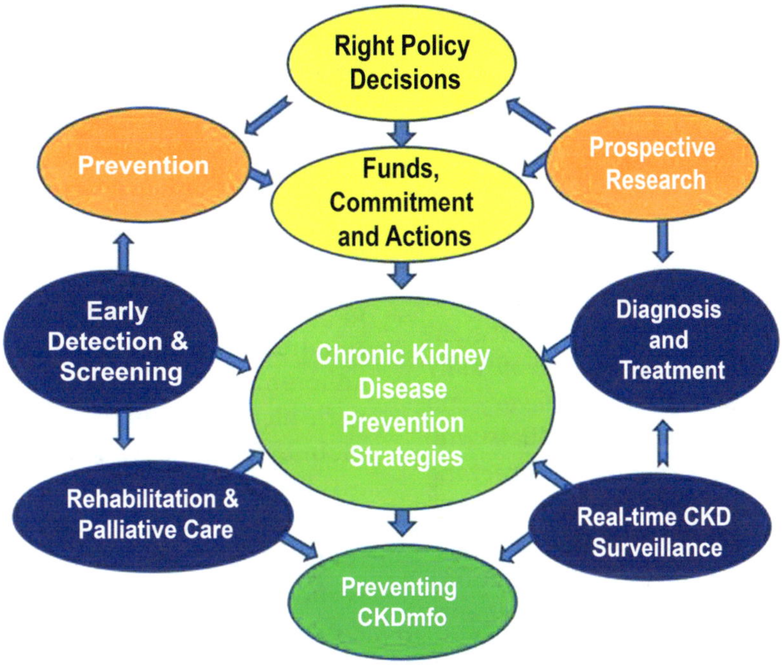

Figure 9.18. Strategies for prevention and control of chronic kidney disease.

Source: https://www.researchgate.net/profile/Sunil-Wimalawansa/publication/282873549/figure/fig4/AS:961434703904779@1606235304223/Strategies-for-prevention-and-control-of-chronic-kidney-disease-of-multifactorial-origin.gif.

9.6.1. Regular Health Screenings

Regular health screening is critical in the early detection and control of CKD, an illness that affects millions worldwide. Screening allows clinicians to identify risk factors and monitor kidney function for follow-up, hence facilitating timely action. For instance, screening individuals with a family history of kidney disease can lead to the early detection of CKD, significantly enhancing patient outcomes. These preventive measures are crucial in regions where CKD is still common, pointing to the necessity of proactive health care. Furthermore, these screenings can also identify underlying diseases such as hypertension and diabetes that are generally comorbid with CKD. Intervening on these risk factors early can diminish the effects of CKD, enhancing the quality of life of individuals at risk for developing or progressing to kidney failure. Targeted health screening is crucial in preventing the global epidemic of CKD, especially in resource-poor settings. It is reported that in developing countries, renal treatment and early detection are suboptimal, leading to a high rate of morbidity and mortality from CKD. For example, regular screening targeting those at risk, such as first-degree relatives of CKD patients, can provide valuable information regarding family trends towards health. The integration of these site-specific screening programs not only detects early cases of CKD but also informs communities about the disease's risk. Cost-effective screening plans in clinics and community health initiatives are also necessary because they can reduce the economic burden of late-stage kidney disease treatment. Such programs are most relevant in countries where the health resources are already short, and prevention rather than treatment is an essential shift. An investment in recurrent screening for health can eventually lead to better systems of healthcare delivery and improved health outcomes for individuals who are at risk of CKD. Comprehensive screening programs need to be culturally sensitive and family-centered to get better participation and promote adherence. By involving the community in such programs, local outreach programs to inform families about the importance of kidney health checks, for example, more individuals will tend to get involved in screenings. First-degree relatives who are potential screening participants are actively included in local outreach programs, and a support group is also encouraged, which facilitates awareness and prevention. As emphasized in studies conducted in Pakistan and elsewhere, when screenings become widely accessible and are focused on high-risk groups, the chances of identification and control of CKD at an early stage are significantly increased, hence relieving pressure on healthcare systems and improving longevity and quality of life for populations at risk (Ilyas et al., 2024; Hoefer et al., 2025).

9.6.2. Dietary Recommendations

Nutritional management of CKD patients is central in curbing the disease and its associated complications. Patients with CKD are likely to have their metabolic status changed; thus, dietary modification is paramount in serving renal function as well as overall health. A coordinated nutritional plan focuses on modifying protein, sodium, potassium, and phosphorus consumption, depending on the stage of CKD in the patients. Minimizing protein consumption reduces the kidneys' workload, and controlling potassium and phosphorus intake helps prevent complications such as hyperkalemia and bone disease. The implementation of these dietary measures poses challenges to healthcare professionals, particularly with respect to adherence and feasibility in daily life; therefore, ongoing patient education and follow-up are required. New approaches to enhancing dietary adherence in CKD patients have come forward, with increasing appreciation for the utility of mobile technology. The KIDNEYTEXT trial is a recent example of the potential of one-to-one text message intervention as a method of realizing dietary behavioral change in long-term hemodialysis patients. By providing individualized dietary recommendations based on renal guidelines and promoting healthy eating habits, this intervention aims to increase adherence to dietary restrictions, ultimately leading to improved overall health outcomes. The research highlights the integration of technology in the care of CKD, particularly since it offers a scalable approach to providing individualized dietary recommendations. Results from such interventions could become the new standard for patient-centered care for chronic disease management. Besides, the significance of personalized nutrition counseling cannot be overstated, as it is tailored to the specific needs of CKD patients. Counseling has to consider the psychological and emotional aspects of dietary restrictions, particularly with the knowledge that CKD is a chronic disease that, in many instances, may disturb many patients. In particular, incorporating patient-centered care aspects into diet planning ensures that patients' lifestyles and preferences are taken into account, resulting in better compliance with dietary advice. As healthcare systems increasingly recognize the role of personalized care, continued research into effective dietary interventions will be imperative. Last but not least, encouraging dietary guideline compliance is not only essential for physical well-being but also for improving quality of life in patients with chronic kidney disease (Brown et al., 2019; Adams et al., 2016).

9.6.3. Management of Underlying Conditions

Proper control of underlying conditions is the cornerstone in preventing CKD progression. The intricate relationship of CKD with comorbid illnesses such as hypertension and diabetes accentuates the imperative of integrative care for patients. Of all these, blood pressure control is the most critical because its increase will enhance kidney damage and cardiovascular complications. Through lifestyle modification, including changes in dietary habits and physical activity levels, and drug treatment involving the use of ACE inhibitors, doctors can significantly enhance their patients' outcomes. Not only do these actions address the acute manifestations of CKD, but also its chronic aspects that contribute to its development, emphasizing the need for tailored treatment programs and ongoing monitoring to further refine interventions according to the specific conditions of individual patients. Moreover, diabetes control can be just as crucial in the CKD environment, and hyperglycemia is directly correlated with deteriorating renal function. Ideal glycemic control can reduce microvascular complications that have an extremely significant influence on kidney function. Management with a multifaceted approach, which may include continuous glucose monitoring, medication adjustments, and counseling of lifestyle choices, keeps the patient active and informed. Second, emphasizing regular screening for renal function can result in the early detection of CKD progression, allowing for early changes in treatment plans to be initiated. Multidisciplinary care by endocrinologists, nephrologists, and primary care physicians can enhance patient compliance with the treatment regimen, which in turn can lead to better diabetes control and maintenance of renal function. Lastly, the importance of lifestyle interventions cannot be overstated in the management of the contributory conditions for CKD. Smoking cessation, alcohol moderation, and healthy weight maintenance are all essential components of a total treatment plan. These lifestyle changes not only lower cardiovascular risk factors but also promote overall kidney function by decreasing the incidence of complications from hypertension and diabetes. Education plays a central role in this aspect, as it enables patients to make informed decisions about their health. Moreover, professional assistance can also ensure adherence to lifestyle modifications, establishing an active plan for managing CKD and related conditions. Thus, knowledge of the interaction between comorbidities and CKD, as outlined in the consensus statement on kidney disease management, is pivotal in enhancing patient outcomes and quality of life, thus addressing short-term and long-term patient needs (Black et al., 2015; Dewitte et al., 2017).

SUMMARY

The dissemination and management of CKD are severe threats to the global healthcare system. Proper coding of CKD cases cannot be stressed enough, as evidenced by recent findings of outrageous rates of uncoded CKD, up to as high as 58.7% in acute medical settings. Not only do missed opportunities in proper coding impede successful patient management, but they also conceal the actual burden of disease on the healthcare system. Enhancing coding standards within secondary care will enable healthcare professionals to detect and treat CKD patients needs better, so that they receive early intervention and treatment accordingly. With a focus on coded quality improvement, healthcare professionals can implement specific interventions that yield better patient outcomes and reduce mortality, ultimately propelling efforts against CKD more aggressively (Dolan et al., 2025). Besides, the integration of newer healthcare technologies, such as telemedicine, has immense potential to revolutionize CKD care. Telemedicine enables real-time observation and remote consultation, providing patients with greater convenience and access to the care process. The approach is particularly promising for dialysis patients, who require constant observation and follow-up due to the nature of the condition. The recent evidence of increased telemedicine adoption amid the COVID-19 pandemic underlines its promise as a sustainable approach to CKD management. Telemedicine, by reducing barriers caused by geographical distance and improving compliance with prescribed treatment regimens among patients, enhances the overall quality of life for survivors of CKD. However, it is essential that the study continues to explore its efficacy compared to conventional models of care and assesses the challenges that will be encountered in implementing it (Santosh et al., 2024). As more is learned about CKD, the medical world must take a holistic perspective towards prevention and treatment. Risk factor modification of diseases such as diabetes and hypertension is crucial to stem the tide of progression of CKD and improve patient quality of life. Furthermore, equipping healthcare providers with the resources and knowledge base to recognize and treat CKD properly will ensure more aggressive care. The development of coding practices, telemedicine, and integrative patient management all demonstrate changing times in dealing with CKD. By adopting these measures and recognizing the supreme importance of systematic healthcare development, it is possible to limit the implications of CKD in patients as well as in healthcare systems, ushering in a future of better health (Santosh et al., 2024; Dolan et al., 2025).

CKD is a significant public health burden, very well recognized for its substantial contribution to morbidity and premature mortality globally. CKD's burden is not just impaired kidney function but also encompasses an array of complications, such as mineral and bone disorders, anemia, and heightened cardiovascular disease risk. Studies indicate that hyperphosphatemia and high fibroblast growth factor 23 (FGF23) concentrations are new independent risk factors for adverse cardiovascular outcomes in CKD patients. Treating these complications is significant because they have a direct effect on the overall quality of life and health outcomes in patients with this condition. Understanding these interconnected factors not only opens the door to improved patient management but also to the development of tailored therapies aimed at mitigating the risks of CKD (Bino et al., 2019). The development of therapeutics like Auryxia® (ferric citrate) underscores the evolving face of CKD management. Approved for its two-pronged advantage, Auryxia serves both as a phosphate binder to control serum phosphate and as an iron replacement therapy to treat iron deficiency anemia in patients with CKD. Its mechanism of action is fascinating in that it offers an alternative solution to the twin challenges of high phosphate and low iron in this patient population. Clinical trials consistently demonstrate the effectiveness of Auryxia, resulting in significant reductions in serum phosphate levels and improvements in iron parameters. As these advancements continue to emerge, it is essential to take note of the long-term impacts that come with Auryxia treatment and its capacity to decrease cardiovascular hazards resulting from CKD-associated complications (Bino et al., 2019). The interrelationship between CKD and cardiovascular disease is multifactorial and elaborate, and research has emphasized a greater significance to the connection beyond traditional risk factors. Of specific interest is increased arterial stiffness and left ventricular hypertrophy, rather than atherosclerosis, as promoters of cardiovascular morbidity in patients with CKD. Living kidney donor studies provide a unique chance to assess the acute effect of low GFR on arterial stiffness and blood pressure, thereby illuminating the causal pathways for renal dysfunction to lead to cardiovascular events. By understanding these factors, future research can better elucidate the interplay between kidney and cardiovascular health, ultimately guiding therapeutic interventions to mitigate the complications of CKD and cardiovascular disease.

CLOSER LOOK

RENAL OSTEODYSTROPHY

Renal osteodystrophy is a severe bone disease that directly occurs from CKD, particularly its end stage. It is the bone component of chronic kidney disease-mineral and bone disorder (CKD-MBD), a complex systemic disorder characterized by disturbances in calcium, phosphorus, parathyroid hormone (PTH), vitamin D metabolism, and bone remodeling. In the healthful subject, the kidneys play a crucial role in mineral homeostasis through the excretion of phosphate, activation of vitamin D, and regulation of calcium absorption. With declining renal function, these regulatory processes break down and disturbances follow that eventually affect bone structure, bone density, and bone remodeling. Renal osteodystrophy is a spectrum of bone lesions that includes high-turnover bone disease (osteitis fibrosa), low-turnover bone disease (adynamic bone disease), osteomalacia, and mixed uremic osteodystrophy, along with their pathophysiologic mechanisms and presentation The pathogenesis of renal osteodystrophy is multifactorial and occurs early during the course of CKD development. The decreased glomerular filtration leads to phosphate retention, which stimulates the release of PTH (secondary hyperparathyroidism). The kidneys, in turn, are unable to activate inactive vitamin D to its active metabolite form (calcitriol), impairing intestinal calcium absorption and leading to hypocalcemia, also causing stimulation of PTH release. Persistent hyperPTH enhances bone resorption and turnover, most prominently in osteitis fibrosa cystica, the prototypic high-turnover lesion of CKD. On the opposite end, a dynamic bone disease is caused by PTH suppression, often due to over-treatment with vitamin D analogs or calcimimetics, and is associated with reduced bone turnover, abnormal bone formation, and increased fracture risk. Osteomalacia with defective mineralization of the bones is typically found in the context of aluminum intoxication (historically) or vitamin D deficiency. In contrast, the mixed uremic osteodystrophy demonstrates both high and low turnover characteristics.Clinically, renal osteodystrophy may present with bone pain, muscle weakness, skeletal deformity, and increased risk of fractures. Growth retardation in children with CKD is an extremely disabling feature. Cardiovascular sequelae also follow extra-skeletal calcification, and especially vascular calcification, which is responsible for the high mortality of CKD. Diagnosis of renal osteodystrophy involves a combination of clinical evaluation, biochemical testing (including serum phosphate, calcium, PTH, alkaline phosphatase, and vitamin D), and imaging. Bone biopsy is the gold standard for definitive diagnosis and classification, but is used rarely due to its invasive nature. Newer modalities, such as dual-energy X-ray absorptiometry (DEXA) and high-resolution peripheral quantitative CT (HR-pQCT), yield data regarding bone density and microarchitecture, but are unable to distinguish between states of turnover.

Management of renal osteodystrophy aims to normalize mineral dysequilibration and suppress PTH to target levels without developing a dynamic bone disease. Management choices include diet phosphate restriction, phosphate binders, vitamin D analogues, and calcimimetics. Parathyroidectomy is an option for resistant secondary hyperparathyroidism. Effective management must be coupled with close monitoring to avoid the problems of hypercalcemia, over-suppression of PTH, and exacerbation of bone disease. In practice, renal osteodystrophy is the deep interconnection of kidney function and skeletal health, and its treatment and prevention are central to the overall management of patients with CKD.

References

1. Ghafar, M. H. A., Al-Junid, S. a. M., Ali, M. S. a. M., Mohamad, F., & Razak, A. H. A. (2025). Chronic kidney Disease diagnostic tools Based on Machine Learning Algorithms: A review. *Journal of Electrical & Electronic Systems Research*, *26*(APR2025), 18–26. https://doi.org/10.24191/jeesr.v26i1.003Adams, L. G., Bartges, J. W., Berent, A. C., Lulich, J. P., et al. (2016). ACVIM Small Animal Consensus Recommendations on the treatment and prevention of uroliths in dogs and cats. https://core.ac.uk/download/323070830.pdf (accessed on 25th June 2025).
2. Ahmed, A., Maisel, A., Alberti, A., Palazzuoli, A., Mebazaa, A., Ammann, P., Ammann, C., et al. (2010). Cardio-renal syndromes: Report from the consensus conference of the Acute Dialysis Quality Initiative. https://core.ac.uk/download/pdf/8389436.pdf (accessed on 25th June 2025).
3. Ahmed, H. H., Ahsan, M., Chowdhury, E., Co, E., Devabhaktuni, S., et al. (2018). Cardiovascular aspects of patients with chronic kidney disease and end-stage renal disease. https://core.ac.uk/download/322432874.pdf (accessed on 25th June 2025).
4. Alam, A., Arena, R., Bahous, S. A., Benetos, A., Blacher, J., Blacher, J., Boudville, N., et al. (2014). Effect of a reduction in glomerular filtration rate after nephrectomy on arterial stiffness and central hemodynamics: Rationale and design of the EARNEST study. https://core.ac.uk/download/19502512.pdf (accessed on 25th June 2025).
5. Alfieri, R., Consoli, S., & Caldiroli, L. (2025). World Kidney Day: A call to action for chronic kidney disease prevention and multidisciplinary care. *Giornale di Clinica Nefrologica e Dialisi*. https://www.semanticscholar.org/paper/a21ef686650a3e2071b8b11cb00f3262b1390e57 (accessed on 25th June 2025).
6. Amann, K., Banerjee, D., Bansal, N., Blankestijn, P. J., et al. (2018). Chronic kidney disease and arrhythmias: Conclusions from a kidney disease: Improving Global Outcomes (KDIGO) Controversies Conference. https://core.ac.uk/download/157581856.pdf (accessed on 25th June 2025).
7. Andant, T., Anderson, J. D., Andersson, C., Badawy, A., Balwani, M., Bissell, D. M., Bissell, D., et al. (2019). Acute hepatic porphyrias: Review and recent progress. https://core.ac.uk/download/323074395.pdf (accessed on 25th June 2025).
8. Anderson, C. A. M., Cavanaugh, K. L., Greene, J. H., Ikizler, T. A., et al. (2015). Results of a novel screening tool measuring dietary sodium knowledge in patients with chronic kidney disease. https://core.ac.uk/download/323065782.pdf (accessed on 25th June 2025).
9. Arnold, W., Johnson, R. J., Kuro-o, M., Lanaspa, M. A., et al. (2018). Novel treatment strategies for chronic kidney disease: Insights from the animal kingdom. https://core.ac.uk/download/150600152.pdf (accessed on 25th June 2025).
10. Astor, B. C., Coresh, J., de Jong, P. E., Eckardt, K. U., et al. (2011). The definition, classification, and prognosis of chronic kidney disease: A KDIGO Controversies Conference report. https://core.ac.uk/download/pdf/82342539.pdf (accessed on 25th June 2025).
11. Awdishu, L., Moore, T., Morrison, M., Trzebinska, J., et al. (2019). A primer on quality assurance and performance improvement for interprofessional chronic kidney disease care: A path to Joint Commission certification. https://core.ac.uk/download/323064308.pdf (accessed on 25th June 2025).

12. Baptista, A., Barroso, E., Ferreira, A. C., Monteiro, M. C., et al. (2012). Orthotopic liver transplantation in familial amyloidotic polyneuropathy is associated with long-term progression of renal disease. https://core.ac.uk/download/71736710.pdf (accessed on 25th June 2025).
13. Benoit, D., Lameire, N., Van Biesen, W., Vanholder, R., et al. (2016). Acute kidney injury in critically ill cancer patients: An update. https://core.ac.uk/download/55807820.pdf (accessed on 25th June 2025).
14. Bino, A., Ganz, T., & Salusky, I. B. (2019). Mechanism of action and clinical attributes of Auryxia® (ferric citrate). https://core.ac.uk/download/323076204.pdf (accessed on 25th June 2025).
15. Black, C., Fluck, N., Marks, A., Mitchell, M., et al. (2015). Long-term prognosis after acute kidney injury (AKI)–What is the role of baseline kidney function and recovery? A systematic review. https://core.ac.uk/download/29151088.pdf (accessed on 25th June 2025).
16. Bohlius, J., Bohlke, K., Castelli, R., Djulbegovic, B., et al. (2019). Management of cancer-associated anemia with erythropoiesis-stimulating agents: ASCO/ASH clinical practice guideline update. https://core.ac.uk/download/225130659.pdf (accessed on 25th June 2025).
17. Brown, M., Campbell, K. L., Chow, C., Craig, J. C., et al. (2019). Targeted, structured text messaging to improve dietary and lifestyle behaviors for people on maintenance hemodialysis (KIDNEYTEXT): Study protocol for a randomized controlled trial. https://core.ac.uk/download/323229018.pdf (accessed on 25th June 2025).
18. Budoff, M. J., Cespedes, A., Choi, T. Y., Li, D., et al. (2011). Mild and moderate pre-dialysis chronic kidney disease is associated with increased coronary artery calcium. https://core.ac.uk/download/323062306.pdf (accessed on 25th June 2025).
19. Costa, D., Patella, G., Provenzano, M., Ielapi, N., Faga, T., Zicarelli, M., Arturi, F., et al. (2023). Hyperkalemia in CKD: An overview of available therapeutic strategies. *Frontiers in Medicine, 10.* https://www.semanticscholar.org/paper/17e43ebc7d6d12c277be3aada84c3a84bb9d16c9 (accessed on 25th June 2025).
20. D'Marco, L., Fernández-Fernández, B., García-Carro, C., Gorgojo-Martinez, J., et al. (2020). GLP-1 receptor agonists and diabetic kidney disease: A call of attention to nephrologists. https://core.ac.uk/download/372708454.pdf (accessed on 25th June 2025).
21. Daschner, C., Kleber, M., Stach, K., Yuecel, G., Husain-Syed, F., Ayasse, N., Berg, A. H., et al. (2024). Association between arterial stiffness, carbamylation, and mortality in patients undergoing coronary angiography with no or mild chronic kidney disease. *Cardiorenal Medicine*, *15*, 83–97. https://www.semanticscholar.org/paper/2b930e1627e8ed69133fa200d299e3c70c7fedeb (accessed on 25th June 2025).
22. De Vincentiis, M., De Virgilio, A., Fusconi, M., Gallo, A., et al. (2016). Clinic manifestations in granulomatosis with polyangiitis. https://core.ac.uk/download/74319070.pdf (accessed on 25th June 2025).
23. Dewitte, A., Ishani, A., Ishani, A., Morden, A., Pai, A. B., Schneider, A. G., Lewington, A. J., et al. (2017). Acute kidney disease and renal recovery: Consensus report of the Acute Disease Quality Initiative (ADQI) 16 Workgroup. https://core.ac.uk/download/84041861.pdf (accessed on 25th June 2025).

24. Dhondt, A., Lameire, N., Van Biesen, W., Vanholder, R., et al. (2015). Prognostic robustness of serum creatinine-based AKI definitions in patients with sepsis: A prospective cohort study. https://core.ac.uk/download/55803944.pdf (accessed on 25th June 2025).

25. Dolan, S., Anand, A., Kalra, P. A., & Stewart, S. (2025). Uncoded chronic kidney disease prevalence in secondary care: A retrospective audit with population health implications. *BMC Nephrology, 26*. https://www.semanticscholar.org/paper/f8edc7f99f4a6f21d64f7dbdb4b7724016dcc2e0 (accessed on 25th June 2025).

26. Eder, M., Omić, H., Gorges, J., Badt, F., Kikić, Ž., Saemann, M., Tong, A., et al. (2021). Influenza vaccination uptake and factors influencing vaccination decision among patients with chronic kidney or liver disease. *PLoS ONE, 16*. https://www.semanticscholar.org/paper/fc8a078593220b752bacf17ac97c6fed476bafa7 (accessed on 25th June 2025).

27. Ekström, T. J., Nordfors, L., Shiels, P. G., Stenvinkel, P., et al. (2017). Current epigenetic aspects the clinical kidney researcher should embrace. https://core.ac.uk/download/84340482.pdf (accessed on 25th June 2025).

28. Ellis, R. J. B., Decker, B. S., Guise, D. M., Johnson, J. R., et al. (2016). Knowledge and awareness among patients with chronic kidney disease stage 3. https://core.ac.uk/download/227054278.pdf (accessed on 25th June 2025).

29. Griveas, I., Sitaras, P., Andriopoulos, C., & Aktsiali, M. (2019). Sucroferric oxyhydroxide: A novel phosphate binder for the management of mineral bone disease in dialysis patients. *Blood, Heart and Circulation*. https://www.semanticscholar.org/paper/076a193f9612694ce3aac37b9eca88b958936315 (accessed on 25th June 2025).

30. Grlić, S., Gregurović, V., Martinić, M., Davidović, M., Kos, I., Galić, S., Fištrek Prlić, M., et al. (2024). Single-center experience of pediatric cystic kidney disease and literature review. *Children, 11*. https://www.semanticscholar.org/paper/831befafc72f05a55381a4def9df63739a7223f9 (accessed on 25th June 2025).

31. Gul, M. H., Waheed, A., Jha, M., Wardak, A. B., Ilma, B., & Khan, U. (2025). Revolutionizing anemia management in dialysis: Unveiling the potential of FDA-approved Vadadustat for chronic kidney disease (CKD) patients. *Annals of Medicine and Surgery, 87*, 1094–1096. https://www.semanticscholar.org/paper/596d67ae1bfa65a844a6dbb3d52823004cbbca8c (accessed on 25th June 2025).

32. Ha, Y., Lee, J., Kim, J., Jeong, C., Lim, Y., Lee, J., & Baek, K. H. (2025). Long-term efficacy and safety of denosumab: Insights beyond 10 years of use. *Endocrinology and Metabolism, 40*, 47–56. https://www.semanticscholar.org/paper/d6ec4843d7af30d8074260f81878690497550525 (accessed on 25th June 2025).

33. Habli, M. M. (2024). Comprehensive insights into diabetic nephropathy: Pathophysiology, clinical features, and emerging treatments. *Journal of The Egyptian Society of Nephrology and Transplantation*. https://www.semanticscholar.org/paper/55f2eac7074464c58c0d322841cc625add4c3e29 (accessed on 25th June 2025).

34. Hoefer, L. T., Weber, N., Jazmati, M., Noack, M. J., Barbe, A. G., & Graf, I. (2025). Chronic kidney disease with related oral health problems and alterations in the tongue microbiome illustrated by a 15-year-old girl: A case report. *Case Reports in Pediatrics, 2025*. https://www.semanticscholar.org/paper/eba247614a6f907f89abc800c9b2c4448ee236f0 (accessed on 25th June 2025).

35. Ilyas, A., & Ali, B. (2024). Screening first-degree relatives of patients with chronic kidney disease (CKD) in Pakistan. *JPMA. The Journal of the Pakistan Medical Association*, *74*(9), 1729. https://www.semanticscholar.org/paper/56e06f32da96f4711101c1fc7efc137eff8802f7 (accessed on 25th June 2025).

36. Jakubowska, W., Kiełkowicz, A., Pactwa, F., Pisera, A., et al. (2023). A review on the classification and current treatment of chronic kidney disease. https://core.ac.uk/download/597985229.pdf (accessed on 25th June 2025).

37. Jardine, A. G., Mark, P. B., & Stoumpos, S. (2014). Cardiovascular morbidity and mortality after kidney transplantation. https://core.ac.uk/download/42353945.pdf (accessed on 25th June 2025).

38. Khalid, A., Khan, M. Z., Mehmood, G., & Qureshi, M. S. (2023). Machine learning hybrid model for the prediction of chronic kidney disease. *Computational Intelligence and Neuroscience*, *2023*. https://www.semanticscholar.org/paper/c59d82b3cb94d689928f18b8cdc03c1c03fc19b6 (accessed on 25th June 2025).

39. Lo, R. H., Narasaki, Y., Lei, S., & Rhee, C. M. (2023). Management of traditional risk factors for the development and progression of chronic kidney disease. *Clinical Kidney Journal*, *16*, 1737–1750. https://www.semanticscholar.org/paper/47c6c964b2de652c8ce8ea66399269d8e8892797 (accessed on 25th June 2025).

40. Marrone, M., Di Lauro, K., Cornali, K., Masci, C., Vanni, G., Vita, C., & Noce, A. (2025). Sustainability and role of plant-based diets in chronic kidney disease prevention and treatment. *Frontiers in Pharmacology*, *16*. https://www.semanticscholar.org/paper/0573986d5260fa567972907467f0848fd5d0ceec (accessed on 25th June 2025).

41. Muryawan, M. H., & Pambudi, A. R. (2015). Karakteristik kejadian penyakit ginjal kronik pada sindrom nefrotik anak. https://core.ac.uk/download/76927633.pdf (accessed on 25th June 2025).

42. Octivani, F., Arsatt, M. I. A., Maulana, A., & Wedayani, A. A. A. N. (2025). Relationship between patients with hypertension stage 2 and chronic kidney disease (CKD) at Harapan Keluarga Hospital. *Jurnal Biologi Tropis*. https://www.semanticscholar.org/paper/770a1f66ab57ce421e519f31f81f9dabbf7058af (accessed on 25th June 2025).

43. Owolabi, M. S., Berinyuy, E., & Abdulkabir, A. O. (2025). The interplay between breast cancer and diabetes mellitus: Shared mechanisms, risk factors, and integrated management strategies. *BIOMED Natural and Applied Science*. https://www.semanticscholar.org/paper/39e6cac1f6a249d605cdfc550d4132fc0ec1fb3f (accessed on 25th June 2025).

44. Ramchandani, S., Mohammed, Y. N., Rahaman, Z., & Khurana, S. (2024). The role of telemedicine in enhancing chronic kidney disease (CKD) management and dialysis care. *Cureus*, *16*. https://www.semanticscholar.org/paper/4fb45dbbae54bc5dadc02f212e8fd221ecd2d362 (accessed on 25th June 2025).

45. Rohr, M., Brandenburg, V., & Brunner-la Rocca, H. (2023). How to diagnose iron deficiency in chronic disease: A review of current methods and potential marker for the outcome. *European Journal of Medical Research*, *28*. https://www.semanticscholar.org/paper/a9ffc8fbbed9a08a8b1d9a49c6e9d59b68512011 (accessed on 25th June 2025).

46. Saeed, Z., Sirolli, V., Bonomini, M., Gallina, S., & Renda, G. (2024). Hallmarks for thrombotic and hemorrhagic risks in chronic kidney disease patients. *International Journal of Molecular*

Sciences, 25. https://www.semanticscholar.org/paper/6945747047f7769e63017a740abb671bc1b62a35 (accessed on 25th June 2025).

47. Shivakumar, M., Kim, Y., Jung, S. H., Woerner, J., & Kim, D. (2024). Frequency of adding salt is a stronger predictor of chronic kidney disease in individuals with genetic risk. *Pacific Symposium on Biocomputing, 30*, 551–564. https://www.semanticscholar.org/paper/fd51558b04e7212923cfb45fcc46a5b3d2d513a7 (accessed on 25th June 2025).

48. Singh, S., Tiwari, M., Kumar, V., & Pandey, A. (2025). Role of Ayurveda in prevention and management of non-communicable diseases: A review. *International Journal of Research in Ayurveda and Pharmacy*. https://www.semanticscholar.org/paper/d36de674e45a4bacb07dabbf6e556b8ebf675b53 (accessed on 25th June 2025).

49. Slee, A. D. (2012). Exploring metabolic dysfunction in chronic kidney disease. https://core.ac.uk/download/17352998.pdf (accessed on 25th June 2025).

50. Ullah, A., Abbasi, M. S. R., Jawad, M., Shah, M. A. U., Zia, W., & Rahat, A. (2025). Pattern of menstrual irregularity in chronic kidney disease (CKD) patients in tertiary care hospital. *Insights–Journal of Health and Rehabilitation*. https://www.semanticscholar.org/paper/9db87a00d4dc5ee15e75a109f20fb295c2f6a1a8 (accessed on 25th June 2025).

51. Wang, N., & Zhang, C. D. (2024). Recent advances in the management of diabetic kidney disease: Slowing progression. *International Journal of Molecular Sciences, 25*. https://www.semanticscholar.org/paper/42ae3a00fea146cd51701f8c1323fc9ed7e353bd (accessed on 25th June 2025).

52. Yadav, A. K., Modi, G. K., Ojha, J. P., Sahay, M., Prasad, N., John, O., Pandey, R., et al. (2017). The Indian Chronic Kidney Disease (ICKD) study: Design and methods. https://core.ac.uk/download/42581977.pdf (accessed on 25th June 2025).

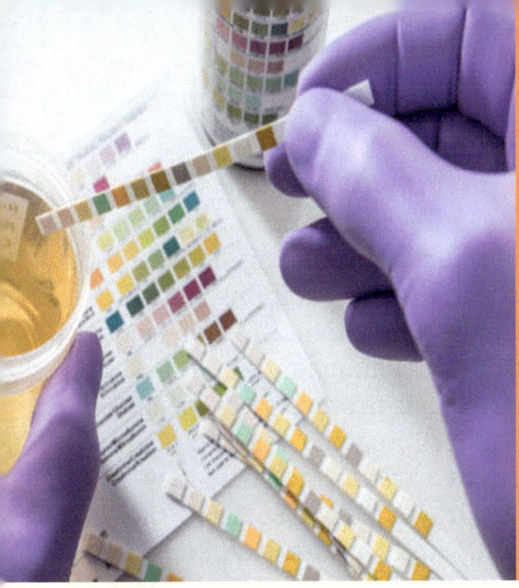

Chapter 10

URINARY TRACT INFECTIONS (UTIS)

Contents

Introduction

Urinary tract infection (UTI) is a significant public health issue among heterogeneous populations with increased prevalence in certain groups, such as women and individuals with specific medical conditions. UTI results from the invasion of the urinary tract by pathogenic microorganisms, whose presentation ranges from mild inflammation to overwhelming systemic illness. As the second most common type of infection in the body, UTIs are a call for continued research and the development of effective treatment strategies. Antibiotic resistance is a component that significantly influences the complications of treating such infections; a thorough understanding of both traditional and alternative treatment methods is essential. With growing antimicrobial resistance due to antibiotic abuse, a new line of treatments is becoming more prominent, indicating that the time is ripe to investigate newer prophylactic interventions to curtail UTIs and enhance patient outcomes. The impact of UTIs also extends beyond temporary physical discomfort, and it has a strong bearing on the quality of life of

UTI sufferers. In some populations, such as the chronically ill, like patients with multiple sclerosis (PwMS), the incidence and burden of UTIs could be high. UTIs have been proven to aggravate underlying neurological conditions, with subsequent complications further reducing quality of life. Effective management of UTIs is therefore essential in these patients. Regulations that are put in place encourage conservative diagnostic strategies through the implementation of urine cultures to confirm infection, as well as treatments that follow some recommendations focused on the specific patient's needs. Clinicians need to be familiar with these protocols to optimize treatment and decrease the burden of UTIs in this population, underlining the importance of multidisciplinary treatment. Recent research suggests novel alternative treatments that may be used to supplement or replace conventional antibiotic treatment to prevent UTIs. Some of these include natural compounds such as D-mannose, N-acetylcysteine (NAC), and *Morinda citrifolia* fruit extract that have been shown prevent bacterial adhesion and biofilm formation and consequently prevent infection. Initial studies have suggested that such alternatives can be on a par with antibiotic effectiveness, particularly in invasive procedures patients, presenting a plausible path to limit the use of antibiotics and combat resistance. With the inclusion of such nutraceutical agents in ongoing research on conventional therapy, the findings support further inquiry into their roles in preventing UTIs. As medicine continues to advance, achieving the proper balance between effective treatment and avoiding antibiotic reliance becomes increasingly essential, paving the way for new forms of UTI treatment that hold great promise for improving patient care and safety in the long run (Figure 10.1).

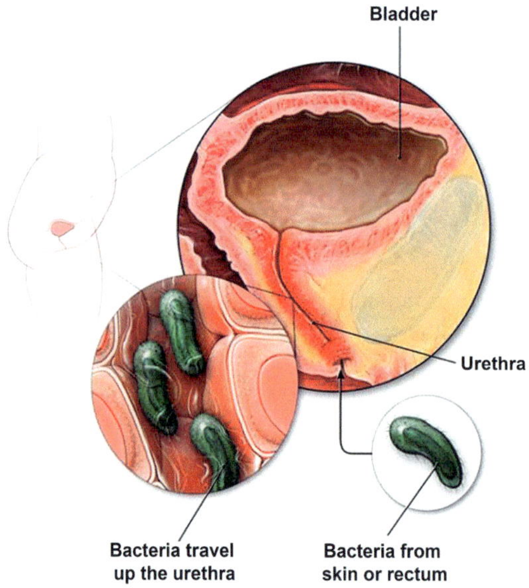

Figure 10.1. Urinary tract infection basics.

Source: https://www.cdc.gov/uti/media/images/uti.jpg.

Definition of Urinary Tract Infections

The term UTIs refers to a collection of clinical syndromes characterized by the presence of pathogenic microorganisms within the urinary tract, that is, the bladder, urethra, ureters, and kidneys. A UTI can manifest in various forms, such as cystitis, which is the inflammation of the bladder, or pyelonephritis, an infection of the kidneys. In reality, UTI diagnosis is based on the identification of frequent signs such as dysuria, frequency, and urgency in addition to laboratory findings. Importantly, the identification of positive urine cultures, i.e., a set of colony-forming units (CFUs) indicative of infection, plays a critical role in diagnosis, particularly when symptoms are present (Chataway et al., 2016). Therefore, the overlap of clinical signs and microbiological data is the basis of UTI diagnosis. In elderly groups, the definition of UTIs is further complicated by the fact that the disease can present in an atypical manner. In such populations, urinary tract infections can occur without typical symptoms or in the presence of nonspecific signs, making the diagnosis even more troublesome. Successful diagnosis relies on the emergence of new urinary symptoms, which may, but do not have to be, accompanied by systemic signs, such as fever (Beveridge et al., 2011). Routine urinalysis remains a valuable tool in this age group; however, results must be interpreted cautiously as the evidence in its favor is limited. In addition, the problem of asymptomatic bacteriuria—the presence of bacteria without symptoms—represents a significant clinical dilemma, as over-treatment can lead to unnecessary consumption of antimicrobials and the development of resistance. Additionally, the definition of UTIs is not merely an infection count; it requires a more nuanced consideration based on the patient's setting, particularly in cases where underlying conditions are present. For instance, patients with multiple sclerosis (PwMS) often experience neurogenic bladder, making them prone to recurring UTIs and interfering with diagnosis (Chataway et al., 2016). Such symptoms in these patients may overlap with neurological symptoms, and therefore, diagnosis and management become a comprehensive process. The need to incorporate urine cultures, along with symptom assessment, reflects an essential distinction between symptomatic and asymptomatic infections, directing clinical management toward more targeted treatments (Beveridge et al., 2011). Ultimately, a thorough comprehension of UTI's definition identifies not just the clinical manifestations but also the crucial contributions of patient history and laboratory confirmation to effective treatment outcomes.

Importance of Studying UTIs

The significance of UTIs also goes beyond the individual health problems they present and into the areas of broad public health. UTIs are among the most frequent bacterial infections, particularly for women due to anatomical and physiological factors. In this case, knowledge of the particular etiologic agents involved, such as various species of Proteus, is necessary, as these pathogens may be responsible for more complex clinical conditions, including urinary stone formation and chronic infections with significant adverse effects on patient quality of life. Specifically, the Proteus species' capacity for biofilm formation, particularly on indwelling catheters, poses a higher risk to long-term care patients, necessitating studies directed towards designing effective prevention and treatment strategies (Drzewiecka et al., 2013). This focus not only mitigates individual suffering but also lowers healthcare costs associated with repeated infection and complications. Moreover, knowledge of UTIs significantly enhances understanding of the functional dysmorphias related to urinary tract anatomy and physiology. UTIs in children, for instance, are often linked with disorders like lower urinary tract dysfunction (LUTD), which can result in serious long-term consequences if not treated thoroughly. It has been proven through research that children with CKD are at higher risk for recurrent UTIs, which increases the risk of rapid loss of renal function. Recognition of LUTD signs in children highlights the intricate interaction between UTIs and other health status conditions, underscoring the need for multidisciplinary management that addresses UTIs as well as the accompanying urinary tract dysfunctions (Öborn et al., 2014). Identifying these connections, healthcare providers can develop targeted interventions that restore renal function and overall health. Finally, the environment of UTI research has implications for public health policy and education. Increased awareness about risk factors for and prevention against UTI encourages knowledge that empowers patients to seek early medical treatment and preventive measures. Secondly, education regarding UTI-related risks, such as those presented by opportunistic organisms like Proteus, reinforces the culture of vigilance among healthcare providers. Such a proactive strategy can lead to quicker diagnosis and more tailored treatment options, hence reducing the health system burden of UTIs. Because UTIs remain a significant issue worldwide, prioritized prevention strategies and research will play a crucial role in reducing their occurrence and enhancing the outcome of patients (Drzewiecka et al., 2013; Öborn et al., 2014). Through exhaustive research studies, the path of UTI research can translate facts into reality, benefiting both individual patients and society (Figure 10.2).

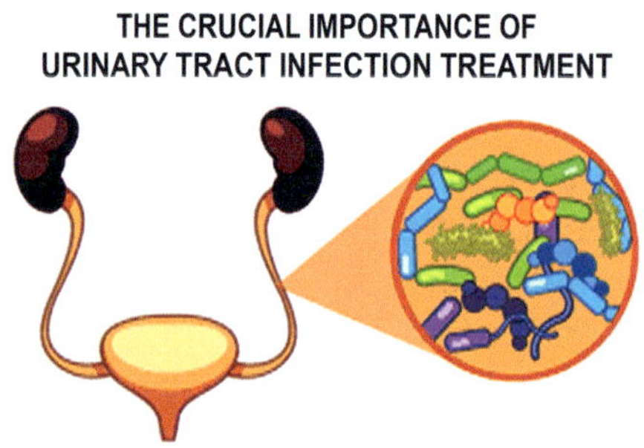

Figure 10.2. The crucial importance of urinary tract infection.

Source: https://encrypted-tbn0.gstatic.com/images?q=tbn:ANd9GcRk4iE5nbxdKsYcCYkxAd2IseJjNzrjxW7Obg&s.

10.1. Anatomy of the Urinary Tract

The anatomy of the urinary system is fundamental to understanding UTIs. The urinary system consists of the kidneys, ureters, bladder, and urethra, all of which play a role in urine creation, transport, and excretion. The kidneys remove waste products from the bloodstream to create urine, which is then transported via the ureters into the bladder. From there, the urine is stored until it is discharged via the urethra. The structural integrity of this system is critical in preventing infection. Anatomical defect or obstruction, such as ureteric duplication and bladder exstrophy, makes an individual susceptible to UTI through manipulation of normal urinary flow and susceptibility to colonization by bacteria, hence emphasizing the importance of knowledge about urinary tract anatomy in prevention and infection management (Baskin et al., 2018). Another essential component of urinary tract anatomy is the bladder, along with its physiological mechanisms. The bladder, being a muscular bag, distends to store urine and contracts during micturition, making its musculature essential for bladder function. Urination is regulated by the coordination of the detrusor muscle and the external sphincter, with there being elaborate nervous system control. Adequacies or dysfunctions of this anatomy can result in inefficient bladder emptying or excessive residual urine, creating an optimal culture medium for bacterial proliferation. Current evidence suggests that factors influencing the anatomy of the bladder during embryonic life, such as mesenchymal-epithelial interactions, have a significant impact on its function (Musa et al., 2025). It is thus of utmost importance to have a complex understanding of bladder anatomy to comprehend the mechanisms underlying UTIs. The anatomy of the urethra is also largely responsible for the occurrence of urinary tract infections. The urethra, being the final passage for urine excretion, is shorter in females than in males and therefore is more prone to UTIs in women. Furthermore, because the opening of the urethra is nearer to the anus, there is a greater risk of contamination by bacteria from the gastrointestinal tract. Stricture or blockage of the urethra can result from anatomical defects or medical conditions, which aggravate the situation by preventing the flow of urine and creating a site for bacterial growth. Moreover, hormonal effects and sexual activity can alter the microenvironment of the urethra, varying infection risk. Thus, advanced knowledge of urethral anatomy and its functional implications is required to comprehend the pathways by which UTIs can progress, justifying the role of anatomical information in both prevention and treatment strategies (Musa et al., 2025) (Figure 10.3).

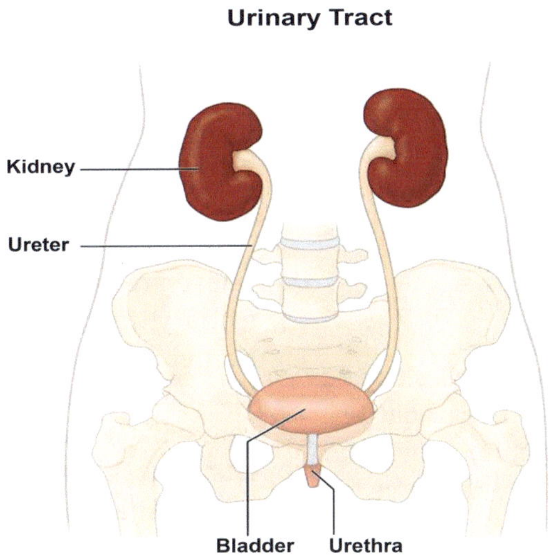

Figure 10.3. The urinary tract.

Source: https://www.niddk.nih.gov/-/media/Images/Health-Information/Urologic/Urinary-Tract-BIG_2064x1895.jpg?imbypass=truc.

10.1.1. Components of the Urinary System

The urinary system comprises several key structures that work together to filter blood, produce urine, and eliminate waste. The kidneys are the primary filtering organs, responsible for removing waste products and excess material from the bloodstream. Each kidney contains approximately one million nephrons, which are functional units that begin the process of generating urine through a complex process that includes filtration, reabsorption, and secretion. Once urine is produced in the kidneys, it moves down through the ureters—muscular tubes that transport urine to the bladder. The bladder is an empty organ that acts as a storage site for urine until it is released from the body. Learning about these parts, it is possible to understand how infections or alterations in this system can lead to conditions such as UTIs that have significant effects on overall health (Kirdis et al., 2011). The urethra is also part of the urinary system, as it is the channel for urine to exit the body. This tube is shorter in females and thus more susceptible to UTIs, as bacteria have an easier time ascending to the bladder from the external environment. The anatomical design of the urethra, as well as the surrounding muscle groups, is vital to urinary continence and regulation of urination. Urethral dysfunction or obstruction will produce stasis, thus predisposing to infection. The interaction between the lining of the urethra and urine is crucial; urothelial cells play a protective role, responding to potential pathogens and contributing to maintaining urodynamic equilibrium (Kesav et al., 2024). Knowledge of the subtleties of the elements of the urinary system is essential in unraveling the mechanisms through which UTIs develop and are maintained. The role of the various anatomical aspects of the urinary system involves significant immunologic considerations. The urothelial lining of the bladder serves as a barrier to pathogens while also triggering immunity. The barrier is situated to detect pathogens through the use of pattern recognition receptors with particular affinity for damage-associated molecular patterns. Once the pathogen has been detected, the urothelium can trigger inflammation, which, while necessary for the defense against infection, may also be responsible for urinary manifestations of UTIs, such as dysuria and urgency. Additionally, the presence of beneficial bacteria in the urinary system can influence the immune response of the urothelium and provide resistance against uropathogens. The study suggests an intricate relationship between these microbes and the host immune responses, as well as the need for further research into the mechanisms by which imbalances in this system can lead to the onset of UTIs (Kirdis et al., 2011; Kesav et al., 2024) (Figure 10.4).

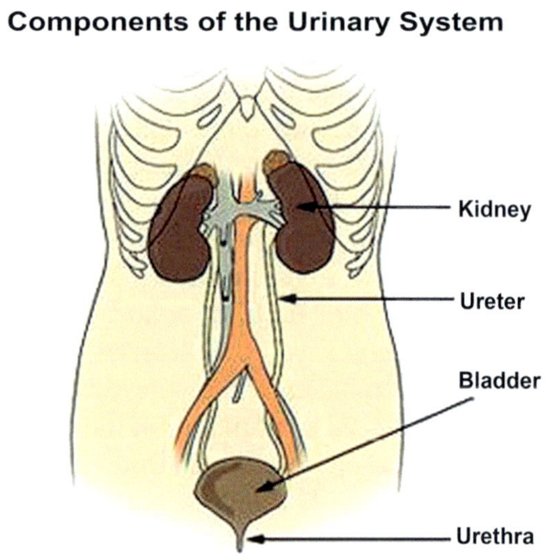

Figure 10.4. Components of the urinary system.

Source: https://training.seer.cancer.gov/images/anatomy/urinary/urinary_system.jpg.

10.1.2. Function of Each Component

There are several anatomical structures in the urinary tract, each playing a role in maintaining homeostasis and preventing infection. The kidneys are the primary organs of filtration, removing waste products and excess material from the blood. The urine is secreted by the kidneys and flows downward in the form of ureters to the bladder. The bladder is a reservoirthat temporarily stores urine, allowing for controlled urination while preventing ongoing leakage. This volume of storage is an important essential since it enables frequent voiding, which helps remove pathogens that find entry into the urinary tract. In addition, the bladder sphincter and urethral sphincter allow for voluntary control of urination, which prevents unnecessary infections due to retrograde urine flow, a condition that is undesirable when pathogenic organisms are involved. The urethra is also the primary contributor to the expulsion of urine, and its design significantly influences susceptibility to UTIs. In females, the urethra is shorter and nearer to the rectum, and therefore more likely to be contaminated with bacteria. The male urethra plays a dual role in both the urinary and reproductive systems. These structural differences permit uropathogens to easily ascend from the urethra to the bladder and kidney, thereby infecting them. For instance, pathogens such as *Escherichia coli* can easily adhere to the bladder epithelium, circumventing the host's immune mechanism. The presence of biofilms, as seen in certain strains, exacerbates this condition by promoting bacterial resistance to therapy and supporting chronic infections, underscoring the importance of anatomical and functional information in UTI pathology (Baho et al., 2019). Excluding anatomical parameters, various microbial pathogens have a significant influence on urinary tract infection processes. These include the genus Proteus, which is essential because it can produce urease and biofilm and can lead to such complications as the formation of struvite stones. Its swarming nature makes Proteus capable of infecting new niches at an alarming rate, e.g., on catheter surfaces, with such infection reservoirs. Their enzymes also degrade the host's defense, paving the way for more virulent infections. Moreover, virulence factors (e.g., fimbriae and flagella) maximize their fitness within urinary niches via motility and adherence. Consequently, understanding these pathogenic processes is necessary to facilitate effective treatment and prophylaxis against complications, and thus the need for future research into anatomical function and pathogen behavior (Drzewiecka et al., 2013).

10.1.3. How Anatomy Relates to UTIs

The anatomy of the urinary tract is also a fundamental cause of susceptibility to UTIs, particularly through its anatomical components. The urinary tract comprises the kidneys, ureters, bladder, and urethra, functioning as a pathway for urine elimination from the body. All the components are aligned in a manner to function together, but whenever any malformation or anatomical anomaly happens, it increases the risk of infection. For instance, the proximity of the urethra to the rectum in women allows for the free transfer of bacteria, such as *E. coli*, from the rectal region into the urinary tract. This anatomical arrangement explains the higher prevalence of UTIs among women compared to men. Additionally, variations in the length and location of the urethra may explain differences in infection rates, illustrating how anatomical features are linked to UTI pathogenesis and have significant clinical significance for prevention and treatment. Additionally, the anatomical features of the bladder itself significantly contribute to its susceptibility to infection. The bladder serves as a reservoir for urine before it is expelled from the body, and its immunological environment is critical to defend against infection. The urothelial lining of the bladder is essential to avert bacterial adherence, and disruption of this barrier results in increased susceptibility to UTIs. In addition, anatomical defects like vesicoureteral reflux, in which urine moves in the wrong direction from the bladder to the kidneys, predispose to more extensive infection. The military-like defense of the bladder, consisting of its muscular wall and reflexive pressure mechanisms, often fails when such defects exist, allowing bacteria to travel upward and multiply. These anatomical dynamics must be understood to create effective interventions for the prevention and treatment of UTI. The anatomical relationships between the organs of the urinary tract and their roles in immune function contribute to the complexity of UTIs. For instance, kidneys not only filter waste products but also have a vital role in producing various substances important in immune defense. They include the production of antibodies and other immune cells that combat infection. There have been demonstrations of relationships between certain types of *E. coli* and their virulence in causing UTIs, highlighting where anatomy and microbial virulence factors intersect in infection contexts.

Strain AIEC, which approximates uropathogenic *E. coli* (UPEC), exhibits such overlap since it can adhere to and invade prostate epithelial cells, thereby increasing the risk of infection among susceptible individuals. Since the anatomically distinct regions of the urinary tract interact with pathogens, an understanding of these interactions sheds light on the etiology and therapeutic complexity of UTIs (Figure 10.5).

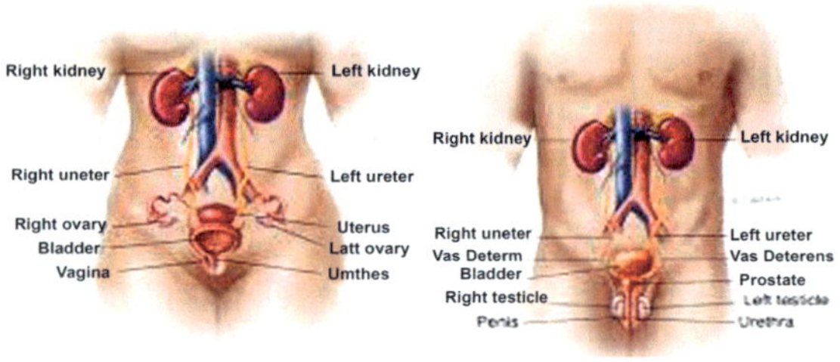

Figure 10.5. How anatomy relates to UTIs.

Source: https://lh6.googleusercontent.com/proxy/jTMn4iOpT8x3VG_SC-MoPyJ0nx17sproXYZVicKWqffonzFnua31z5aDyBc4jjFjfn7voIr2du2MvwodXTTKFsE-Yyq5Fydn3BmJI3TAP64zgTZyE0BA4ULLOw.

10.2. Causes of Urinary Tract Infections

The etiology of UTIs is predominantly bacterial, with *Escherichia coli* being the single most frequent causative agent. The Gram-negative rod is responsible for about 80-90% of community-acquired UTIs primarily because it is capable of adhering to the uroepithelium, of enhancing biofilm formation, and of evading the host's immune mechanisms. In addition, risk factors such as sexual activity, diaphragm use, and recent antibiotic therapy increase the vulnerability to acquiring a UTI, highlighting the importance of having a thorough knowledge of both microbial virulence and host susceptibility. Additionally, antimicrobial resistance complicates the treatment profile, with E. coli strains exhibiting increased resistance patterns due to the excessive prescription and misuse of antibiotics, necessitating regular monitoring of antibiotic sensitivity profiles to guide effective therapy. Therefore, knowledge of the causative factors is crucial in applying appropriate preventive measures and treatment protocols. Exposure to healthcare is significantly responsible for the causation of UTIs, particularly within a hospital environment. From one surveillance study of *E. coli* cases of bacteremia, prior treatment for urinary tract infection was identified as the most significant independent risk factor, implying that infections can be at an elevated risk of recurrence in already infected patients. Furthermore, nearly half of the cases presented involved a history of healthcare exposure, with procedures such as urinary catheterization being common among them. These findings highlight a significant point of intersection between hospital procedures and the incidence of UTIs, underscoring the role of healthcare-associated infections in the broader epidemiology of this disorder. This cluster requires stricter clinical practices, centered around liberal use of urinary catheters and risk management strategies to minimize the recurrence of UTIs in susceptible groups due to healthcare-associated factors that can significantly add to the morbidity of these infections. Demographic factors also play a significant role in determining the prevalence and risk of urinary tract infections. Women, particularly those of childbearing age, are much more at risk than their male counterparts, predominantly due to some anatomical characteristics that facilitate bacterial invasion into the urinary system. As indicated by evidence that UTI is a strong predictor of dysuria and elevated body temperature, detection of these clinical symptoms can permit early diagnosis and treatment, which in turn can minimize complications. Second, the universal application of antibiotics in the treatment of febrile illness in children has the potential to obscure underlying causes of UTI symptoms, as seen in studies of increasing rates of multidrug-resistant *E.*

coli. This points to the necessity of clinicians embracing comprehensive diagnostic approaches to differentiate UTIs and other febrile illnesses to ensure appropriate management of urinary tract infection patients, like those that are being investigated in recent research (Dzeing-Ella et al., 2012; Claxton et al., 2016) (Figure 10.6).

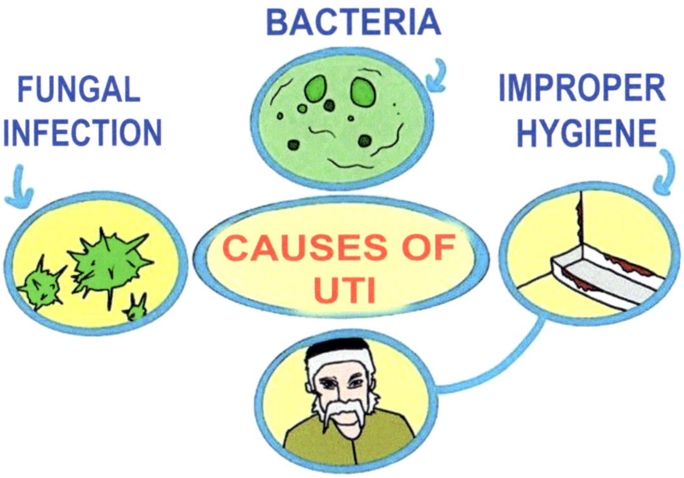

Figure 10.6. Causes of urinary tract infections.

Source: https://nuawoman.com/blog/wp-content/uploads/2019/09/causes-of-uti2.jpg.

10.2.1. Bacterial Pathogens Commonly Involved

Bacterial pathogens are most commonly implicated in the etiology of UTIs, with *Escherichia coli* being the primary causative agent. The Gram-negative rod causes approximately 80% of all uncomplicated UTIs due primarily to its ability to adhere to uroepithelial cells and evade host defense. Uropathogenic *E. coli* strains possess specialized fimbriae and adhesins that facilitate colonization of the urinary tract, resulting in inflammation and infection. In addition to *E. coli*, other pathogens, such as Klebsiella pneumoniae, Proteus mirabilis, and Enterococcus faecalis, also cause UTIs. The prevalence and distribution of these pathogens vary based on the patient population and health status, highlighting the need for targeted diagnostic and treatment measures to effectively treat the infection. In recent years, the sudden onset of antibiotic resistance among pathogens responsible for UTIs has posed unprecedented challenges to clinical management. *E. coli* strains have been increasingly resistant to commonly employed antimicrobial agents, and treatment has become more difficult. This increasing resistance is primarily due to the indiscriminate or unwarranted use of broad-spectrum antibiotics, which can have a selective pressure for the development of resistant strains. A review of studies found poor compliance with UTI treatment guidelines was particularly low, at merely 40%, a situation that may be fueled by physician prescribing behavior and patient factors (Alvarez et al., 2005). Poor conformity to standard treatment guidelines results in therapy failure and ultimately leads to increased morbidity among UTI patients. Secondly, understanding the epidemiologic patterns of the causative bacterial pathogens for UTIs is essential for driving public health response and antimicrobial stewardship. Although E. coli remains the most prevalent pathogen, rising rates of multidrug-resistant organisms necessitate ongoing monitoring and research into new treatments and preventive measures. The use of rapid tests can facilitate the earlier detection of causative pathogens and resistance patterns, ultimately leading to improved patient outcomes. Additionally, public health interventions aimed at educating patients and healthcare providers about the appropriate use of antimicrobials and infection control are necessary to curb the emergence of resistant strains (Chew et al., 2012). Ultimately, a comprehensive multimodal strategy that combines rigorous diagnosis, personalized treatment, and stringent public health measures is necessary to effectively manage UTIs and counter the threat of resistant bacterial pathogens (Figure 10.7).

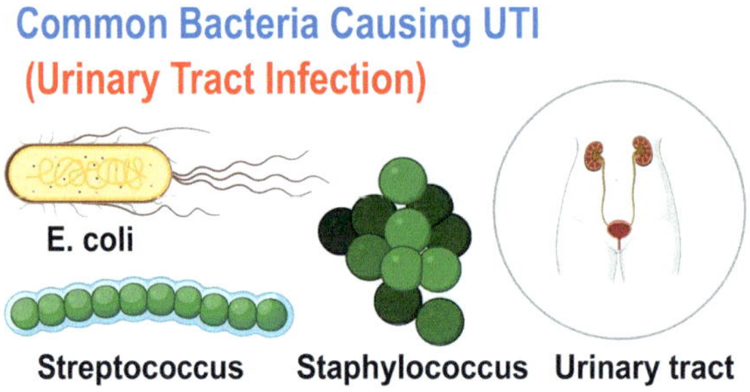

Figure 10.7. Common bacteria causing UTI.

Source: https://microbenotes.com/wp-content/uploads/2022/05/Common-Bacteria-Causing-UTI-Urinary-Tract-Infection.jpeg.

10.2.2. Risk Factors for Developing UTIs

The prevalence of UTIs is influenced by several risk factors that significantly increase susceptibility. Among these, physiological and anatomical factors are of utmost significance, particularly in females. The female urethra is shorter, and bacterial movement from the outside to the bladder is a simple affair, thereby making them more prone to infection. In men, UTIs occur mainly due to obstructive states or prostatic disease hindering the free passage of urine. Urinary catheter use is also a high-risk factor among both men and women because the catheters provide an easy pathway for germs to flow up the system and infect. Environmental factors, such as poor hygiene practices, also contribute to this risk factor, making education and preventive interventions essential in preventing cases of UTI. Second, certain medical conditions and treatment regimens are significant contributors to the potential for contracting UTIs. Patients undergoing chemotherapy and radiotherapy, particularly those intended for malignancies affecting the pelvic region, are highly susceptible to developing complications like infection. Research indicates that intensity-modulated radiotherapy cervical cancer patients experience a 32.5% incidence of UTIs, with *Escherichia coli* and Enterococcus species as the predominant pathogens (Yao et al., 2025). Also, co-morbidities such as diabetes mellitus weaken the immune system, such that the patient is prone to infections like UTIs. The degree of complexity involved in caring for these patients extends beyond managing first-order medical conditions to instituting measures that prevent secondary infections, which can complicate their treatment course. Lastly, sexual intercourse and hydration status are also integral parts of the etiology of UTIs. More instances of UTI episodes are also reported among sexually active females, with microbial introduction during intercourse facilitating high infection rates. Furthermore, inadequate fluid consumption can lead to concentrated urine, which in turn can facilitate the development of bacteria-infested urinary habitats. A risk factor assessment in multidisciplinary hospitals revealed that variation in hydration status was a factor influencing the growth of UTI, demonstrating the role lifestyle plays in increasing infection risk (Sursyakova et al., 2022). Minimizing the occurrence of UTI in high-risk individuals is imperative and must be met with education and behavioral interventions to modify these risk factors. Together, appreciating the various facets of these risk factors is essential to the successful prevention and management of urinary tract infections.

10.2.3. Role of Hygiene and Sexual Activity

The articulation of sexual acts and hygiene practices is pivotal in the prevention and control of UTIs. Inadequate personal hygiene, especially in women, has been associated with an increased risk of acquiring UTIs because of the anatomic closeness of the urethra to the rectum. Adequate hygiene before and after sexual intercourse is essential in the prevention of bacterial access into the urinary system. Research has demonstrated that easy-to-adopt practices, like urinating before and after sex and proper washing of the genital area, can significantly contribute to the prevention of UTIs.

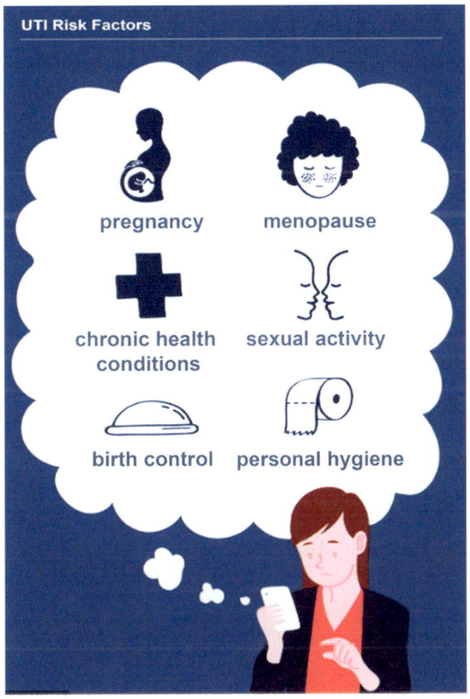

Figure 10.8. Role of hygiene and sexual activity in urinary tract infections.

Source: https://miro.medium.com/v2/resize:fit:1400/0*wJMBLH2sAyAaW0iR.png.

Public health interventions to educate people about these habits of cleanliness, therefore, have the potential to achieve a lot in the way of both health and wellbeing among groups at risk of developing UTIs. Sex is known to be a risk factor for UTIs, particularly in women, who are predisposed to recurrent infection. During intercourse, the urethra is vulnerable or can become subjected to trauma during intercourse and thus can serve as a pathway by which bacteria may migrate up the urinary tract. In addition, sexual lubricants and other such sexual health products may carry bacteria that would disrupt the natural balance of the urogenital flora, posing a challenge to preventing UTIs. Sexually active individuals need to be aware of these risks. These risks need to be negated by the inclusion of hygiene tips for their sex. Educational emphasis placed on safe sex, in addition to increased awareness of hygiene, can reduce the incidence of UTIs but enhance healthier sexual relationships. Alternatives to antibiotics have been proposed for UTI prevention, and the practice of hygiene has emerged as the most effective approach. Specific hygienic habit, including genital cleaning before and after sexual intercourse, has been identified by research as essential to reducing the risk of infection. While other treatments, such as cranberry juice and immunization, have been shown to be ineffective in preventing UTIs in a sporadic but consistent manner, their work indicates an increasing interest in non-antibiotic measures. First and foremost, the recognition of hygiene as a protective measure stems from studies demonstrating its safety and efficacy, particularly in high-risk groups such as pregnant women. The results also concur with the appeal for a survey of the holistic method of hygiene education and its practice as an intervention of first-line measure in preventing UTIs (Bonnici et al., 2014; Flower et al., 2018) (Figure 10.8).

10.3. Symptoms of Urinary Tract Infections

Symptoms of UTIs can vary profoundly across patients, thereby leading to misdiagnosis and confusion with other health conditions. Typically, patients report dysuria, which is defined as painful urination or burning micturition, which is painful and distressing. In children, symptoms may be even less obvious, as their vocabulary skills are often limited in expressing pain. Additionally, suprapubic pain and lumbar pain are also frequently reported, representing the symptoms of urinary tract and bladder inflammation and irritation. It is also important to note that systemic symptoms, such as fever and vomiting, may occur, particularly in complicated cases, representing probable complications that must be treated urgently (Bartoszewicz et al., 2022). Clinicians must therefore remain vigilant in detecting these symptoms to avoid misinterpretation and ensure prompt treatment. The toilet anxiety associated with urinary tract infections in older populations should also be managed, as the symptoms may present differently compared to younger patients. In older patients, the diagnosis of a UTI requires the identification of new urinary symptoms, which can coexist with systemic findings such as fever and nonspecific malaise (Beveridge et al., 2011). This group may present with atypical symptoms, which can lead to diagnostic challenges; therefore, healthcare providers should be vigilant for even slight changes in urinary patterns. In this context, reliance on urinalysis is common; however, a paucity of evidence exists regarding its utility in diagnosing UTIs in older individuals. Thus, a comprehensive review of both physical and urinary symptoms plays a crucial role in determining the correct diagnosis and treatment protocols. Urinary tract infections also significantly impede the quality of life, particularly in patients with recurrent infections. The infections are characterized by increased frequency and urgency of micturition, where patients experience a compulsive urge to pass urine with little output of urine, accompanied by pain. This cycle of repetitive cravings can detrimentally affect normal day-to-day activities and social interactions, inducing psychological stresses such as anxiety and frustration. Moreover, patients with indwelling catheters are also at a higher risk for catheter-associated urinary tract infections, which underscore the need for alternative treatment methods for catheters to mitigate infection threats (Beveridge et al., 2011). Given that knowledge of the symptoms and their implications for patient health is the most critical, attention to educating patients on preventive actions can also diminish the impact of UTIs on one's welfare (Figure 10.9).

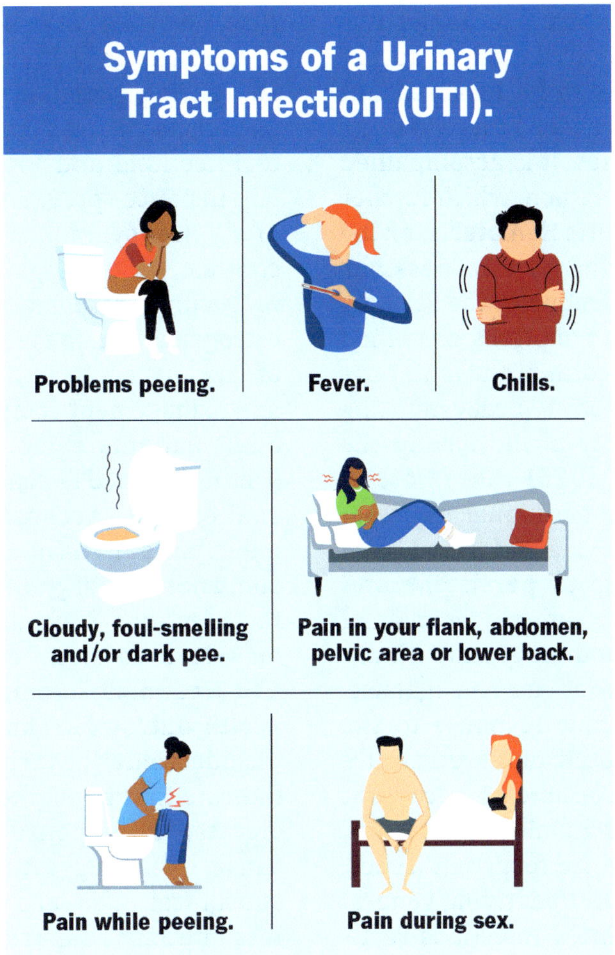

Figure 10.9. Symptoms of urinary tract infections.

Source: https://my.clevelandclinic.org/-/scassets/images/org/health/articles/9135-urinary-tract-infection.

10.3.1. Common Symptoms Experienced

The symptomatology of UTIs is characteristic and often epidemic, causing great distress for all who suffer from it. One of the typical symptoms is dysuria, a painful burning when they urinate. Patients will complain of an urgent need to urinate, one that is usually followed by the emission of small amounts of urine. This sensation is exacerbated by the presence of inflammation in the urinary system, making the experience all the more discomforting. Additionally, patients may experience an increased need to urinate, which, coupled with pain, can enormously impair activities of daily living. These symptoms not only herald the onset of an infection but also prompt individuals to seek medical attention for treatment, thereby initiating the diagnostic investigation necessary to diagnose and treat the infection successfully (Anton et al., 2025). A second frequent symptom from UTI patients is pain or discomfort in the lower abdomen. The cause of pain is inflammation of the bladder wall, also referred to as cystitis, and can range from mild irritation to severe cramping. The pain tends to be localized but can radiate, providing a broader sphere to one's general well-being. At times, it is accompanied by pain in the suprapubic region, which further enhances the clinical picture. Hematuria, or the presence of blood in urine, is also possible, which is a worrisome indication of the severity of the infection. All these symptoms combined affect not only physical health but also impose psychological trauma, thereby typically inducing anxiety and loss of quality of life among the infected (Bahari et al., 2025). Chronic and recurrent UTIs introduce additional layers of symptomatology. Patients may be faced with recurring bouts, leading to persistent and cyclical pain. In some cases, patients complain of symptoms extending beyond the typical urinary tract complaints, such as fatigue and malaise, and may portend a systemic response to the infection. It should be noted that women are usually particularly susceptible to recurrent infection, due in part to anatomical differences. Still, men also can experience recurrent issues, especially when there is an underlying general medical condition. That these infections recur may be a source of considerable distress and necessitate frequent medical intervention, which may include the use of prolonged antibiotic prophylaxis. A clear understanding of the entire array of symptoms associated with UTIs is crucial for developing effective management and prevention strategies (Anton et al., 2025).

10.3.2. Symptoms in Different Demographics

The manifestation of UTI symptoms may vary significantly among groups, depending on a complex interplay of biological, behavioral, and socioeconomic influences. Females tend to report the classic symptoms of UTIs, including dysuria, frequency, and urgency, due to their anatomic differences, specifically a shorter urethra that facilitates the ascent of pathogens. Also, women are bound to have varying symptomatology at various times in their lives, i.e., during pregnancy or menopause, where endocrine changes may influence susceptibility to infections and presentation of symptoms. For instance, pregnant patients will complain of atypical symptoms or increased urgency. In contrast, postmenopausal females will complain of recurrent infections because of reduced estrogen affecting the vaginal flora and integrity of the urinary tract, hence making diagnosis and management complicated. Conversely, older adult patients exhibit distinctive patterns of symptoms in UTI that make proper diagnosis challenging. According to clinical studies, older patients have atypical symptomatology; confusion, lethargy, or even falls are attributed to infection. Such an atypical presentation may lead to significant delays in diagnosis and treatment, ultimately resulting in poorer health outcomes. The findings of studies that included older participants aged 60 and above indicate that biomarkers of inflammation were elevated in response to microorganisms that cause UTIs, suggesting a high prevalence of subclinical infections within this age category. It is of utmost importance to understand these nuances, as standard criteria for diagnosis will underreport cases of UTIs in the elderly, and this age group requires more focused and specific clinical responses to treatment (Haley et al., 2024). Furthermore, demographic factors such as gender and injury status can significantly influence the incidence and nature of UTIs in groups with specific vulnerabilities, i.e., spinal cord injury patients. Indications are that patients with spinal cord injury suffer unnecessarily high rates of UTIs, mainly as a result of neurogenic bladder dysfunction and bladder management practices employed. For instance, users of intermittent catheterization have much higher rates of UTIs compared to other practices applied in bladder management. The most frequently isolated bacteria in such cases are *Escherichia coli* and Proteus mirabilis, necessitating targeted therapeutic interventions. Various populations of individuals with varying presentations of UTI emphasize the need to adopt individualized management to mitigate the risk of infection and enhance patient outcomes (Milicevic et al., 2024). Policies that target tailoring interventions to demographic information will most likely lead to more successful health pathways in affected individuals.

10.3.3. Complications from Untreated UTIs

UTIs can have a variety of complications when left untreated, particularly among vulnerable groups such as pregnant women. UTIs left untreated can extend from cystitis that is localized to severe infections such as pyelonephritis that could lead to systemic disease. Pyelonephritis is a serious health risk, with renal scarring and permanent kidney damage, but it also threatens maternal and fetal health. It can result in life-threatening conditions like preterm labor and low birth weight, emphasizing the importance of early detection and treatment during pregnancy. It is necessary in prenatal management to screen for asymptomatic bacteriuria (ASB) basis to avoid complications due to untreated UTIs, since ASB prevalence among pregnant women can range from 2-10%, according to clinical guidelines (Jajczak et al., 2025).

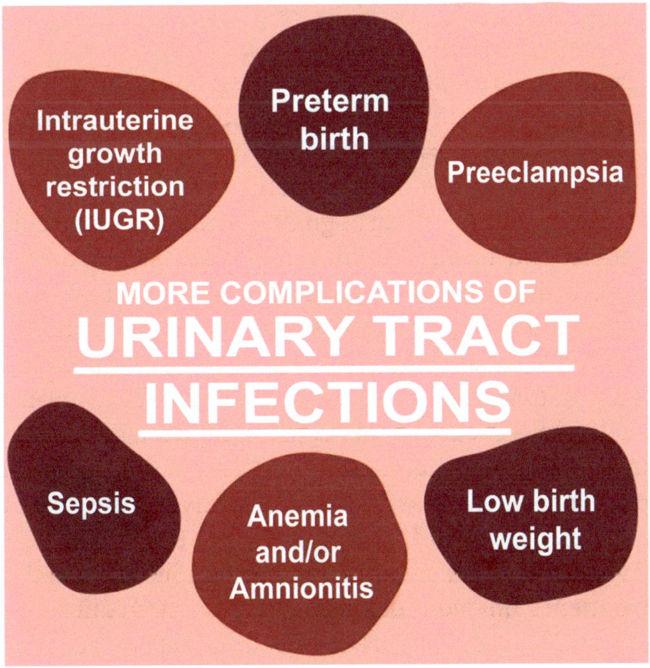

Figure 10.10. Complications from untreated UTIs.

Source: https://cdn-bnmhg.nitrocdn.com/kqzVLedydBgqCxIUpThxMOBZVWYWAftP/assets/images/optimized/rev-0fdd27d/www.abclawcenters.com/wp-content/uploads/2023/10/UTI4.jpg.

An untreated UTI may also cause serious systemic sequelae beyond the urinary tract. Acute kidney injury in such instances occurs when the kidneys are unable to clear waste products and maintain fluid balance due to infection-induced swelling and fibrosis. It may progress to chronic kidney disease (CKD) and place patients at risk for additional cardiovascular complications and renal impairment. In addition, evidence exists that untreated uncomplicated UTIs have the potential to cause life-threatening maternal morbidity, such as sepsis, an extreme response to infection that can result in multi-organ dysfunction. Because the broad-based effects of untreated infection on long-term well-being are so dramatic, the medical profession must emphasize the need for early intervention and appropriate treatment protocols to prevent disease exacerbation (Wassenaer et al., 2012). Moreover, the untreated UTI complications are heightened healthcare costs, driven by hospitalization and extended care for consequent conditions. Not only does delayed treatment heighten the chances of hospitalization because of more complicated infections, but it also necessitates extensive therapy for consequent chronic ailments resulting from initial UTIs. For instance, maternal pyelonephritis is not only a cause of acute health concerns like labor instability. Still, it may also increase the risk of neonatal complications to some extent, impacting both short-term and long-term health determinants for both the mother and newborn. Regular screenings and early antibiotic therapy—along with pregnancy-based considerations for safety—are thus essential parts in curbing the adverse consequences associated with UTIs (Wassenaer et al., 2012; Jajczak et al., 2025) (Figure 10.10).

10.4. Diagnosis of Urinary Tract Infections

Diagnosis of UTIs heavily relies on both clinical presentation and laboratory workup. Dysuria, urinary frequency, and urgency are reported symptoms in most cases. These usually prompt individuals to seek medical evaluation. Clinical presentation by itself might not always be sufficient to establish a diagnosis, particularly in atypical cases or in patients with co-morbidities, i.e., MS or diabetes. Diagnosis in the laboratory is typically made through urinalysis and urine culture, where the presence of nitrites, leukocyte esterase, and bacteria indicates a UTI. Proper diagnosis is significant since improper diagnosis can lead to inappropriate treatment and can further deteriorate the causative condition of urinary dysfunction. Urine culture is the gold standard for diagnosing UTIs, as it enables the identification of pathogens and determination of antibiotic sensitivity. Accuracy of urine cultures can be influenced by some factors, including the timing when urine is obtained and the patients' hydration. The use of clean-catch midstream samples as advised reduces contamination, hence making results more accurate. Other tests, such as rapid antigen tests, can also be used in diagnosis, providing quicker reporting but with lower sensitivity compared to standard culture. It is essential to comprehend the intricacies of UTI diagnosis, not only for the effectiveness of treatment but also to prevent complications such as recurrent infections or the development of antibiotic resistance. Education of patients on their disease and the importance of follow-up visits is also crucial in the management of UTIs. For recurrent infection, among other conditions, including MS, issues relating to continuation of treatment modalities like clean intermittent catheterization (CIC) need to be understood. Research indicates that ongoing support from healthcare providers and significant symptomatic improvement can aid compliance with CIC guidelines, eventually lowering the risk of UTIs. Additionally, addressing psychological obstacles and providing explicit instructions on infection prevention could encourage patient involvement and compliance. As evident from Elders et al. (2018), the interaction between effective self-management and outcome discloses the necessity of a comprehensive strategy in diagnosis and ongoing management of urinary tract infection (Figure 10.11).

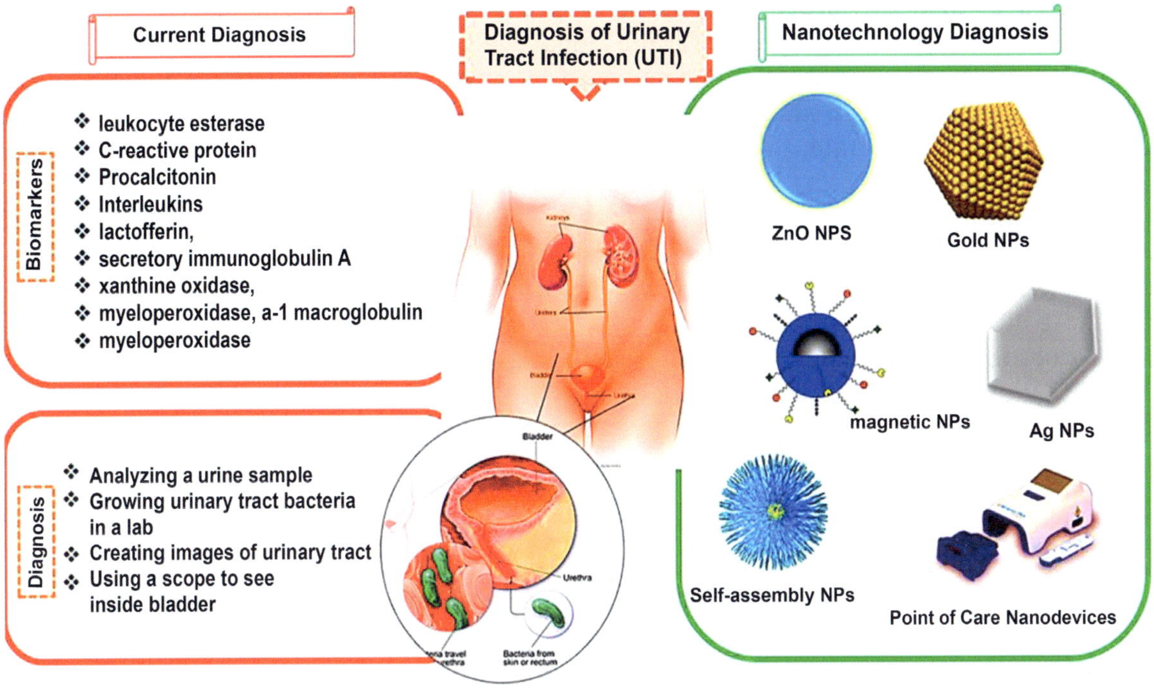

Figure 10.11. Diagnosis of urinary tract infections.

Source: https://www.mdpi.com/nanomaterials/nanomaterials-11-00546/article_deploy/html/images/nanomaterials-11-00546-g001.png.

10.4.1. Methods of Diagnosis

The diagnosis of UTI is mainly reliant on urine analysis by laboratory testing and clinical assessment. Historically, a constellation of symptoms, including dysuria, frequency, urgency, and flank pain, directs the clinician to a presumptive diagnosis. The urinalysis is then followed by assays for the presence of leukocyte esterase, nitrite, and hematuria. While these point-of-care tests may be utilized fairly frequently, they have variable sensitivity and specificity, resulting in both false negatives and false positives, particularly in high-risk populations, such as renal transplant patients. Contreras-Sanz et al. (2014) determined that conventional urinalysis methods may significantly undercount UTI prevalence, considering the necessity for more accurate diagnostic methodologies in this vulnerable population. With the evolution of the epidemiology of UTIs, improving diagnosis remains a critical area of focus in enhancing patient outcomes. In addition to routine urinalysis, urinary culture remains the gold standard in confirming the diagnosis of UTIs. The procedure involves cultivating the urine to identify the bacterial organism that causes the infection and its sensitivity to antibiotics. Although it is the gold standard, the process can be time-consuming, taking 24 to 48 hours to produce a result. Such a delay may interfere with early treatment, particularly for severe cases that necessitate prompt action. New techniques are also emerging on the horizon that could potentially be a speedier and more sensitive method for detecting infections, including the measurement of urinary ATP levels. For instance, research suggests that applying ATP measurement along with intracellular detection of bacteria in urothelial cells can significantly enhance diagnostic validity, potentially identifying infections that would otherwise go undetected by standard procedures (Contreras-Sanz et al., 2014). This change in diagnostic testing would quite fundamentally transform UTI management, particularly for populations at high risk of chronic infection. Research has also recently examined the application of non-antibiotic prophylactic agents in the treatment of UTI and emphasized careful diagnostic practices that inform treatment. To illustrate, the efficacy of N-acetylcysteine and D-mannose versus standard antibiotic therapy for preventing UTIs following urodynamic tests was compared in a clinical trial. The results indicated that there was no statistically significant difference in the incidence of UTI between the two prophylactic interventions, suggesting that these nutraceutical substances could be viable alternatives in specific contexts. As resistance to conventional antibiotics continues to increase, the incorporation of non-antibiotic options into diagnostic and treatment protocols may eventually become unavoidable. Thus, diagnostic methods not only need to confirm the presence of UTIs but also address the broader issue of antimicrobial resistance and the emergence of alternative therapeutic strategies, effectively redirecting the UTI management paradigm in practice.

10.4.2. Importance of Urine Culture

Urine culture is the foundation of the diagnostic evaluation in the treatment of UTIs, enabling clinicians to isolate pathogens with crystal-clear precision. Traditional approaches tend to employ urinalysis, which may be non-specific, particularly in cases of individuals presenting in a non-characteristic fashion, e.g., the elderly. Urine culture becomes necessary when the initial clinical assessment suggests a UTI, especially in cases involving nonspecific or absent symptoms. In the absence of specificity from urine culture results, treatment is inappropriately given, leading to overdiagnosis and unjustified antimicrobial exposure. According to Beveridge et al. (2011), it is vital to know the causative microorganism in order to make decisions regarding effective therapeutic regimens and guide correct antimicrobial stewardship. The utility of urine culture extends beyond determining the evidence of infection; it also forms the foundation for determining antimicrobial susceptibility. All infections must be treated using an evidence-based intervention to avoid promoting antibiotic resistance. This is particularly relevant in light of the rising trend in multidrug-resistant organisms, making UTI complicated. The local resistance pattern can be demonstrated using urine cultures, which are necessary for formulating individual treatment protocols. According to Beveridge et al. (2011), the application of local guidelines to urine culture results can enhance the efficacy of treatment regimens and reduce the risk of resistance by utilizing narrow-spectrum antimicrobial agents. Thus, the role of urine culture is twofold: to identify pathogens and assist the clinician's decision-making process in providing an intentional response to cases of UTI. Also, periodic urine culture analysis becomes imperative in specific patient populations, including chemotherapy-treated animals, as noted by a study among canines suffering from transitional cell carcinoma (TCC). In such situations, the incidence of UTIs is high, and the impact of the underlying disease may become crucial to the outcome of clinical conditions. Close follow-up of UTIs in these patients is necessary because it facilitates early treatment and management of potential complications from untreated infections. The findings of identify some determinants, such as sex and primary site of tumor, that influence the likelihood of positive cultures, which highlights the need for an individualized course of treatment. Therefore, urine cultures not only guide treatment but also provide information regarding patient-specific risk and hence contribute to patient benefit in the management of UTI (Figure 10.12).

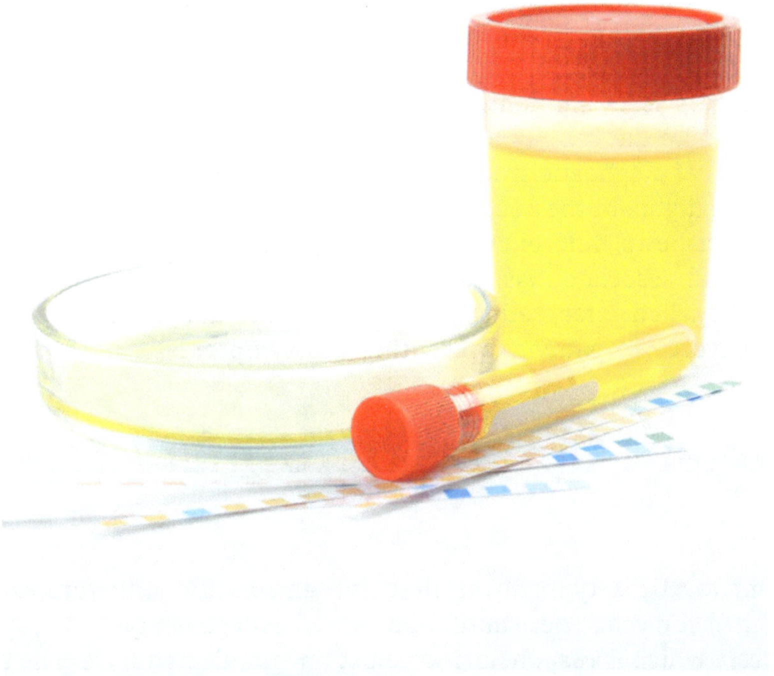

Figure 10.12. Importance of urine culture of urinary tract infections.

Source: https://myfloridalab.com/cdn/shop/files/uro_800x.webp?v=1707021795.

10.4.3. Differential Diagnosis Considerations

Differential diagnosis of UTI is necessary to ensure appropriate management and treatment. UTIs can present with a myriad of symptoms overlapping other conditions, and hence, proper diagnosis is essential. STIs, pyelonephritis, and even appendicitis, for instance, may be accompanied by such symptoms as dysuria and flank pain. Hence, the clinician must conduct a comprehensive assessment based on the patient's history, physical examination findings, and relevant laboratory tests. Proper differentiation of these conditions not only guides ideal treatment strategies but also avoids inappropriate intervention, which might follow in the case of a wrong diagnosis. As the sequelae of untreated UTIs, such as renal scarring and systemic infection, are of concern, differential diagnosis is a key area of management of patients. This necessitates a formal process to expedite the establishment of a correct diagnosis as early as possible. The use of rapid diagnostic tests has also emerged as a key factor in the differential diagnosis of UTIs, particularly among children. It has been found that the combination of dipstick testing for nitrite and leukocyte esterase can provide helpful information in excluding or including a diagnosis of UTI. For instance, both leukocyte esterase and nitrite dipstick test results strongly elevate the odds of UTI, supported by pooled likelihood ratios (LR^+). Conversely, a negative result on these tests is reasonable to exclude a diagnosis of UTI and trigger consideration for other illnesses such as STIs or other urinary tract diseases. Because accelerated testing can potentially significantly accelerate diagnosis and facilitate enhanced clinical decision-making, accelerated testing is nevertheless an integral aspect of the differential diagnostic process. Therefore, implementing these diagnostic approaches to clinical practice can improve outcomes by enabling timely and successful interventions in suspected cases of UTI (Doley et al., 2005). Additionally, the importance of methodological quality in diagnostic research cannot be overstated, particularly in the process of differential diagnosis for UTIs. The majority of diagnostic approaches rely on weak research methodology, and could even bias the effectiveness of diagnostic tests unintentionally. Using firmly established tools, such as QUADAS, helps practitioners evaluate the validity of research informing their differential diagnosis practice. Variations in the quality of diagnostic studies affect the reliability of conclusions about differential diagnosis, and therefore highlight the need for a critical appraisal of current evidence. As evidenced from recent systematic reviews, different diagnostic tests may behave differently based on the stage of clinical conditions and associated issues of quality (Biggi et al., 2005). This evidence informs clinicians to be vigilant when interpreting the results of the diagnostic tests, thereby enhancing the quality of care delivered to patients presenting UTI symptoms.

10.5. Treatment Options for Urinary Tract Infections

The initial treatment for UTIs typically is first-line antibiotics, nitrofurantoin, trimethoprim-sulfamethoxazole, and fosfomycin. These antibiotics work best against typical uropathogenic bacteria such as *Escherichia coli*, which is responsible for most uncomplicated UTIs. The choice of antibiotic is typically based on local resistance patterns and the patients' medical history, such as allergies and previous efficacy. However, the emergence of antibiotic resistance in uropathogens complicates treatment regimens. Thus, caregivers need to be up-to-date with alternative treatment strategies and resistance patterns to modify management practices accordingly. Finally, the deployment of appropriate first-line treatments is crucial in minimizing UTI morbidity, achieving optimal treatment outcomes, and preventing the development of enhanced resistance. In more advanced situations or in instances where first-line therapy is unsuccessful, second-line therapy in the guise of ciprofloxacin or levofloxloxacin may be employed. These fluoroquinolones have increased activity against multiply resistant bacteria and are particularly useful in the treatment of pyelonephritis or recurrent infection. The effectiveness of these agents is typically offset by potential side effects, including tendonitis and gastrointestinal discomfort, as well as concerns regarding their contribution to the development of resistance. Recent research suggests that combination therapies, specifically those involving colistin and other medications, can enhance outcomes for drug-resistant infections. Clinicians need to be aware of the implications of prescribing broader-spectrum drugs, balancing effective care with the risk of resistance (Angelis et al., 2017). Thus, a successful treatment of UTI should maximize both immediate efficacy and ultimate control. Furthermore, novel therapeutic methods are being developed as integral components of UTI therapy, particularly in the cases of multidrug-resistant pathogens. One of the more promising areas of research is bacteriophage therapy, founded on the viruses that selectively target bacteria, with the prospect of offering a novel means to combat resistant pathogens. In addition to bacteriophages, novel combinations of licensed antibiotics, such as meropenem and colistin, are being explored to enhance treatment efficacy against resistant infections (Angelis et al., 2017). Notably, nephrotoxicity issues with agents like colistin underscore the need for clinicians to balance risks versus benefits. With advancing research, the identification and utilization of novel antibiotics and other therapies emphasize the need to remain vigilant against the increasing microbial resistance as a background, ensuring that effective therapeutic interventions continue to be at hand for patients (Figure 10.13).

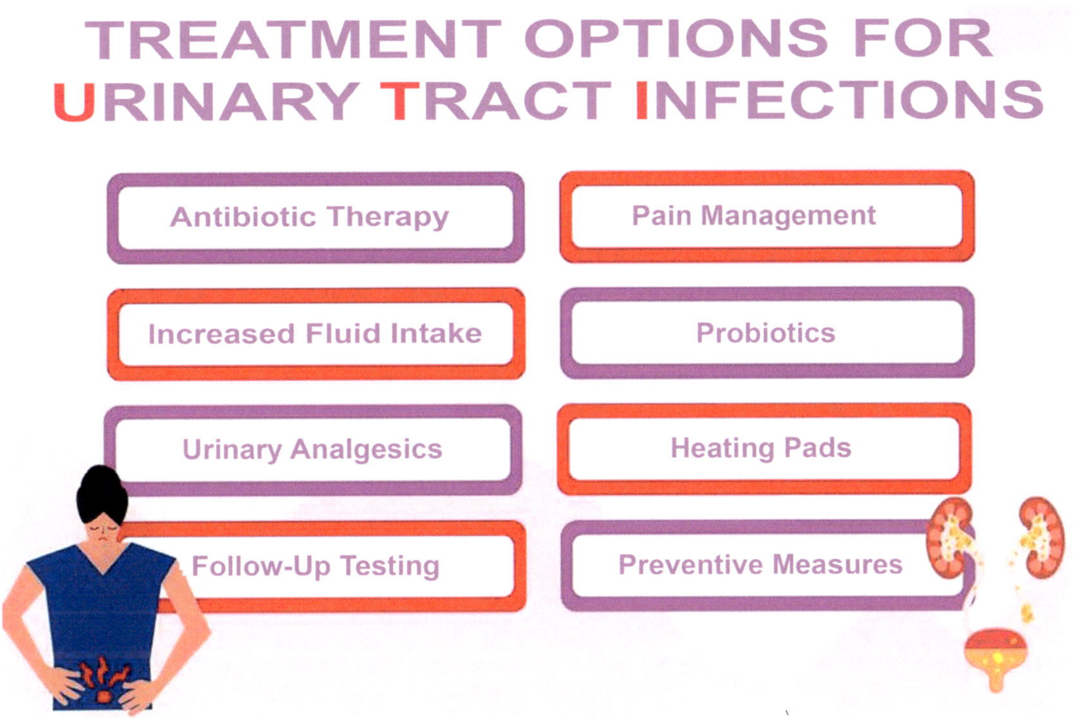

Figure 10.13. Treatment options for urinary tract infections.

Source: https://www.gardenobgyn.com/cdn-cgi/image/format=webp,width=1200,height=630/https://www.gardenobgyn.com/sms/dashboard/blog_img/1081254613.png.

10.5.1. Antibiotic Therapies

Antibiotic therapy is of paramount importance in UTI management, particularly in the setting of bacterial resistance complications. The selection of effective antimicrobials is typically guided by the susceptibility of the pathogens causing the infection. Trimethoprim-sulfamethoxazole and nitrofurantoin are often utilized as first-line antibiotics for uncomplicated UTIs due to their activity against most of the common uropathogens, such as *Escherichia coli*, for example. However, the emergence of multidrug-resistant pathogens necessitates individualized therapy. As seen in recent studies, infections with resistant strains, such as carbapenemase-resistant Klebsiella pneumoniae, require more aggressive treatment strategies, including combination therapy or newly licensed antibiotics that can overcome resistance barriers (Angelis et al., 2017). Local knowledge of resistance patterns is therefore crucial in achieving maximum therapeutic outcomes. Apart from the increasing rates of resistance, the preferred choice of antibiotic therapy should also consider patient factors, such as renal function and potential drug interactions. One study indicates that aminoglycoside monotherapy can be linked with higher mortality rates in specific circumstances, most importantly carbapenem-resistant Pseudomonas aeruginosa infections (Britt et al., 2018).

This indicates that combination regimens must be utilized in particular patient populations, particularly those afflicted with complicated UTIs. In general, as the leading treatment for UTIs, the trend is toward combining new drugs that can target resistant organisms without increasing side effects. New antibiotic development aims to provide clinicians with more powerful tools with which to fight the challenge posed by resistant organisms. Lastly, the approach to antibiotic therapy for UTIs is one of balancing efficacy and safety, particularly with respect to resistance patterns. Prescribers must maintain a sharp eye for making effective therapy selections, utilizing antimicrobial susceptibility testing and best practice guidelines. The advent of new drugs, like ceftazidime-avibactam, against resistant pathogens is a welcome advance in UTI treatment in the face of multidrug-resistant organisms. Furthermore, ongoing research on adjunctive therapies and other treatment regimens is necessary, as it provides new avenues for combating chronic and resistant infections. The quest to optimize antibiotic therapy for UTIs is thus a daily challenge that still requires ongoing adjustments and innovations in clinical practice (Figure 10.14).

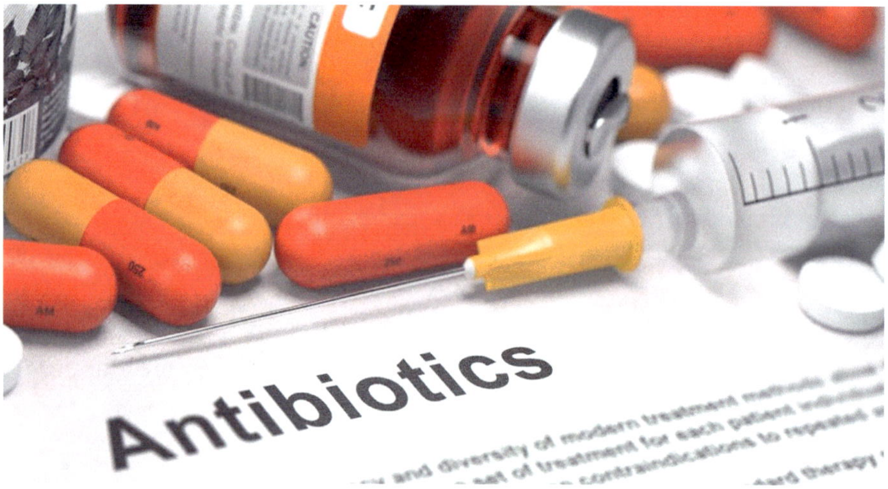

Figure 10.14. The role of antibiotics in UTI treatment.

Source: https://www.drrajeshdhakeurologist.com/wp-content/uploads/2023/06/antibiotic_resistance-9780-1024x538.jpg.

10.5.2. Home Remedies and Lifestyle Changes

Home remedies as well as lifestyle modifications are essential in preventing as well as managing UTIs. Increasing fluid intake, especially water, is a beneficial approach. The dilution of urine occurs, forcing the kidneys to urinate at shorter intervals and flushing out possible pathogens from the urinary tract, thereby decreasing the likelihood of infection. Additionally, natural diuretics such as cranberry juice have been brought into the limelight for their alleged function in preventing bacteria from adhering to the bladder lining of the urinary tract, but more research is needed to confirm this in full. Incorporating such home remedies into their lives can help individuals find a holistic alternative to the traditional medical interventions, addressing UTIs from preventive and therapeutic angles. Lifestyle modifications also play a tremendous role in UTI recurrence and overall urinary health. Frequent habits of cleanliness, especially after intercourse, play a key role in preventing the introduction of bacteria into the urinary tract. Wiping from front to back and voiding after coitus can also decrease the risk of infection. Additionally, wearing cotton undergarments over synthetic materials can reduce moisture accumulation and create an unfavorable environment for bacterial growth. Incorporating probiotic food in the diet also serves to strengthen the gut, which in its turn influences the balance of bacteria within the urogenital area. These actions demonstrate the interrelation between general health and the body's susceptibility to infection, emphasizing the importance of holistic interventions in maintaining health. Apart from dehydration and hygiene, stress management is another significant aspect of urinary health. Stress can impact the immune system, therefore potentially making an individual more susceptible to infections like UTIs. Engaging in stress-reducing practices, such as meditation, yoga, and regular physical exercise, can help ensure overall health and improve immune function. Moreover, proper rest is also crucial since it allows the body to heal and rejuvenate, increasing vigor and resistance to infection. The inclusion of these lifestyle changes may provide a considerable cornerstone towards avoiding UTIs as well as improving overall well-being. As such, lifestyle adjustments coupled with home remedies should not be overlooked in the overall cure and prevention of urinary tract infections (Alewijnse et al., 2016; Abdel-Fattah et al., 2018).

10.5.3. Preventative Measures

Preventive efforts are key in preventing the occurrence of UTIs, especially among high-risk groups like pregnant women. As research points out, the heavy use of antibiotics during pregnancy contributes to antimicrobial resistance (AMR) and necessitates a revision of preventive interventions. Involving patients in learning about their health and the consequences of antibiotic use is imperative. The majority of women also reported low self-efficacy in performing actions to maintain their health (Bandura et al., 2020). This suggests that educational interventions focused on self-management and behavioral change, targeting factors such as staying hydrated and maintaining hygiene, could be effective in reducing UTI episodes. Knowledge of the importance of water use, for instance, empowers individuals to take charge of their health and perhaps reduce demand for antibiotic therapy. In addition to behavioral interventions, public health interventions aiming at the broader setting within which UTIs occur are also essential. A UK national survey highlighted the importance of infection prevention programs in healthcare facilities, reporting that healthcare-associated infections (HAIs) continue to burden both patients and healthcare systems, with urinary tract infections (UTIs) being one of the primary concerns (Cairns et al., 2018). Integrating evidence-based infection control measures with education to focus on healthcare workers can significantly reduce the incidence of HAIs, including UTIs. Through educating the health workers with the capability of executing prevention practices, antibiotic overreliance can be minimized. Such holistic approaches can enhance patient outcomes while simultaneously addressing the significant rise in AMR. Furthermore, community hygiene and awareness campaigns for UTI risk factor promotion can also help in overall prevention practices. Educational programs that bring to the attention of the public the importance of proper wiping and toileting, the relevance of good hydration, and the impact of certain lifestyle conditions, such as the use of ventilation-friendly undergarments, are beneficial. Based on existing literature, most individuals lack awareness of their susceptibility to UTIs or healthy behaviors that can minimize their infection risk (Bandura et al., 2020). Hence, the development of specially crafted educational materials for distinct population groups, such as pregnant women and other at-risk groups, is crucial. Through the instillation of awareness and active health management, communities can come together to reduce the incidence of UTIs and ultimately their contribution to individual and community health (Figure 10.15).

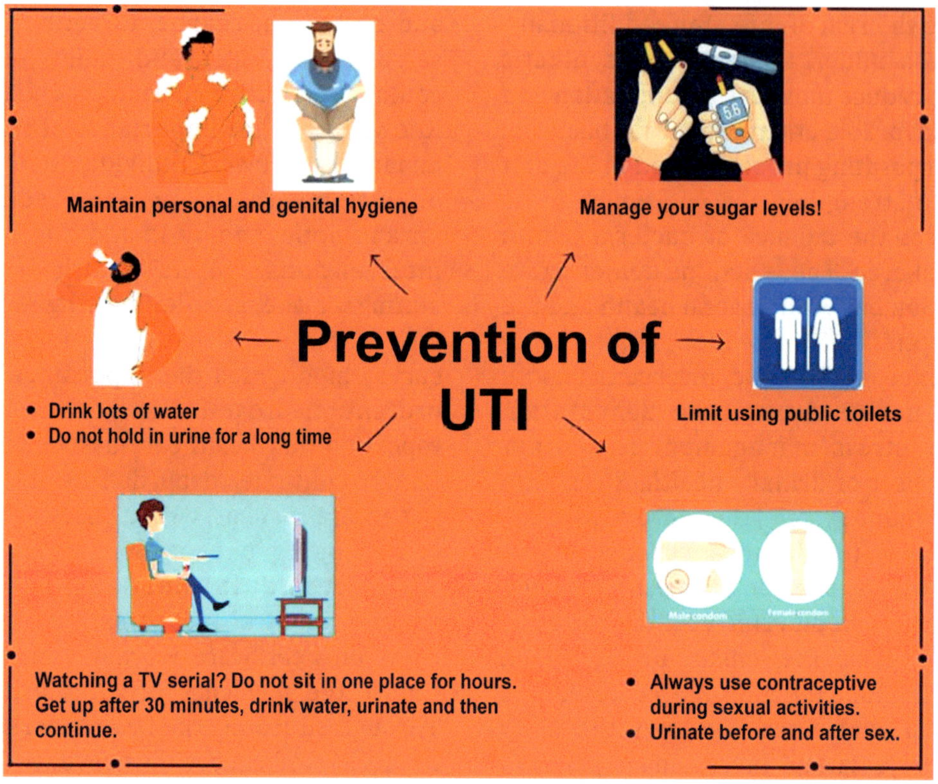

Figure 10.15. Preventative measures for urinary tract infections.

Source: https://cdn-ilaccmh.nitrocdn.com/DZJxrPEKJWZxQPoxxzOnTWilWyPSbula/assets/images/optimized/rev-4c15682/nhcancerclinics.com/wp-content/uploads/2024/05/asdq34234-1024x819.png.

10.6. Impact of Urinary Tract Infections

UTIs are a public health concern affecting patient health and healthcare spending. The pathogenesis of UTIs typically begins with bacterial colonization, which progresses to the development of mild to severe symptoms, including pyelonephritis. Because UTIs are more common among women due to anatomical factors, they often result in recurrent infections that can lead to increased healthcare use. Evidence shows that patients with recurrent UTIs usually experience a lower quality of life due to the severity of their chronic symptoms and the anxiety about possible future infections. Additionally, the economic burden of recurrent UTIs, including outpatient visits, laboratory assessments, and treatments, indicates the importance of effective management and prevention to minimize this common issue. The association between urinary catheter use and UTI is most challenging in hospitalized patients, especially in intensive care. Indwelling urinary catheters, although often necessary for patient monitoring and care, are associated with a significant risk of catheter-associated urinary tract infections (CAUTIs). There is evidence to suggest that the use of nurse-initiated orders for catheter removal can help reduce the incidence of CAUTIs in the intensive care unit. For instance, a piece of research revealed a 29% reduction in CAUTI cases after the implementation of protocols, demonstrating that systematic interventions can contribute to better patient outcomes. Although the findings lacked statistical significance for the general reduction, fewer CAUTIs mean shorter stays in hospitals, reduced antibiotic utilization, and lower healthcare costs, proving that stricter protocol refinement is necessary to minimize these infections among patients at most significant risk (Eckert-Davis et al., 2017). Resistance to antimicrobials is also a key factor in the management of UTIs. Most patients are treated with broad-spectrum antibiotics for UTI, a process that, while being focused towards acute patient care, is contributing to the emerging problem of antibiotic resistance. Compliance with practice guidelines for the treatment of UTI was seen to be shockingly low in one study, with 40% guideline practice adherence. This digression not only complicates the treatment scenario but can even lead to adverse outcomes in patients, including treatment failure and chronic infection. Further, culture results are a double-edged sword; while they may enhance compliance in some cases, it has been reported to decrease compliance with prescriptions for UTI. This multifactorial interaction highlights the importance of educating healthcare professionals about the significance of guideline implementation and appropriate antimicrobial use in efforts to reverse resistance and improve patient safety (Alvarez et al., 2005) (Figure 10.16).

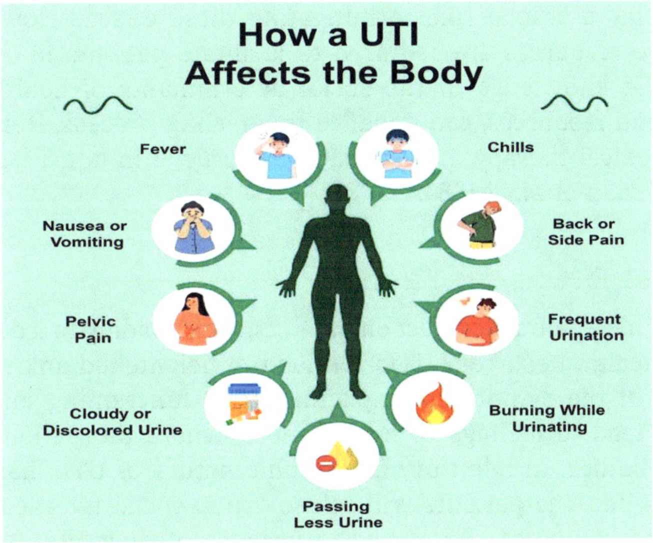

Figure 10.16. Impact of urinary tract infections.

Source: https://images.everydayhealth.com/images/seo-graphic-content-initiative/eh-how-a-uti-affects-the-body-seo-graphics.png?sfvrsn=e0ca9469_3.

10.6.1. Physical Health Implications

It is essential to learn about the physical health effects of UTIs because such infections could have a detrimental impact on a patient's overall health. UTIs are usually caused by the invasion of bacteria in the urinary tract, leading to symptoms such as pain, burning sensations during urination, and frequent urination. Such infections could advance to the kidneys unless treated, leading to more complex conditions such as pyelonephritis. In addition, systematic reviews have indicated that recurrent UTIs can significantly decrease a person's quality of life, with physical health consequences extending far beyond the urinary system. The discomfort and associated symptoms can lead to reduced physical activity, increased anxiety, and overall poor health outcomes. Therefore, early intervention, coupled with effective management strategies, should be emphasized to avoid these physical health dangers (Abdel-Fattah et al., 2018). Furthermore, UTIs have also been linked to systemic effects that can exacerbate existing medical conditions. For instance, those whose immune systems are already compromised are particularly vulnerable to the adverse impacts from UTIs, since the infection can further weaken their immune system and predispose them to disease. Recent studies have suggested that the body's immune reaction to a UTI may contribute to an exacerbation of chronic diseases, thereby producing an aggravated risk for such patients. This confluence of UTIs with other sickness concerns indicates the necessity for a comprehensive treatment approach, one that addresses not only the infection itself but also considers the broader implications for physical well-being. Failure to properly treat a UTI can result in an increased risk of future complications, underscoring the importance of understanding the systemic impact of such infections (Jenkinson et al., 2008). Further, the physical effects of UTIs also extend to lifestyle and behavioral factors affecting management and recovery. Recurrent UTI patients often report a significant alteration in their lifestyle, with school or work absenteeism, higher health costs, and productivity loss. Behavioral adjustments, such as enhanced fluid intake and adherence to antibiotic dosing schedules, can play a crucial role in mitigating these effects. However, both educational materials and healthcare resources are required to facilitate patients in managing the condition effectively. Education and knowledge of the social determinants of health, in conjunction with appropriate education and resources, can enhance the healing process. Hence, a multidisciplinary response comprising medical therapy and education is crucial in addressing the physical health effects of UTIs (Abdel-Fattah et al., 2018).

10.6.2. Psychological Effects on Patients

Psychologically, UTIs can have a notable effect on patients, often leading to a decrease in psychological well-being and mental health. Recurrent UTIs can lead to heightened anxiety and distress related to the unpredictability of the symptoms, impacting daily functioning and social relationships. Uncertainty is likely to lead to feelings of helplessness, where the patient feels they have little control over their own bodies. In addition, the chronic nature of UTIs has a debilitating impact on feelings of loneliness because patients will refuse group social interaction or close contact to prevent sudden pain or humiliation. From this experience of their illness, it is evident that the psychological aspect is not a secondary effect of physical discomfort but is instead a primary factor that plays an immense role in their overall condition and sense of quality of life. In examining the interactions between states of mind and physical health, research has indicated that psychiatric disorders such as adjustment disorder can be a contributing factor to the causation and severity of urinary infections. In one study among patients with adjustment disorder, there was found to be a higher rate of infection overall, along with urinary tract infection also being reported as more common among women than men. The findings confirm the complex interaction between psychological well-being and susceptibility to infection, with the stress of adjustment disorders being claimed to weaken immune systems and lead to adverse health outcomes. The link suggests considering mental health as well as physical health in treating patients, since ignoring the psychological nature of a patient's UTI experience may detract from treatment effectiveness and rehabilitation. In addition, the management and treatment of UTIs must also involve interventions that cater to the mental health aspects of patients. Interventions involving mental health care, such as cognitive-behavioral therapy, can help equip individuals with coping strategies and resilience to ease the cognitive load of UTI recurrences. Stress-reduction therapies have been shown not only to improve psychological symptoms but also to lower infection rates by strengthening the immune system. The incorporation of more comprehensive care modalities that address both physical and emotional symptoms gives patients more control and can lead to greater health improvement. The identification of the emotional effects on patients suffering from UTIs enables healthcare providers to provide more comprehensive interventions that acknowledge the multidimensional nature of human health and its resulting impact on treatment success.

10.6.3. Economic Burden of UTIs

The economic burden of UTIs is substantial, affecting both patients and healthcare systems. UTI is the most common healthcare-associated infection, representing approximately 17.9% of all acute hospital inpatient healthcare-associated infections, according to recent evidence. In addition to highlighting the clinical importance of UTIs, this prevalence underscores their significant economic costs, including diagnostic testing, therapeutic interventions, and potential hospitalization. The financial cost extends beyond immediate healthcare costs because recurrent UTIs can cost long-term use of healthcare services, which will mean overall higher costs to both patients with these infections and healthcare systems. In addition to direct costs, such as treatment and hospitalization, UTI financial costs also involve indirect costs attributed to lost productivity. Its victims experience chronic lack of work or school attendance, and consequently lose wages and diminished quality of life. UTIs also cause complications such as pyelonephritis, which require more intense treatment and hospitalization and therefore indirectly raise costs. The economic burden of these infections is not limited to the acute setting; non-acute hospitals also experience a high incidence of UTIs, with these infections accounting for 28.1% of healthcare-associated infections in the non-acute hospital setting (Allardice et al., 2008). The broad incidence in over one healthcare setting confirms that interventions must be implemented to reduce UTIs. Preventive measures and prompt treatments would significantly lower the economic impact attributed to UTIs. Increased expenditure on education, including proper hygiene methods and safe drinking practices, may reduce infection rates and thereby alleviate the burden on healthcare resources. In addition, increased progress in more efficient prophylactic treatments would reduce recurrence rates, hence reducing the cost of continuing healthcare. To combat the economic burden of UTIs, therefore, requires a multi-faceted approach based on consideration of prevention, treatment optimization, and best practice facilitation in hospitals and outpatient facilities (Abdel-Fattah et al., 2018). The spread of UTIs can not only benefit individuals but also alleviate healthcare systems' financial costs, resulting in a greater emphasis being placed on UTI management campaigns.

SUMMARY

A critical analysis of UTIs underscores the need for increasing treatment and diagnostic quality. UTI burden extends beyond the symptomatic care alone; it impacts patient quality of life, cost in hospitals, and patterns of antibiotic use. As evidence from recent studies demonstrates, there are tremendous rates of inappropriate antibiotic prescribing, particularly among emergency medicine physicians. Ineffective treatment not only fails to effectively treat infections but also contributes to the rapid development of antibiotic-resistant bacterial strains, thus underscoring the need for evidence-based compliance (Chardavoyne et al., 2020). Lastly, the effective treatment of UTIs requires a multi-step approach that involves proper diagnostic procedures, individualized treatment protocols, and ongoing education of healthcare professionals. In addition to improving antibiotic stewardship, additional research is needed on the normative UTI investigation routines, particularly in children. Available evidence suggests that routine investigations are largely ineffective in improving long-term outcomes, such as reducing the risk of renal scarring (Biggi et al., 2005). This is an argument for reevaluating common procedures used when treating UTIs in children in favor of more efficient and less invasive methods. Original research on the subject is the greatest demand, for it is by way of sound research that medical practitioners can establish protocols that address not just immediate symptoms but also shield against future repercussions. For truly revolutionizing the management of UTI, there must be a convergence of efforts from healthcare practitioners, researchers, and policy-makers. This could be achieved through the development of holistic training programs with an orientation towards evidence-based principles, as well as public awareness programs targeting urinary tract health among the general public. Furthermore, policies to encourage judicious use of diagnostics and therapeutic interventions are necessary to combat the looming threat of antibiotic resistance. By establishing an environment dedicated to evidence-based practices, it is possible to create a path towards improved health and reduced UTI occurrence in both the short and long term. By collaborating on these efforts, the medical community can strive to significantly reduce the prevalence of UTIs among patient populations.

UTIs are a critical public health issue, particularly when taking into account how often they occur in certain groups, such as women, who become infected more frequently than men. Such frequency is caused by anatomical and physiological factors, such as the fact that in females, the urethra is shorter and narrower. Additionally, the risk factors for UTI go beyond anatomical details and encompass lifestyle, cleanliness habits, and intercurrent conditions such as diabetes or urinary retention. It is crucial to understand these concepts, as they can influence not only prevention but also treatment strategies, ultimately leading to better outcomes in affected patients. Understanding the multifaceted nature of UTIs is essential for developing targeted education programs that reduce incidence rates and improve health literacy among vulnerable populations. Further, another critical aspect of management of UTIs is the relevance of understanding implications in patients receiving clean intermittent catheterization (CIC), especially patients with chronic illnesses such as multiple sclerosis. Research has shown a number of factors influence the abandonment or continued use of CIC, including the frequency of urinary tract infections experienced during CIC administration, and learning. Infections due to this can psychologically discourage patients from continuing with CIC, forming the possibility of an infection complication loop. Therefore, healthcare professionals must prioritize establishing intensive care systems, which can include educational components on infection prevention and symptom management. This way, the healthcare professionals will be able to promote substantial compliance with CIC and consequently enhance the quality of life in infected patients (Elders et al., 2018). In addition, interventions aimed at reducing UTI incidence during the adaptation period of CIC are also critical. Proactive measures, such as patient-specific education and supportive follow-up, can help provide a more assistive experience for individuals making the transition to CIC. Through research, there is an emphasis on ongoing clinical support and individualized care planning to reduce the risk of infection at this pivotal time. Additionally, developing measures to assess a patient's readiness and willingness to adopt CIC can be invaluable in facilitating a smoother transition. These strategies, aside from offering solutions to the immediate healthcare issues associated with UTIs, also empower patients with information and confidence to handle their condition effectively (Abdel-Fattah et al., 2018). To conclude, a combined approach to understanding and treating UTIs has the potential to improve overall health outcomes and patient satisfaction.

CLOSER LOOK

VESICOURETERAL REFLUX (VUR)

VUR is a urologic anomaly in which urine abnormally drains backward from the bladder into one or both ureters and, in the presence of severe VUR, into the kidneys. The retrograde flow inappropriately interferes with the standard one-way urinary drainage system. It puts the patient, particularly children, at risk for recurrent UTIs and also potential long-term renal damage. VUR occurs as a failure of the VUJ—the area where the ureter enters the bladder—to function as an adequate valve. Usually, the ureter passes over the bladder wall in a curved fashion, and with bladder filling and contraction, pressure on the ureter closes it off to prevent backflow. In VUR, either the anti-reflux mechanism is congenitally inadequate or is compromised by acquired disease, leading to pathological reflux of urine.

VUR is of two types: primary and secondary. Primary VUR is more common and is secondary to a ureterovesical junction birth defect, resulting in a short intramural ureter and an incompetent valve. It has a familial tendency and presents with a diagnosis made in infancy or early childhood as part of screening for febrile UTIs. Secondary VUR, on the other hand, is typically acquired and results from increased bladder pressure secondary to obstruction or abnormal voiding, such as posterior urethral valves or a neurogenic bladder. VUR is also graded I to V based on severity and grade of reflux, as seen on a voiding cystourethrogram (VCUG). Grade I is backflow into a non-dilated ureter, and Grade V is extreme dilation and coiling of the ureter and renal pelvis with obliteration of papillary impressions.

VUR children can be clinically seen with recurrent febrile UTIs, a cause of concern for pyelonephritis by ascending infection and scarring of the kidney. In some cases, it may be diagnosed after a chance detection of hydronephrosis in prenatal or postnatal imaging. Symptoms may be fever, irritability, poor feeding, abdominal or flank pain, and enuresis. Ultimately, if not treated or severe, VUR can progress to renal damage, hypertension, proteinuria, and chronic kidney disease, especially if the diagnosis is late or if treatment is inadequate.

Diagnosis of VUR is established by imaging studies such as renal ultrasound to evaluate for hydronephrosis and scarring, and VCUG to diagnose and quantify the reflux. A nuclear medicine scan, like DMSA (dimercaptosuccinic acid), in some cases is used to look for renal scarring. Treatment depends on the severity of the reflux, the patient's age, UTI status, and renal status. Mild grades (Grades I–III) naturally resolve with increasing age, and are managed conservatively with watchful waiting and prophylactic antibiotics for UTIs. Severe grades (Grades IV–V) or complicated by recurrent infections or renal injury can be handled by surgical correction by means of ureteral reimplantation or minimally invasive endoscopic injection with bulking agents like Deflux.

References

1. Pickard, R., Chadwick, T., Oluboyede, Y., Brennand, C., Von Wilamowitz-Moellendorff, A., McClurg, D., Wilkinson, J., Ternent, L., Fisher, H., Walton, K., McColl, E., Vale, L., Wood, R., Abdel-Fattah, M., Hilton, P., Fader, M., Harrison, S., Larcombe, J., Little, P., . . . Thiruchelvam, N. (2018). Continuous low-dose antibiotic prophylaxis to prevent urinary tract infection in adults who perform clean intermittent self-catheterisation: the AnTIC RCT. *Health Technology Assessment, 22*(24), 1–102. https://doi.org/10.3310/hta22240Abdel-Fattah, M., Brennand, C., Chadwick, T., Fader, M., et al. (2018). Continuous low-dose antibiotic prophylaxis for adults with repeated urinary tract infections (AnTIC): A randomized, open-label trial. https://core.ac.uk/download/293885024.pdf (accessed on 25th June 2025).

2. Al Rawashdah, S., Al Salhi, Y., Carbone, A., Coppola, G., et al. (2017). Prospective study to compare antibiosis versus the association of N-acetylcysteine, D-mannose and *Morinda citrifolia* fruit extract in preventing urinary tract infections in patients submitted to urodynamic investigation. https://core.ac.uk/download/98337961.pdf (accessed on 25th June 2025).

3. Aleandri, M., Ambrosi, C., Conte, A., Conte, M., et al. (2016). The adherent/invasive *Escherichia coli* (AIEC) strain LF82 invades and persists in human prostate cell line RWPE-1 activating a strong inflammatory response. https://core.ac.uk/download/54536849.pdf (accessed on 25th June 2025).

4. Alewijnse, A., Alhasso, A., Alves, S., Amaro, J. L., Balshem, H., Bastian, H., et al. (2016). Conservative interventions for urinary incontinence in women: An overview of Cochrane systematic reviews. https://core.ac.uk/download/293881644.pdf (accessed on 25th June 2025).

5. Allardice, G. M., Coubrough, S., Noone, A., Reilly, J., et al. (2008). Results from the Scottish national HAI prevalence survey. https://core.ac.uk/download/9023284.pdf (accessed on 25th June 2025).

6. Alvarez, A., McCaig, D. J., Bearden, D. T., Ibrahim, E. H., Brown, E. M., European Antimicrobial Resistance Surveillance System, Haaijer-Ruskamp, F. M., et al. (2005). Limited effect of patient and disease characteristics on compliance with hospital antimicrobial guidelines. https://core.ac.uk/download/pdf/12919553.pdf (accessed on 25th June 2025).

7. Angelis, M. D., Mascellino, M. T., & Oliva, A. (2017). Multi-drug-resistant Gram-negative bacteria: Antibiotic-resistance and new treatment strategies. https://core.ac.uk/download/227029142.pdf (accessed on 25th June 2025).

8. Anton, C. I., Ștefan, I., Zamfir, M., Ghiațău, C. F., Sima, C., Osman, C. L., Ștefan, T. A., et al. (2025). Etiology and risk factors of recurrent urinary tract infections in women in a multidisciplinary hospital in Romania. *Microorganisms, 13*. https://www.semanticscholar.org/paper/1c234faea8d86f3987269746da8d228b5cbcb375 (accessed on 25th June 2025).

9. Bahari, H., Tajik, A., Doostparast, A., Shahrokh Abadi, R. N., Javanshir, S., Aliakbarian, M., & Khodashahi, R. (2025). Antibiogram pattern of recurrent urinary tract infections in kidney transplant patients: A single-center cohort study. *Clinical Transplantation and Research*. https://www.semanticscholar.org/paper/79f84613831d9c9480835d059d782a116d9e7421 (accessed on 25th June 2025).

10. Baho, S., Czapnik, P., & Samarasinghe, S. (2019). Preliminary analysis of the anti-biofilm efficacy of manuka honey on extended spectrum β-lactamase producing *Escherichia coli* TEM-3 and *Klebsiella pneumoniae* SHV18, associated with urinary tract infections. https://core.ac.uk/download/228189014.pdf (accessed on 25th June 2025).
11. Bandura, A., Elzayat, M. A., Ghouri, F., Luszczynska, A., Ogden, J., et al. (2020). 'There is no choice apart from antibiotics...': Qualitative analysis of views on urinary infections in pregnancy and antimicrobial resistance. https://core.ac.uk/download/288346181.pdf (accessed on 25th June 2025).
12. Bartoszewicz, J., Gorajek, A., Grądzik, A., Kudan, M., et al. (2022). Urinary tract infections in children–A review. https://core.ac.uk/download/587245945.pdf (accessed on 25th June 2025).
13. Baskin, L., Cao, M., Cunha, G. R., Liaw, A., et al. (2018). Development of the human bladder and ureterovesical junction. https://core.ac.uk/download/323311351.pdf (accessed on 25th June 2025).
14. Beveridge, L. A., Davey, P. G., McMurdo, M. E. T., Phillips, J., et al. (2011). Optimal management of urinary tract infections in older people. https://core.ac.uk/download/20450519.pdf (accessed on 25th June 2025).
15. Biggi, A., Fretzayas, A., Gervaix, A., Haberlik, A., Hitzel, A., Hitzel, A., Piepsz, A., et al. (2005). Further investigation of confirmed urinary tract infection (UTI) in children under five years: A systematic review. https://core.ac.uk/download/57941.pdf (accessed on 25th June 2025).
16. Biggi, A., Fretzayas, A., Gervaix, A., Haberlik, A., Hitzel, A., Hitzel, A., Hoberman, A., et al. (2005). How does study quality affect the results of a diagnostic meta-analysis? https://core.ac.uk/download/57953.pdf (accessed on 25th June 2025).
17. Bonnici, J. J. (2014). Urinary tract infections in the community. https://core.ac.uk/download/46603064.pdf (accessed on 25th June 2025).
18. Britt, N. S., Burnham, C. A. D., Durkin, M. J., Hampton, N., et al. (2018). Importance of site of infection and antibiotic selection in the treatment of carbapenem-resistant *Pseudomonas aeruginosa* sepsis. https://core.ac.uk/download/212861648.pdf (accessed on 25th June 2025).
19. Budreckis, D. M., Byrne, B. A., Pollard, R. E., Rebhun, R. B., et al. (2015). Bacterial urinary tract infections associated with transitional cell carcinoma in dogs. https://core.ac.uk/download/323071867.pdf (accessed on 25th June 2025).
20. Cairns, S., Gibbons, C., King, H., Llano, M., et al. (2018). Results from the third Scottish National Prevalence Survey: Is a population health approach now needed to prevent healthcare-associated infections? https://core.ac.uk/download/293863931.pdf (accessed on 25th June 2025).
21. Chardavoyne, P., & Kasmire, K. E. (2020). Appropriateness of antibiotic prescriptions for urinary tract infections. https://core.ac.uk/download/305124072.pdf (accessed on 25th June 2025).
22. Chataway, J., Curtis, C., Haslam, C., Pakzad, M., et al. (2016). Urinary tract infections in multiple sclerosis. https://core.ac.uk/download/79505036.pdf (accessed on 25th June 2025).
23. Chew, D. J., Daniels, J. B., Irom, S., Keil, D., et al. (2012). Evaluation of the efficacy and safety of high-dose short-duration enrofloxacin treatment regimen for uncomplicated urinary tract infections in dogs. https://core.ac.uk/download/323068657.pdf (accessed on 25th June 2025).

24. Claxton, A., Kirby, A., Mifsud, A., Rodgers, A., Johnson, A. P., Abernethy, J., Barbadoro, P., et al. (2016). Epidemiology of *Escherichia coli* bacteremia in England: Results of an enhanced sentinel surveillance programmed. https://core.ac.uk/download/74235355.pdf (accessed on 25th June 2025).

25. Contreras-Sanz, A., Farmer, C. K., Peppiatt-Wildman, C. M., Courtneidge, H. R., Malone-Lee, J., Durodie, J., Kelley, R., et al. (2014). Urinary ATP and visualization of intracellular bacteria: A superior diagnostic marker for recurrent UTI in renal transplant recipients? https://core.ac.uk/download/30706795.pdf (accessed on 25th June 2025).

26. Doley, A., Hoberman, A., Hoberman, A., Hoberman, A., Weinberg, A. G., Rodriguez Caballero, A. M., Aronson, A. S., et al. (2005). Rapid tests and urine sampling techniques for the diagnosis of urinary tract infection (UTI) in children under five years: A systematic review. https://core.ac.uk/download/57944.pdf (accessed on 25th June 2025).

27. Drzewiecka, D., Kwil, I., Maszewska, A., Moryl, M., Ostrowska, K., et al. (2013). *Proteus* sp. – An opportunistic bacterial pathogen–Classification, swarming growth, clinical significance and virulence factors. https://core.ac.uk/download/71976791.pdf (accessed on 25th June 2025).

28. Dzeing-Ella, A., Rougemont, A., Murray, B., Wolf, B. H. M., Olaleye, B. O., Guerra, C. A., CLSI, et al. (2012). Prevalence and predictors of urinary tract infection and severe malaria among febrile children attending Makongoro Health Centre in Mwanza City, North-Western Tanzania. https://core.ac.uk/download/pdf/11307801.pdf (accessed on 25th June 2025).

29. Eckert-Davis, L. (2017). The impact of a nurse-driven Foley catheter removal protocol on catheter associated urinary tract rates in critical care areas. https://core.ac.uk/download/213032097.pdf (accessed on 25th June 2025).

30. Elders, A., Buckley, B., Bugge, C., Creswell, J. W., McClurg, D., Fowler, C. J., Moore, K. N., et al. (2018). Factors affecting continuation of clean intermittent catheterization in people with multiple sclerosis: Results of the COSMOS mixed-methods study. https://core.ac.uk/download/293885223.pdf (accessed on 25th June 2025).

31. Farkas, D. K., Galea, S., Gradus, J. L., Jiang, T., et al. (2020). Associations between adjustment disorder and hospital-based infections in the Danish population. https://core.ac.uk/download/288432803.pdf (accessed on 25th June 2025).

32. Flower, A., Hollywood, A., Mercer, B. M., Costelloe, C., Towers, C. V., Wing, D. A., Department of Health, et al. (2018). A systematic review of non-antibiotic measures for the prevention of urinary tract infections in pregnancy. https://core.ac.uk/download/156784544.pdf (accessed on 25th June 2025).

33. Haley, E., Luke, N., Mathur, M. C., Festa, R. A., Wang, J., Jiang, Y., Anderson, L. A., et al. (2024). The prevalence and association of different uropathogens detected by M-PCR with infection-associated urine biomarkers in urinary tract infections. *Research and Reports in Urology*, *16*, 19–29. https://www.semanticscholar.org/paper/65d5b4d6585d5ceeb27ebbe3fa11b1cecb1648cd (accessed on 25th June 2025).

34. Hamid, R., & Losco, G. (2014). Pelvic organ prolapse-associated cystitis. https://core.ac.uk/download/29410932.pdf (accessed on 25th June 2025).

35. Jajczak, M., Jesionek, S., Kałuziak, P., Kaźmierczak, A., et al. (2025). Review of urinary tract infections in pregnancy: Risks, complications and management. https://core.ac.uk/download/636385688.pdf (accessed on 25th June 2025).

36. Jenkinson, D., Englyst, H., Hamidon, S., Kwan, J., Kammersgaard, L., Vassallo, M., et al. (2008). Systemic infections after acute stroke. https://core.ac.uk/download/293885223.pdf (accessed on 25th June 2025).

37. Kesav, N. R. (2024). Development of a urothelial cell line expressing a caspase-1 biosensor to measure cellular inflammatory responses to potential uropathogens. https://core.ac.uk/download/621510305.pdf (accessed on 25th June 2025).

38. Kirdis, H. (2011). Development of novel methods for microbiological evaluation of urology products. https://core.ac.uk/download/622419122.pdf (accessed on 25th June 2025).

39. Milicevic, S., Sekulić, A., Nikolić, D., Tomašević-Todorović, S., Lazarević, K., Pelemis, S., Petrovic, M., et al. (2024). Urinary tract infections in relation to bladder emptying in patients with spinal cord injury. *Journal of Clinical Medicine, 13.* https://www.semanticscholar.org/paper/278e657600227917800c99a718afee81f8a85f94 (accessed on 25th June 2025).

40. Musa, S., & Rrustemi, Q. (2025). Urinary tract infections classification and nursing management. https://core.ac.uk/download/656543434.pdf (accessed on 25th June 2025).

41. N'Dow, J., & Wilt, T. J. (2008). Benign prostatic hyperplasia: Part 2–Management. https://core.ac.uk/download/4193265.pdf (accessed on 25th June 2025).

42. Öborn, H. (2014). Lower urinary tract dysfunction in children with chronic kidney disease: Before and after renal transplantation. https://core.ac.uk/download/70341161.pdf (accessed on 25th June 2025).

43. Sauerwein, D., Trudeau-Vanhems, E., Tanagho, E. A., Van Kerrebroeck, E. V., Egon, G., Wielink, G., Creasey, G. H., et al. (2003). A 7-year follow-up of sacral anterior root stimulation for bladder control in patients with a spinal cord injury: Quality of life and users' experiences. https://core.ac.uk/download/pdf/11480324.pdf (accessed on 25th June 2025).

44. Sursyakova, T. V., Safyanova, S., Dronov, D. Y., & Kozlov, D. Y. (2022). Assessment of the influence of risk factors for the development of urinary tract infections as a form of ISMP on the example of large multidisciplinary hospitals in the Altai Territory. *Sanitarnyj Vrač (Sanitary Doctor).* https://www.semanticscholar.org/paper/f9882ad296fcb68bced72b93c9654f407efc91fe (accessed on 25th June 2025).

45. Van Wassenaer, A., Ott, A., Macejko, A. M., Bedford Russell, A. R., Mol, B. W. J., Anderson, B. L., Kazemier, B. M., et al. (2012). Costs and effects of screening and treating low-risk women with a singleton pregnancy for asymptomatic bacteriuria, the ASB study. https://core.ac.uk/download/pdf/15477453.pdf (accessed on 25th June 2025).

46. Yao, Y., Tao, L., Ma, L., Fan, Y., Zheng, D., Wang, J., & Chen, W. (2025). Etiological factors and development of a predictive model for urinary tract infections in cervical cancer patients undergoing intensity-modulated radiotherapy. *Infection and Drug Resistance, 18*, 1637–1645. https://www.semanticscholar.org/paper/df4851040921ea31a8d50199df890e3dff7d50b9 (accessed on 25th June 2025).

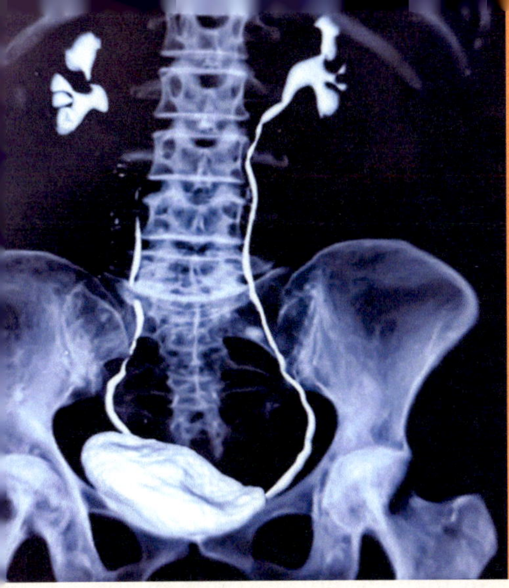

Chapter 11

OBSTRUCTIVE UROPATHY AND UROLITHIASIS (KIDNEY STONES)

Contents

Introduction

The development of obstructive uropathy and urolithiasis, which are often in the form of kidney stones, represents a significant urological health concern. Obstructive uropathy is the presence of an obstruction within the urinary tract that disrupts the normal flow of urine. The condition can be brought about by a variety of etiologies, like anatomical abnormalities, tumors, or the presence of kidney stones, crystalline formations secondary to alterations in metabolism. Although the presence of these stones can be solitary, their role as a contributory cause to obstructive uropathy is very suspicious. The coexistence of the two conditions usually supports a clinical presentation, and hence morbidity and potentially renal failure in cases of poor management. Obstructive uropathy and urolithiasis can be diagnosed and detected using state-of-the-art diagnostic apparatus. Traditional methods, such as intravenous urography, have been the norm in this field; however, increased knowledge of their limitations has prompted an examination of alternative imaging modalities. Ultrasound, for example, has appeared as a method that does not expose the patient to ionizing radiation while still sufficiently illustrating the presence or absence of calculi and approximating obstruction in the urinary tract. In addition, the combination of kidneys, ureters, and bladder (KUB) X-rays with ultrasound provides higher detection rates for ureteral stones, as suggested by the fact that this technique is superior to IVU in isolation (Ismail et al., 2001). Thus, the shift toward more efficient diagnostic techniques is part of a broader movement to improve patient care within urological practice. The latest literature presents Doppler ultrasound as a valuable aid in diagnosing urinary obstruction, thereby expanding the scope for non-invasive evaluation. For instance, intrarenal arterial Doppler studies can effectively identify both obstructed and unobstructed kidneys. A cohort study of 54 patients confirmed a significant elevation of resistivity index (RI) values between obstructed and normal kidneys, attesting to the efficacy of this method (Mohamed et al., 2018). This enhancement of diagnostic accuracy not only makes obstructive uropathy easier to manage but also minimizes the risks associated with more intrusive imaging modalities, such as CT scans. With continued progress in understanding urolithiasis and obstructive uropathy, the integration of state-of-the-art diagnostic interventions is essential for achieving optimal patient outcomes and enhancing overall urological health (Figure 11.1).

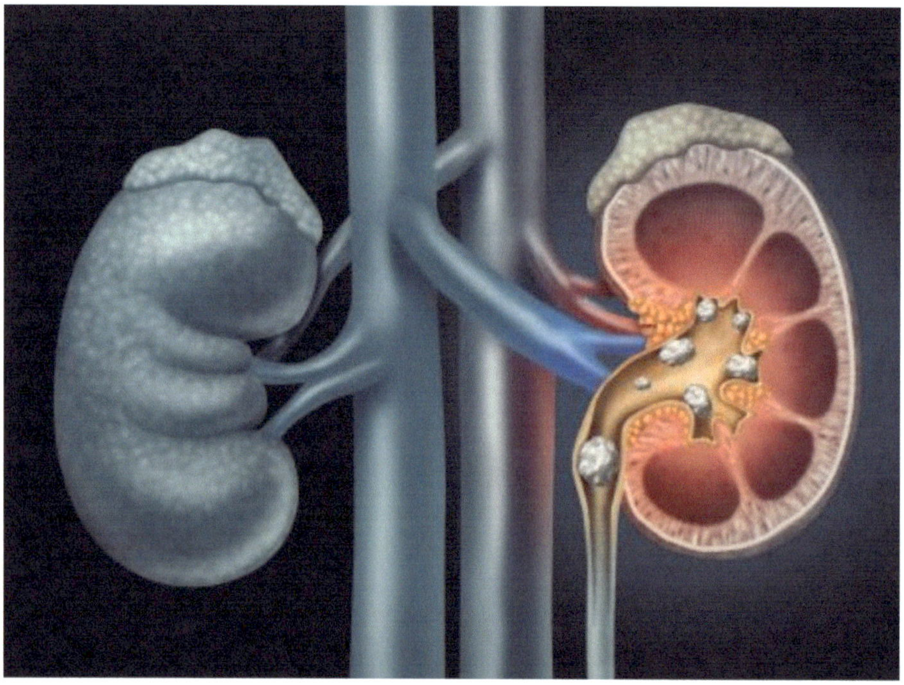

Figure 11.1. Obstructive uropathy and urolithiasis (kidney stones).

Source: https://www.aapc.com/codes/webroot/upload/articles_pdf/2023/uca/Art2_p3.webp.

Definition of Obstructive Uropathy

Obstructive uropathy is a serious clinical condition characterized by impairment of urine flow through the urinary tract, resulting in detrimental changes to renal function. Obstruction can occur in various segments of anatomy, ranging from the kidneys themselves to the ureters, bladder, or urethra. The common causes include urolithiasis, stricture, tumor, and prostatic hypertrophy, which can all lead to impairment in the normal drainage of urine. Consequently, the affected kidneys are likely to undergo renal pelvis and calyces dilation, a condition referred to as hydronephrosis, that can jeopardize renal parenchyma and cause irreparable damage if not managed. Furthermore, the duration and magnitude of the obstruction play a critical role in determining the degree of renal impairment that the patient will experience. Thus, diagnosis and early treatment of obstructive uropathy are necessary to preserve renal function. Clinical manifestations of obstructive uropathy are more than mere anatomical obstruction; they typically result in profound physiological changes in renal architecture. If the urine cannot drain normally, increased intraluminal pressure stresses the renal tissues, which can produce inflammatory and fibrotic responses. This process can later result in acute renal failure, for which early diagnosis and treatment become a necessity. In patients of urolithiasis, several factors can predispose them to the formation of obstructive uropathy, including a history of urinary tract infections and the presence of other comorbidities. For instance, studies highlight the manner in which female gender and urinary tract infections significantly increase the risk of complications such as sepsis or acute pyelonephritis in the event of ureteral stones (Asero et al., 2022). It is thus crucial to understand the multifaceted nature of obstructive uropathy so that effective therapeutic strategies can be developed. Obstructive uropathy is typically diagnosed with the assistance of newer imaging modalities to ascertain the severity and location of the obstruction. Ultrasound remains a first-line imaging modality, with the ability to demonstrate hydronephrosis and other structural disease. In certain circumstances, Doppler ultrasonography can provide information on renal vascular flow patterns. Studies have indicated that elevated values of the resistivity index (RI) in obstructed kidneys can be good predictors of severe obstruction (Mohamed et al., 2018). This non-invasive technique not only aids in the diagnosis and confirmation but also allows for direction of the urgency and mode of treatment from conservative care to surgery. An appreciation for the central role of early diagnosis in obstructive uropathy helps further to emphasize the interrelatedness of the disease with urolithiasis, further illustrating the necessity for holistically managed regimens in those thus affected.

Overview of Urolithiasis (Kidney Stones)

Urolithiasis, or more commonly referred to as kidney stones, is a prevalent disease characterized by the existence of solid mineral deposits in the renal system. Kidney stones vary in size, make-up, and clinical presentation, and will tend to induce obstructive uropathy if left untreated. The pathophysiology is multifaceted and arises as a consequence of complicated biochemical changes leading to supersaturation of the urine with stone-forming substances such as calcium, oxalate, uric acid, and phosphate. Risk factors for stone development include dehydration, unhealthy eating habits, metabolic disorders, and certain genetic predispositions. Notably, the incidence of kidney stones is on the rise worldwide, and it is particularly significant because the recurrence rate can be greater than 50% in five years following a first episode, highlighting the need for adequate prevention and patient education. Diagnosis of urolithiasis typically involves a combination of laboratory examinations and imaging modalities to determine stone composition and assess urinary tract obstruction. Traditionally, intravenous urography was the gold standard for diagnosing nephrolithiasis; however, this method has limitations, including exposure to ionizing radiation and the use of contrast media, which can be harmful to patients (Ismail et al., 2001). As a counter measure, non-invasive diagnostic imaging modalities such as plain abdominal X-rays and ultrasound are rapidly gaining popularity because of their safety and efficacy in the detection of renal calculi. To a greater extent, the combination of ultrasound and KUB X-rays significantly enhances the detection rates of calculi, especially in cases suspected of ureteral involvement. This shift toward safer diagnostic techniques reflects the evolving outlook on these diseases and the importance of accurate diagnosis in the effective treatment of urolithiasis. In recent years, studies have sought to elucidate the potential of medical prophylaxis for preventing recurrent kidney stones, particularly with novel therapeutic agents. One of the research targets is sodium/glucose cotransporter isoform 2 inhibitors, which have been shown to produce a 30%-50% reduction in stone rates in diabetic patients (Bally et al., 2022). Why this has the effect it does is not clear, and therefore, their application must be studied in non-diabetic stone formers too. As can be deduced from trials such as the SWEETSTONE trial, researchers aim to quantify how drugs like empagliflozin can affect urinary supersaturation levels, thereby reducing stone event recurrences in non-diabetic subjects. Ultimately, this is a response to the necessity of a comprehensive treatment approach for urolithiasis, involving not only pharmacotherapy but also lifestyle modifications to alleviate the disease burden (Figure 11.2).

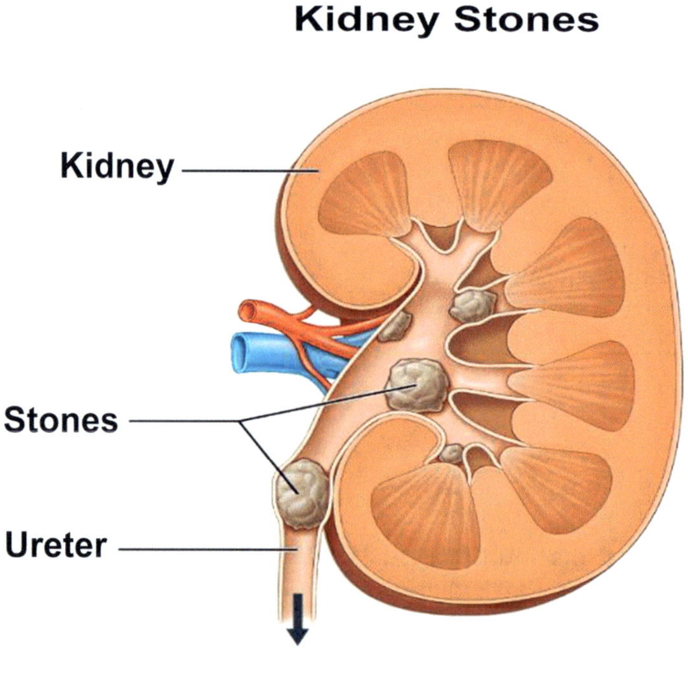

Figure 11.2. Overview of urolithiasis.

Source: https://www.niddk.nih.gov/-/media/Images/Health-Information/Urologic/Kidney-stones-English-labels.jpg?imbypass=true.

Importance of Understanding These Conditions

A proper understanding of urolithiasis and obstructive uropathy is needed for effective clinical management and patient care. Physicians familiar with these conditions can diagnose and initiate corrective interventions at an early stage, thus avoiding complications such as chronic kidney disease or renal failure. Obstructive uropathy must be diagnosed early, as prolonged obstruction can lead to irreversible injury to the kidneys. In addition, various methods of diagnosis, such as ultrasound or Doppler ultrasound, enhance the ability to accurately evaluate kidney function, as seen with the utility of the RI in assessing vascular resistance in obstructed kidneys. Understanding the mechanisms and consequences of these diseases enables medical experts to apply the appropriate treatments on time, thereby facilitating a favorable prognosis and lifestyle for patients. Furthermore, knowledge of the pathophysiology of urolithiasis enables targeted prevention, significantly advancing public health. Recognizing risk factors such as dietary intake, fluid intake, and hereditary predisposition, health professionals can advise patients on how to implement lifestyle changes to reduce the likelihood of forming stones. For instance, the implantation of the requirement for adequate fluid consumption that helps dilute urine is critical in preventing supersaturation of the minerals responsible for creating the stones. Preventive interventions, with a deeper understanding of the condition, may lead to fewer emergency treatments and hospitalizations later on, thus reducing healthcare costs and promoting a healthier populace overall. Such a shift from reactionary to proactive treatment highlights the importance of understanding the intricate nature of obstructive uropathy and urolithiasis in clinical practice. It is vital to place research and education front and center on these conditions, as developments in therapeutic techniques and diagnostic technology continue to evolve. Understanding the diagnostic utility of alternative imaging modalities, such as Doppler ultrasonography and KUB, as referenced by recent publications, allows for a more precise definition of obstructive pathology with reduced unnecessary ionizing exposures (Ismail et al., 2001). In addition, studies comparing intrarenal arterial Doppler recordings in obstructive and non-obstructive kidneys (Mohamed et al., 2018) highlight the critical role of novel modalities in enhancing diagnostic accuracy. While highlighting ongoing research provides clinical information with added depth, it also lays the foundation for more sophisticated treatment methods, ultimately leading to improved patient care for the treatment of obstructive uropathy and urolithiasis.

11.1. Anatomy of the Urinary System

The urinary system is essential in keeping the body's homeostasis in check through the regulation of fluid balance, electrolytes, and the excretion of wastes. Consisting of the kidneys, ureters, bladder, and urethra, each organ is involved in the systematic process of urine creation and expulsion. The kidneys are bean-shaped organs located retroperitoneally, and they filter the blood, reabsorb vital substances, and excrete the waste products as urine. In the kidney, the nephron is the functional unit in which glomerular filtration initiates the process of urine formation. This dynamic setup highlights the importance of studying urinary anatomy, particularly in cases of obstructive uropathy and urolithiasis, as any disruption in this system can lead to severe clinical complications. With obstructive uropathy, the anatomy of the urinary tract may be significantly altered, bringing about unfavorable effects if not addressed. Obstruction can occur anywhere along the path of the urinary system, such as at the ureters, where stones in the kidneys are most commonly lodged. Renal pelvis and calyceal dilatation will typically follow as a result to an obstruction and may be visually assessed with ultrasound techniques. Of interest here, the evolution of modalities used for diagnosis, such as ultrasound and KUB, has enhanced renal colic and obstructive uropathy evaluation. A study identified that integrating KUB with ultrasound enhances detection rates of calculi considerably, demonstrating the use of these imaging modalities in understanding the contribution of urinary anatomy towards obstructive conditions (Ismail et al., 2001). RI is also a significant diagnostic biomarker in the evaluation of obstructive uropathy. Intrarenal arterial Doppler ultrasound was used to distinguish between obstructed and nonobstructed kidneys in a study conducted among patients with unilateral acute renal colic. The mean RI is significantly higher in obstructed kidneys compared with normal ones, highlighting the physiological changes associated with obstruction. An RI greater than 0.7 offers extremely high specificity and sensitivity in the diagnosis of acute renal obstruction, thereby avoiding potentially risky CT scans and minimizing patient exposure to ionizing radiation. These findings confirm the role of Doppler ultrasound in assessing the anatomical and functional status of the urinary system, providing key information for the management of urolithiasis and obstructive uropathy (Mohamed et al., 2018).

11.1.1. Structure and Function of the Kidneys

The kidneys are highly developed organs that play a crucial role in maintaining homeostasis in the human body. The anatomy of a kidney comprises an outer renal cortex and an inner renal medulla, both of which are organized into functional units known as nephrons. Each nephron contains a glomerulus for filtration and a tubule for reabsorption and secretion. The kidneys regulate electrolyte balance, fluid balance, and waste elimination through a complex filtering process. Therefore, any defect in the kidney structure or function will lead to severe health conditions, which primarily are obstructive uropathy and urolithiasis. They mainly lead to an impairment of the urinary tract, leading to renal damage and reduced ability to filter, which is crucial to consider when it comes to kidney pathology and how it impacts overall well-being. The functional capability of the kidneys is then evaluated using other imaging techniques, such as Doppler ultrasonography. This non-invasive method assesses blood perfusion through the renal vasculature and enables the diagnosis of obstructive uropathy based on the measurement of renal artery RI. In a prospective study of patients presenting with unilateral acute renal colic, it was demonstrated that obstructed kidneys demonstrated a significantly higher mean RI compared to unobstructed kidneys, with correlation to elevated perfusion pressure in obstructed segments (Mohamed et al., 2018). This correlation suggests that the kidneys' capacity to regulate intrarenal blood supply is impaired in obstruction, a condition that can lead to ischemia and further nephron injury if left untreated. Understanding the structure and function of the kidneys is valuable, especially in the case of kidney stones, which can lead to obstructive uropathy.

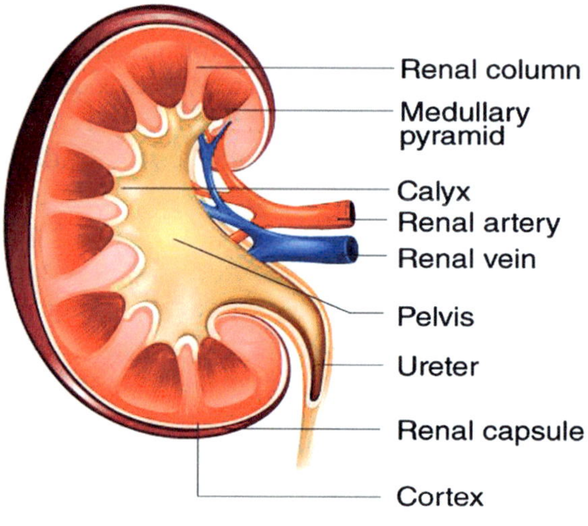

Figure 11.3. Structure and function of the kidneys.

Source: https://cdn1.byjus.com/wp-content/uploads/2022/06/kidney-diagram.png.

The formation of kidney stones, or urolithiasis, occurs in the renal tubules, where precipitation of crystalline material due to supersaturation and altered urine composition leads to the formation of kidney stones. The impact of stones on renal function can be considerable as they can obstruct the flow of urine and lead to hydronephrosis, a dilatation of the renal pelvis and calyces (Ding et al., 2009). Both obstructive uropathy and kidney stones require a thorough understanding of renal anatomy and physiology to devise effective treatment strategies that eliminate obstruction and restore kidney function, highlighting the interconnection between these clinical conditions (Figure 11.3).

11.1.2. Role of the Ureters and Bladder

The ureters and bladder play crucial roles in the removal and storage of urine, making them vital components of the urinary system. Ureters are muscular tubes that are employed to transport urine from the kidneys to the bladder by peristaltic movements. This ensures homeostasis by ensuring the adequate removal of waste products and excess fluid from the body. In urolithiasis and obstructive uropathy, these structures can be compromised by obstructions caused by stones in the kidney or by other disease processes. Such obstructions have the potential to cause increased pressure in the urinary tract and the subsequent formation of hydronephrosis, an accumulation of retained urine in one kidney. It is essential to address these obstructions promptly to prevent permanent damage to the kidneys and overall health. The bladder is a temporary storage reservoir for urine, leading to urination. The bladder's capacity for urine storage allows intermittent, rather than continuous, elimination, which is crucial for social function. The detrusor muscle, which is the smooth muscle of the bladder, contracts during micturition to force urine out of the bladder down the urethra. However, diseases like obstructive uropathy can have a significant impact on bladder function, which is most often reflected in symptoms of decreased capacity and frequency of micturition. Such impairment can be an additional clinical challenge in the context of urolithiasis if ureteric stones lead to obstructive pathology in the bladder. Benign etiology of obstructive uropathy is seen to be more prevalent in some studies, and therefore, there must be early management to prevent such complications. Knowledge of the behavior of kidney stones in the ureters and bladder is crucial to individuals who treat such conditions. More recent imaging modalities, such as CT urography, have revolutionized our approach to the bladder and ureters in the context of obstructive uropathy. Imaging tests enable the evaluation of the entire urinary tract, providing visualization of structural and functional ureteric abnormalities.

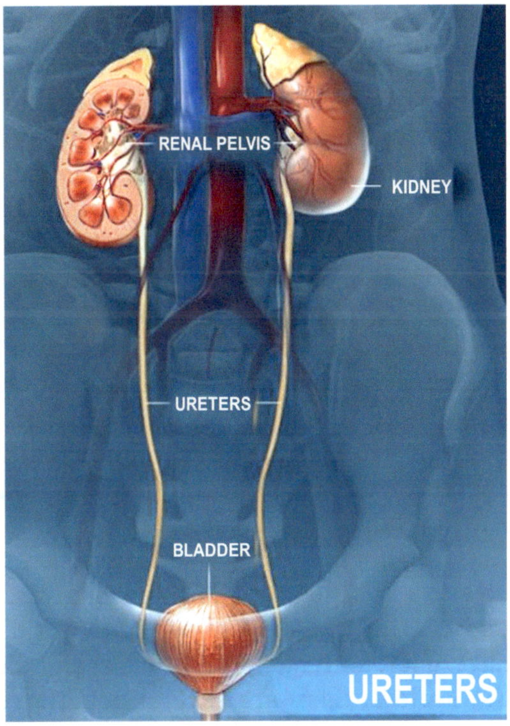

Figure 11.4. Role of the ureters and bladder.

Source: https://dreminozbek.com/wp-content/uploads/2024/08/Ureter.jpg.

To demonstrate, CT urography can characterize ureteral obstructions, providing useful information on the site, type, and severity of the obstruction. Exhaustive studies have reported a predominance of benign causes for obstruction, whereas malignant causes contributed significantly to high-grade hydronephrosis. The relevance of such technologies cannot be overstated, as they enable timely diagnoses and inform treatment planning. The nuanced findings from such imaging studies not only contribute to the management of kidney stone patients but also provide additional information regarding the interdependencies of the ureters, bladder, and extensive urinary system, affirming their critical contribution to renal function (Ismail et al., 2001; Kaginalkar et al., 2024) (Figure 11.4).

11.1.3. Pathways of Urine Flow and Potential Obstruction Points

Urine flows from the renal system in a specific path that originates from the kidneys and terminates at the bladder. After blood is filtered by nephrons in the kidneys, it forms urine, which moves into the renal pelvis and subsequently to the ureters. Urine is transported to the bladder by a peristaltic wave through muscular tubes. Obstructive uropathy, however, can occur anywhere along this pathway, rendering urine flow futile and potentially harmful. Obstruction can result from anatomical abnormalities, strictures, or, most significantly, kidney stones, which have the potential to clog the ureters. Obstruction not only hampers normal excretion but is also associated with heightened intrarenal pressure, with consequent permanent kidney damage, if left untreated (Wagenius et al., 2021). In the ureters, there are several notable sites of obstruction that are particularly prone to obstruction. As an illustration, the ureteropelvic junction, the site where the renal pelvis transitions into the ureter, is a common location for congenital or calculous obstruction. Similarly, the mid-ureteral segment and ureterovesical junction are essential locations that become obstructed by stone development or by extrinsic pressure of nearby tissue. Such obstructions carry clinical importance, one of which is hydronephrosis—a dilation of the renal pelvis due to urine unable to escape. With greater pressure from such obstructions, the risk of infection and ultimate renal compromise is dramatically increased, emphasizing the urgency of medical intervention to abate normal urine flow (N/A, 2022).

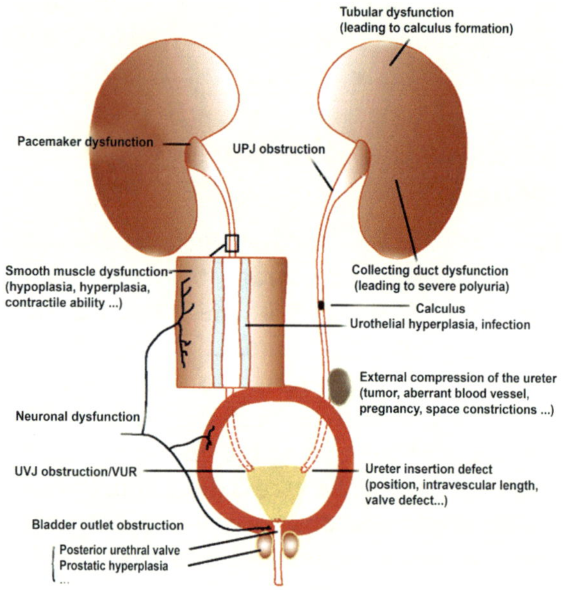

Figure 11.5. Pathways of urine flow and potential obstruction points.

Source: https://media.springernature.com/lw685/springer-static/image/art%3A10.1007%2Fs00467-008-1072-y/MediaObjects/467_2008_1072_Fig1_HTML.gif.

Clinical implications of obstructive uropathy underscore the importance of identifying these pathways and their potential sites of obstruction. When it comes to urolithiasis treatment planning, doctors must be specific and particular regarding the size and location of kidney stones since different-sized stones at specific sites of obstruction are more at risk for complications such as elevated infections and renal failure. Emergent treatments, such as ureteroscopy or lithotripsy, may be used in the management of obstructions, particularly for stones near fragile anatomical junctions. Also, research into newer techniques of urinary stenting may potentially provide alternative interventions for maintaining urine flow in patients with recurrent obstruction. As knowledge about such pathways and sites of obstruction increases, so does the potential for improved patient outcomes for the management of obstructive uropathy and its complications (Figure 11.5).

11.2. Causes of Obstructive Uropathy

The pathogenesis of obstructive uropathy is extensive and can be caused by numerous anatomical and pathological reasons. Most likely, the most frequent cause is urolithiasis or the presence of urinary stones that can occur anywhere in the urinary system. When the stone obstructs the ureter, it restricts the drainage of urine from the kidney, leading to increased pressure within the urinary tract. This backflow can result in hydronephrosis, an enlargement of the kidney caused by urine reflux. However, it is not just mechanical blockages that cause uropathy; cancerous growths also play their role. Neoplastic processes may invade or compress the ureters, further interfering with urinary drainage and adversely impairing renal function.

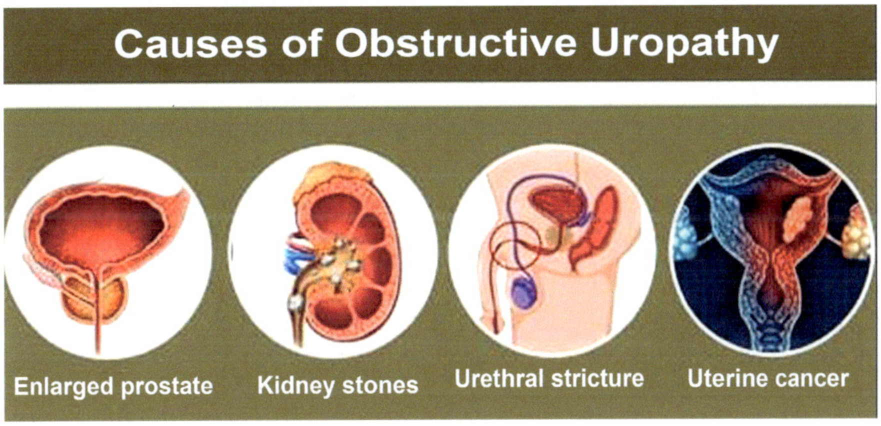

Figure 11.6. Causes of obstructive uropathy.

Source: https://images.medindia.net/patientinfo/450_237/causes-of-obstructive-uropathy.jpg.

A second crucial cause of obstructive uropathy arises from external sources, such as pelvic masses or other systemic processes that impinge upon the urinary system. Pregnancy is a condition that produces temporary obstruction as the expanding uterus compresses the ureters. Further, BPH in older men is a common benign cause of urethral obstruction. Prostate enlargement can impede the flow of urine and produce analogous effects to stone obstruction. It is important to recognize such extrinsic causes early because they may require urgent intervention to avoid permanent damage to the kidneys or worsening morbidity. Proper imaging and careful clinical evaluation are necessary to determine the etiologies and develop effective management plans. On a more somber note, malignant ureteral obstruction (MUO) is particularly challenging for physicians, given the complexity involved with treating the same. Advanced cancers may usually cause MUO and would need personalized treatment timetables because of the unique presentation and with each case presenting different complications. The limited clinical data available are insufficient for establishing standardized protocols in treating MUO, hence supporting personalized assessment. Based on research, the early resolution of obstructive conditions is crucial as it directly affects the preservation of renal function and patient prognosis (Brînză et al., 2018). In addition, the application of ureteral stenting in the alleviation of obstruction has also been practical in preserving kidney function following relief, demonstrating the need for early intervention (Danarto et al., 2019). Management of the cause of obstructive uropathy is essential in maintaining renal function and optimizing patient benefit (Figure 11.6).

11.2.1. Anatomical Abnormalities

Anatomical defects play a significant part in the pathogenesis of obstructive uropathy and urolithiasis. The defects may manifest as congenital malformation, for example, ureteropelvic junction (UPJ) obstruction or pelvic renal ectopia, and may cause blockade in the free flow of urine from the kidneys. Obstruction poses a threat to urinary stasis, leading to the development of kidney stones due to the accumulation of minerals and salts in the urine. The occurrence of these anatomical abnormalities not only increases the complexity of anatomy but also in clinical management. It is crucial to be aware of the implications of these conditions in order to plan proper treatment, as anatomically abnormal patients may require specialized endourological or surgical correction to restore urinary flow without leading to other complications, such as infection or renal injury. Calyceal rupture, secondary to urinary tract obstruction, is a classic demonstration of the profound effect of anatomical defects on kidney function. Resulting from the extravasation of urine from the kidney calyces, this condition occurs most frequently as a result of increased intrapelvic pressure due to anatomical defects that cause obstruction. The ruptures set the stage for serious complications in the form of infection and the formation of perinephric urinomas, which act to exacerbate renal damage. Early diagnosis and treatment of calyceal rupture are necessary to avert such risks. A proper imaging investigation, such as non-contrast CT scans, is for diagnosis and the assessment of the severity of the condition in patients who have had past nephrolithiasis or other anatomical defects. Such interventions not only play a role in diagnosis but also guide therapeutic interventions, which ultimately lead to positive patient' outcomes. The management of patients with anatomical defects in urolithiasis and obstructive uropathy also underscores the need for a multidisciplinary management approach. Radiologists, urologists, and nephrologists must collaborate to develop an overall treatment plan that addresses both the stone disease and the underlying pathology. For instance, endourological minimal-invasive procedures have proven useful in managing renal stones with anatomical abnormalities, allowing for the extraction of the stone without impairing renal function. Long-term follow-up management is also an essential in monitoring the recrudescence of the stones and the potential development of secondary complications due to the original anatomical defects. Thus, the detection and management of anatomical deviations are crucial for improving outcomes and providing efficient, patient-focused care for patients with obstructive uropathy and urolithiasis.

11.2.2. Tumors and External Compression

The tumor-extrinsic compression interaction has significant implications for obstructive uropathy, a condition that arises when there is an obstruction to urinary outflow. Tumors in the pelvis or adjacent organs can compress the ureters, causing them to fail to transport urine from the kidneys to the bladder. Obstruction can lead to backpressure and secondary renal complications such as hydronephrosis. The clinical assessment of this condition would often involve the use of imaging techniques, such as ultrasound or CT scans, to establish the presence and extent of tumors that may be producing urinary obstruction. Care should be taken that the various types of tumors, benign or malignant, with similar obstructive presentations, are recognized by healthcare workers, since management and treatment would primarily be based on the nature and aggressiveness of the tumors. In uropathy due to obstruction, the role of extrinsic compression is not restricted to neoplastic masses but involves many structural malformations and disease processes that are capable of diverting normal urinary tracts. To illustrate, supplanting cysts or benign prostatic hyperplasia can cause severe ureteral obstruction. Not only do such compressive forces disrupt normal urinary flow, but they can, if not alleviated, cause chronic renal injury. Physiologic reactions to such increasing pressures include renal parenchymal alterations that can be measured quantitatively by advanced imaging modalities, such as shear-wave elastography. It has been proven that elevated intrapelvic pressure has been found to correlate with increased shear-wave speed in renal parenchyma, indicating an increase in stiffness by both benign and malignant tumor obstructions (Saffari et al., 2018). Understanding these dynamics is crucial for developing effective diagnostic and treatment strategies. In addition, proper diagnosis of the obstructive uropathy secondary to tumors or compression necessitates a multidisciplinary opinion by urologists, oncologists, and radiologists. Due to the heterogeneity of the underlying causes of urinary obstruction, a successful treatment program must be designed to address both the immediate effects of the obstruction and the underlying pathology. External compression can require surgical intervention, particularly when there are tumors. On the other hand, pharmacotherapy can be an adjunct once long-term interventions are under consideration. The internal medicine manual recommends following systematic algorithms to guide management in the case of obstructive uropathy (Bielosludtseva et al., 2017). By adopting these measures, medical practitioners have the potential to substantially enhance patient outcomes, thereby emphasizing the importance of early detection and intervention in conditions that arise secondary to tumors and external compression (Figure 11.7).

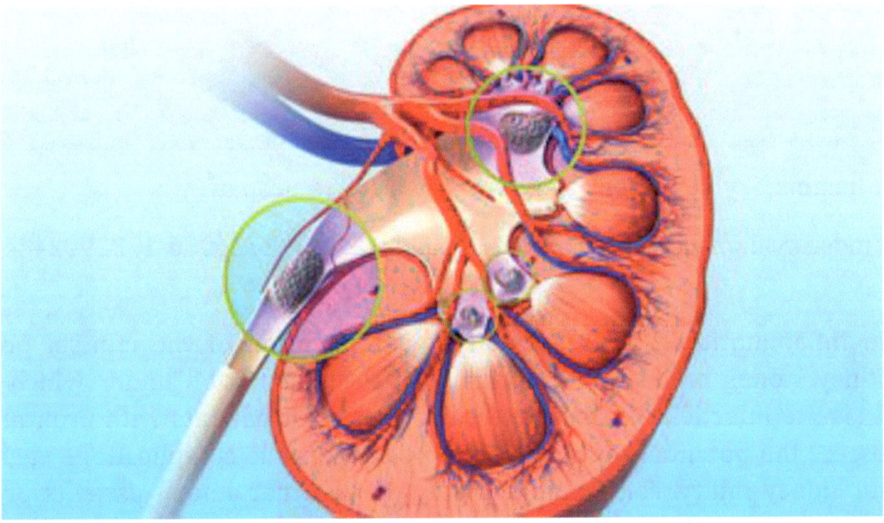

Figure 11.7. Tumors and external compression of obstructive uropathy.

Source: https://www.pediatriconcall.com/master/bucket-img/253-obstructive-uropathy/obstructive-uropathy-1.jpg.

11.2.3. Inflammatory Conditions and Infections

Obstructive uropathy's associated inflammatory diseases are an essential factor in the pathophysiology and treatment of urolithiasis. In the context of kidney stones, inflammation can ensue as a secondary response to the obstruction caused by the stone itself and lead to increased intraluminal pressure and resultant tissue edema. This inflammatory response can enhance pain and make the clinical picture more complex by allowing the formation of further stones, as the accumulation of debris and inflammatory mediators has the potential to crystallize and cause the rocks to grow. Furthermore, treatment interventions are usually effective only if both the stones and the accompanying inflammation are addressed, demonstrating a two-fold therapeutic focus. These are significant in the management of obstructive uropathy, where successful management of inflammation can lead to enhanced urinary flow and recovery of symptoms.

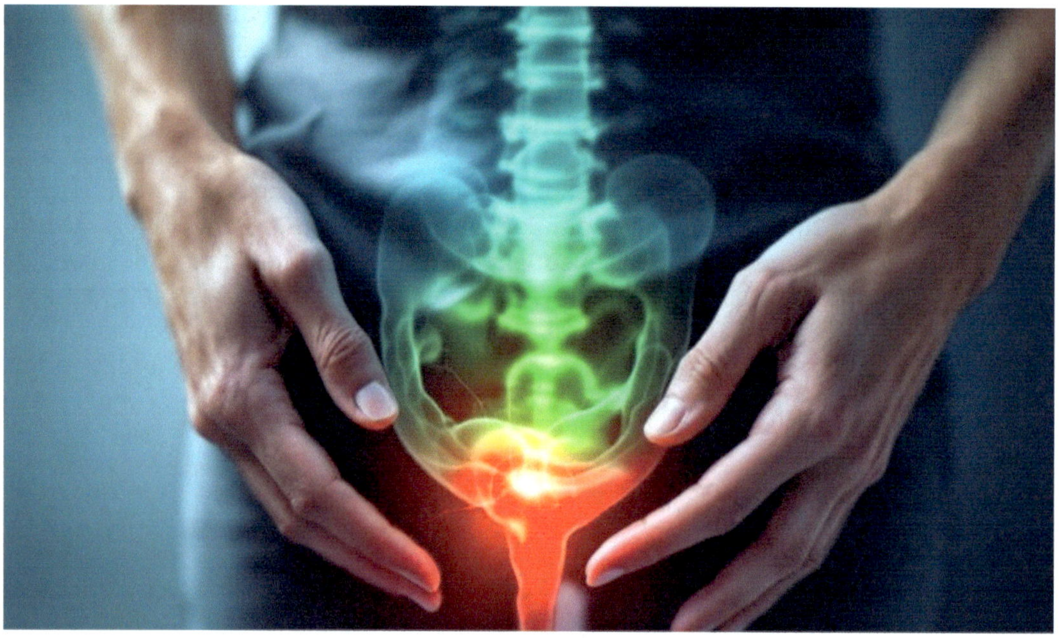

Figure 11.8. Inflammatory conditions linked to obstructive uropathy.

Source: https://mdsearchlight.com/wp-content/uploads/2024/11/26086-1732902444494-728x420.jpg.

Aside from inflammation, UTI is a frequent complication of the clinical presentation of urolithiasis. Kidney stones predispose to urinary stasis, a condition under which bacteria may proliferate and lead to infection. Research indicates that most patients with urolithiasis will have UTIs, which possess the potential to increase the risk of serious complications such as uroseptic shock and acute kidney injury. For example, a study found that among patients presenting with UTIs, those with urolithiasis had a greater risk of serious outcomes. These conditions are more severe among patients in whom the intervention is delayed, hence justifying the need for timely diagnosis and treatment. As such, an awareness of the interaction between UTIs and urolithiasis is crucial for efficient clinical practice. The diagnostic strategy for treating obstructive uropathy-related inflammatory conditions and infections has undergone a significant transformation with the use of advanced imaging modalities. Methods such as intravenous urography have been in use for a long time; however, they are limited by factors including longer examination times, higher costs, and exposure to ionizing radiation and contrast media. New evidence supports the use of alternatives, such as ultrasound and KUB imaging, which can also accurately detect calculi and identify the level of obstruction without posing the same risks. Evidence indicates a combination of KUB and ultrasound yields better detection rates of urinary calculi, particularly at the ureteral level. This shift in diagnostic strategy highlights an increasingly recognized need for safe, effective, and patient-friendly methods in the management of inflammatory conditions associated with obstructive uropathy and urolithiasis, with a focus on improving patient outcomes in this complex field (Figure 11.8).

11.3. Types of Kidney Stones

Kidney stone development, or urolithiasis, is a multifactorial process influenced by numerous biochemical and physiologic determinants. Of all kidney stones, the most prevalent are calcium oxalate stones, which account for approximately 80% of cases. They typically form when urine concentrations of calcium and oxalate are elevated, which is frequently dependent on diet and metabolic status. Hypercalciuria, a common condition among the patients who develop these stones as well, can be due to genetic factors or secondary factors such as renal tubular acidosis, and lead to an increase in calcium in the urine. Additionally, the interaction of urine pH with inhibitors such as citrate plays a major role in stone formation, making the treatment of calcium oxalate stones a complex clinical issue (Ismail et al., 2001).

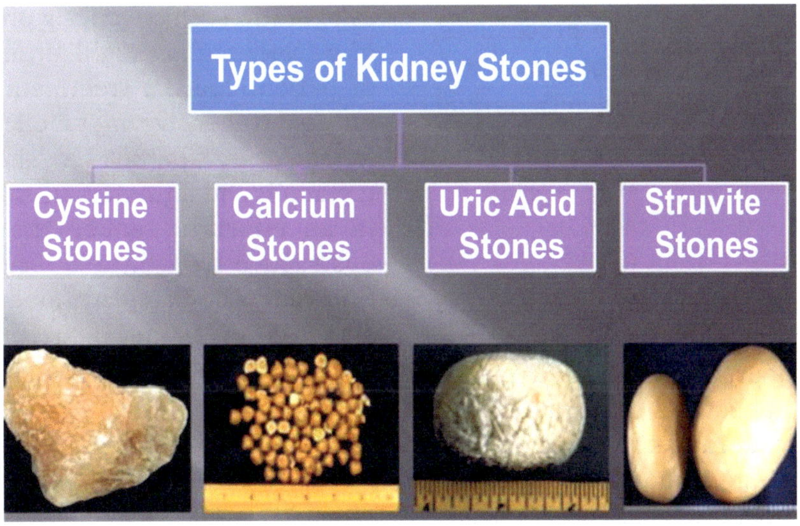

Figure 11.9. Types of kidney stones.

Source: https://urolife.in/wp-content/uploads/2012/07/kidney_stones_4.png.

Another significant form of kidney stones is the struvite stones, which occur most frequently in patients with urinary tract infections caused by urease-producing organisms. Struvite stones are composed of magnesium ammonium phosphate and are bigger and more likely to obstruct other stones. They develop due to the alkaline urine environment created by the infection, which supports the deposition of urinary minerals. Struvite stone patients are predisposed to complicated renal conditions like obstructive uropathy, which may need to be surgically treated. Therapy for struvite stones also involves addressing the concurrent infection to prevent recurrence, highlighting an integral approach in the management of other forms of urolithiasis (Fuster et al., 2018). Uric acid stones represent another distinctive form of kidney stone formation, which is mostly common in conditions of acid urine. These stones can occur in conditions such as gout, where urine supersaturation is caused by high levels of uric acid. Uric acid stones account for 5-10% of all kidney stones and are associated with high metabolic syndrome risk factors. They can also indicate overall metabolic abnormalities. Unlike calcium stones, uric acid stones are dissolvable with dietary changes and drugs that alkalinize urine, providing patients with a non-surgical management option over surgical procedures. The identification of the type of stone will significantly improve treatment options and patient outcomes in urolithiasis (Fuster et al., 2018) (Figure 11.9).

11.3.1. Calcium Stones

The development of calcium stones, which are largely calcium oxalate and calcium phosphate, is a common form of urolithiasis. The stones are formed as a result of several different factors, such as metabolic derangements, diet, and urinary tract status. The pathophysiologic basis for the development of calcium stones typically involves supersaturation of calcium or oxalate in the urine, accompanied by concomitantly low citrate levels, which would otherwise prevent crystallization. Dietary factors, such as over-ingestion of foods rich in oxalate or excessive sodium, can also exert an additive effect to promote stone formation. More recent evidence demonstrates a strong association between inflammatory bowel disease (IBD) and the formation of calcium oxalate stones. Research has established that individuals with IBD have a higher risk of nephrolithiasis due to variations in gut absorption and increased urinary excretion of calcium and oxalate (Ganji-Arjenaki et al., 2017). Thus, understanding these mechanisms is crucial in designing effective prevention programs for patients susceptible to calcium stone disease. Treatment of calcium stones generally entails a multidisciplinary regimen tailored to the individual patient. Treatment may initially involve dietary modification, including the restriction of high-oxalate food consumption and proper hydration, to allow for the dilution of substances that are likely to form stones in the urine. Medical therapy may also involve thiazide diuretics to reduce urinary calcium excretion, particularly in patients with hypercalciuria. Potassium citrate supplements are also often used to increase urinary citrate levels and inhibit crystal formation. As clinical trials emphasize, early and appropriate intervention can effectively preclude recurrence of calcium stones, highlighting the importance of patient-specific treatment protocols based on comprehensive metabolic work-up (Ganji-Arjenaki et al., 2017). Therefore, treating metabolic and lifestyle causes becomes essential in an effort to reduce the burden of both obstructive uropathy and recurrent urolithiasis. Knowledge of diagnostic modalities for calcium stones is vital in the management of obstructive uropathy. Imaging techniques are essential for the detection of the existence and location of stones in the urinary tract. Traditional methods, such as intravenous urography, although effective, have been associated with higher risks of ionizing radiation and increased costs (Ismail et al., 2001). Over the last few years, ultrasonography has gained momentum as a first-line, non-invasive approach with real-time assessment of renal anatomy and the potential for detecting obstruction by stones. The use of a combination of KUB X-rays and ultrasound has been shown to enhance stone detection significantly. It comes in handy in patients with renal colic, where obstructive stones can be diagnosed early and guide prompt therapeutic measures, avoiding sequelae like hydronephrosis or renal failure. Management with the best diagnostic methods helps health practitioners take proper care of patients with a predisposition to the development of calcium stones and their complications (Figure 11.10).

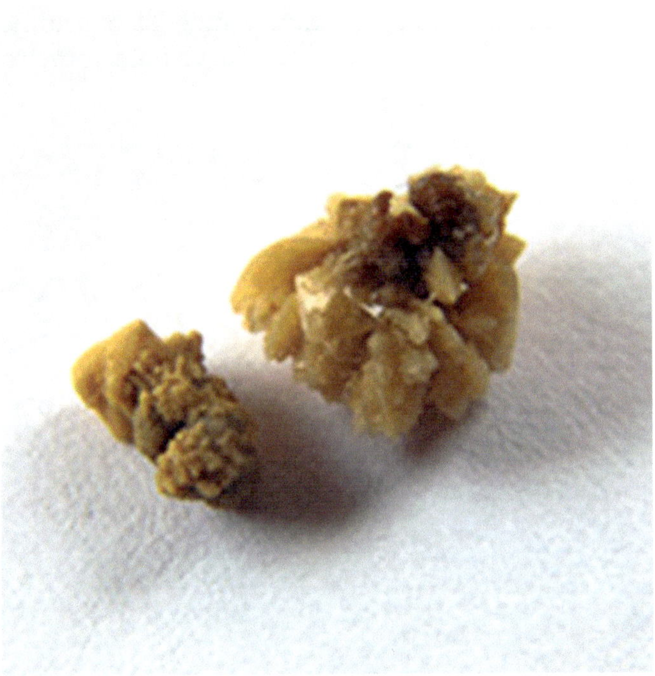

Figure 11.10. Calcium stones.

Source: https://kidneycop.com/wp-content/uploads/2021/02/calcium-oxalate-kidney-stone-different-type-kidney-crystals.jpg.

11.3.2. Struvite Stones

Struvite stones, or infection stones, are one of the most prevalent kidney stones associated with UTIs. They are typically made of magnesium ammonium phosphate and tend to form in alkaline urine. The UTI-causative bacteria, such as Proteus mirabilis, are urease-positive, which raises the urine pH by hydrolyzing urea into ammonia. This biochemical reaction leads to the precipitation of the struvite crystals, which have a high growth rate and may contribute to the formation of large calculi. Struvite stones are clinically relevant because, in addition to causing obstructive uropathy, they may lead to recurrent infection and other consequences if left untreated. The clinical picture of struvite stones is often associated with characteristic signs of urinary obstruction, including flank pain, hematuria, and fever, particularly in the presence of an associated infection. Imaging modalities provide the mainstay of diagnosis, the traditional ones being intravenous urography. However, this method has drawbacks, including increased examination time and exposure to ionizing radiation. As noted, the two together (KUB X-ray and ultrasound) are beneficial as they can adequately detect both stone presence and consequent dilation of the pelvicalyceal system and is a more patient-friendly alternative without the risk of intravenous urography (Ismail et al., 2001).

Struvite stones are typically best treated by a multi-dimensional regimen that treats the stone along with the accompanying urinary tract infection. Surgical intervention, such as percutaneous nephrolithotomy or ureteroscopy, is sometimes required to address the larger calculi, notably as these calculi can cause significant obstruction. Treatment after surgery involves antibiotic therapy to eliminate the bacterial infection and prophylactic measures designed to prevent recurrence, such as avoiding alkaline urine. An understanding of the underlying condition causing the formation of struvite stones will also guide treatment. For instance, strategies to acidify urine can help manage such stones in the long run, thereby lowering the risk of developing other complications, including obstructive uropathy and urolithiasis (Figure 11.11).

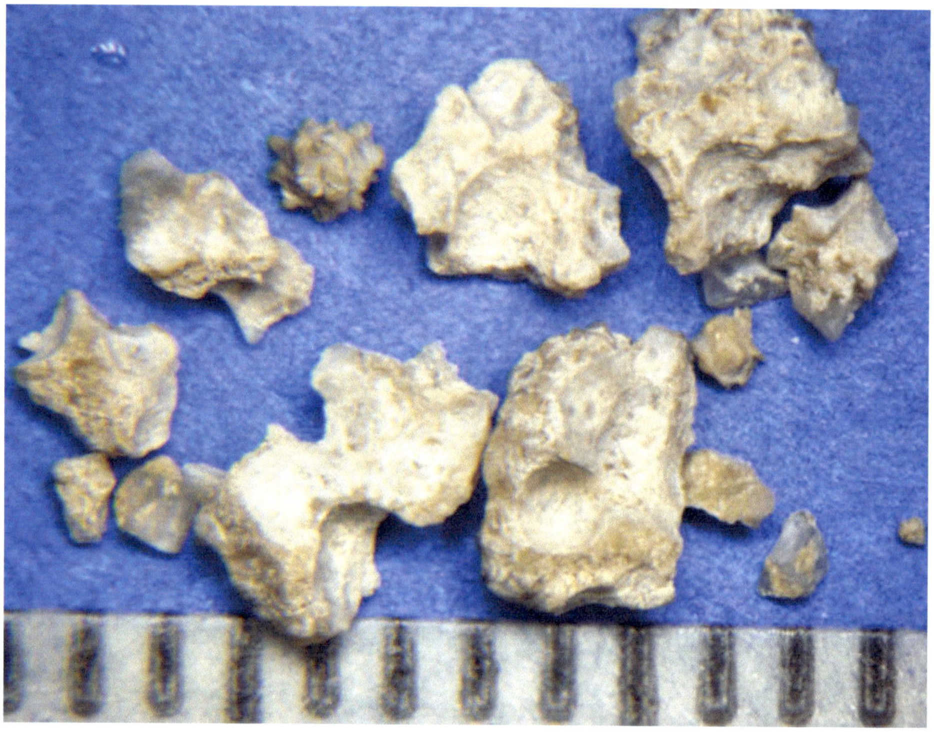

Figure 11.11. Struvite stones.

Source: https://vetmed.umn.edu/sites/vetmed.umn.edu/files/styles/folwell_half/public/2022-11/figure_2.jpg?itok=sAx9kdOb.

11.3.3. Uric Acid Stones

Uric acid stones are a significant category of kidney stones that have unique pathophysiologic mechanisms that distinguish them from other stone varieties. They are present predominantly in hyperuricemic conditions, where elevated blood uric acid levels lead to its crystallization in the renal tubules and the urinary tract. Etiologies of hyperuricemia include obesity, dehydration, a high-purine diet (in organ meat and certain seafood), and some metabolic disorders. Urine's acidic pH is also a significant consideration, as acidic urinary pH enhances uric acid crystallization. Because uric acid stones are highly prevalent in patients with underlying metabolic disease, awareness of these factors is imperative in the prevention and management of urolithiasis, particularly in high-risk groups for obstructive uropathy. Diagnosis of uric acid stones typically involves a thorough evaluation, including both biochemical tests and imaging studies. Ultrasound and KUB radiography are also found to be beneficial in the diagnosis of urinary stones, with ultrasound being more favored due to its lack of ionizing radiation and its ability to verify the presence of any co-existing hydronephrosis secondary to obstruction (Ismail et al., 2001). Furthermore, biochemical analysis of the urine can reveal a low urinary pH and decreased citrate levels, both of which are predictors of vulnerability to uric acid stone development. This evaluation is significant, as the management of underlying metabolic diseases—such as renal tubular acidosis or hyperuricemia—can successfully decrease the risk of recurrent stone formation. Identification and management of these metabolic derangements—those conditions closely associated with uric acid stone formation—ultimately lead to successful therapeutic management of obstructive uropathy in such involved patients. Treatment regimens for uric acid stones focus on both recurrence prevention and alleviation of signs and symptoms of acute obstructive uropathy. Treatment options can involve dietary modifications to lower the concentration of uric acid, for example, increased fluid intake, reduced intake of purine-rich foods, and a focus on alkaline-forming foods for the improvement of urine pH. In different scenarios, drugs like allopurinol are prescribed to inhibit uric acid synthesis, hence preventing stone formation. Observational data indicate that achievement of a urinary pH of greater than 6.0 dissolves uric acid stones, illustrating the importance of urine alkalinization in therapy (Fuster et al., 2018). Clinical management, however, must address individual patients with a multiparameter strategy, properly managing precipitating metabolic states as well as their contribution to obstructive uropathy to optimize patient outcomes (Figure 11.12).

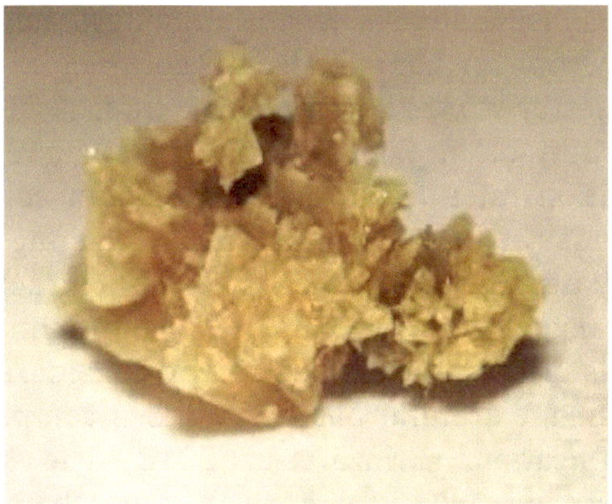

Figure 11.12. Uric acid stones.

Source: https://3.imimg.com/data3/FH/PX/MY-9282724/uric-acid-stones.jpg.

11.4. Symptoms and Diagnosis

Symptomatology of obstructive uropathy typically occurs in a range of painful symptoms that can significantly affect the quality of a patient's life. These involve loin pain, hematuria, dysuria, and anuria on exceptionally severe occasions. Anorexia and asthenia have similarly been reported by research to be present alongside these urinary abnormalities more often than not, illustrating a systemic presentation due to renal impairment. For instance, among 37% of patients who had the presentation of loin pain and among 15% who experienced anuria in a cross-sectional analysis, the variety of clinical presentations of the disease is indicated. Urinary tract infection is another serious complication that can worsen symptoms, further increasing the need for immediate clinical intervention. For this reason, early recognition of these signs is crucial to prevent renal failure through early diagnosis and treatment. Obstructive uropathy can typically be diagnosed by a careful clinical assessment complemented with advanced imaging techniques. During the initial evaluation, doctors may perform ultrasound studies, which are painless and reliable in identifying kidney dilation and obstructive patterns. Computed tomography (CT) scans further enhance the accuracy of diagnosis by providing clear visualization of obstructing masses or stones in the urinary tract. According to clinical study research, patients of obstructive uropathy often present with significant renal function impairment, reflected in their glomerular filtration rates (GFR) and hemoglobin concentrations (Brînză et al., 2018). Proper diagnosis is necessary to establish the etiology, ranging from urolithiasis to neoplasms such as prostatic cancer. Early detection of the character of obstructions not only facilitates effective therapeutic measures but also plays a pivotal role in improving patients' outcomes. Obstructive uropathy treatment needs an individualized strategy considering the unique situation of every patient. For instance, malignant ureteral obstruction is a complex condition due to its complex nature and potential complications (Brînză et al., 2018). The therapeutic goal is the restoration of renal and urinary flow function because delay can exacerbate injury and compromise survival potential. Where there is adequate urinary drainage, studies suggest that various interventions such as nephrostomy and ureteral stenting yield prompt relief of symptoms. The prognosis, however, varies significantly with etiology. While intervention could beneficially influence benign etiologies, malignancies are usually compounded by poorer prognosis with increased mortality and complications requiring close monitoring. It is thus becoming essential to develop some strategies in an attempt to improve renal recovery and patient survival from this feared condition (Figure 11.13).

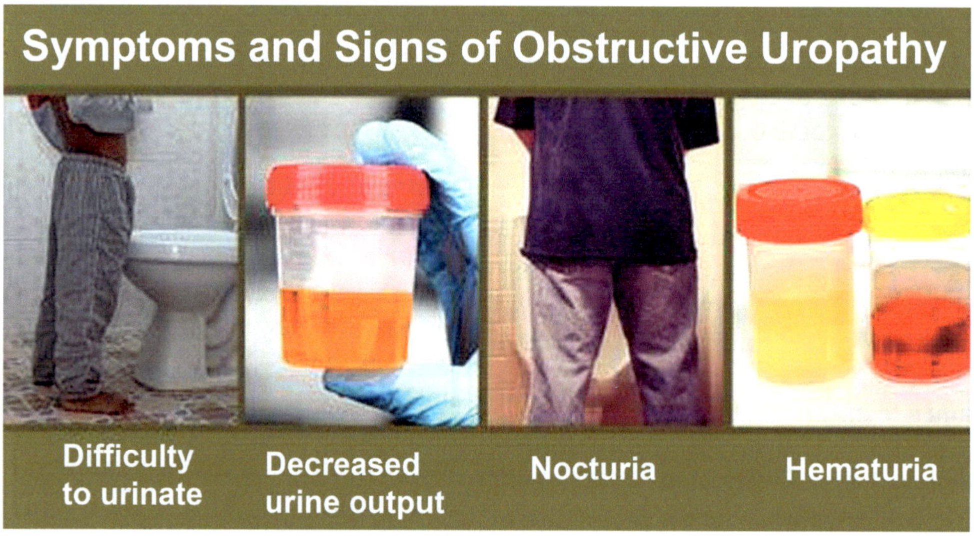

Figure 11.13. Symptoms and diagnosis of obstructive uropathy.

Source: https://images.medindia.net/patientinfo/450_237/symptoms-and-signs-of-obstructive-uropathy.jpg.

11.4.1. Common Symptoms of Obstructive Uropathy

Obstructive uropathy refers to the blockage of urine flow along the urinary tract, resulting in a symptom complex that is crucial for diagnosis and management. The central symptom is flank pain, characterized as sharp and colicky, located in the side or back and typically corresponding to the site of obstruction. The patients can define this pain as it is intermittent and stabbing, which tends to cause distress and difficulty lying down. In addition to flank pain, the patient may present with hematuria or blood in the urine, which can be indicative of trauma to the lining of the urinary tract caused by the obstruction. Also, obstructive uropathy may lead to urinary retention with secondary infection, which presents as fever, chills, and dysuria, necessitating early diagnosis and treatment. Obstructive uropathy in the majority of cases occurs coincidentally with conditions such as urolithiasis, leading to other complications. For instance, kidney stones can lead to an abrupt increase in the severity of symptoms because stones can form partial or even total obstruction of the urinary apparatus, thereby complicating clinical presentations. A significant percentage of patients with ureterolithiasis present with obstructive uropathy, and 81% of patients present with degrees of obstructed urine flow, particularly second-degree uropathy (Düber et al., 2023). This one with obstructive uropathy and kidney stones demonstrates the importance of recognizing what symptoms, such as having trouble urinating, frequent urination, and urgency, may be produced due to the pressure buildup in the renal pelvis and ureters secondary to obstruction. The resultant heightened pressure within the urinary system from obstructive uropathy can have the ability to cause systemic effects, such as nausea and vomiting, which are usually underreported in initial complaints. Gastrointestinal symptoms can be caused by stress related to acute pain or infection from obstruction. Moreover, once kidney function begins to decline, patients may exhibit signs of renal compromise, such as fatigue, loss of appetite, and changes in mental status. This multifaceted symptomatology necessitates thoughtful clinical evaluation to differentiate obstructive uropathy from other pathologies as early treatment is essential to prevent permanent renal injury. Effective techniques, such as percutaneous nephrostomy (PCN) and Double J Stenting, have proven beneficial in alleviating these symptoms and restoring normal function (Ali et al., 2020).

11.4.2. Symptoms Associated with Kidney Stones

Symptoms of kidney stones are highly variable depending on the size, site, and composition of the stone in the urinary tract. One of the most classic symptoms is pain, also referred to as renal colic. Pain is typically colicky, radiating from the flank or lower back and down to the abdomen and groin. It is often described as being one of the worst pains one can experience. With said pain may come bouts of nausea, vomiting, and hematuria, which represent the presence of blood in the urine. These symptoms not only typify kidney stones but also strongly suggest an underlying obstructive uropathy, highlighting the similarities between these two medical conditions (Ali et al., 2020). In addition to acute pain, the patient will also experience disruptions in urinary routines, from frequency to urgency to urinate. Dysuria or painful urination is also a highly prevalent symptom that manifests itself as the stone jams into the urinary tract, inflaming the lining of the urethra. The occurrence of these symptoms can result in extreme discomfort and disruption to the patient's routine. Furthermore, the severity of these symptoms is typically correlated with the size of the stones and degree of obstruction, with bigger stones or complete obstruction expected to exacerbate these conditions of the urinary system. As many as 81% of patients with ureterolithiasis are said to present with symptoms of obstructive uropathy, with varying levels of intensity and concomitant symptoms, a factor that underscores the importance of early diagnosis and management (Düber et al., 2023). Chronic cases of kidney stones can have additional complications if not treated. Because the stones can cause long-term blockage, they can lead to kidney damage or infection, which is characterized by fever, chills, and persistent pain. In addition, the extended back pressure as a result of blockage can lead to severe renal impairment because the kidneys' filtration mechanism is compromised. These complications not only extend the duration of suffering but also heighten the demand for medical care. It is thus imperative to learn about the various symptoms associated with kidney stones to enable appropriate management and prevention of long-term damage. The application of these timely treatment techniques, including interventions such as Percutaneous Nephrostomy or Double J stenting, can alleviate these risks and facilitate normal urinary function, as seen in recent research exploring emergency treatment techniques of obstructive uropathy caused by urolithiasis (Ali et al., 2020) (Figure 11.14).

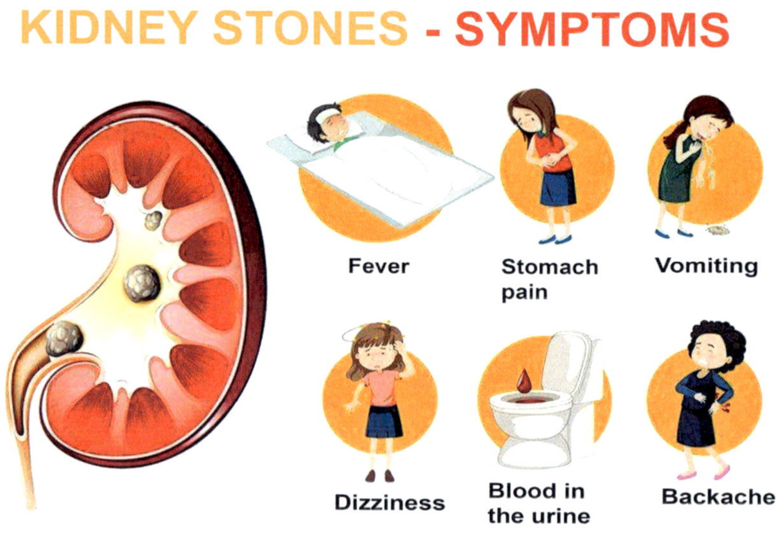

Figure 11.14. Symptoms associated with kidney stones.

Source: https://max-website20-images.s3.ap-south-1.amazonaws.com/10_Symptoms_of_Kidney_Stones_7de1597701.jpg.

11.4.3. Diagnostic Methods (Imaging, Urine Tests)

Imaging modalities play a central role in evaluating urolithiasis and obstructive uropathy, as they provide a comprehensive overview of the underlying pathology. CT has emerged as the gold standard in urinary tract imaging due to its high sensitivity and specificity for detecting obstructions and calculi. There is evidence that CT imaging not only identifies the stones but also evaluates the severity of related complications such as hydronephrosis and renal parenchymal damage. This suggests that early identification can have a significant effect on the success of treatment. For example, in xanthogranulomatous pyelonephritis, CT scans correctly diagnosed the condition preoperatively in the majority of patients, providing valuable information regarding the severity of obstruction and the condition of surrounding tissues (Al-Ghazo et al., 2006). Imaging is thus a critical instrument employed in the treatment of obstructive uropathy. Urine examination, both urinalysis and culture, is also a required diagnostic test used to assess obstructive uropathy secondary to urolithiasis. Urine examination can yield important information regarding the presence of red and white blood cells, crystals, and bacteria in the urine, thereby helping to identify the etiologies of urinary tract obstruction. For instance, a positive urine culture is most commonly suggestive of infection, which is typically secondary to obstructive pathology. Studies have shown that in xanthogranulomatous pyelonephritis, the majority of patients have urine culture-positive results, suggesting a relationship between infection, obstruction, and derangement of renal function (Al-Ghazo et al., 2006). This is important because it is used to formulate the appropriate type of treatment, whether lithotripsy, stenting, or surgery. Hence, analysis of urine complements imaging by providing a broader clinical context necessary for effective management. In addition to imaging and urinalysis, an interdisciplinary team is typically required to enhance diagnostic rates and outcomes of therapy in patients with urolithiasis and obstructive uropathy. Cooperation among urologists, radiologists, and laboratory technicians enables a comprehensive evaluation, facilitating the timely detection of potential complications. For example, hydronephrosis, which is secondary to obstructive uropathy, is generally well managed by treatment with ureteral stenting or percutaneous nephrostomy to relieve the obstruction and prevent renal injury. The application of various diagnostic agents facilitates the stratification of patient risk, especially in patients with more complex situations where underlying malignancies are also responsible for urinary obstruction. Lastly, a methodical and careful diagnostic approach is essential to optimize patient outcomes and prevent long-term harmful effects of obstructive uropathy (Figure 11.15).

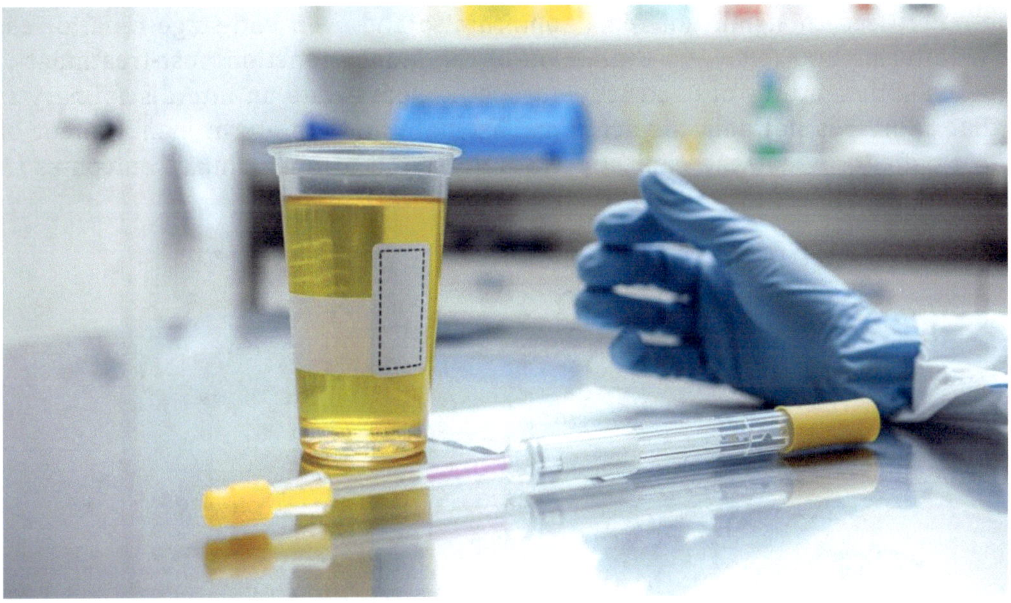

Figure 11.15. Diagnostic methods (imaging, urine tests).

Source: https://referrallabs.in/wp-content/uploads/2024/12/image-2-1024x585.jpeg.

11.5. Treatment Options for Obstructive Uropathy

Treatment of obstructive uropathy is individualized in terms of the cause, the level of obstruction, and the patient's factors. Relief of obstruction and prevention of complications secondary to renal injury is usually the initial treatment. Procedures such as urethral or suprapubic catheterization are widely utilized for temporary relief of symptoms, particularly for those caused by bladder outlet obstruction by a cause like benign prostatic hyperplasia or bladder cancer. Additionally, nephrostomy may be employed in situations where catheterization is either insufficient or impossible. Such initial interventions are crucial in stabilizing renal function and serving as a window for further definitive treatments, as the literature supports the success of urinary diversion before more aggressive interventions in obstructive nephropathy (Abdullahi et al., 2018). Treatment modalities for obstructive uropathy thereafter rely on the management of the underlying etiology. For instance, urolithiasis or kidney stones, which are one of the most common causes of obstructive uropathy, require specialized interventions such as ureteroscopy and lithotripsy for breaking down the stones. Surgery may also include percutaneous nephrolithotomy or open surgery for extremely large or complicated stones. When malignancy is the etiology, chemoradiation therapy may be needed to reduce tumor masses that are obstructing the flow of urine and facilitate urinary drainage. Surgical interventions, such as ureteroneocystostomy, may become necessary to bypass the obstruction in patients with obstructive uropathy, illustrating the multidimensional nature of treatment strategies required to overcome these complications (Düber et al., 2023). The fate of patients with obstructive uropathy is mainly dependent on the promptness and appropriateness of the treatment administered. Early detection and treatment are critical to preventing permanent kidney injury and avoiding mortality risks due to acute complications. For instance, patients of high-grade ureterolithiasis typically present with obstructive uropathy, and failure to clear the obstruction might lead to significant renal compromise and even end-stage renal disease. Thus, consistent monitoring and follow-up evaluation of the kidney function post-treatment is crucial. In general, the subtle features of obstructive uropathy necessitate an interdisciplinary treatment approach that addresses not only the acute management and long-term management options of the individual patient's needs and clinical presentations but also maximizes outcomes (Abdullahi et al., 2018) (Figure 11.16).

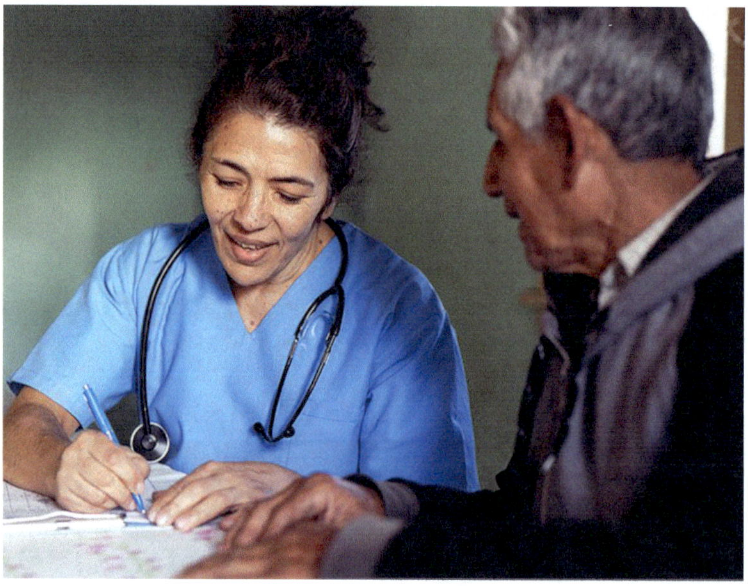

Figure 11.16. Treatment options for obstructive uropathy.

Source: https://media.post.rvohealth.io/wp-content/uploads/sites/3/2024/07/obstructive-uropathy-GettyImages-2161560677-Thumb.jpg.

11.5.1. Surgical Interventions

Surgical intervention is an essential component of the care of obstructive uropathy and urolithiasis in the presence of complications that mandate immediate intervention or failure of conservative management. Ureteroscopy and percutaneous nephrolithotomy are the most common surgical methods of evacuation of kidney stones producing significant obstruction. Ureteroscopy gives direct access to ureter stones and is usually less invasive than percutaneous nephrolithotomy, which is reserved for more complex or larger stones located in the renal pelvis or calyces. The treatment applied depends on a number of variables like the size of the stone, site, patient anatomy, and overall health status. The effectiveness of these interventions not only alleviates urinary obstruction but also significantly reduces the risk of eventual complications of neglected kidney stones and obstructive uropathy. For patients who require surgical treatment, early diagnosis and management are crucial. Inability to intervene in a timely fashion can lead to severe complications like rupture of the calyceal system, which increases urinary obstruction and creates a high-risk environment for infection and renal damage. Calyceal rupture typically occurs due to increased intrapelvic pressure resulting from urinary obstruction, necessitating urgent intervention to prevent severe consequences, such as urinary extravasation or urosepsis (Bui et al., 2024). Early recognition of symptoms and imaging modalities assists in avoiding complications from increasing by ensuring that intervention is carried out before they become severe. Thus, inclusion of surgical intervention in a total management plan is essential for avoiding complications and obtaining optimal patient outcomes with obstructive uropathy. Furthermore, managing the underlying causes of obstructive uropathy, such as strictures or anatomical defects, is crucial for long-term success following surgery. In patients with recurrent nephrolithiasis, thorough evaluations can reveal anatomical defects that must be corrected with surgical procedures in addition to stone removal. Prevention of morbidities, such as urosepsis, depends on effective surgical management (Musalmani et al., 2018). Urosepsis can occur as a severe complication of urinary infection and obstruction, emphasizing the intervention role of surgical procedures in correcting normal urinary flow and relieving obstruction. Thus, inclusion of surgery in the treatment plan not only eliminates the immediate issue of obstructive uropathy but also addresses the long-term issues of health regarding recurrent stone disease (Figure 11.17).

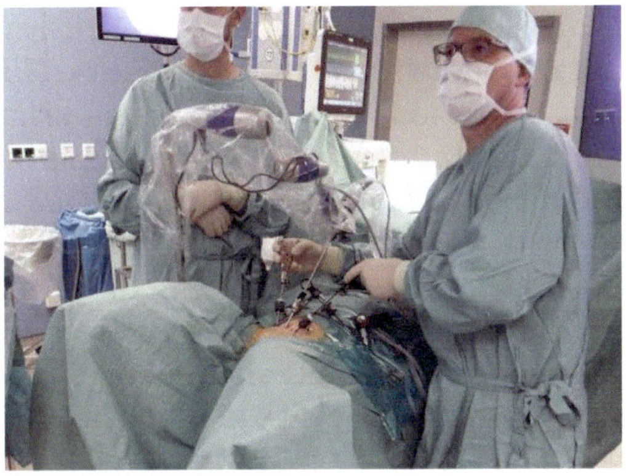

Figure 11.17. Surgical interventions for obstructive uropathy.

Source: https://www.mdpi.com/children/children-09-00298/article_deploy/html/images/children-09-00298-g001.png.

11.5.2. Medical Management and Medications

The clinical treatment of obstructive uropathy and urolithiasis primarily focuses on symptom relief, reducing stone formation, and managing the underlying cause of obstructive episodes in the urinary tract. The majority of the time, patients initially present with acute pain in the flank, hematuria, or retention of urine, necessitating a sensitive assessment that can include radiologic imaging and laboratory tests.

Adequate pain relief is of paramount significance; nonsteroidal anti-inflammatory agents (NSAIDs) and opioids are usually employed for pain relief. Patients in whom spontaneous passage of stones is anticipated are usually advised to increase their fluid intake to enhance excretion. Additionally, drugs such as alpha-blockers are found to be beneficial for relaxing the ureteral smooth muscles and facilitating stone passage. Depending on the underlying etiology, further medical treatment may include thiazide diuretics to inhibit calcium stone formation or potassium citrate to correct metabolic acidosis in cases of uric acid stones. Further, treating patients with complicated urolithiasis also involves a very intimate awareness of the patient's medical history and associated conditions, most significantly inflammatory bowel disease (IBD). IBD has been most closely linked with urinary complications, particularly nephrolithiasis, with various types of stone, including uric acid and calcium oxalate, observed in affected individuals. In fact, evidence exists to the extent that urinary complications may arise in as many as 22% of IBD sufferers, and therefore, individualized medical management strategies become an imperative. Medical intervention is often directed toward the monitoring of electrolyte balance and correction of some of the metabolic derangements due to bowel disorders, placing patients at risk of stone formation. The strategy of a multilateral approach not only successfully treats urolithiasis but also improves the quality of life by preventing recurrent occurrences and their complications, such as obstructive uropathy (Ganji-Arjenaki et al., 2017). Where medical management is suboptimal or complications arise, operative measures are needed. Minimally invasive strategies such as ureteroscopy and shock wave lithotripsy are applied routinely for stone extraction or fragmentation, particularly where obstruction and infection exist. Surgical intervention is also warranted in recurrent stone formers or in those with severe comorbidities, such as calyceal rupture, which can result in severe consequences if left untreated. The importance of early diagnosis of such conditions cannot be overstated; prompt operative intervention will prevent progression to severe complications, including renal failure or sepsis. Additionally, post-op care typically includes diuretics, pain management protocol, and patient education regarding lifestyle modifications and diet modification therapy for recurrence prevention with a holistic modality for obstructive uropathy and urolithiasis management. The multifaceted intervention encompasses both short-term symptom relief and long-term interventions aimed at preserving urinary health and preventing recurrence (Bui et al., 2024).

11.5.3. Lifestyle Modifications and Preventive Measures

Preventative measures and lifestyle modifications are crucial in controlling obstructive uropathy risk as well as urolithiasis. Key measures include maintaining proper hydration to dilute urinary substances that contribute to stone formation. Evidently, increased fluid intake has been proven to significantly decrease kidney stone prevalence, as higher urine volumes help reduce supersaturation of stone-forming salts. Additionally, lower the sodium content to decrease calcium excretion and consequently lower the risk of calcium stones. Patients with metabolic disorders should also follow individualized dietary plans, tailored to reduce specific substances relevant to their condition, thereby enhancing renal health. These pre-emptive lifestyle changes not only help prevent the recurrence of stones but also minimize the uropathic morbidity of obstructive uropathy, thereby maximizing overall renal function. The incorporation of regular exercise into one's lifestyle also turns out to be an equally crucial step in preventing urolithiasis. Regular exercise has been associated with numerous general health benefits, including weight regulation and increased metabolic rates. Notably, obesity has been adequately proven to be a causative risk factor for kidney stones since it is linked with deranged calcium metabolism and hyperexcretion of stone-forming substances in urine. An orderly, regulated aerobic and anaerobic exercise program can enhance metabolic function, thereby reducing the risk of renal calculi formation. In addition, exercises improve the quality of urinary flow, which may prevent urinary stasis andconsequently, bacterial colonization is the primary component of the pathogenesis of obstructive uropathy. Thus, developing an exercise habit guarantees long-term renal health and reduces complications associated with kidney stones. Moreover, understanding the role of prophylactic pharmacologic interventions can be supplementary to lifestyle changes in the management of kidney stones. Some medications may be prescribed to correct underlying metabolic abnormalities that are responsible for stone formation, such as hyperuricemia or hypercalcemia. Thiazide diuretics, for instance, can be beneficial in reducing urinary excretion of calcium in patients predisposed to calcium stones. Some medications, however, are capable of modifying the pH of urine, making the environment less conducive to stone growth. However, these pharmacological maneuvers should be considered in addition to routine lifestyle modifications, supporting the overall prevention strategy. By incorporating personalized dietary habits, physical activity, and pharmacological treatment, it is feasible to significantly reduce the risk of urolithiasis and its associated complications, including obstructive uropathy, leading to improved renal function and quality of life.

11.6. Treatment Options for Urolithiasis

Urolithiasis, or kidney stones, is a multi-modal treatment that relies on the size, nature, and location of the stones, as well as the overall health of the patient. Initial conservative management often involves hydration and pain control, of which the latter is mainly accomplished via the administration of nonsteroidal anti-inflammatory drugs (NSAIDs) to decrease pain. For the smaller stones, particularly those of <5 mm in diameter, spontaneous passage is probable, and conservative monitoring could be an appropriate strategy. However, with the increasing size of the stone or complications such as obstructive uropathy, more forceful maneuvers may become necessary. For instance, patients with acute ureterolithiasis may, in certain cases, be managed using interventions such as ureteroscopy, where a small scope is employed to visualize and remove stones, thereby ceasing the obstruction and preventing renal damage, according to prevalence and treatment studies (Düber et al., 2023). Where stones fail to pass naturally or where obstructive characteristics become more pronounced, surgical interventions are necessary. Extracorporeal shock wave lithotripsy (ESWL) is one of the non-invasive treatments which are commonly applied, utilizing acoustic waves to shatter the stones into fragments that can be easily passed. This is particularly beneficial for individuals with stones in the renal pelvis or upper ureter. However, this method of treatment may be compromised by the presence of greater and denser stones, or in patients with certain anatomical flaws. In these instances, percutaneous nephrolithotomy is an adequate option; the minimally invasive procedure allows surgeons to directly approach the kidney via small incisions to remove large stones, not only addressing the stones themselves but also the blockages they cause. Overall, these surgical options effectively capture the demand for individualized treatment strategies in the management of urolithiasis (Abdullahi et al., 2018). Additionally, the importance of addressing the underlying causes of stone formation cannot be overstated in the treatment of urolithiasis. Patients typically are encouraged to adopt life modifications that will prevent recurrence, such as diet modification, hydration, and, in some cases, medication for individuals with specific metabolic abnormalities. For instance, in calcium oxalate stones, one can be aided by reducing dietary oxalate and increasing calcium intake, because, surprisingly, dietary manipulation can help prevent stone formation. Additionally, pharmacological therapy can be applied in some cases, for instance, potassium citrate for the prophylaxis of stones and thiazide diuretics in patients with calcium-sodium stones. Effective management of urolithiasis, therefore, relies not only on stone treatment but also on preventive measures to prevent future complications of obstructive uropathy (Düber et al., 2023) (Figure 11.18).

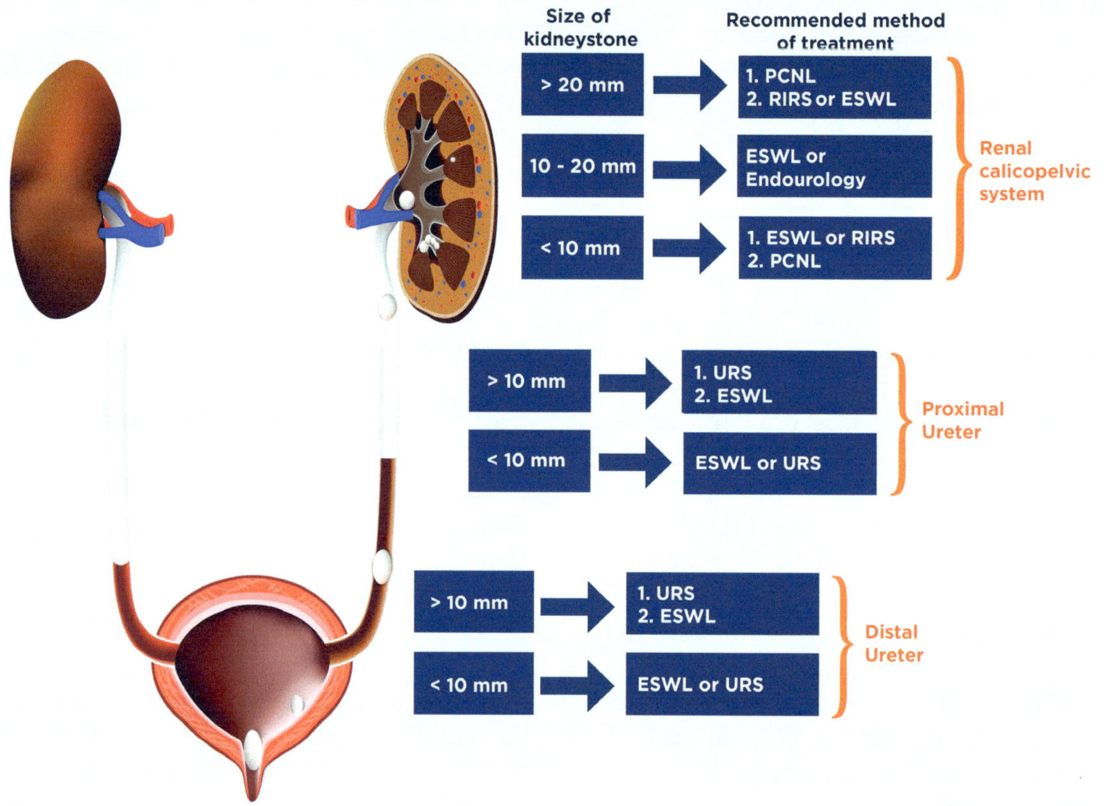

Figure 11.18. Treatment options for urolithiasis.

Source: https://www.dornier.com/wp-content/uploads/sites/2/2018/01/Recommended-Stone-Treatment-ENG.jpg.

11.6.1. Extracorporeal Shock Wave Lithotripsy (ESWL)

ESWL is now a focal noninvasive treatment for patients with obstructive uropathy and urolithiasis, particularly for renal calculi. The procedure achieves its goal by delivering high-energy shock waves to shatter kidney stones into small fragments that may be easily eliminated from the urinary tract. Not only does ESWL eliminate the need for surgical methods, but it also reduces recovery time and associated complications. Nevertheless, its effectiveness can be influenced by various factors, including the composition, size, and location of the stones in the urinary system. Where there are large or irregular stones, additional treatment may be required to remove them entirely, thus necessitating a comprehensive understanding of ESWL as part of a multidisciplinary approach to treatment (Fathurrahman et al., 2020). Investigations have demonstrated that, while relatively safe, ESWL does have risks, namely to the renal parenchyma. One investigation assessing the hemodynamic effects of ESWL reported no significant change in renal cortex blood flow but noted an elevation in the resistive index (RI) in hydronephrotic kidneys post-treatment. This emphasizes the necessity of careful patient selection because patients with existing renal impairment or obstruction are at risk of developing increased renovascular resistance after the procedure (Chuang et al., 2005). Hence, healthcare professionals need to carefully weigh the benefits of ESWL against the risk of inducing vascular changes that might further complicate existing renal disease. Proper imaging techniques and careful preoperative evaluation can be employed to minimize such risks and enhance patient outcomes. Moreover, it is worth considering the combination of ESWL with other endourological procedures, particularly in cases of complex obstructive uropathy or a heavy stone burden. For instance, multimodal approaches combining ESWL with ureteroscopy or percutaneous nephrolithotomy can enhance the overall stone removal success rates while allowing individualized treatment strategies based on individual patient needs. These robust management strategies are more effective in treating stone encrustation and obstruction, resulting in improved overall renal health. As seen in research on abandoned DJ stent cases, applying a combination of therapies—such as using ESWL—is highly beneficial in inpatient care while minimizing morbidity from conventional surgery (Fathurrahman et al., 2020). In conclusion, ESWL is a cornerstone technology in the treatment of urolithiasis, requiring ongoing research and refinement to optimize its application in the clinical setting (Figure 11.19).

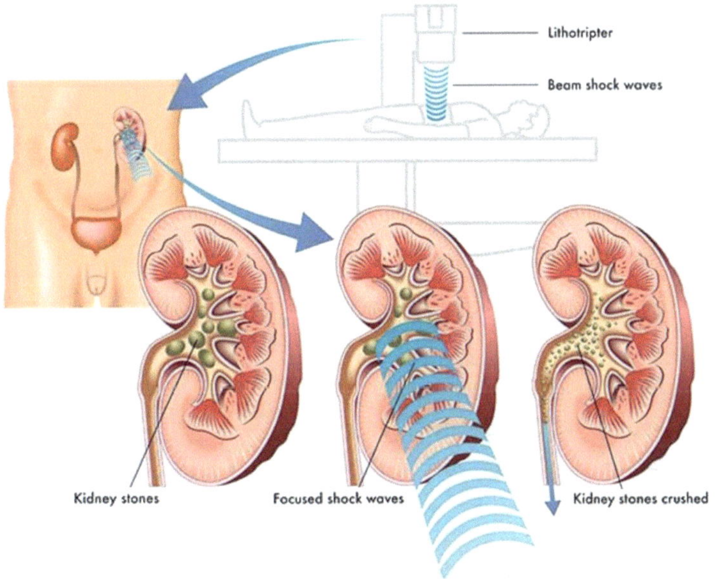

Figure 11.19. ESWL-extracorporeal shock wave lithotripsy treatment for kidney stones.

Source: https://www.drvamsikrishna.com/wp-content/uploads/2019/04/Extracorporeal-shock-wave-lithotripsy-demonstration-Dr.-Vamsi-Krishna.png.

11.6.2. Ureteroscopy and Laser Lithotripsy

Ureteroscopy is a minimally invasive procedure that has become the gold standard of treatment of urolithiasis, especially in cases of obstructive uropathy caused by kidney stones. Through the passage of a thin, flexible tube equipped with a built-in camera, ureteroscopy provides direct visualization of the ureter and kidney. The obstruction can be diagnosed and stones cleared with high precision through this method. Due to its high success rate, ureteroscopy is often combined with laser lithotripsy, a device that utilizes focused laser energy to fragment stones into smaller, more easily passable pieces. The integration of these techniques has resulted in significant improvements in treatment outcomes. Therefore, it is also a preferred choice for patients with ureteral stones and complications, thereby minimizing the risk of re-obstruction or renal functional impairment, as highlighted in several clinical studies. Laser lithotripsy with the Holmium YAG laser has been found highly effective in treating stones of various sizes and compositions. The versatility of this technology will enable it to target stones safely in challenging anatomical structures, with a high likelihood of achieving a high stone-free rate after the operation. Evidence has demonstrated that complications and recovery time are less with ureteroscopy and laser lithotripsy compared to traditional surgery. For instance, one study showed significantly higher rates of stone clearance when the procedure was compared with the conventional methods, such as pneumatic lithoclast (Awan et al., 2024). Furthermore, the reduced operative time of laser lithotripsy contributes to its appeal as a modern treatment alternative, as it enables patients to return to normal much earlier and more effectively. Obstructive uropathy secondary to kidney stones necessitates a multidisciplinary treatment plan including not only surgical procedures, but also complete assessment and postoperative care of the patient. Following ureteroscopy and laser lithotripsy, careful surveillance for infection or complications of urinary tract obstruction is required. Postoperative stenting is a common procedure that assists in the flow of urine and prevents obstruction as the renal system heals. Long-term outcomes have shown that patients undergoing ureteroscopy and laser lithotripsy exhibit greater levels of satisfaction, symptom relief, and reduced rates of stone recurrence (Fathurrahman et al., 2020). This emphasizes the need for further research and refinement of these techniques, ultimately leading to best practices for the acute and chronic presentations of urolithiasis.

11.6.3. Dietary and Fluid Intake Recommendations

Hydration and dietary control are at the heart of both the prevention and treatment of urolithiasis and obstructive uropathy. Individuals at risk of developing kidney stones must prioritize adequate hydration as a cornerstone of prevention. An increase in water intake helps dilute the urinary concentration of chemicals recognized to form stones, reducing the likelihood of crystal precipitation. Elevated urinary output of over 2.5 liters per day has been shown to significantly reduce the incidence of stone formation. Other than water, several other fluids such as lemonade, a citrus juice, also raise urinary citrate. Citrate inhibits stone formation and is therefore a beneficial addition to dietary treatment in patients with urolithiasis. Maintaining a balance in fluid intake and regular physical activity is essential to prevent stagnation of the urinary tract and ensure the body's normal functioning. In addition to increasing fluid intake, lifestyle changes can significantly impact the management of kidney stones. For example, restricting foods rich in oxalate, i.e., spinach, nuts, and chocolate, especially in those at risk of developing calcium oxalate stones, is a good idea. Additionally, lowering sodium intake is also beneficial, as excessive salt intake increases urine calcium excretion, thereby predisposing the individual to stone development. For patients with uric acid stones, it is advisable to reduce protein intake, especially from animal sources, as this can lead to heightened uric acid levels in the urinary tract. The addition of a balanced diet made of fruits, vegetables, and whole foods not only improves overall health but also aids in maintaining urinary contents at their optimal level. Understanding one's nutritional needs is essential for effective management. The composition of the diet also interacts with environmental and genetic risk factors for stone formation. Metabolic factors have been highlighted in recent times, particularly in children, as more kidney stones have been reported globally (Filler et al., 2010). Individualized nutritional advice, including adequate quantities of calcium—often mistakenly believed to be a risk factor for stone formation—can diminish the risk, as dietary calcium chelates oxalate within the gastrointestinal tract and lessens its absorption. Health education, particularly in ensuring a proper balance of fluid intake with a healthy diet, can make a substantial contribution to reducing the occurrence of obstructive uropathy and kidney stones. It is essential that health practitioners collaborate with nutritionists to develop personalized programs that consider not only metabolic disorders but also individual preferences, allowing for an active approach towards resolving this multifaceted urological disorder (Bui et al., 2024).

SUMMARY

The evaluation of obstructive uropathy and urolithiasis shows that efficient and timely intervention is crucial for patient outcomes. The therapeutic option for obstructive uropathy due to kidney stones, including PCN and DJ stenting, has been viewed as an effective measure to normalize increased serum urea and creatinine levels. Comparative research indicated that both procedures gave comparable times to normalize serum, with average durations of 97.654 hours for PCN and 106.453 hours for DJ stenting, displaying the versatility of treatment modalities available to clinicians in dealing with such complicated cases (Ali et al., 2020). This information indicates the importance of personalizing patient management, as variability in response can lead physicians to the optimal intervention strategy. Further, the data on the prognosis of obstructive uropathy portrays additional intricacy in the clinical management of the patients. The most common etiologies, like urolithiasis, benign prostatic hypertrophy, and malignancies, portray the multifactorial etiology of obstructive uropathy. The findings of a study in Cameroon showed severe impairment of renal function among the patients, high mortality and morbidity rates and severe underlying ill conditions (Ebana et al., 2016). This emphasizes not only the requirement for emergency surgical intervention but also comprehensive, multidisciplinary care approaches involving underlying illnesses, promising to improve renal recovery and long-term survival among affected patients. Finally, the thread running through the studies enumerated is that timely diagnosis and effective management of obstructive uropathy are of critical importance. As the findings demonstrate, renal function deteriorates at a rate that is alarming if treatment is delayed, resulting in undesirable consequences. This necessitates that some steps be taken to create awareness about the symptoms and consequences of kidney stones as well as obstructive uropathy among healthcare professionals and society in general. In general, improvements in timely access to effective treatments, as well as better patient education, may lead to better health outcomes and significantly reduce the impact of obstructive uropathy and its associated complications. The use of clinical guidelines and ongoing patient follow-up remains central to the management of this complex medical issue.

Urolithiasis and obstructive uropathy, also known as kidney stones, are medical conditions that require proper diagnosis and treatment. The pathophysiology of such conditions is crucial to understand because it clarifies how urinary obstruction can lead to renal injury and CKD. When there's a blockage in the urinary tract, e.g., due to kidney stones, the urine usually flows normally; however, it may get interrupted, which may result in elevated pressure, renal ischemia, and decreased function of the kidneys. Thus, therapeutic approaches must not only target prompt relief of the blockage but also avoid late complications, e.g., progression to ESRD (Lin et al., 2017). Specific information about mechanisms, risk factors, and management regimens is vital for practitioners in the management of these urinary conditions. Obstructive uropathy and urolithiasis treatment has evolved over the years, with early treatment being central to preventing permanent kidney damage. Analgesics, hydration, and dissolution stone medications are used in conservative treatment; however, in complicated cases, surgery becomes necessary. Methods such as extracorporeal shock wave lithotripsy or ureteroscopy are used to eliminate stones and restore the urinary flow. Additionally, recent studies have investigated novel therapeutic interventions for mitigating renal injury resulting from urine obstruction. Hydrogen sulfide (H_2S), for instance, has been found to be a protective agent that prevents renal injury and facilitates the recovery of kidney function after decompression (Lin et al., 2017). These gains in therapy demonstrate a continued focus on optimizing patient outcomes, most notably the prevention of additional renal complications. The broader public health significance of obstructive uropathy extends beyond the outcome of individual patients and underscores the need for prevention and early detection public health campaigns. As CKD is present in over 10% of the global population, understanding the interconnectivity among urinary obstructions, kidney stones, and CKD is crucial for maximizing healthcare strategies (Jakubowska et al., 2023). Public health educational programs can increase awareness of risk factors, such as hydration levels, dietary habits, and genetic predisposition to kidney stones, leading to early diagnosis and control. Long-term management of obstructive uropathy is multidisciplinary and involves dietary guidance, regular monitoring of renal function, and patient education to minimize recurrence. Lastly, the management of obstructive uropathy and urolithiasis requires a thorough understanding of its pathophysiology, early intervention, and effective prevention.

CLOSER LOOK

HYDRONEPHROSIS

Hydronephrosis is an abnormality where the renal pelvis and calyces are distended or stretched as a consequence of an obstruction or defect in urinary drainage from the kidney to the bladder. It can affect one (unilateral) or two (bilateral) kidneys and can be caused by an extensive range of congenital or acquired conditions. Hydronephrosis is not a disease, but rather a radiologic and clinical finding indicating an abnormality of the urinary tract. The degree of dilatation can vary from mild to severe and, if left untreated in its early stages, can result in progressive renal parenchymal atrophy. This condition may be diagnosed prenatally on routine ultrasounds or can manifest later in life with abdominal mass, flank pain, UTIs, hematuria, or impaired kidney function.

The pathophysiology of hydronephrosis is based on the imbalance between outflow and urine output. Due to obstruction, there is insufficient drainage of urine, leading to increased pressure within the renal collecting system. This, with time, causes renal pelvis and calyces stretching and thinning that compresses renal tissue and hampers its ability to filter blood properly. The common obstructive causes include ureteropelvic junction (UPJ) obstruction, ureterovesical junction (UVJ) obstruction, kidney stones, tumors, strictures, or congenital malformations such as posterior urethral valves in males. Vesicoureteral reflux (VUR), with backflow of the urine from the bladder into the ureters and kidneys, or pregnancy caused by mechanical compression from the expanding uterus, may cause hydronephrosis.

Hydronephrosis is most often diagnosed using imaging modalities, with ultrasonography being the most commonly utilized due to its non-invasive nature and ability to detect renal dilation. Further assessment may be a voiding cystourethrogram (VCUG) for identification of VUR, or a diuretic renogram (MAG3 scan) to differentiate between obstructive and non-obstructive etiology and to assess renal function. In others, CT or MRI may be utilized for more accurate anatomical evaluation. The grading systems, such as the Society for Fetal Urology (SFU) classification or Onen grading system, help determine the severity and guide treatment choices.

Treatment of hydronephrosis depends on the etiology, extent of dilation, and presence or absence of symptoms or renal impairment. Mild or non-obstructive hydronephrosis, particularly in infants, often resolves spontaneously and may require only observation with repeated imaging. Where there is obstruction and renal function is threatened, surgical relief may be achieved through pyeloplasty (in the case of UPJ), stenting, or nephrostomy drainage to restore normal urine flow and preserve renal tissue. Infection with hydronephrosis is managed with antibiotics, and secondary etiologies such as stones and tumors are treated directly.

References

1. Muhammad, A. S., Abdulwahab-Ahmed, A., Agwu, P. N., Abdullahi, K., & Mungadi, I. A. (2018). Management of obstructive nephropathy in a tertiary hospital in North West Nigeria: A five-year review. *East and Central African Journal of Surgery*, *22*(3), 42. https://doi.org/10.4314/ecajs.v22i3.6Al Musalmani, M., Chanda, A., Ganaw, A., Hassan, M., et al. (2018). Urosepsis: Flow is life. https://core.ac.uk/download/322440132.pdf (accessed on 25th June 2025).
2. Al-Ghazo, M. A., Al-Kaisi, N. S., Ghalayini, I. F., Khader, Y. S., et al. (2006). Xanthogranulomatous pyelonephritis: Analysis of 18 cases. https://core.ac.uk/download/pdf/82368488.pdf (accessed on 25th June 2025).
3. Ali, L., Khan, F. H., Khan, S., Orakzai, M., et al. (2020). Comparison of percutaneous nephrostomy and double J stent in early normalization of renal function tests in patients with obstructive uropathy due to urolithiasis. https://core.ac.uk/download/551320508.pdf (accessed on 25th June 2025).
4. Andrzejak, A., Kowalczyk, E., Olszewski, H., Stolarek, J., et al. (2024). Hydronephrosis associated with cervical cancer: Case report on pathophysiology, diagnosis, and management. https://core.ac.uk/download/620863389.pdf (accessed on 25th June 2025).
5. Asero, V., Autorino, R., Basran, S., Belladelli, F., Bologna, E., Brown, D. R., Cho, H. J., et al. (2022). Characteristics of sepsis or acute pyelonephritis combined with ureteral stone in the United States: A retrospective analysis of large national cohort. https://core.ac.uk/download/566464001.pdf (accessed on 25th June 2025).
6. Awan, A. S., Haider, A., Asadullah, M., Quddus, M. B., El Khalid, S., & Memon, W. A. (2024). Comparing Holmium (Ho): YAG laser with pneumatic lithoclast for treatment efficacy of ureteric stones. https://core.ac.uk/download/616635519.pdf (accessed on 25th June 2025).
7. Bally, L., Cereghetti, G., Faller, N., Fuster, D., et al. (2022). Impact of the SGLT2 inhibitor empagliflozin on urinary supersaturations in kidney stone formers (SWEETSTONE trial): Protocol for a randomised, double-blind, placebo-controlled cross-over trial. https://core.ac.uk/download/527935244.pdf (accessed on 25th June 2025).
8. Bielosludtseva, K., Botvinikova, L., Dmytrychenko, V., Fesenko, N., et al. (2017). *Essential Practical Skills in Internal Medicine*. https://core.ac.uk/download/pdf/196150200.pdf (accessed on 25th June 2025).
9. Brînză, A., Lupu, S., Marcu, D., Maxim, D., et al. (2018). A brief review of the literature on the malignant ureteral obstruction. https://core.ac.uk/download/216809655.pdf (accessed on 25th June 2025).
10. Bui, L., Cruz, G., Heer, M. S., Jones, C., et al. (2024). Calyceal rupture secondary to nephrolithiasis: A case report emphasizing early diagnosis and management. https://core.ac.uk/download/652333730.pdf (accessed on 25th June 2025).
11. Chen, T. H., Chen, Y. Y., Hsiao, C. Y., Hsiao, M. C., et al. (2019). Urolithiasis is a risk factor for urosepsis shock and acute kidney injury in patients with urinary tract infection. https://core.ac.uk/download/275933286.pdf (accessed on 25th June 2025).
12. Chuang, S. M., Huang, C. H., Juan, Y. S., Li, C. C., et al. (2005). Evaluation of intrarenal blood flow by Doppler ultrasonography immediately after extracorporeal shock wave lithotripsy

on hydronephrotic kidney. https://core.ac.uk/download/pdf/81106820.pdf (accessed on 25th June 2025).

13. Danarto, R. (2019). Patient prognosis after relief of obstruction. https://core.ac.uk/download/297187272.pdf (accessed on 25th June 2025).

14. Ding, J. (2009). Childhood urinary stones induced by melamine-tainted formula: How much we know, how much we don't know. https://core.ac.uk/download/pdf/82222181.pdf (accessed on 25th June 2025).

15. Dosani, M. T., Moir, J., Rix, D., Soomro, N., et al. (2011). Endourological management of urolithiasis in donor kidneys prior to renal transplant. https://core.ac.uk/download/pdf/8630277.pdf (accessed on 25th June 2025).

16. Düber, C., Halfmann, M. C., Jorg, T., Mager, A., et al. (2023). Structured reporting in radiology enables epidemiological analysis through data mining: Urolithiasis as a use case. https://core.ac.uk/download/621759390.pdf (accessed on 25th June 2025).

17. Ebana, H. F., Ekane, G. H., Halle, M. P., Nzuobontane, D., et al. (2016). The profile of patients with obstructive uropathy in Cameroon: Case of the Douala General Hospital. https://core.ac.uk/download/478430243.pdf (accessed on 25th June 2025).

18. Fathurrahman, H., Hasroni, H., & Hakim, L. (2020). Endourologic management in neglected double J stent at Soetoro Hospital Surabaya: Retrospective-descriptive study, period 2013–2016. https://core.ac.uk/download/297829211.pdf (accessed on 25th June 2025).

19. Filler, G., & Sharma, A. P. (2010). Epidemiology of pediatric urolithiasis. https://core.ac.uk/download/534389889.pdf (accessed on 25th June 2025).

20. Fuster, D. G., & Moe, O. W. (2018). Incomplete distal renal tubular acidosis and kidney stones. https://core.ac.uk/download/212380677.pdf (accessed on 25th June 2025).

21. Ganji-Arjenaki, M., Nasri, H., & Rafieian-Kopaei, M. (2017). Mephrolithiasis as a common urinary system manifestation of inflammatory bowel diseases: A clinical review and meta-analysis. https://core.ac.uk/download/143840259.pdf (accessed on 25th June 2025).

22. Ismail, H. S. (2001). Comparative study between ultrasound & KUB and IVU in renal colic patients in Kelantan. https://core.ac.uk/download/85127303.pdf (accessed on 25th June 2025).

23. Ismail, H. S. (2001). Comparative study between ultrasound and KUB and IVU in renal colic patients in Kelantan. https://core.ac.uk/download/132566828.pdf (accessed on 25th June 2025).

24. Jakubowska, W., Kiełkowicz, A., Pactwa, F., Pisera, A., et al. (2023). A review on the classification and current treatment of chronic kidney disease. https://core.ac.uk/download/597985229.pdf (accessed on 25th June 2025).

25. Kaginalkar, V. R., Titare, P., & Suraparaju, P. V. (2024). Characterization of ureteric obstructive lesions using single bolus CT urography: A single center study. https://core.ac.uk/download/635338274.pdf (accessed on 25th June 2025).

26. Kumar, T. S. (2011). Urolithiasis associated with renal insufficiency: Factors predicting outcome – Prospective study. https://core.ac.uk/download/235658849.pdf (accessed on 25th June 2025).

27. Lin, S. (2017). Daily hydrogen sulfide treatment enables early recovery of renal function and mitigates renal injury following the relief of prolonged urinary obstruction. https://core.ac.uk/download/85003089.pdf (accessed on 25th June 2025).

28. Mohamed, S. K. (2018). Doppler sonographic evaluation of intrarenal arteries in acute renal obstruction. https://core.ac.uk/download/235668643.pdf (accessed on 25th June 2025).

29. N/A. (2022). Urinary stents. https://core.ac.uk/download/534897932.pdf (accessed on 25th June 2025).

30. Saffari, A., Mehrabi, A., Wühl, E., Muttray, J., Schenk, J. P., Meyburg, J., Hafezi, M., et al. (2018). ARFI shear-wave elastography with simulation of acute urinary tract obstruction in an *ex vivo* porcine kidney model. https://core.ac.uk/download/581832838.pdf (accessed on 25th June 2025).

31. Wagenius, M. (2021). Complications and treatment aspects of urological stone surgery. https://core.ac.uk/download/479542435.pdf (accessed on 25th June 2025).

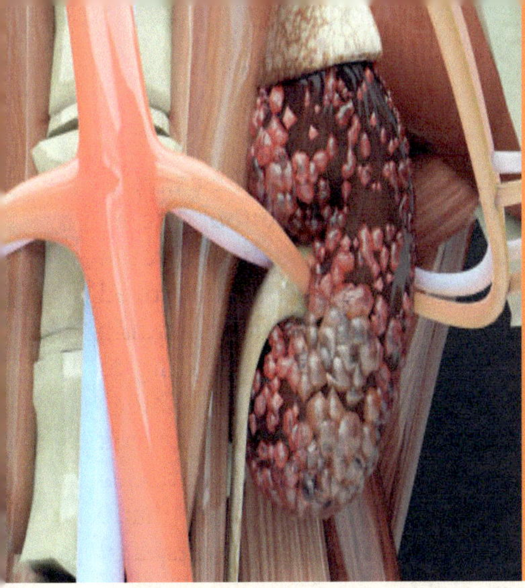

Chapter 12

RENAL AND UROTHELIAL TUMORS

Contents

Introduction

The biological intricateness of urothelial and renal tumors creates significant challenges in practice and research in oncology. These neoplasms develop from the urinary tract and kidney and account for an impressive fraction of cancer morbidity and mortality worldwide. The discovery of the underlying fundamental mechanisms of tumor growth and development is thus crucial for formulating proper prevention and treatment strategies. The histologic and molecular variability of these cancers necessitates a broader investigation to determine their biological behavior, genetic predisposition, and correlation with patient survival. The studies can potentially identify new biomarkers and therapeutic targets that can enhance the prognosis and survival rate of patients, a need that is crucial in oncology. Later studies have also explored the role of LDL receptor-related proteins (LRPs) in cancer, identifying that they have critical functions in the biology of renal and urothelial carcinomas. Research conducted using the Cancer Genome Atlas (TCGA) examined the expression profile of thirteen LRPs across a number of malignancies and observed that expression of LRP1 correlated with survival in specific cancers, such as bladder urothelial carcinoma. Interestingly, elevated LRP1 mRNA levels were found to be associated with compromised survival rates, suggesting its potential use as a prognostic indicator. Additionally, LRP2 had the opposite effect, with elevated expression being associated with improved survival in renal clear cell carcinoma. These findings highlight the importance of understanding LRP signaling pathways and their role in modulating cancer behavior, ultimately contributing to the overall goal of enhancing patient care and outcomes in renal and urothelial tumors (Gilder et al., 2017). Except the genetic factor, the clinical presentation of renal and urothelial tumors is of great significance in diagnosis and management. Case studies also highlight the subtleties involved in diagnosing urothelial carcinomas, particularly in challenging cases of local lymphatic and distant metastasis. Proper clinical workups, such as blood examinations, imaging tests, and histopathology, are necessary for accurate diagnosis and effective treatment planning. To put this into perspective, in one reported case, a post-mortem found extensive metastasis, which underscores the aggressive nature of such tumors and the need for early detection strategies. As the field of renal and urothelial tumor studies continues to evolve, the integration of molecular information with clinical data remains crucial for advancing therapeutic strategies and improving patient outcomes (Clercq et al., 2011) (Figure 12.1).

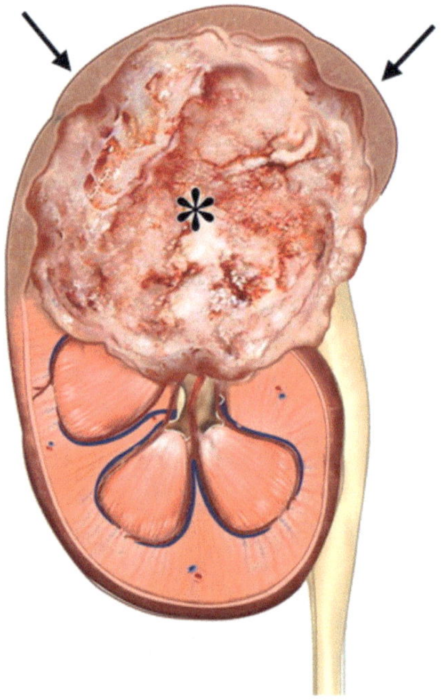

Figure 12.1. Urothelial cancer.

Source: https://pubs.rsna.org/cms/10.1148/rg.306105501/asset/images/medium/105501fig03a.jpeg.

Definition of Renal and Urothelial Tumors

The field of renal and urothelial neoplasms is a broad category of malignant growths from the kidneys and bladder. Renal tumors most often are of renal parenchymal origin and may be present in one of several forms, the most prevalent being renal cell carcinoma (RCC). This particular type of tumor accounts for a large percentage of kidney cancers and is known for its highly variable clinical course and response to treatment. Urothelial tumors, however, occur in the urothelium, the transitional epithelium of the bladder and upper urinary tract. The tumors, especially transitional cell carcinoma, are a serious public health issue due to their prevalence and rates of recurrence and progression. Understanding these definitions is crucial for clinicians and scientists alike to properly diagnose, manage, and study these cancers in the interest of improving patient outcomes. Contributing to the complexity of the renal and urothelial tumor universe are the distinct biological behaviors and treatment concerns of each tumor type. Renal cell carcinoma, for instance, has several histological subtypes, such as clear cell, papillary, and chromophobe carcinoma, each with characteristic molecular features and variable drug sensitivity. Among the urothelial carcinoma spectrum, further classification and grading significantly influence the treatment approach. As emphasized in the 2nd International Consultation on Bladder Cancer proceedings, accurate classification and grading of urothelial neoplasia are crucial in determining prognosis and management. The recommendations made highlight the importance of pathologist expertise in identifying lesions, recurrence, and the use of contemporary terminologies, which enable easy understanding in histopathological examination (Al-Ahmadie et al., 2015). The association between renal and urothelial tumors is also stressed because of their possible shared etiology and overlapping risk factors. Studies have shown that bladder urothelial carcinoma patients have elevated risks of developing upper tract urothelial carcinoma (UTUC), which may represent a clonal association secondary to intraluminal metastasis or independent oncogenic processes driven by environmental and inherited factors. A systematic review examining the relationship indicated that intravesical recurrence following radical nephroureterectomy for UTUC differs widely among patients, highlighting the complex interaction between the two types of tumors (Aben et al., 2020). This fact emphasizes the necessity of having a profound understanding of the behavior of both renal and urothelial malignancies and how it influences patient surveillance, screening, and treatment in practice (Figure 12.2).

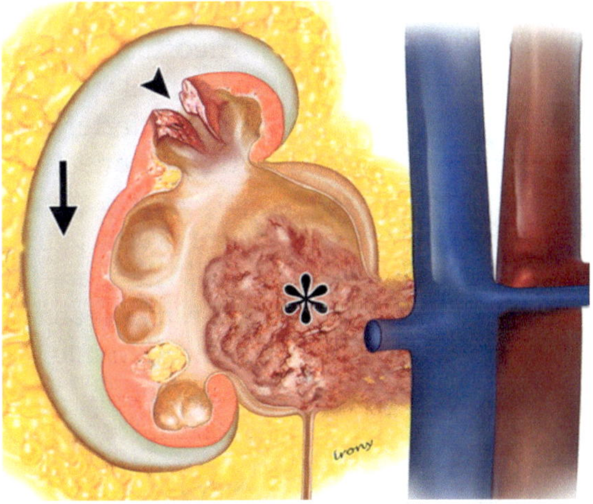

Figure 12.2. Urothelial cancer of the renal pelvicalyceal system.

Source: https://external-content.duckduckgo.com/iu/?u=https%3A%2F%2Fpubs.rsna.org%2Fcms%2F10.1148%2Frg.306105501%2Fasset%2Fimages%2Fmedium%2F105501fig07a.jpeg&f=1&nofb=1&ipt=522c9c0cf0e8382f8180778a9019147ca358a6dd64b74dd1d4302c969a76ffcb.

Importance of Studying These Tumors

The study of RCCs and urothelial tumors is of utmost importance due to the rising incidence and overwhelming effects on public health. RCC, the most common kidney cancer, has become more widespread globally and underscores the need for targeted research. With the advancement in genomics, studies have isolated diverse molecular mechanisms that contribute to tumor initiation, indicating that a holistic understanding of such tumors would portend paradigm shifts in tumor treatment. By identifying the gene expression alterations behind renal tumors, scientists can identify candidate biomarkers that can be used to enhance early detection and improve patient outcomes. The conclusions from this research will be able to guide clinical strategies specific to renal and urothelial cancer patients and, therefore, meet an urgent need for tailored treatment protocols. Also critical is the exploration of new treatments for urothelial carcinoma, especially because bladder cancer remains among the most prevalent in the United States. Despite this historically limited success in developing novel therapies for non-muscle invasive bladder cancer (NMIBC), clinical evidence is increasingly becoming recognized of the potential of immunotherapy and molecular targeted therapy. The NCI Bladder Cancer Task Force extended an invitation to collaborate in advancing clinical trial designs for these novel treatments, recognizing the intricacies of bladder cancer's molecular characteristics (Abrams et al., 2016). With a focus on the unique biological features of bladder tumors, researchers can reveal accurate targets for treatment so that they can make significant improvements in the effectiveness of their treatments, which will be vital to improving survival and quality of life for patients with bladder cancer. Examining how integrins work in cancer biology is another critical research area in renal and urothelial tumors. Integrins are primarily implicated in cell adhesion, migration, and extracellular matrix remodeling, which contribute to tumor metastasis and angiogenesis (Arun et al., 2018). The identification of overexpression of integrin subunits in such cancers can be useful in identifying the driving force behind cancer development. This information would be tantamount to the development of integrin antagonists as therapeutic drugs, and this would be a significant advancement in the field of cancer medication paradigms. Integrin high-affinity ligands, in turn, could result in the targeted delivery of therapeutic molecules to tumor sites with increased efficacy of medication and minimal side effects. As such, the value of research on these tumors extends beyond fundamental research; it encompasses new methods of intervention that could potentially transform clinical practice in oncology.

12.1. Anatomy and Physiology of the Urinary System

The urinary system of the body, primarily responsible for waste elimination and homeostasis regulation, is formed by several anatomical structures that are essential, like the kidneys, ureters, bladder, and urethra. Located retroperitoneal to the kidneys, filtration of the blood is performed by them, resulting in waste products being eliminated in the form of urine. There are functional units referred to as nephrons in each kidney wherein glomeruli act as filtration and tubules perform reabsorption and secretion. This intricate function is not only essential for waste removal but also crucial for regulating electrolyte balance, blood pressure, and acid-base homeostasis. Given that urothelial neoplasms can occur in the urinary tract, it is essential to understand the anatomy and physiology of the organs, as any disturbance could predispose individuals to oncogenic events and resultant tumor formation in these organs, thereby relating urinary system anatomy directly to renal and urothelial tumor pathology. The anatomy of the urinary system has an intrinsic connection with its physiology, supporting efficient filtration and excretion activities. Blood is forced through the nephron, which produces a filtrate with necessary nutrients and waste products. Selective reabsorption of water and solutes occurs primarily in the proximal convoluted tubule, with the loop of Henle responsible for concentrating urine. The subtle physiological process is essential in regulating proper fluid balance and homeostasis, which are vital to good health. Dysfunction in these mechanisms can lead to pathophysiological states, hence predisposing to renal and urothelial tumors. Awareness of normal urinary system function forms the basis for an appreciation of the impact of structural changes, such as tumor growth, on kidney and urinary tract function, as well as the importance of early diagnosis. Urothelial tumors, arising in the lining of the urinary tract, present unique pathological challenges due to their complex relationship with the underlying physiological mechanisms of the urinary system. Urothelium, being one of the more slowly cycling epithelia, is susceptible to cellular alterations that can lead to tumorigenesis upon the occurrence of oncogenic mutations. As has been observed, activation of the receptor tyrosine kinase pathway due to genetic mutations can trigger urothelial carcinomas, demonstrating a possible connection between anatomical susceptibility and physiological alterations that lead to tumor development. Investigations into these mechanisms in murine models have provided important insights into urothelial tumor initiation and progression pathways, reinforcing the importance of both anatomy and physiology in cancer investigations. This integration of biological principles is crucial for identifying putative drug targets and predicting clinical responses in patients with renal and urothelial cancers, thereby reinstating the relevance of holistic learning in these domains (Chapelle et al., 2009) (Figure 12.3).

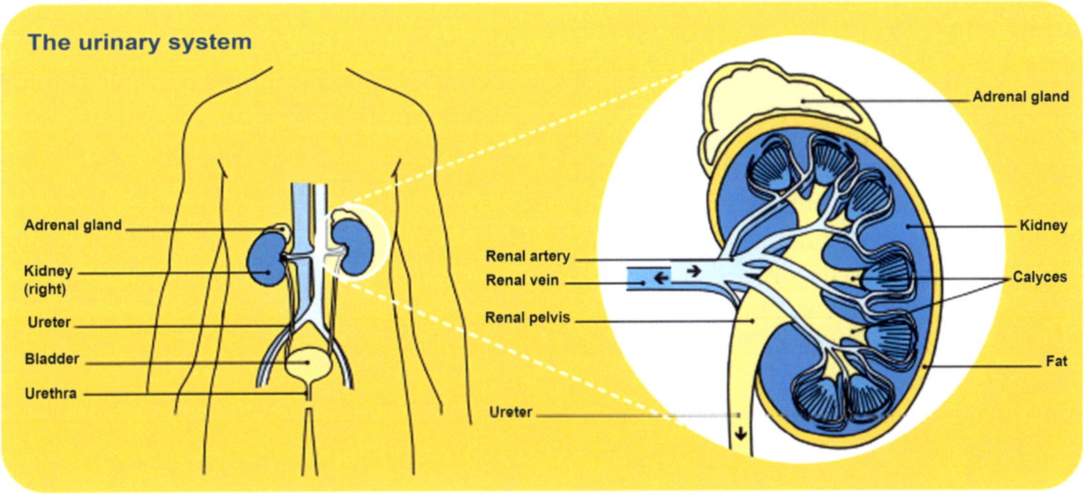

Figure 12.3. Anatomy and physiology of the urinary system urothelial tumors.

Source: https://external-content.duckduckgo.com/iu/?u=https%3A%2F%2Fwww.cancervic.org.au%2Fimages%2Furinary-system.PNG&f=1&nofb=1&ipt=2bece74d8660678fd9ecc3f61224b2f07684d9153867406530d383882f8bbdf0.

12.1.1. Structure of the Kidneys

The kidneys are well-developed and vital for the body's homeostatic mechanisms, including the elimination of wastes and electrolyte balance. A capsule envelops the kidney and consists of the outer cortex and inner medulla containing the renal pyramids. The anatomy of the kidney is conducive to its physiological function; the nephron, the functional unit, is into strategically positioned segments. Made of glomerulus and tubular apparatus, nephrons facilitate blood filtration and selective reabsorption of essential substances. Understanding renal architecture not only aids in comprehending normal kidney function but is also relevant in defining pathological changes involving renal and urothelial neoplasms, particularly because renal cell arrangement may influence tumor behavior and prognosis (Cody et al., 2002). In the renal cortex, the glomeruli play a key role in filtering the blood to produce urine. The complex process involves the passage of blood through special capillary beds, allowing for the selective elimination and removal of waste products while preserving essential proteins and cells. The renal tubules, extending into the medulla, further modify the filtrate by processes such as reabsorption and secretion. The collecting ducts and loop of Henle are particularly significant in concentrating urine and osmolarity regulation. Alterations in these structures can have a impact on kidney function and tumor formation. Research has pointed out the molecular profile of neoplastic transformation of renal cells, which verifies that structural alterations closely foretell specific tumor entities, such as clear cell and chromophobe carcinomas (Trapani et al., 2010). The renal vascular input is the other vital component of their structure, aiding blood flow to enable filtration and metabolic functions. Renal arteries branch from the abdominal aorta and provide blood through the renal hilum into the arcuate and interlobar arteries. The developed venous drainage system of the renal veins maintains an efficient return of blood into systemic circulation. This vascular network maintains renal function and plays a crucial role in the case of tumors, as neovascularization is a common property of tumors, which enhances growth and metastasis. Advances in molecular profiling emphasize the importance of the dynamics of blood supply to tumors in tumor biology, and it is suggested that understanding kidney structure is the most critical step towards developing effective therapeutic intervention against renal and urothelial tumors (Cody et al., 2002).

12.1.2. Function of the Urinary Tract

The urinary system is vital to homeostasis in the human body through the production, transport, and excretion of urine. It comprises the kidneys, ureters, bladder, and urethra, all of which play a role in the efficiency of waste removal and fluid regulation in total. The kidneys are the primary organs of filtration, cleansing blood to remove excess waste products, toxins, and fluids. Through processes such as glomerular filtration, tubular secretion, and reabsorption, the kidneys facilitate the salvaging of essential nutrients like electrolytes and glucose while removing waste products. As renal and urothelial malignancies disrupt these processes, awareness of the anatomy and physiology of the urinary tract is necessary to fully understand the total impact of such cancers on renal function and overall physiological balance. Ureters transport urine from the kidneys to the bladder through rhythmic contractions of muscles, known as peristalsis, for efficient transport. The mechanism is not only essential for waste removal but also for preventing reflux, which can occur due to their location. The bladder serves as a storage reservoir, storing varying volumes of urine until it is deliberately excreted via the urethra. Whereas in the case of renal and urothelial tumors, the urinary tract's functioning can be drastically impaired. Obstructions resulting from tumors within the renal parenchyma or urothelium can disrupt urine flow and complicate the situation with hydronephrosis or infection. In fact, upper tract urothelial carcinoma can be linked with advanced disease stages and impact renal function, as highlighted by a recent study that reviews the predictive roles of such cancers (Amirian et al., 2014). Furthermore, proper functioning of the urinary tract is vital in metering and applying homeostatic mechanisms such as blood pressure regulation and acid-base balance. The complex regulating functions of the kidneys define the overall metabolism and fluid balance of the body. Aberrant states such as renal tumors grossly disrupt such functions, predisposing to systemic disease manifestations. For instance, research has established that the methylation status of certain genes might be pivotal in identifying recurrence of upper tract urothelial carcinoma and may define treatment (Ci et al., 2015). Because the ability of the urinary tract to rid the body of waste and maintain internal balances is a prerequisite for health, the impact of tumors in this area emphasizes the importance of vigilance in preserving renal function and the integrity of the urinary tract (Figure 12.4).

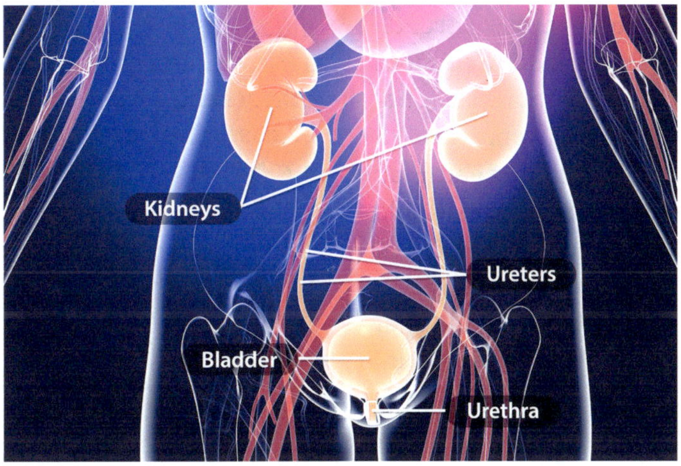

Figure 12.4. Function of the urinary tract urothelial tumors.

Source: https://img.lb.wbmdstatic.com/vim/live/webmd/consumer_assets/site_images/article_thumbnails/BigBead/urinary_tract_infections_bigbead/1800x1200_urinary_tract_infections_bigbead_alt.jpg.

12.1.3. Role of Urothelium in the Urinary System

The urothelium, a specialized epithelial layer that lines the urinary tract, plays a vital role in maintaining the function and integrity of the bladder and urinary tract. Made up of several layers of cells, this transitional epithelium is a key element of the barrier that protects against toxic substances and pathogens traversing from the urine to subjacent tissues. This selectivity is necessary, as the urinary bladder is exposed to various types of waste materials that could otherwise trigger inflammatory responses or damage to nearby tissues. Sensory function is also contributed by the urothelium, helping in bladder filling and voiding control by its nerve fibers, which transmit messages to the central nervous system upon urgency. It is critical to understand the multifunctional roles of the urothelium, particularly in urothelial tumors, as any impairment of its structure or function can predispose an individual to malignancies. In considering the importance of urothelial pathology, it is essential to understand the malignancy risk associated with various pathological conditions of the urothelium. Diseases like neurogenic bladder may lead to radical alterations in urothelial health, fostering a conducive environment for developing bladder cancer. Advances in the area of stem cells have highlighted the promise of regenerative therapy, offering a potential pathway for bladder reconstruction.

Current practices opt to utilize intestinal tissues for such procedures, which harbor unwanted consequences, including metabolic disturbances and increased rates of complications. The search for stem cell-based urothelial tissue can reverse these threats, paving the way for improved and safer treatment interventions. This area of work highlights the functional and intact requirement of a urothelium for maintaining urinary health, as well as for managing bladder malignancies. Aside from its sensory and physical barrier functions, the urothelium is now also a unifying topic in bladder cancer pathology debates. International Consultations on Urological Diseases, with its strictly evidence-based approach, emphasized the importance of refining the resolution of urothelial neoplasia grading and classification.

The proceedings of the 2nd International Consultation on Bladder Cancer highlight a systematic approach to identifying various bladder lesions, including papillary and inverted tumors, which tend to present challenges both in diagnosis and management.

The ability of the urothelium to regenerate and accommodate such pathologies implies its dynamic nature. With the increasing knowledge of urothelial tumors, there is a growing need for stringent guidelines and diagnostic criteria to achieve the ultimate objective of improving patient outcomes and optimizing clinical practices in bladder cancer therapy (Al-Ahmadie et al., 2015).

12.2. Types of Renal Tumors

Kidney cancers are divided into several heterogeneous types, each with specific biological characteristics and clinical behaviors. Renal cell carcinoma (RCC) is the most common type and comprises several subtypes, including clear cell, papillary, and chromophobe carcinomas. Clear cell renal cell carcinoma accounts for approximately 70-80% of RCC cases and is characterized by a characteristic morphology and specific genetic mutation, primarily the VHL tumor suppressor gene. Papillary renal cell carcinoma, on the other hand, occurs in approximately 10-15% of cases and has a characteristic histological appearance associated with mutations within the MET gene. This feature is crucial because it significantly impacts treatment and prognosis. Furthermore, ongoing research studies are utilizing genomic characterizations to gain a deeper understanding of these various renal tumor subtypes and to enhance patient outcomes and treatments. Other than renal cell carcinoma, other interesting renal tumors that exist include Wilms tumor, which predominantly occurs in children, and renal sarcomas, which are rare but extremely virulent neoplasms. Wilms tumor or nephroblastoma is the most common kidney cancer in children and is often associated with chromosome 11 abnormalities. The prognosis for Wilms tumor is excellent when it is detected early, due to improvements in surgical techniques and chemotherapy. On the other hand, renal sarcomas like leiomyosarcoma are more challenging due to their aggressive nature and resistance to standard treatments. Proper diagnosis and definition of these isolated renal tumor forms are crucial for implementing successful treatment protocols and improving survival rates in affected patients, underscoring the need for continued research in the field. Increased complexity in molecular and genomic evaluation of cancer has also demystified the role of specific biomarkers for renal tumors. For example, research on LDL receptor-related proteins (LRPs) has been able to detect probable correlations between the expression levels of these proteins and survival rates in patients with various cancers, including renal tumors (Gilder et al., 2017). This research highlights how the differential expression of these proteins can impact tumor behavior and the response to treatment. Moreover, the genomic classification of renal tumors provides a framework for elucidating their biology and treatment response, with the potential for more personalized therapy for patients (Bossé et al., 2017). As the landscape of renal oncology continues to evolve, it is increasingly important to utilize these discoveries to optimize patient treatment and outcomes in renal cancer (Figure 12.5).

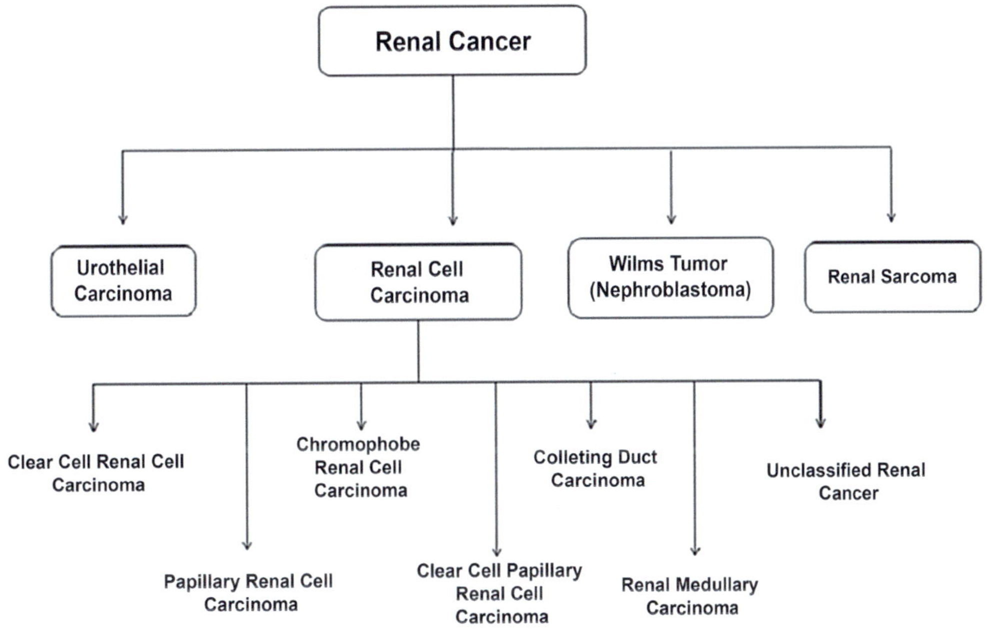

Figure 12.5. The classification of renal cancer.

Source: https://external-content.duckduckgo.com/iu/?u=https%3A%2F%2Fwww.researchgate.net%2Fpublication%2F366138694%2Ffigure%2Ffig2%2FAS%3A11431281106009927%401670577308812%2FThe-classification-of-renal-cancer.png&f=1&nofb=1&ipt=4db188008eb7454b2a3fdb44011580eb02a64e5c8e57778ba648e44c7b4f4e94.

12.2.1. Renal Cell Carcinoma (RCC)

RCC is the most frequent kidney cancer that arises from the renal epithelium and accounts for over 90% of kidney neoplasms. RCC pathogenesis is multifactorial, with genetic susceptibilities, lifestyle, and underlying disorders playing important roles in the development of RCC. Notably, RCC in its early stages is often asymptomatic, and early diagnosis and prompt therapy are therefore complex. When they occur, symptoms may present in the form of hematuria, flank pain, and a palpable abdominal mass, often indicative of advanced disease. As RCC progresses, its molecular biology is germane information, particularly in terms of individualized therapies. Recent studies have pinpointed the likely significance of certain gene expressions, and these have contributed to the understanding of tumor behaviors and patient survival rates, with findings revealing differential roles in RCC versus other cancers (Gilder et al., 2017).

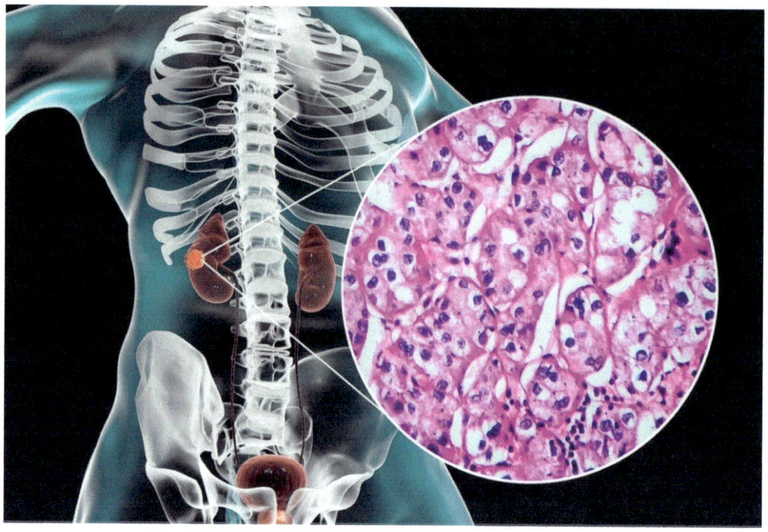

Figure 12.6. Renal cell carcinoma.

Source: https://external-content.duckduckgo.com/iu/?u=https%3A%2F%2Fd2jx2rerrg6sh3.cloudfront.net%2Fimages%2Fnews%2FImageForNews_737951_16756916615796854.jpg&f=1&nofb=1&ipt=eb1b0b6aaf004a2bcb81ca8ee375358d27e3ac27d0aaedf166672056ccab48d3.

Renal cell carcinoma treatment is a clinical approach that involves multidisciplinary practice, combining surgery, targeted therapy, and immunotherapy. Historically, radical nephrectomy has been the treatment of choice for localized RCC, with nephron-sparing approaches being utilized more commonly to preserve renal function. In metastatic disease, targeted agents have revolutionized patient outcomes, notably those directed against the VEGF and mTOR pathways. Despite advances, metastatic RCC remains a challenging disease to treat effectively. Notably, the prognostic utility of biomarkers is an area of great interest within the research community since they have the potential to guide treatment decisions as well as optimize patient stratification. The identification of biomarkers that correlate with patient survival, particularly in renal clear cell carcinoma, is imperative for adopting a more personalized treatment approach (Gilder et al., 2017). In examining the overlap between urothelial tumors and renal cell carcinoma, overlap in pathways has to be given consideration, as well as treatment approaches. Presenting urothelial carcinoma metastatically could complicate RCC treatment in cases where concomitant distal organ and lymphatic dissemination are involved. The detection of lymphatic metastases in an assumed urothelial carcinoma, for example, highlights the overlap of diagnostic and clinical considerations that must be taken into account when treating the patient. Combining cutting-edge imaging techniques and histopathological examinations enhances diagnostic accuracy, which is crucial for the creation of therapeutic strategies. Second, the dynamic nature of immunohistochemistry and molecular identification signals a shift toward a more advanced understanding of tumor microenvironments and their implications for survival and treatment responses, calling for further investigation into how these tumors function biologically (Figure 12.6).

12.2.2. Wilms Tumor

Wilms tumor or nephroblastoma is the most frequent kidney cancer in children between the ages of 2 and 5. It is a tumor that arises from immature mesenchymal cells of the embryonic kidney, typically with genetic predispositions in the form of syndromes like WAGR (Wilms tumor, Aniridia, Genitourinary abnormalities, and Range of developmental delays) and Beckwith-Wiedemann syndrome. The presentation of Wilms tumor clinically also often includes an abdominal mass, hematuria, and abdominal pain, which provokes further imaging investigations or biopsy. The prognosis of Wilms tumor has dramatically improved over the past decades due to advances in multi-modal treatment strategies like surgery and chemotherapy, a reflection of a deep understanding of the tumor biology and behavior in children.

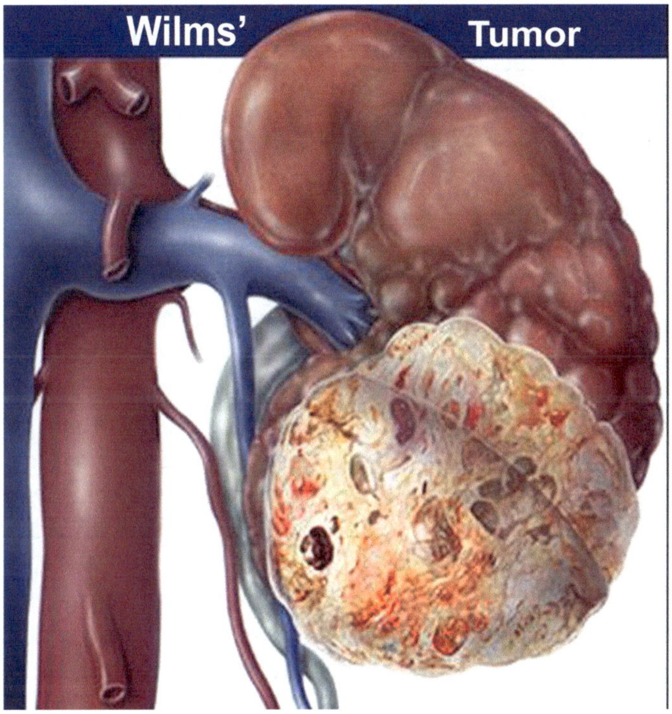

Figure 12.7. Wilms tumor.

Source: https://external-content.duckduckgo.com/iu/?u=https%3A%2F%2F1.bp.blogspot.com%2F-Qmlk-GVaqlo%2FVxUxEc3wYNI%2FAAAAAAAAA30%2FKmq27Pd1c5kLB5p-srKdx5lyW_Z5AvUqQCLcB%2Fs1600%2FKevin-Somerville.png&f=1&nofb=1&ipt=ea539138cc4055f477ce96d063a12703ac2f46c56d606dcfc0e2a217e84a7a19.

The molecular profile of Wilms tumor reveals significant information about its pathogenesis. Current studies of nephroblastomas have highlighted the restricted involvement of specific mutations in initiating tumor development, particularly with receptor tyrosine kinases such as KIT, PDGFRα, and EGFR. These results indicate that mutations within these genes do not play an essential role in nephroblastoma pathogenesis despite specific patterns of protein expression. Interestingly, a correlation has been identified wherein certain high-risk tumors express immunohistochemical KIT, which offers the potential for targeted therapies that would exploit such markers. In seeking more specific treatment strategies, insights into these molecular pathways remain at the core of optimizing patient outcomes in high-risk disease subgroups (Aslanidis et al., 2018). In contrast to Wilms tumor, clear cell adenocarcinoma (CCA) of the urinary tract is a distinctive pathology with poor prognosis and aggressive character. Being predominantly in the female urethra, this rare malignancy has fascinated scientists with its elusive molecular profile. Investigation studies have examined genetic defects, such as driver mutations and pathway anomalies, that are responsible for CCA. Through the use of whole-exome sequencing and bioinformatics, researchers have begun to define the mutational spectrum, which provides for candidate genes that contribute to oncogenesis and tumor suppression. These discoveries not only enrich our knowledge regarding CCA's etiology but also delineate auspicious therapeutic targets, thereby placing it within more widely accepted renal tumors within the overall discussion of renal and urothelial cancers (Figure 12.7).

12.2.3. Renal Sarcomas

Of all the renal tumors, renal sarcomas are among the most uncommon and most virulent groups and constitute a challenge to clinicians due to their atypical presentation and poor prognostic outcomes. The tumors originate in the renal parenchyma or associated soft tissue structures and include several subtypes, such as leiomyosarcoma and rhabdomyosarcoma. A 43-year-old patient came in with macroscopic hematuria and was diagnosed with leiomyosarcoma of the distal ureter, as one key report indicates (Bonello et al., 2016). Sarcomas in the genitourinary tract are undertreated due to their rarity, and due to their rarity, there is a minimal amount of work contained within the literature, thereby complicating existing management options for health practitioners. Therefore, it is necessary to value the clinical behavior and therapeutic potential of renal sarcomas so that the patient's outcome can be maximized. Diagnosis of renal sarcomas tends to be multidimensional, and often it begins with imaging studies, which may not be discriminative enough for distinguishing between benign and malignant lesions. The use of needle biopsy has become a valuable diagnostic tool, more so, providing rich histopathological details necessary to determine the nature of a renal mass. According to studies, even small renal masses, those smaller than 4 cm, are challenging to distinguish from benign pathology, resulting in a significant fraction (de Leval et al., 2018). The success of needle biopsy allows the clinician to adequately assess not only the risk of malignancy but also to acquire beneficial information regarding the primary vs. secondary nature of the lesion. Thus, accurate diagnosis heavily dictates the subsequent treatment and prediction, highlighting the importance of complete pretherapeutic evaluation. Renal sarcomas treatment generally is multimodal and includes surgery, chemotherapy, and sometimes radiotherapy, in line with the nature and stage of the tumors. Surgical removal is the primary treatment and plays a crucial role in achieving a cure, particularly when the cancer is localized and resectable. However, due to advanced presentation disease, the majority of patients will suffer a poor outcome, with rates being significantly impacted by factors such as tumor type and histological grade. Furthermore, innovation in the development of new therapeutic modalities is driving a re-evaluation of management protocols, highlighting the need for individualized treatment protocols based on precise pretherapeutic diagnoses (de Leval et al., 2018). Due to the multifactorial interactions affecting renal sarcoma outcomes, further study into their biology, as well as into treatment options, is of the utmost importance to maximize survival and quality of life for affected patients (Figure 12.8).

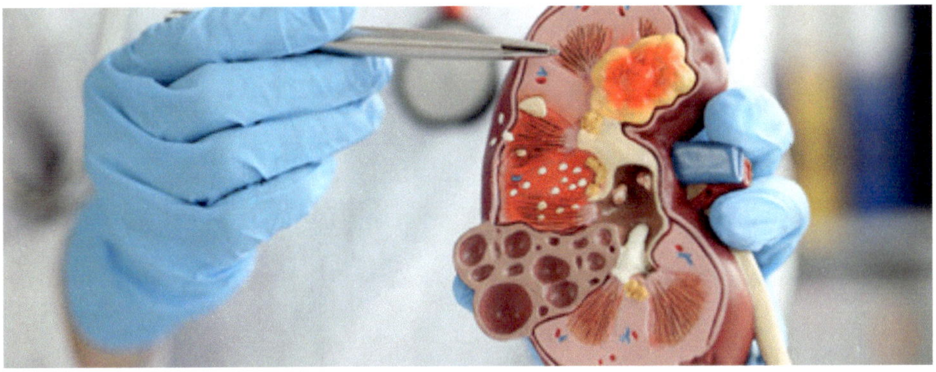

Figure 12.8. Renal sarcoma.

Source: https://www.netmeds.com/images/cms/magefan_blog/nmslite/1702276934_renal-sarcoma_480x180.jpg.

12.3. Types of Urothelial Tumors

Urothelial neoplasms, the majority of which originate from the urothelium of the bladder, ureter, and renal pelvis, are highly variable in their histologic appearances and biological behavior. The most common is transitional cell carcinoma (TCC), showing variable differentiation from low-grade papillary neoplasms to highly aggressive carcinomas. This variability influences prognosis and treatment planning because well-differentiated tumors are less virulent. In contrast, poorly differentiated tumors have a propensity to metastasize and are associated with worse patient outcomes. Furthermore, it is worth noting that both genetic predisposition and environmental exposures contribute to the incidence and development of these tumors, and therefore, more comprehensive studies are needed to investigate their etiology and pathophysiology. A second crucial urothelial tumor category is squamous cell carcinoma and adenocarcinoma, both less common than TCC but of special clinical significance. Squamous cell carcinoma typically arises on the background of chronic irritative lesions, such as schistosomiasis or chronic catheterization, while adenocarcinoma may arise from glandular urothelial structures or due to the involvement of adjacent tissue. Their prevalence can vary geographically and usually represents local public health concerns, such as endemic diseases. Comprehensive studies have shown that in contrast to TCC, clinic management of these tumors also differs quite sharply, with the necessity of specific treatment modalities, e.g., neoadjuvant chemotherapy and tumor type and stage-specific surgery (Halpern et al., 2018). Recent advances in biomolecular science are most crucial for deciphering the nuances of urothelial tumors and their respective prognoses. It has been demonstrated that specific genetic alterations and expression patterns serve as biomarkers for patient stratification, informing treatment and outcome. For instance, the regulation of LDL receptor-related proteins is linked to patient survival in bladder urothelial carcinoma, indicating the significance of personalized medicine in cancer (Gilder et al., 2017). Moreover, evolving imaging techniques, such as novel PET/MRI tools, enhance diagnostic capabilities for the identification of initial tumors and precise staging, which are crucial for effective management. Thus, the integration of molecular data with emerging imaging modalities can improve the clinical management of urothelial neoplasms and benefit patients (Figure 12.9).

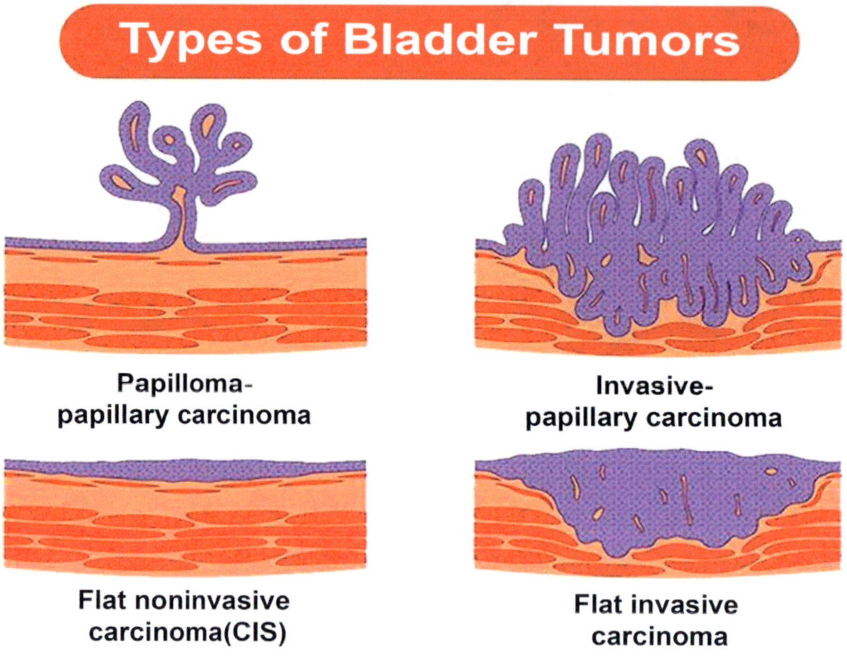

Figure 12.9. Types of urothelial tumors.

Source: https://www.medicalindiatourism.com/wp-content/uploads/2022/03/Types-of-Bladder-Cancer-in-Men.jpg.

12.3.1. Transitional Cell Carcinoma (TCC)

TCC, or urothelial carcinoma, is the most frequent bladder cancer and also exists in the renal pelvis and in the ureter. Its urothelial derivation characterizes it and is particularly significant due to its multifocality and recency. TCC pathology can range from a broad spectrum of morphologic features, including papillary and flat growth patterns, to varying prognostic features. Notably, highly graded cases of TCC can be shown to have aggressive behavior and invade the vessel, as in the unusual case of IVC invasion. Significant studies have reported such occurrences, indicating that those tumors of advanced stages have been found to invade lymph nodes and local tissues, citing the importance of early diagnosis and multimodal treatment measures to improve patient survival and cure rate (Raed et al., 2017). The presenting clinical symptom of transitional cell carcinoma can be extremely nonspecific, and the ensuing difficulty in diagnosis is not unusual. A lot of the patients present with vague, easily confused symptoms like abdominal pain, hematuria, or even weight loss, which highlights the importance of proper clinical workup and imaging studies. In a single case of a 71-year-old male, the application of sophisticated imaging revealed a complex appearance of renal hypertrophy and IVC thrombus, ultimately to raise the possibility of renal cell carcinoma until further pathology yielded high-grade TCC. Such atypical presentations require a discerning differential diagnosis, as the superimposed signs in renal and urothelial neoplasias may lead to mismanagement. Clinicians should exercise caution during their assessment, particularly in suspicious imaging findings, to enable appropriate interventions (Raed et al., 2017). Metastatic transitional cell carcinoma poses additional challenges, particularly when it metastasizes beyond the urinary tract. Imaging evidence of metastases to organs in distant locations, such as the lungs or liver, introduces significant complexity to clinical management, as revealed through documented case presentations where patients had both lymphatic and distant metastases. This dissemination poses staging and treatment paradigm choice problems. After all, total approaches are key to managing both the primary tumor and metastatic disease. Histopathologic study and immunohistochemical evaluation remain key in establishing metastatic TCC, providing critical details on therapeutic targets and prognostic variables. Understanding the multifaceted nature of transitional cell carcinoma and the means to develop better early detection methods will subsequently enable more effective management methods and patient outcomes for renal and urothelial tumors (Figure 12.10).

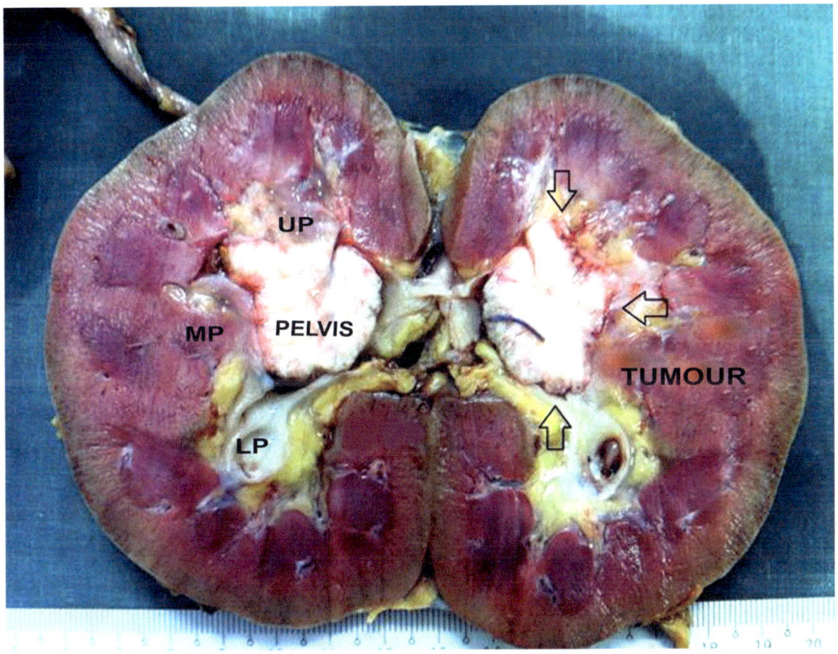

Figure 12.10. Transitional cell carcinoma.

Source: https://prod-images-static.radiopaedia.org/images/6228349/b47167d10451965410ca227ab65bff_big_gallery.jpg.

12.3.2. Squamous Cell Carcinoma (SCC)

SCC is a significant category of neoplasms that can occur in numerous organ systems, including the renal and urothelial systems. Characterized by squamous cell growth, SCC typically occurs as a result of chronic irritation or inflammation, which is part of its pathogenesis in the urothelium. The relationship between SCC and susceptibility risk factors, such as exposure to carcinogens, compromised immune response, and chronic inflammation, has been well described. As SCC metastasizes to local lymph nodes and distant organs such as lungs and liver, early detection and diagnosis are imperative to improve the patient's prognosis. Interestingly, some patterns in the SCC histopathology have been reported by research studies, which are essential in distinguishing it from other malignancies and thus determining appropriate therapeutic choices (Clercq et al., 2011). For urothelial and renal tumors, therapeutic decisions for squamous cell carcinoma have significantly altered regarding targeted therapy and immunotherapy. Recent advancement highlights the role of fibroblast growth factor (FGF) signaling pathways in oncogenesis, with specific mention of SCC induction. Aberrant FGF signaling is typically implicated in neoplastic transformation, influencing tumor growth and metastasis (Helsten et al., 2015). The incidence of FGFR mutations and amplifications has led to the identification of pharmacological molecules that inhibit FGF/FGFR signaling. Such agents also include selective inhibitors that can combat not only SCC but also a variety of other carcinomas, indicating the broad clinical application of this therapy. This has opened up new avenues for individualized treatment regimens targeting the same feature: genetic alterations in squamous cell carcinomas. Further, the occurrence of squamous cell carcinoma in the renal and urothelial tracts also points towards the need for thorough investigation of the molecular mechanisms involved in such tumors. Awareness of the genetic and epigenetic alterations in SCC can aid in the detection of novel biomarkers that enhance screening and diagnostic specificity. Furthermore, ongoing clinical trials testing FGF/FGFR inhibitors hold promise for optimizing therapeutic outcomes, particularly in cases of treatment resistance. The incorporation of molecular biology into daily practice will further advance the management of squamous cell carcinoma towards personalization, ultimately benefiting patient management of renal and urothelial malignancies. Treatment of these advanced interactions between treatment response and genetic processes will be of prime importance in advancing outcomes in patients diagnosed with this virulent form of cancer (Figure 12.11).

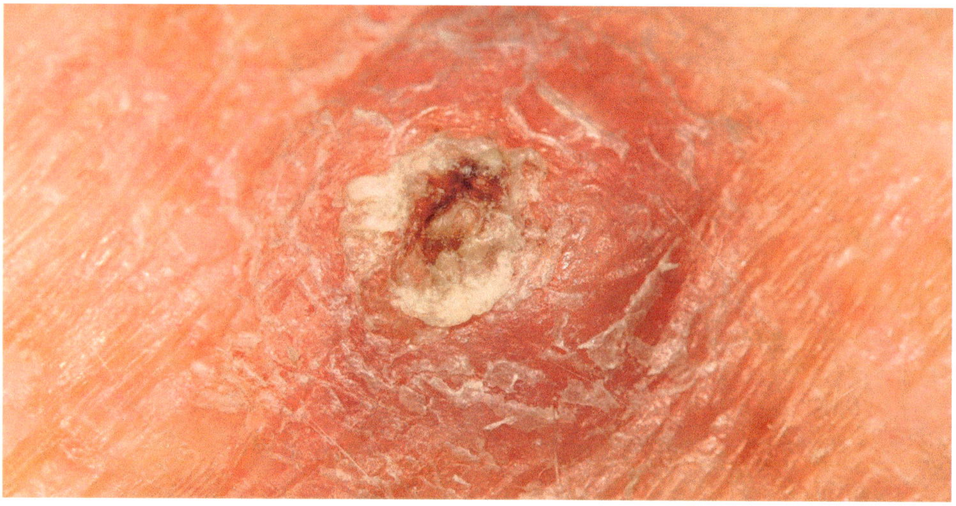

Figure 12.11. Squamous cell carcinoma.

Source: https://external-content.duckduckgo.com/iu/?u=https%3A%2F%2Fqdermatology.com.au%2Fapp%2Fuploads%2F2019%2F05%2FQ-Dermatology_Web-Banners_29.jpg&f=1&nofb=1&ipt=ecb147746068eccd1da45407d759825cdcd05bb834a6e459b3e536045c8421f9.

12.3.3. Adenocarcinoma

Adenocarcinoma, a malignant tumor originating from glandular epithelial cells, plays a significant role in the renal and urothelial tumor profile. With its glandular structure, adenocarcinoma can occur in diverse tissues, such as the kidney, bladder, and prostate. In renal oncology, renal cell carcinoma (RCC), specifically identified as clear cell carcinoma, is the most prevalent kidney malignancy and quintessentially represents the clinical subtlety associated with adenocarcinomas. The heterogeneity and variability of RCC in histopathologic features are the cause of its complexity. It takes profound knowledge to diagnose and manage it appropriately. Furthermore, the metastatic nature of renal adenocarcinomas makes it clinically significant because these tumors have the potential to metastasize to lymph nodes, lungs, and other locations. Thus treatment regimens and patient outcomes are problematic. The relationship with other cancers of the urinary tract is emphasized by the frequent occurrence of synchronous neoplasias, as seen clinically. Particularly noteworthy is that it has been found that patients who present with coexistent bladder carcinomas in association with renal adenocarcinomas necessitate a multidisciplinary approach to treatment. As an illustration, there was a report of a patient with rectal adenocarcinoma and synchronous bladder cancer, proposing a potential link through shared oncogenic pathways like PIK3CA gene mutations (Colombino et al., 2013). The diagnosis and treatment of such patients become particularly challenging, as the presence of multiple primary cancers requires precise evaluation to ascertain global treatment strategies to be adopted. High-intensity investigations, such as high-level imaging and histopathological analysis, are crucial in determining the spectrum of disease and informing clinical intervention. Due to the increasing prevalence and variability of adenocarcinoma within the renal and urothelial context, early detection and molecular analysis are critical. The use of techniques such as biopsy and genomic sequencing has now become an integral diagnostic tool for the identification of mutations to be applied in guiding targeted therapy. For example, the detection of PIK3CA pathway mutations may indicate a high-risk profile for progression, warranting more aggressive treatment (Clercq et al., 2011). Both the surgical therapy of the localized disease and the medical treatment of advanced disease must be tailored to the individual tumor biology and patient considerations. As technology advances, it is of utmost importance to integrate evidence from studies aimed at understanding the molecular causes of adenocarcinoma to further inform us and encourage the development of more effective treatment schemes for renal and urothelial cancers (Figure 12.12).

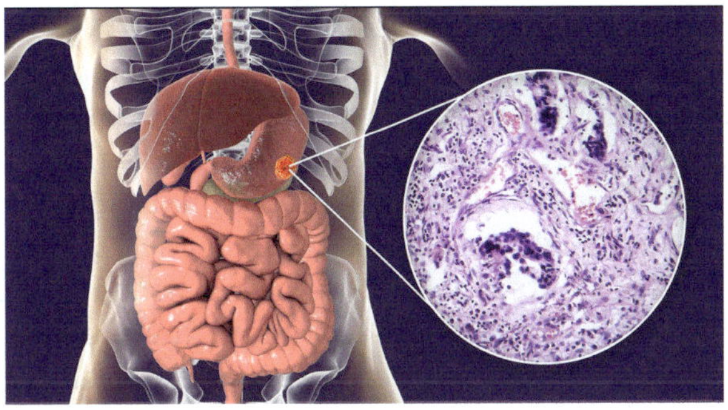

Figure 12.12. Adenocarcinoma.

Source: https://external-content.duckduckgo.com/iu/?u=https%3A%2F%2Fghealth121.com%2Fwp-content%2Fuploads%2F2021%2F01%2FAdenocarcinoma-Image-1.jpg&f=1&nofb=1&ipt=0b559cce7a183849deed54ada0cdf5e06b14841c161757964aeeb5a905124868.

12.4. Risk Factors and Epidemiology

The epidemiology of renal and urothelial tumors exhibits a complex interplay of multifactorial risk factors that profoundly influences patient outcomes. RCC, which is the most prevalent kidney cancer, exhibits variability in incidence among geographic and demographic groups. Among these, smoking is identified as an established risk factor for RCC and UCB. Not only does cigarette smoking increase the likelihood of developing these cancers, but smoking is linked with poorer prognoses following diagnosis as well. Furthermore, the epidemiologic features of those afflicted generally indicate elevated frequencies among older persons and males, advocating the use of targeted screening practices in those who are at higher risk. It is crucial to recognize these population differences in an effort to design effective prevention programs and an overall management strategy that considers the unique needs of diverse patient populations. UTUC is an example of why it is essential to distinguish between different urinary tract cancers due to their varied epidemiological profiles. Though smoking remains a prevailing risk factor with UCB, UTUC is uniquely affected by aristolochic acid toxicity and mismatch repair defects, and is less commonly involved in bladder cancer. These are critical risk factors to recognize for the initiation of effective prevention and early detection strategies. In addition, the rarity of UTUC reflects its understudied compared to other urothelial cancers. Promotion of vigorous research efforts and inter-institutional coordination is essential not only in the detection of high-risk patients but also to optimize therapeutic approaches that may lead to maximal results. This risk factor disparity dictates intense consideration in handling renal and urothelial cancer epidemiology. The significance of modern imaging technology and advances in cancer biology cannot be overstated in promoting an understanding of risk stratification and the management of renal and urothelial cancers. Advanced imaging modalities such as CT and MRI have transformed the way these tumors are diagnosed, albeit with some limitations of sensitivity for staging, particularly in UTUC, where conventional imaging may be insufficient. Striving to optimize these approaches, along with the development of new biomarkers, leads to the improvement of prognostic capability, thereby facilitating individualized therapeutic methods. Additionally, total tumor resection has also been emphasized in high-risk cases, where radical nephroureterectomy remains the standard practice. These advances in imaging and therapy underscore the ongoing need for research focused on refining risk assessment methods to the fullest extent for patient benefit, especially in light of the advancing understanding of renal and urothelial tumor pathogenesis, as cited in Halpern et al. (2018) and Bensalah et al. (2015) (Figure 12.13).

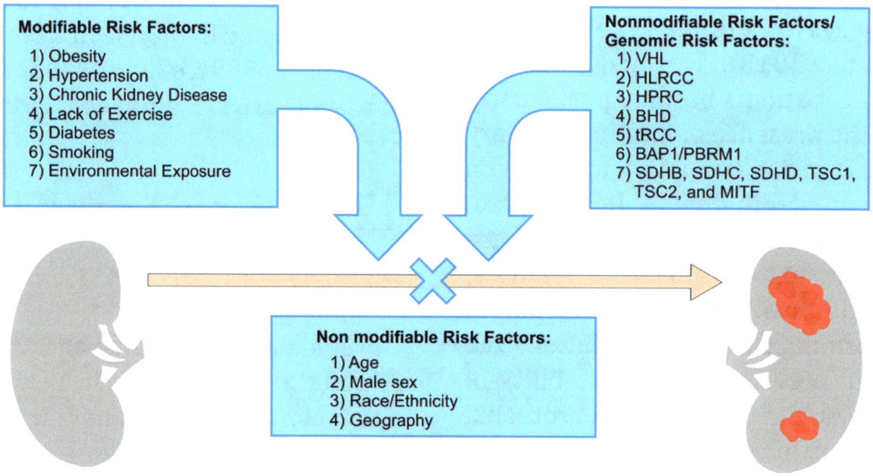

Figure 12.13. The epidemiology of renal and urothelial tumors.

Source: https://www.europeanurology.com/cms/10.1016/j.eururo.2022.08.019/asset/92d75279-b6df-4a0a-8069-af8433d55f9d/main.assets/gr5_lrg.jpg.

12.4.1. Genetic Predispositions

Genetic predispositions need to be understood in the study of renal and urothelial tumors, as inherited elements are crucial in determining an individual's susceptibility to developing these cancers. Lynch syndrome, a common genetic disorder, is also closely associated with various cancers, including urothelial carcinomas. Individuals with this syndrome have mutations in the mismatch repair genes, which predispose them to the development of such tumors. Identifying patients with Lynch syndrome through genetic screening is crucial, as it enables anticipatory surveillance and early intervention. Recent observations reinforce that mutation in these repair genes confers a higher risk of bladder cancer and emphasize the ongoing need for research into other inherited patterns of urothelial carcinogenesis. This finding is notable for highlighting the importance of genetic testing and counseling in optimizing management strategies within high-risk populations (Cheng et al., 2018). Apart from Lynch syndrome, the field is also seeing growing interest in the application of next-generation sequencing to detect genetic risk for renal and urothelial malignancies. Its application in identifying oncogenic drivers in patients and enhancing treatment regimens through personalized medicine significantly enhances treatment options. Unexpectedly, it has been shown that certain genetic alterations, such as activating mutations in KRAS, occur in non-malignant diseases. This finding is crucial because it expands the history of the genetic environment beyond cancer to suggest a complex interaction between heritable traits and cancer susceptibility. The effect of a greater understanding of these genetic markers can make screening and prevention processes more efficient in targeting each individual based on their own specific genetic profile, enabling a holistic approach to treating renal and urothelial tumors (Adashek et al., 2020). Combined, the addition of genetic susceptibility to the model of renal and urothelial tumor research is revolutionizing what is understood about and how to manage these conditions. With increased understanding of the cancer heritable factors, there is a trend toward personalized therapeutic approaches. For example, patients with certain genetic mutations can be treated with agents tailored to their molecular profile, showing success in some cases. Furthermore, research that examines the coincidence between genetic syndromes and sporadic cases provides valuable information on tumorigenesis. Therefore, the continuous evolution of genetic testing and its integration into clinical practice underscores the significant role of genetics in cancer therapy and prevention. The implementation of these advancements will lead to improved patient outcomes and increased understanding of the advanced biology of renal and urothelial tumors (Cheng et al., 2018; Adashek et al., 2020).

12.4.2. Environmental Exposures

Environmental exposure is very crucial in the causation and pathogenesis of renal and urothelial malignancies, primarily by the action of a variety of carcinogenic agents found in the environment. Tobacco smoke is one of the most significant etiologic factors for these cancers. There is evidence to suggest that tobacco smoke, which contains a blend of chemicals with carcinogenic effects, has very substantial correlations with bladder cancer (BC) and RCC formation. For instance, the relative risk (RR) of BC incidence in all smokers has been reported at 2.57, increasing up to 3.37 for current smokers, with former smokers still having a higher risk of 1.98. Such evidence highlights the predominant effect of smoking on cancer risk. It emphasizes tobacco cessation as the key to curbing mortality from such tumors, thus locating environmental exposure as a focal concern of cancer epidemiology (Begg et al., 2016). Aside from tobacco, environmental toxins such as heavy metals are another principal risk factor for renal and urothelial cancers. The etiology of cancer associated with heavy metal exposure is complex and often difficult to establish definitively. Some studies, however, have indicated that noxious chemicals like mercury, lead, and cadmium can activate oncogenic pathways, leading to tumorigenesis. Model animal studies have shown that higher levels of heavy metals correlate with an increased frequency of tumors, and this points to a deleterious interaction of the metals with genes for cancer risks. Further, some studies have shown that excess metals induce a setting for cancer advancement by interfering with cellular signaling pathways and causing oxidative stress that can result in the formation of renal and urothelial tumors (Trapani et al., 2010). The consequences of these exposures guide environmental policy and public health. Efforts to minimize exposure to carcinogenic agents, particularly in areas with high pollution or previous contamination, are vital not only for avoiding cancer but also for realizing additional benefits for health. Environmental monitoring programs established to track the prevalence of toxic elements and heavy metals in the environment can inform more efficient regulatory choices that reach vulnerable populations. Moreover, increased public sensitization about the risks of tobacco smoke and environmental poisons is likely to improve healthier lifestyle practices and improve community health initiatives. Overall, the integration of environmental health aspects into cancer control strategies is pivotal in solving the etiologic causes of renal and urothelial neoplasms (Trapani et al., 2010; Begg et al., 2016) (Figure 12.14).

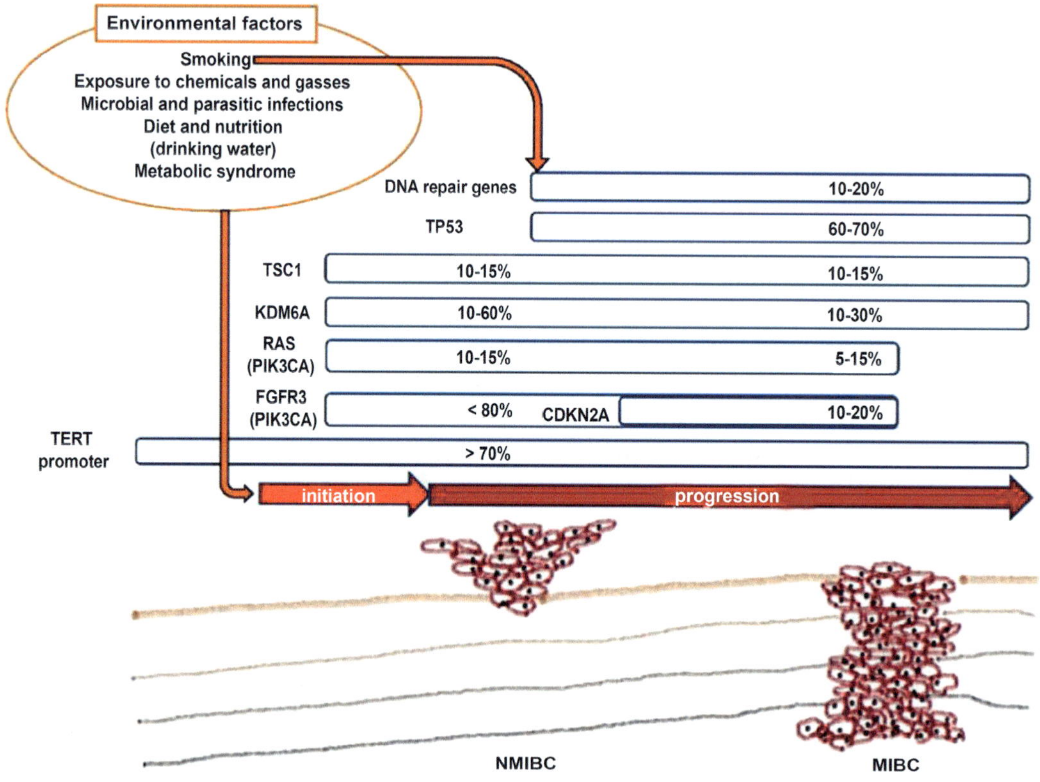

Figure 12.14. Environmental exposures of renal and urothelial tumors.

Source: https://pub.mdpi-res.com/ijms/ijms-21-06072/article_deploy/html/images/ijms-21-06072-g001.png?1598188951.

12.4.3. Lifestyle Factors

The lifestyle factors implicated in the pathogenesis of renal and urothelial neoplasms are as diverse as they are complex. Among the most significant lifestyle-related risk factors for their development is tobacco smoking, which has been repeatedly associated with both renal cell carcinoma and bladder cancer risk. The carcinogenic substances found in cigarette smoke can contribute to the genetic mutations of the cells lining the urinary tract, allowing for the development towards malignancy. Moreover, obesity has also been identified as a key factor in this, and research has shown that excess body weight causes changes in hormone levels as well as inflammation markers, both of which are involved in tumorigenesis. Understanding these lifestyle factors is significant when it comes to organizing prevention and intervention strategies, particularly considering that modification of these habits can drastically reduce cancer risk among high-risk populations. Diet also plays a pivotal role in the pathogenesis of renal and urothelial neoplasms. Higher consumption of fruits and vegetables is associated with a reduced risk of cancer, possibly due to their rich antioxidant, vitamin, and phytochemical content that neutralizes oxidative stress. Conversely, high consumption of processed foods and sodium is associated with elevated risk for urothelial tumors. Moreover, adequate hydration, particularly water consumption, may help to dilute any carcinogens present in the urine and also ensure urinary tract health. Healthy eating habits education programs could be potential ways of reducing the cancer incidence rates among the population. The inclusion of nutrition awareness into public policy can potentially yield significant long-term returns in cancer reduction. Physical exercise is an integral aspect of lifestyle that, regardless of dietary considerations, has been shown to influence cancer risk. Regular exercise is associated with numerous health benefits, including maintaining weight and improving metabolic function, both of which can help reduce cancer risks. Physical inactivity, however, has been seen to have greater risks for a variety of cancers, including renal and urothelial system cancers. According to emerging trends, highly physically inactive populations might see a rise in cancer diagnoses. Engaging in routine exercise not only strengthens the immune system but also may make newer treatments more successful, as research emphasizes the benefits of incorporating lifestyle modification into conventional therapies (Botticelli et al., 2018). Moreover, the search for knowledge on genomic alterations in malignancies and non-malignancies highlights the importance of holistic approaches to cancer prevention, which involve lifestyle factors as well as the understanding of precision medicine (Adashek et al., 2020).

12.5. Symptoms and Diagnosis

The symptoms of renal and urothelial tumors are often non-specific, making it challenging in the early stages to diagnose them. Patients may experience nonspecific symptoms, such as hematuria, flank pain, and weight loss. Hematuria, or the presence of blood in urine, is particularly indicative, occurring in approximately 65% of ureteral urothelial carcinoma patients, which makes it a significant diagnostic marker (Raed et al., 2017). Flank pain can arise from tumor growth or obstruction with resultant hydronephrosis. In addition, systemic symptoms such as fatigue and unintentional weight loss may further complicate presentations. These nonspecific symptoms are common to several diseases and not unique to renal cancer, making differential diagnosis critical to avoid symptom misattribution to less sinister conditions. Thus, awareness of these clinical presentations is crucial in advancing early intervention and improving patient outcomes. Diagnosis of renal and urothelial cancers is multi-modal and includes imaging, laboratory tests, and biopsies. Initial imaging tests, for example, ultrasound, CT scans, or MRI, are typically used to detect abnormal masses within the kidneys or the urinary tract. For example, CT scans can not only detect tumors but also assess lymph node status and metastasis (Raed et al., 2017). Laboratory investigations, such as urinalysis, can aid in the detection of hematuria and renal function abnormalities. If a tumor is found, it is necessary to perform a biopsy to confirm malignancy. Percutaneous and surgical biopsies can be applied, particularly in cases of suspected vascular invasion. Diagnosis is crucial, and treatment planning and prognostication depend only on the type of tumor, stage, and patient. Staging and grading of renal and urothelial neoplasms also give additional guidance to the management plan and prognosis. The American Joint Committee on Cancer (AJCC) tumor classification system is the most widely used to categorize tumors based on size, local invasiveness, and the presence of distant metastasis. Early-stage tumors, for instance, tend to have better prognoses and can be treated successfully using nephroureterectomy, whereas advanced-stage tumors have poor prognoses (Chang et al., 2005). Tumor grade, a measure of the degree of cellular differentiation, is equally essential in survival prognosis. High-grade tumors tend to be associated with high degrees of cellular aggressiveness and high recurrence rates, supporting the necessity of careful pathological examination following diagnosis. Knowledge of these staging and grading systems not only aids in treatment planning but also facilitates communication between treatment teams and patients regarding results and treatment options (Figure 12.15).

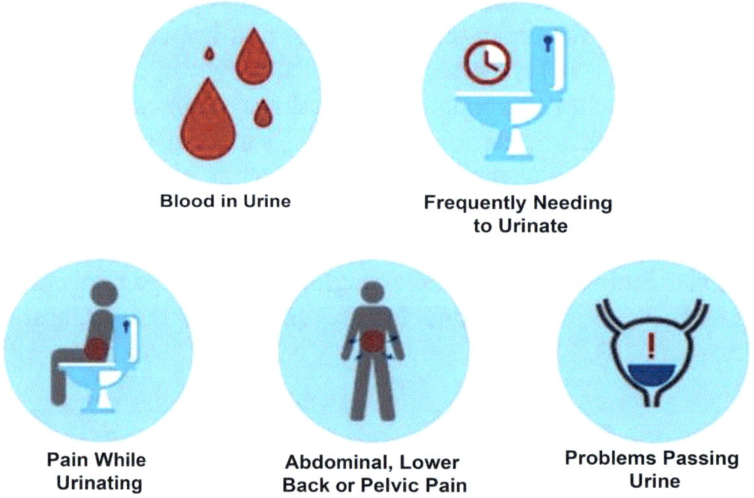

Figure 12.15. The symptoms of urothelial tumors.

Source: https://surjithospital.com/wp-content/uploads/2024/08/WhatsApp-Image-2024-08-21-at-18.13.25_aa0b2cdb.jpg.

12.5.1. Common Symptoms of Renal Tumors

The appearance of renal tumors is primarily defined by a range of signs that vary quite considerably among patients. In the majority of patients, one of the most terrifying signs is hematuria, or blood in urine, which occurs in quite a considerable number of patients. This symptom may occur intermittently, leading the patients to underestimate its significance initially. When combined with other atypical presenting symptoms such as abdominal or flank pain, hematuria may be indicative of a serious underlying disease, typically requiring further clinical evaluation. Early identification of the symptoms is necessary, as renal neoplasms may have an indolent course with no apparent symptoms until advanced stages, when treatment options may be grossly impaired. Identification and understanding of these initial signs can greatly enhance patient outcomes by enabling early intervention and management regimens.

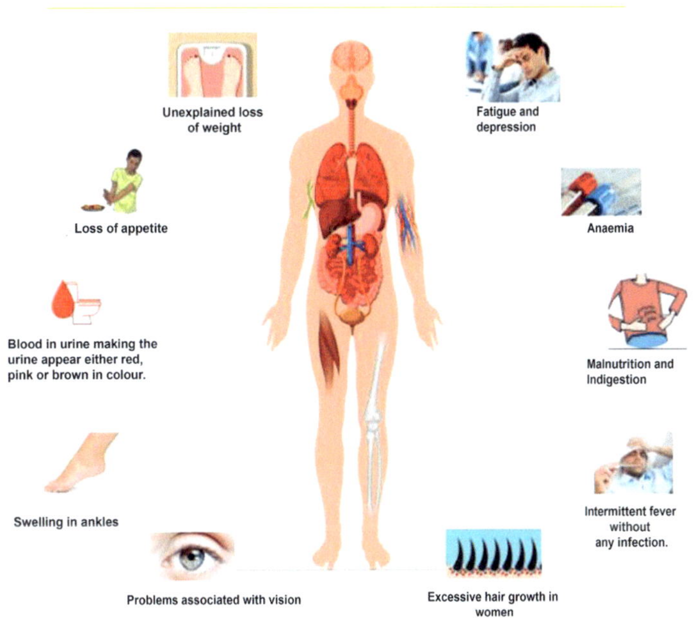

Figure 12.16. Symptoms of renal tumors.

Source: https://www.nirujahealthtech.com/wp-content/uploads/2020/04/Renal-Cancer_-Signs-Symptoms-1.png.

In addition, systemic manifestations such as fever, loss of weight, and fatigue may also accompany renal tumors, reflecting the more widespread impact on the patient's health. Symptoms typically manifest as the body responds to the presence of the tumors, resulting in metabolic alterations and immune responses. Notably, while such systemic presentations are not necessarily specifically characteristic of renal tumors—typically occurring in concert with other pathological processes—they contribute to a clinical presentation requiring careful investigation. Notably, the presence of hematuria, along with systemic symptoms, raises the need for further diagnostic testing to establish the etiology. This in-depth knowledge of symptom identification helps clinicians differentiate between renal tumors and other possible pathologies with identical clinical presentationssuch as urinary tract infection or lower urinary tract symptoms addressed in , such as urinary tract infections or lower urinary tract symptoms, as addressed in the literature on inverted papilloma (Chang et al., 2011). Patients can also develop localized symptoms depending on the size and location of the tumors, e.g., chronic backache and changed urinary habits. For instance, patients with a renal mass may present with increased frequency or urgency of urination, typically without relation to benign conditions. However, as in clinical practice, some patients present with obstructive uropathy and concomitant problematic symptoms such as flank or abdominal pain that also complicate diagnosis (Aggarwal et al., 2012). Recognition of the local signs along with systemic symptoms plays a role in the proper diagnosis and treatment plan. In the end, appropriate knowledge about the common symptoms of renal tumors helps in appropriate medical intervention on time, enhanced patient care, and potentially a better survival rate (Figure 12.16).

12.5.2. Symptoms Associated with Urothelial Tumors

Urothelial neoplasms, most commonly found in the bladder and upper urinary tract, have a vast spectrum of manifestations that can have a significant effect on the quality of life of patients. Hematuria, or blood in the urine, is the most frequent symptom associated with these neoplasms and is present in a high proportion of patients. Hematuria is either gross, i.e., grossly visible to the naked eye, or microscopic, detectable only on laboratory examination. Other than hematuria, patients will similarly complain of dysuria, frequency, and urgency, presenting with evidence of bladder obstruction or irritation. These symptoms and signs will prompt people to visit their physician, followed by investigations such as imaging and cystoscopy to identify the underlying cause. Ultimately, detection of such clinical features is essential in an effort to introduce early intervention and management to improve the outcomes of patients with urothelial tumors. In rare instances, urothelial neoplasms can be combined with other malignancies so that presentations and diagnoses are complex. For example, a case report described a patient with multiple tumors, like bladder carcinoma and colorectal adenocarcinoma, who presented with macrohematuria and rectal tenesmus, and the interdependent nature of presentations in patients with multiple foci of malignancy. Symptoms like rectal bleeding and alteration of bowel habits can first mislead clinicians and lead them to underestimate a possible urothelial malignancy. Therefore, thorough assessments that include symptoms from multiple systems continue to play an essential role in making the right diagnosis. The probability of co-occurrence of multiple tumors underscores the need to thoroughly assess symptoms, as early diagnosis is critical to implementing effective management protocols and improving overall survival rates among urothelial carcinoma patients, particularly in cases involving multifactorial conditions (Colombino et al., 2013). Survival in patients with urothelial cancers can be highly heterogeneous, depending on a multitude of varied factors such as grade, stage, and initial presentation. Research suggests that meticulous documentation of initial presentation, either as hematuria or high-grade ureteral obstruction, can be an important prognostic indicator. For example, gross hematuria is listed as the primary presenting symptom in about 65% of urothelial carcinoma cases, forming a significant correlation between severity of disease and symptomatology. Tumor stage diagnosis remains an important factor in determining the treatment regimen and prognosis afterwards, where early tumors are generally found to have a higher percentage of successful treatment and survival. Notably, the type and grade of tumor can significantly influence recurrence and survival, underscoring the importance of early symptom recognition and prompt treatment to optimize the survival prospects of urothelial tumor-presenting patients (Chang et al., 2005).

12.5.3. Diagnostic Imaging and Procedures

The role of diagnostic imaging in assessing renal and urothelial neoplasms has been revolutionized, enabling early detection and accurate staging. Techniques such as ultrasound, computed tomography (CT), and magnetic resonance imaging (MRI) play a crucial role in imaging the structures of the kidney and detecting potential malignancies. Ultrasound, often as a first-line test, may provide a tool for the detection of masses and abnormalities. However, CT remains the gold standard, especially in determining the extent of the disease and planning for surgery. Particularly, CT urography provides crucial information on the renal pelvis and ureters, which is invaluable in understanding the entire extent of urothelial tumors. As emphasized by recent studies, imaging not only guides diagnosis but also informs the therapeutic plan, influencing the decision-making process between radical nephroureterectomy and alternative treatments, which is an important factor in treating such tumors. This highlights the interaction between imaging modalities and clinical outcomes. Factual knowledge of imaging-pathological correlation is crucial in the effective management of urothelial tumors. Research indicates that preoperative imaging can serve as a predictive marker for disease stage. The relationship between preoperative hydronephrosis and the pathological stage after nephroureterectomy has garnered attention in clinical settings. In particular, radiographic evidence of ipsilateral renal obstruction has been analyzed to determine its association with tumor advancement. To illustrate, a study revealed that 31.7% of patients presented with locally advanced disease, highlighting an essential feature of disease staging through imaging methods. This salient finding provides valuable feedback for clinicians, as knowing the correlation between imaging information and the ultimate pathological stage enables more rational treatment planning, responding to the requirement for accurate diagnostic imaging in modern uro-oncology practice. In addition, the use of serial procedures such as ureteroscopy continues to enhance diagnostic specificity in patients with suspected urothelial carcinoma. Ureteroscopy is a valuable modality in biopsies for the diagnosis of conditions such as carcinoma in situ (Cis) or upper tract urothelial carcinoma (UTUC) in cases where imaging findings are indeterminate.

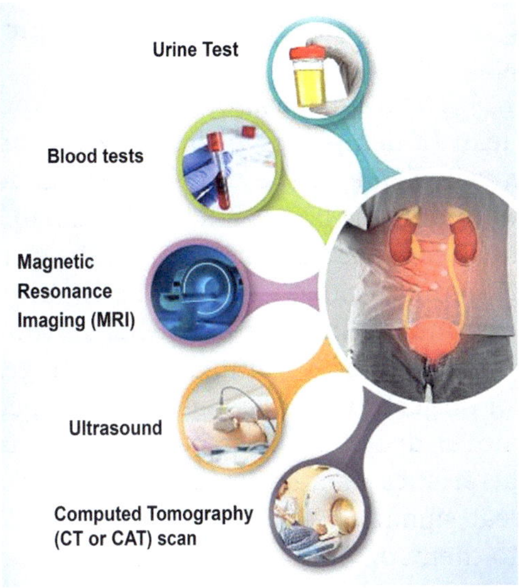

Figure 12.17. The role of diagnostic imaging in the assessment of renal and urothelial tumors.

Source: https://saphaltaincancercare.com/blog/wp-content/uploads/2023/02/What-are-symptoms-of-kidney-cancer-info.jpg.

Study exemplifies this paradigm, demonstrating that following initial adverse imaging, further ureteroscopic assessment can lead to definitive diagnoses in a significant percentage of patients. Particularly in challenging situations, serial ureteroscopy can furnish critical information on tumor presence and extent and guide future therapy. As implied, only 42% of clinically suspected UTUC patients were eventually diagnosed with the disease, witnessing the complexities involved in accurately diagnosing renal and urothelial tumors through imaging and procedural intervention. This also highlights the importance of incorporating diverse diagnostic approaches in optimizing patient outcomes within the uro-oncology treatment paradigm (Figure 12.17).

12.6. Treatment Options

The therapeutic landscape of renal and urothelial cancers has been radically transformed with the advent of immunotherapy, which uses the host's immune machinery to attack cancer. The most promising of the novel therapeutic strategies is the utilization of checkpoint inhibitors, particularly those against programmed cell death-1 (PD-1) and programmed cell death ligand-1 (PD-L1). The mechanism by which checkpoint inhibitors work is through blocking the interactions that lead to dampening of immune responses and hence allowing T-cells to destroy cancer cells effectively. Some of these agents are under investigation in numerous clinical trials, and some, including pembrolizumab and nivolumab, have already been licensed by the FDA for advanced urothelial carcinoma. The most recent of these developments is the development of durvalumab, a high-affinity monoclonal antibody, which promises significant benefits for advanced disease and non-muscle-invasive urothelial carcinoma, thereby offering additional therapeutic options for patients with more favorable disease stages (Chamie et al., 2018). Apart from immunotherapy, the role of targeted therapies has also emerged in the treatment of renal and urothelial malignancies. The novel drugs are designed to specifically target cancer cells by exploiting novel molecular characteristics that are usually overexpressed in tumors. A prime example is integrins, which are of great significance in terms of cell adhesion and motility, and have become significant targets due to their role in tumor growth and metastases. Several integrin antagonists are currently being developed and have shown promise in inhibiting tumor invasion and metastasis, thereby offering new targets for therapeutic intervention. In addition, biomarker profiling using TCGA-derived data identified some of the integrin subunits that are overexpressed in various forms of solid cancers, further delineating potential targets for targeted therapies of renal and urothelial malignancies. This precision medicine approach is employed to tailor treatment, optimizing patient outcomes (Arun et al., 2018). The application of these disparate treatments highlights the multifaceted nature of the approach required for the successful treatment of renal and urothelial tumors. The combination of immunotherapy with targeted therapies holds promise for improving therapeutic outcomes and survival rates. Existing trials seek to test these combinations, deciphering their synergistic uses. For example, clinical trials evaluating the use of durvalumab with standard chemotherapy are ongoing to ascertain whether its combination will enhance efficacy in the treatment of advanced urothelial carcinoma. Additionally, the design of ligands to target overexpressed integrins offers new strategies for locally delivering therapeutic agents to the site of cancer, with the potential to enhance treatment efficacy while reducing systemic toxicity. As research continues, the future of renal and urothelial tumor therapy is also poised to evolve, depicting the shift toward individualized and targeted oncology (Chamie et al., 2018; Arun et al., 2018).

12.6.1. Surgical Interventions

Surgical treatment is an essential component of renal and urothelial cancer management, providing targeted therapy with the capability to alter the course of the disease in patients profoundly. Operations such as nephrectomy, or excision of a kidney, are a standard treatment for localized renal cancer. In addition to removing cancerous tissue, this operation provides staging information to guide subsequent treatment. In addition, partial nephrectomy is increasingly a favored option in patients with small-sized tumors to keep renal function intact and still effectively treat malignancy. Surgical procedure selection typically relies on tumor size, location, and the overall status of the patient, thus requiring individualized treatment protocols in clinical settings. Radical cystectomy is another essential surgical operation, primarily utilized in the case of urothelial bladder tumors. This procedure involves the complete excision of the bladder and overlying tissue, based on the degree of tumor invasion.

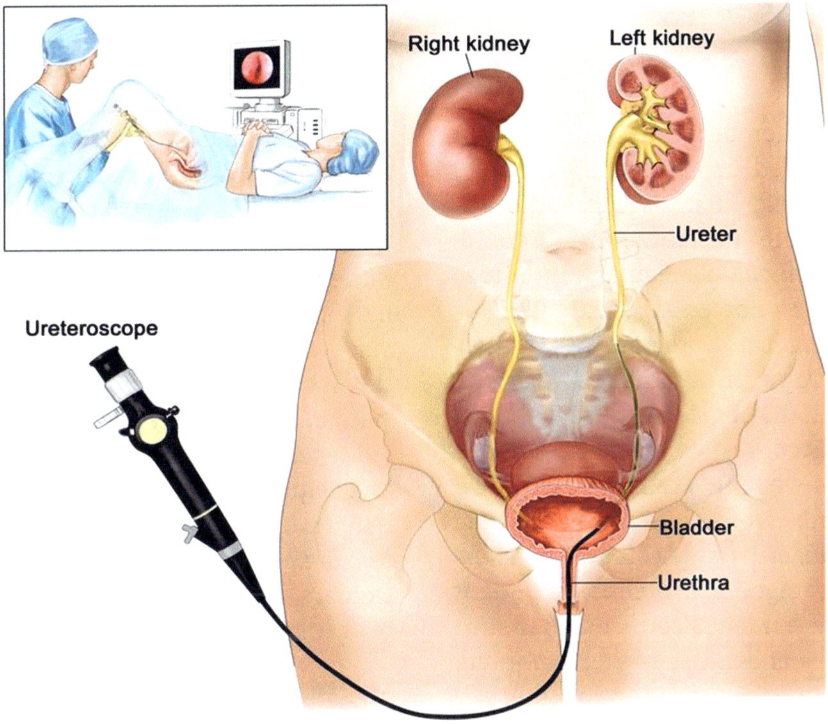

Figure 12.18. Surgical interventions for renal and urothelial tumors.

Source: https://oxfordurologyassociates.uk/wp-content/uploads/2014/03/ureteroscopy-1.jpg.

Radical cystectomy is a multifaceted surgery that needs careful selection of a patient and thorough preoperative evaluation to avoid postoperative morbidity in the form of infection and dysfunction. Minimally invasive techniques, such as laparoscopy and robot-assisted procedures, are increasingly being employed by urologists to achieve enhanced recovery times and reduced hospital stays. However, despite enhanced surgical skills, the psychological impact of such severe anatomical modification should have regular support services to enable patients to deal with various challenges following surgery. Secondly, the implementation of multidisciplinary teams in the surgical treatment of renal and urothelial cancers has to be utilized to optimize patient care. These teams may include urologists, oncologists, pathologists, and radiologists, who collaborate to develop personalized treatment strategies tailored to address the specific needs of each patient. For example, the addition of neoadjuvant treatments, including preoperative chemotherapy, can enhance the effect of surgical treatments and improve long-term survival. Research has shown that controlling lifestyle issues, including the cessation of smoking, is an essential factor in optimizing surgical outcomes and lowering recurrence rates among these patients. However, existing guidelines vary in their advice on this topic (Agrawal et al., 2015). Lastly, the combined approach that considers both surgical and adjuvant treatment can yield improved outcomes in individuals with renal and urothelial cancer (Burity et al., 2014) (Figure 12.18).

12.6.2. Chemotherapy and Radiation Therapy

The application of chemotherapy and radiation therapy has increased in the management of renal and urothelial malignancies. Chemotherapy plays a critical role in managing muscle-invasive bladder cancer, particularly in those individuals who are not good candidates for surgery, such as radical cystectomy. Platinum-based chemotherapy and radiation therapy have been demonstrated to be more effective in enhancing outcomes in patients. These combinations improve in tumor size, local control, and responsiveness in a considerable number of patients, providing a bladder-sparing alternative that can significantly enhance patient quality of life. New evidence confirms that such multimodal regimens achieve higher complete response rates compared to radiation therapy as a monotherapy, demonstrating the necessity of final treatment regimens that consider both efficacy and patient health. Furthermore, new immunotherapy modalities are revolutionizing the treatment of urothelial carcinoma. Recent research has laid the foundation for several immune checkpoint inhibitors targeting key tumor escape mechanisms. Specifically, PD-1 and PD-L1 inhibitors have been identified as promising therapies that enable the immune system to regain its efficacy against cancer cells, resulting in improved patient survival rates. The FDA has also approved a number of agents, including nivolumab and pembrolizumab, highlighting their potential application in combination with traditional treatments to enhance treatment options for urothelial carcinoma at later stages. The shift towards the incorporation of immunotherapies provides a new dimension in the management of renal and urothelial malignancies, propelling steady clinical trials to evaluate their full potential, combined with established modalities such as chemotherapy and radiation therapy (Chamie et al., 2018). The efficiency of multimodal chemotherapy and radiotherapy is also increased with the integration of regional deep hyperthermia among patients with high-risk bladder cancer. This combination therapy, based on studies, not only results in improved local tumor control but also enhances survival rates overall compared to standard treatment. In a cohort study, patients who underwent chemotherapy and radiotherapy had a significantly increased five-year overall survival rate, demonstrating the effectiveness of these combined therapies (Bertz et al., 2019). With ongoing research continually offering more evidence to support the optimal combinations and sequencing of these treatments, it is certain that an individualized strategy will be required to advance treatment in renal and urothelial cancers, ultimately positioning patients for the best long-term outcomes (Figure 12.19).

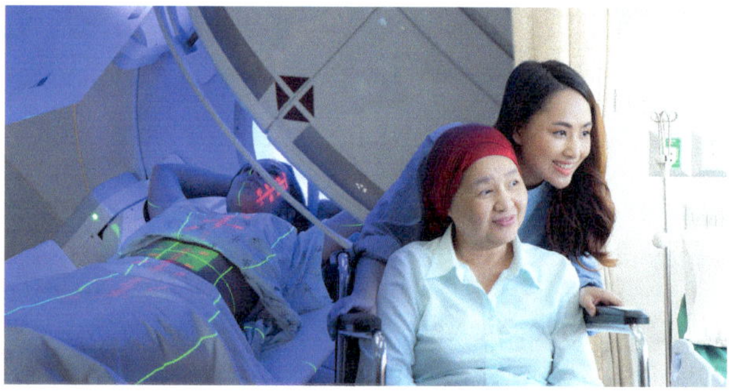

Figure 12.19. Chemotherapy and radiation therapy.

Source: https://www.makatimed.net.ph/wp-content/uploads/2023/07/MMC-_-Blog-Banner-1200x628-opt-2-3.png.

12.6.3. Emerging Therapies and Clinical Trials

The aspect of therapy for renal and urothelial malignancies is rapidly evolving, driven over the past year by advances in molecular biology and immunotherapy. As the understanding of tumors has been improving, new directions for therapy have emerged that focus on targeting the specific genetic and epigenetic differences. For instance, recent advances in NMIBC have changed the approach to clinical trials for immunotherapy and molecular-targeted therapy. These trials primarily focus on personalized medicine approaches, enabling treatment schedules to be tailored to the unique tumor characteristics of each patient. The initiatives that emanated from the NCI Bladder Cancer Task Force Clinical Trials Planning Meeting highlight the imperative of collaboration among clinical researchers, regulatory agencies, and industry to reengineer the therapeutic environment in NMIBC and bring new therapies to maturity to improve outcomes for patients and raise the survival rates (Abrams et al., 2016). Additionally, trial concepts emerging from partnership meetings highlight the novel approaches currently under development. One such recommendation is the Phase 0 window of opportunity trial, wherein an FGFR3 inhibitor is investigated at the early stages of clinical study. Such designs are valuable not merely in assessing the activity of novel drugs but also in providing insight into the biological mechanisms of tumor responses to therapy. Another trial design expresses the need to combine traditional modalities, such as Bacillus Calmette-Guérin (BCG) therapy, with immunomodulatory agents. Such multi-stage, multi-arm trials are imperative for determining the best approach to treating patients who experience recurrence after initial treatments. As bladder cancer is very immunogenic, these emerging strategies are likely to surpass the limitations of existing therapies and usher in revolutionary advances in the practice of clinical medicine (Abrams et al., 2016). For renal cancer, the discovery of targeted therapies highlights the potential benefits of combining therapeutic modalities to optimize therapeutic impact. The complexity of the tumor microenvironment necessitates a strategic approach that encompasses both established pharmacologic therapies and novel agents tailored to the patient's unique cancer signature. As exemplified in recent controversies, the identification of common immune targets provides an opening for innovative combination regimens designed to enhance clinical responses. Experiments seeking the synergistic potential of these therapies are called for, as they aim to maximize therapeutic gain with minimal toxicity. The clinical community recognizes that introducing these new therapies into the treatment process is necessary for remodeling conventional therapy in renal tumors and enhancing patient care. Implementation of this comprehensive therapeutic approach is necessary, as the field of therapy for renal and urothelial tumors continues to evolve.

SUMMARY

In conclusion, the study of renal and urothelial tumors is warranted due to the complexities of their diagnosis, therapy, and management. These cancers are special challenges because they can undermine patient outcomes if not handled properly. The combination of several diagnostic methods, including imaging and cytology, is crucial in finding the customized characteristics of these tumors. For instance, the use of fine-needle aspiration (FNA) has played a progressively critical role in renal mass evaluation, as demonstrated by a study that cited an 83% correlation between FNA and follow-up core biopsies in terms of nuclear grades. This reflects the shift in policy towards receiving earlier and more accurate diagnoses, which has the potential to result in timely intervention and, consequently, impact prognosis. Moreover, clarifying the biological behavior of renal and urothelial neoplasms is crucial in developing effective management programs. Pathophysiologic mechanisms underlying these cancers typically define their malignancy, thus naturally influencing the selection of therapeutic modalities. Post-mortem examination, along with histopathological examination, is significant since it demonstrates the metastatic potential of tumors, for instance, in cases where they metastasize to lymphatic sites and distant organs, such as the lungs and liver. Critical evaluation of such results provides a greater degree of understanding of tumor growth, thereby allowing researchers and clinicians to counter therapy methods that in some way resonate with the individual characteristics of each type of tumor. Finally, the contribution of extensive research and clinical investigations on renal and urothelial tumors cannot be overstated. Cooperation is necessary to enhance the knowledge of these tumors, particularly in view of ever-evolving treatment algorithms and diagnostic protocols. Multimodal approaches have to take center stage in future investigations to optimize diagnostic precision while investigating treatment efficacy through personalized medicine. These approaches hold promise for enhanced patient care and improved survival, particularly in patients with high-grade malignancies. With the adoption of a deeper insight into tumor behavior and the employment of advanced diagnostic modalities, the medical community can make gigantic strides in efficiently dealing with renal and urothelial tumors, ultimately resulting in enhanced clinical results for patients.

Subclassification of renal and urothelial tumors reveals high genomic heterogeneity between the cancer types, showing that the treatment needs to be considered in a multidimensional way. Comprehensive recent work has identified nine major genomic subtypes of urologic cancers, categorized according to their molecular characteristics, including DNA methylation and RNA expression profiles. These subtypes indicate shared biological processes, encompassing not only biology-related tumor behavior but also the influence of the tumor microenvironment on the cancer. It is essential to understand these subtypes to be able to tailor therapy and enhance patient outcomes since disparities in survival rates and pathway activation, including immune checkpoints and metabolism, are seen between these different groups (Bossé et al., 2017). Hence, this genomic data promises to increase our collective understanding of therapeutic implications for most urologic malignancies. The study of non-muscle invasive bladder cancer (NMIBC) highlights the need for new therapeutic strategies, particularly through molecular-targeted and immune-based therapies. As revealed at a recent NCI Bladder Cancer Task Force workshop, an interactive network of research and clinical partners aims to develop a roadmap for new clinical trials to address NMIBC. The lack of ongoing trials within the National Clinical Trials Network (NCTN) highlights the urgent need to address this prevalent cancer subtype, particularly in the context of a freeze in FDA approvals since 1998, with the notable exception of Valrubicin. Despite the increasing availability of genomic data for bladder cancer, the clinical application of these findings to develop effective treatments remains challenging (Abrams et al., 2016). The identification of main translational questions forms the backbone of advancement in NMIBC management and will help direct design of future trials to incorporate next-generation therapeutics. Furthermore, the new knowledge regarding the genomic profile of NMIBC highlights the need to develop targeted therapies in conjunction with immune modulation approaches in the near future. The workshop focused on innovative concepts in trials, such as a Phase 0 window of opportunity trial with FGFR3 inhibitors and a multi-arm trial with BCG therapy plus immunomodulatory agents. These initiatives reflect the potential of personalized medicine to individualize treatments based on the patient's tumor genealogy and immune signature. The inherent immunogenicity of bladder cancer is both a risk and an opportunity because certain tumors may evade the host immune response. Thus, the integration of this genomic information with innovative therapeutic approaches permits dynamic treatment regimens that may be adaptable to the biological features of renal and urothelial cancers, which ultimately enhance the patient's prognosis and his/her quality of life (Abrams et al., 2016).

CLOSER LOOK

UROTHELIAL NEOPLASIA

Urothelial neoplasia refers to a spectrum of abnormal tumors that develop from the urothelium, the specialized epithelial lining of the urinary tract, ranging from the renal pelvis and ureters to the bladder and proximal urethra. It is most commonly associated with the urinary bladder, where urothelial carcinoma (UC) constitutes over 90% of all bladder cancers. They range from benign papillomas to very aggressive invasive carcinomas. Urothelial neoplasia encompasses several histologic grades and stages, with key differences between papillary urothelial neoplasm of low malignant potential (PUNLMP), low-grade urothelial carcinoma, and high-grade urothelial carcinoma. Risk factors for the onset of urothelial tumors include cigarette smoking (most significant), occupational exposure to aromatic amines (e.g., dye and rubber factory workers), chronic urinary tract infection, long-term analgesic abuse, and exposure to certain chemotherapeutic drugs such as cyclophosphamide. Schistosomiasis, particularly in endemic regions, is also encountered with squamous differentiation and carcinoma. Genetically, TP53 and FGFR3 mutations are commonly implicated in high-grade and low-grade tumors, respectively, suggesting alternate molecular tumorigenesis pathways. Clinically, patients present with painless hematuria, which may be gross or microscopic, although irritative voiding symptoms may occasionally be observed. Diagnostic evaluation includes urine cytology, cystoscopy, and imaging studies, such as CT urography. Histopathological examination through biopsy remains the gold standard for establishing a definitive diagnosis and grading. Treatment depends on the grade and stage of the disease. Low-grade non-invasive tumors are initially treated with transurethral resection (TURBT) followed by intravesical therapy, most often Bacillus Calmette–Guérin (BCG) or mitomycin C. High-grade or muscle-invasive disease usually needs radical cystectomy with systemic chemotherapy or immunotherapy. Bladder-sparing with TURBT, chemotherapy, and radiation in some cases is employed. Surveillance is necessary with high rates of recurrence, particularly for non-muscle invasive tumors. Cystoscopy and urine cytology follow-up are essential components of post-treatment surveillance. Histologically, detection of architectural and cytologic alterations permits differentiation between reactive atypia, dysplasia, CIS, and invasive carcinoma. CIS is an elevated, high-grade lesion with a high rate of progression and requires intensive treatment. Over the past few years, advances in immunohistochemistry and molecular diagnostics have enhanced the ability to classify tumors and predict their behavior. Cytokeratin 20, p53, and Ki-67 are some of these markers and have useful information on tumor proliferation and aggressiveness. Divergent differentiation (squamous, glandular, micropapillary, and plasmacytoid) of urothelial carcinoma also has both therapeutic and prognostic implications. In addition, the establishment of immune checkpoint inhibitors against PD-1/PD-L1 in metastatic or platinum-resistant disease is a hallmark of systemic therapy. Multidisciplinary management by urologists, oncologists, pathologists, and radiologists is crucial for managing urothelial neoplasia. Educating patients about modifiable risk factors and early symptoms can aid in timely diagnosis and a better prognosis. As science evolves, targeted therapy and genomic profiling-based personalized medicine strategies will increasingly form the cornerstone of treating this heterogeneous, complex family of tumors.

References

1. Van Doeveren, T., Van De Werken, H. J., Van Riet, J., Aben, K. K., Van Leeuwen, P. J., Zwarthoff, E. C., & Boormans, J. L. (2020). Synchronous and metachronous urothelial carcinoma of the upper urinary tract and the bladder: Are they clonally related? A systematic review. *Urologic Oncology Seminars and Original Investigations*, *38*(6), 590–598. https://doi.org/10.1016/j.urolonc.2020.01.008Abrams, P., Acquaviva, F., Apolo, A. B., Atkins, M. B., Babjuk, M., Balbas-Martinez, V., et al. (2016). Summary and recommendations from the National Cancer Institute's Clinical Trials Planning Meeting on novel therapeutics for non-muscle invasive bladder cancer. https://core.ac.uk/download/42626599.pdf (accessed on 25th June 2025).

2. Adashek, J. J., Kato, S., Kurzrock, R., Lippman, S. M., et al. (2020). The paradox of cancer genes in non-malignant conditions: Implications for precision medicine. https://core.ac.uk/download/323064613.pdf (accessed on 25th June 2025).

3. Aggarwal, B., Bhargava, P., Ghonge, N. P., Jain, M., et al. (2012). Urologic manifestations of inflammatory pseudotumor: Report of 2 cases and review of the literature. https://core.ac.uk/download/323075582.pdf (accessed on 25th June 2025).

4. Agrawal, S., Bogdanovica, I., Britton, J., Gregory, S., et al. (2015). What is the quality of smoking cessation advice in guidelines of tobacco-related diseases? https://core.ac.uk/download/76974057.pdf (accessed on 25th June 2025).

5. Al Nazer, M., Ball, M. W., Bishop, K. D., Blute, M. L., Campbell, S. C., Dagher, C., Delahunt, B., et al. (2018). World Health Organization (WHO)/International Society of Urological Pathology (ISUP) grading in fine-needle aspiration biopsies of renal masses. https://core.ac.uk/download/227054318.pdf (accessed on 25th June 2025).

6. Al-Ahmadie, H. A., Algaba, F., Ali, S., Alvarado-Cabrero, I., et al. (2015). Update for the practicing pathologist: The International Consultation on Urologic Disease-European Association of Urology consultation on bladder cancer. https://core.ac.uk/download/84830990.pdf (accessed on 25th June 2025).

7. Alturki, R. A. (2017). Upper tract urothelial tumor with renal vein and inferior vena cava thrombus: Case report. https://core.ac.uk/download/144728993.pdf (accessed on 25th June 2025).

8. Amirian, M. J., Bagley, D. H., Healy, K. A., Hubosky, S. G., et al. (2014). The significance of functional renal obstruction in predicting pathologic stage of upper tract urothelial carcinoma. https://core.ac.uk/download/46975169.pdf (accessed on 25th June 2025).

9. Araki, M., Ebara, S., Kobayashi, Y., Nasu, Y., et al. (2017). Diagnostic ureteroscopy for cases clinically suspected of carcinoma *in situ* of the upper urinary tract. https://core.ac.uk/download/83616182.pdf (accessed on 25th June 2025).

10. Arun, A. S., Lam, K. S., & Tepper, C. G. (2018). Identification of integrin drug targets for 17 solid tumor types. https://core.ac.uk/download/323071824.pdf (accessed on 25th June 2025).

11. Aslanidis, C., Bihl, M., Briner, J., Bruder, E., et al. (2018). *KIT*, *PDGFRα* and *EGFR* analysis in nephroblastoma. https://core.ac.uk/download/159149675.pdf (accessed on 25th June 2025).

12. Begg, C., Benichou, J., Borzym-Kluczyk, M., Bosetti, C., Burger, M., La Vecchia, C., Chavan, R., et al. (2016). The role of tobacco smoke in bladder and kidney carcinogenesis: A

comparison of exposures and meta-analysis of incidence and mortality risks. https://core.ac.uk/download/30272852.pdf (accessed on 25th June 2025).

13. Bensalah, L., Lucca, M., Mathieu, R., Mbeutcha, A., et al. (2015). Upper urinary tract disease: What we know today and unmet needs. https://core.ac.uk/download/77157189.pdf (accessed on 25th June 2025).
14. Bertz, S., Fietkau, R., Gall, C., Haderlein, M., et al. (2019). Long-term experience of chemoradiotherapy combined with deep regional hyperthermia for organ preservation in high-risk bladder cancer (Ta, Tis, T1, T2). https://core.ac.uk/download/323075812.pdf (accessed on 25th June 2025).
15. Bonello, F., Busuttil, G., & Matocks, S. (2016). Leiomyosarcoma of the distal ureter: A case report. https://core.ac.uk/download/83020783.pdf (accessed on 25th June 2025).
16. Bossé, D., Chen, F., Choueiri, T. K., Creighton, C. J., et al. (2017). Pan-urologic cancer genomic subtypes that transcend tissue of origin. https://core.ac.uk/download/129069439.pdf (accessed on 25th June 2025).
17. Botticelli, A., Marchetti, P., Nuti, M., Rughetti, A., et al. (2018). The ambitious role of anti-angiogenesis molecules: Turning a cold tumor into a hot one. https://core.ac.uk/download/188823002.pdf (accessed on 25th June 2025).
18. Burity, J., Belo da Fonte, I., Bandeira de Melo, P. (2014). Radiological Society of North America (RSNA) 3D printing Special Interest Group (SIG): Guidelines for medical 3D printing and appropriateness for clinical scenarios. https://core.ac.uk/download/212867900.pdf (accessed on 25th June 2025).
19. Chamie, K., Crosetti, A. M., Cummings, A. L., Drakaki, A., et al. (2018). Durvalumab: An investigational anti-PD-L1 monoclonal antibody for the treatment of urothelial carcinoma. https://core.ac.uk/download/323076325.pdf (accessed on 25th June 2025).
20. Chan, Y. Y., Kurzrock, E. A., Osborn, S. L., Sandlin, R. D., et al. (2017). The current use of stem cells in bladder tissue regeneration and bioengineering. https://core.ac.uk/download/323068966.pdf (accessed on 25th June 2025).
21. Chang, L. S., Chang, Y. H., Chen, K. K., Chen, M. T., et al. (2005). Primary urothelial carcinoma of the ureter: 11-year experience in Taipei Veterans General Hospital. https://core.ac.uk/download/pdf/82607306.pdf (accessed on 25th June 2025).
22. Chang, Y. H., Chen, K. K., Chiang, Y. T., Huang, C. H., et al. (2011). Urothelial inverted papilloma of the lower urinary tract—A benign lesion or a precursor of malignancy? https://core.ac.uk/download/pdf/82028646.pdf (accessed on 25th June 2025).
23. Chapelle de la, A., Cristofano Di, A., Flesken-Nikitin, A., Garcia-Espana, A., Sun, A., Suzuki, A., Vidal, A., et al. (2009). Biology of urothelial tumorigenesis: Insights from genetically engineered mice. https://core.ac.uk/download/pdf/8361992.pdf (accessed on 25th June 2025).
24. Cheng, L., Cheng, M., Kaimakliotis, H. Z., Koch, M. O., et al. (2018). Inherited forms of bladder cancer: A review of Lynch syndrome and other inherited conditions. https://core.ac.uk/download/161627377.pdf (accessed on 25th June 2025).
25. Ci, W., Fang, D., He, Z., Li, H., et al. (2015). Contralateral upper tract urothelial carcinoma after nephroureterectomy: The predictive role of DNA methylation. https://deepblue.lib.umich.edu/bitstream/2027.42/110306/1/13046_2015_Article_120.pdf (accessed on 25th June 2025).

26. Cody, T., Gieseg, M. A., Kaldjian, E. P., Madore, B., et al. (2002). Expression profiling of human renal carcinomas with functional taxonomic analysis. https://core.ac.uk/download/pdf/3227141.pdf (accessed on 25th June 2025).

27. Colombino, M., Cossu, A., Paliogiannis, P., Palmieri, G., et al. (2013). Molecular analysis of appendiceal mucinous cystadenoma and rectal adenocarcinoma in a patient with urothelial carcinoma: A case report. https://core.ac.uk/download/18621964.pdf (accessed on 25th June 2025).

28. De Clercq, D., Deprez, P., Ducatelle, R., Maes, S., et al. (2011). Transitional cell carcinoma of suspected ureteral origin, with intra-abdominal and distant metastases in two horses. https://core.ac.uk/download/55849269.pdf (accessed on 25th June 2025).

29. de Leval, L., & Lhermitte, B. (2018). Interpretation of needle biopsies of the kidney for investigation of renal masses. https://core.ac.uk/download/159146723.pdf (accessed on 25th June 2025).

30. Gilder, A. S., Gonias, S. L., Karimi-Mostowfi, N., Mantuano, E., et al. (2017). Expression of LDL receptor-related proteins (LRPs) in common solid malignancies correlates with patient survival. https://core.ac.uk/download/153366552.pdf (accessed on 25th June 2025).

31. Halpern, E. J., Kim, S., Salmanoglu, E., Thakur, M., et al. (2018). A glance at imaging bladder cancer. https://core.ac.uk/download/227055407.pdf (accessed on 25th June 2025).

32. Helsten, T., Kurzrock, R., & Schwaederle, M. (2015). Fibroblast growth factor receptor signaling in hereditary and neoplastic disease: Biologic and clinical implications. https://core.ac.uk/download/323066798.pdf (accessed on 25th June 2025).

33. Trapani, F. (2010). *Osservazioni Sull'attivazione Del Recettore Arilico (Ahr) In Correlazione Alla Contaminazione Ambientale da Metalli Pesanti in Tumori Spontanei di Cani Della Regione Campania. Correlation Between Aryl Hydrocarbon Receptor (AhR) Expression and Environmental Heavy Metals Contamination in Canine Tumors.* https://core.ac.uk/download/11918592.pdf (accessed on 25th June 2025).

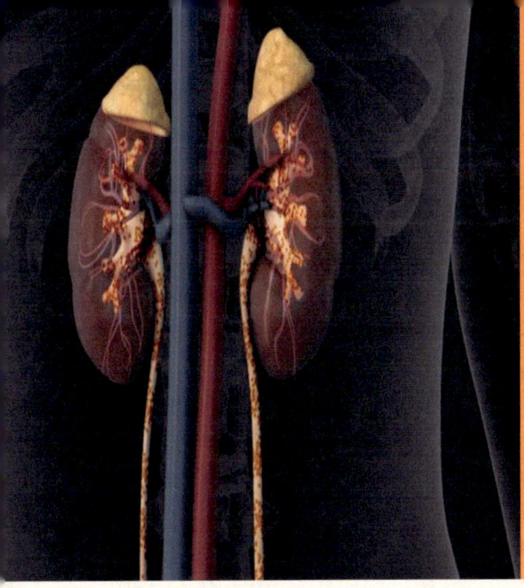

Chapter 13

ELECTROLYTE AND ACID-BASE DISORDERS IN KIDNEY DISEASE

Contents

Introduction

The intricate reciprocal relationship between acid-base and electrolyte derangements and renal disease exists as an actual clinical problem, with an impact on patient outcomes and management. The kidneys play a crucial role in maintaining homeostasis, particularly through the regulation of essential electrolytes such as sodium, potassium, calcium, and bicarbonate. With worsening kidney function, these electrolytes lose their balance, and their possible complications may negatively impact patients' health. Understanding of these disorders is essential, for not only do they make the clinical course of kidney disease complex but also dictate management approaches. In this context, a thorough understanding of the pathophysiology and clinical course of electrolyte and acid-base derangements is crucial for clinicians seeking to enhance care in patients. The most commonly encountered disorders of electrolytes in patients with kidney disease include hyperkalemia, hyponatremia, and metabolic acidosis, and each presents different challenges. For instance, hyperkalemia, or the presence of high potassium levels, is fraught with grave danger, such as cardiac arrhythmias. Likewise, metabolic acidosis is caused by the kidneys' impaired ability to remove hydrogen ions and produce bicarbonate, which can result in additional complications if left untreated. Furthermore, the interaction of the disorders tends to have a combined effect on a patient's condition, requiring a multi-angled assessment and management plan. The many-faceted aspect of such imbalances underscores the necessity of heightened awareness and active surveillance on the part of clinicians in the management of patients with renal disease, since early intervention can considerably reduce morbidity and mortality with such disorders. The consequences of disturbances in electrolytes and acid-base status extend beyond the direct immediate physical aspects, often to psychological and social behaviors in the life of the patient. These disturbances may lead to increased hospitalization, additional healthcare costs, and a reduced quality of life because the patient is unable to manage their condition effectively. Apart from that, these management plans for these disturbances require an interdisciplinary team, with contributions from nephrologists, dietitians, and the nursing team, to promote holistic care. Effective communication among these professionals is necessary in delivering customized treatment plans that address both physiological and psychosocial needs of patients. In understanding the applicability of acid-base and electrolyte disturbances in renal disease, it becomes evident that correcting these issues is not merely a matter of clinical practice, but an act towards achieving improved whole-patient care within the healthcare system (Figure 13.1).

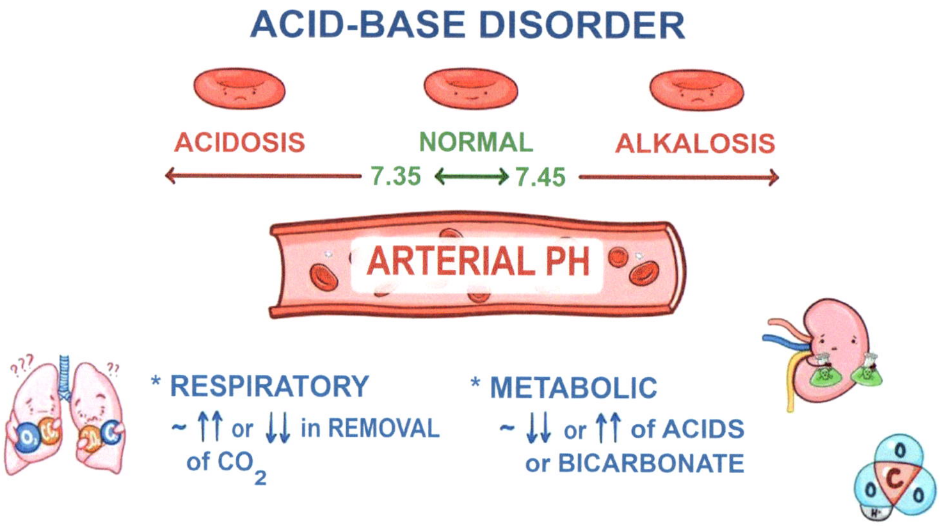

Figure 13.1. Acid-base disorders.

Source: https://d16qt3wv6xm098.cloudfront.net/ghwiv0rgQB64rHHx_rFv6pTmR8OHJ3rf/_.jpg,

Definition of Electrolyte Disorders

Electrolyte imbalances encompass a range of imbalances in the body's essential ions, such as sodium, potassium, calcium, and magnesium, that are crucial to physiological functions. Electrolyte imbalance typically stems from diverse underlying pathologies, particularly those affecting the kidneys. The kidneys play a through crucial mechanisms that regulate electrolytes, maintain homeostasis via filtration, reabsorption, and excretion. When kidney disease does manifest, as in conditions like acute kidney injury (AKI), the mechanisms of control fail, and an abnormal concentration of electrolytes ensues with significant impacts on metabolic and cardiac functions. Additionally, electrolytes have a close relation with acid-base disturbances, making it pertinent for general awareness of such disturbances in patients, particularly in intensive care, where disturbances can lead to severe consequences. The relationship between kidney disease and electrolyte disturbances is also made complex by the presence of comorbid conditions, such as diabetes. Clinical data have indicated that diabetic patients can present with elevated levels of variation from their normal electrolyte levels, including lower sodium and higher potassium and chloride levels compared to non-diabetic patients.

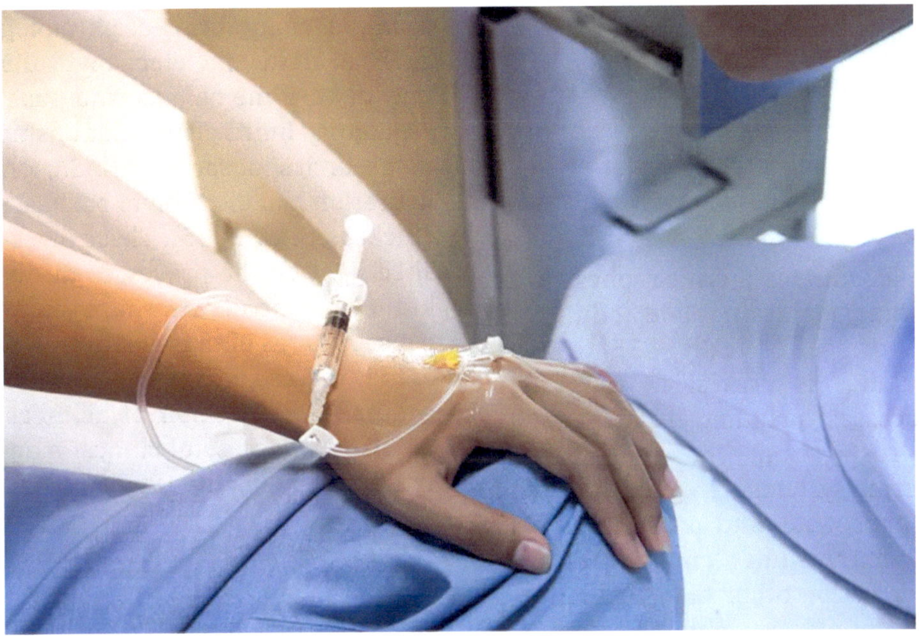

Figure 13.2. Electrolyte disorders in kidney disease.

Source: https://pharmaceutical-journal.com/wp-content/uploads/2022/08/electrolytes-lead-927x617.jpg.

This highlights the inherent complexity of managing and treating electrolyte disorders, as changes in ion concentrations can both cause and result from functional alterations in renal function. Moreover, successful management plans must also account for the interrelationship between the disorders, where not considering one aspect may exacerbate another, ultimately influencing patient prognosis. The understanding of pathophysiologic relationships among diabetes, kidney disease, and electrolyte abnormalities enables a more targeted therapeutic approach, moving beyond empiric treatment to individualized therapy tailored to the patient's specific needs. The challenge in diagnosing and managing electrolyte derangements of kidney disease is also highlighted by evolving classification algorithms for kidney injury, such as RIFLE and KDIGO criteria. Variations in these definitions reflect the need for greater standardization in clinical practice, a requirement underscored by the impact of electrolyte imbalances on prognosis and treatment response. For instance, the successful treatment of AKI and related electrolyte imbalances requires timely intervention and careful monitoring of biomarkers, such as serum creatinine and newer markers like cystatin C. These developments underscore the need for a personalized treatment approach, controlling life-threatening complications, including hyperkalemia and hypertension, in an attempt to preserve renal function. Adopting a multi-component strategy incorporating both traditional and new approaches is essential in mitigating the adverse effects associated with electrolyte imbalances in the context of kidney disease, resulting in improved patient outcomes (Adedoyin et al., 2013; Abdullah et al., 2018) (Figure 13.2).

Overview of Acid-Base Balance

Acid-base homeostasis is a critical physiologic mechanism that maintains body fluid pH within a tight range, typically 7.35 to 7.45. Acid-base balance is crucial in numerous metabolic processes, including enzyme activity and cellular respiration. The body utilizes multiple buffering systems to regulate pH, with bicarbonate, phosphate, and proteins serving as significant extracellular and intracellular buffers. Any deviation other than this renders the body's functioning severely handicapped, and acid-base disorders may also emerge in renal disease patients. Acid-base balance is regulated by complex interactions among renal, respiratory, and metabolic systems; an in-depth understanding of this topic is essential for effectively managing electrolyte disturbances in renal failure. The kidneys play a crucial role in maintaining acid-base balance by excreting hydrogen ions and reabsorbing bicarbonate from the urine. This intricate process occurs in the renal collecting duct, where the epithelial barrier, primarily composed of claudins, allows for effective ion and solute exchange across the membrane. Research highlights that impairment in the functioning of such tight junctions can lead to defective blood pressure and water homeostasis, exacerbating acid-base disorders (Leiz et al., 2019). Secondly, renal excretion control interaction exhibits the coordinated response of the body towards changes in acid-base balance. Disturbances in either system can lead to complications such as metabolic acidosis or alkalosis, conditions that are frequently encountered in patients with chronic kidney disease. Grasping the subtleties of acid-base balance also involves the extrarenal determinants of renal function and the consequent electrolyte disturbances. For example, many forms of physiological stress—such as fluid and electrolyte disturbances—may disturb the balance and push the kidneys' regulatory limits. This relationship is apparent in research sponsored by NASA, which examines hydration and electrolyte balance during stress (Dickson et al., 2025). These investigations also shed light on the processes through which the kidneys control acid-base balance and the consequences of these on overall well-being. As kidney disease often deteriorates renal function, a detailed evaluation of acid-base balance is crucial for successful clinical management and treatment regimens (Figure 13.3).

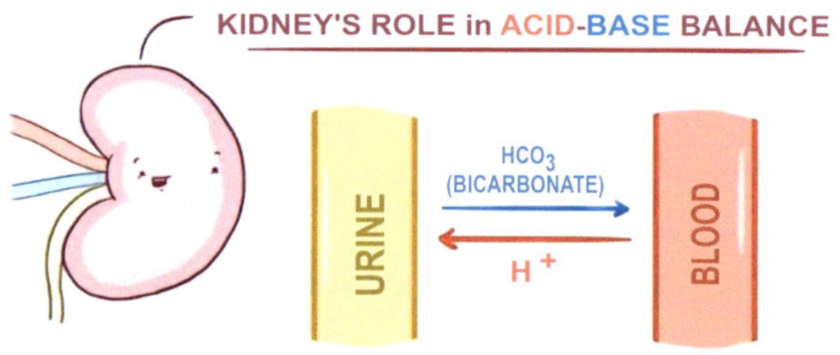

Figure 13.3. The role of the kidney in acid-base balance.

Source: https://d16qt3wv6xm098.cloudfront.net/14FtKRHCSaSe7CscXhXSTd62TKy_rNPJ/_.jpg.

Importance of Studying these Disorders in Kidney Disease

It is imperative to learn about electrolyte and acid-base disturbances in renal disease primarily because of their central function in homeostasis.

The kidneys are vital organs that filter the blood, eliminate waste products, and regulate essential electrolytes, including sodium, potassium, and bicarbonate. As the kidney function fails, the body's ability to regulate these substances is compromised, typically leading to severe disturbances that impact health very severely. Understanding such disorders facilitates the formulation of appropriate interventions that restore balance, thereby reducing the risk of arrhythmias, muscle weakness, and metabolic acidosis. Detailed exploration of these disorders is thus required to improve treatment options and outcomes in patients with chronic kidney disease and other renal impairment. Another critical feature of electrolyte and acid-base disturbances analysis in kidney disease is their association with morbidity and mortality rates in general among the affected individuals. Research indicates that electrolyte imbalance and acid states, such as acidosis, occur frequently among patients with impaired kidneys, obscuring clinical presentation and complicating the treatment approach. Such imbalances can precipitate potentially life-threatening conditions like cardiac complications or respiratory arrest, thereby augmenting the necessity for electrolyte monitoring as part of routine patient care. With the reduction of such potentially life-threatening complications through systematic research and prompt treatment, medical professionals can significantly improve survival rates, as well as create an elevated quality of life for patients suffering from renal disease. Furthermore, familiarity with the pathophysiology underlying electrolyte and acid-base disturbances is necessary to advance treatment alternatives. For instance, insight obtained through the investigation of transport systems and their physiologic functions may provide new treatment modalities that can focus on these pathways more specifically. Monitoring and counterbalancing technologies are continually being refined; therefore, ongoing research in these fields is crucial to optimizing therapy effectiveness. Additionally, since kidney disease often overlaps with other diseases, studying these disorders may also provide insight into general medical principles, thereby adding to the overall body of knowledge for medical practitioners. By dedicating time and resources to studying these disorders, the field of medicine can develop innovations that enhance renal care and aid in improved outcomes in many healthcare settings.

13.1. Role of the Kidneys in Electrolyte Regulation

Kidneys play a vital role in maintaining electrolyte balance, a characteristic essential for the homeostasis of the human body. The kidneys serve as a buffer, maintaining important electrolytes such as sodium, potassium, and calcium within narrow ranges that are essential for physiological processes to occur. By filtration of the blood through the nephron unit complex, the kidneys regulate electrolyte levels in a complex interplay of filtration, reabsorption, and excretion. For instance, excess sodium is often removed in the urine, while potassium is closely regulated to ensure normal muscle function and nerve transmission. In performing these functions, kidneys not only assist in maintaining fluid balance and blood pressure but also enable crucial biochemical and physiological processes within the renal microenvironment. Beyond this, the kidneys also play a role in the intricate regulation of acid-base balance, with an intimate relationship with the control of electrolytes. The kidneys produce pH levels that are important for optimizing cellular function via processes such as bicarbonate reabsorption and the excretion of hydrogen ions. Regulation is particularly vital in the scenario of acid-base disturbances that accompany kidney disease. After renal function is lost, the kidneys' ability to manage these processes is lost, leading to a systemic imbalance. For instance, metabolic acidosis can arise due to the failure of the kidneys to effectively excrete acids, and the consequent reduced bicarbonate levels and other abnormalities in electrolytes. The importance of these diseases extends beyond renal physiology to influence other organ systems, highlighting the kidneys' function as central regulators of homeostasis in the body. In the context of electrolyte and acid-base imbalances, it is significant to consider the interaction between different factors, particularly drugs and diet, on renal function. Some drugs, like non-steroidal anti-inflammatory drugs, have an effect on renal electrolyte handling, changing the balance of fluid and electrolyte management. The delicate balance maintained by the kidneys is easily disrupted, with dehydration, salt intake, and comorbid conditions of hypertension, among others, being some of the etiologies of dysregulation. As cited in research, electrolytic balance disturbances can compromise reproductive health, highlighting the far-reaching consequences of renal function beyond fluid balance and metabolic homeostasis (Araujo et al., 2022). Thus, the maintenance of kidney function is not only crucial for electrolyte and fluid balance, but also for overall physiological well-being, thereby illustrating the organ's vital role in maintaining systemic as well as reproductive health (Figure 13.4).

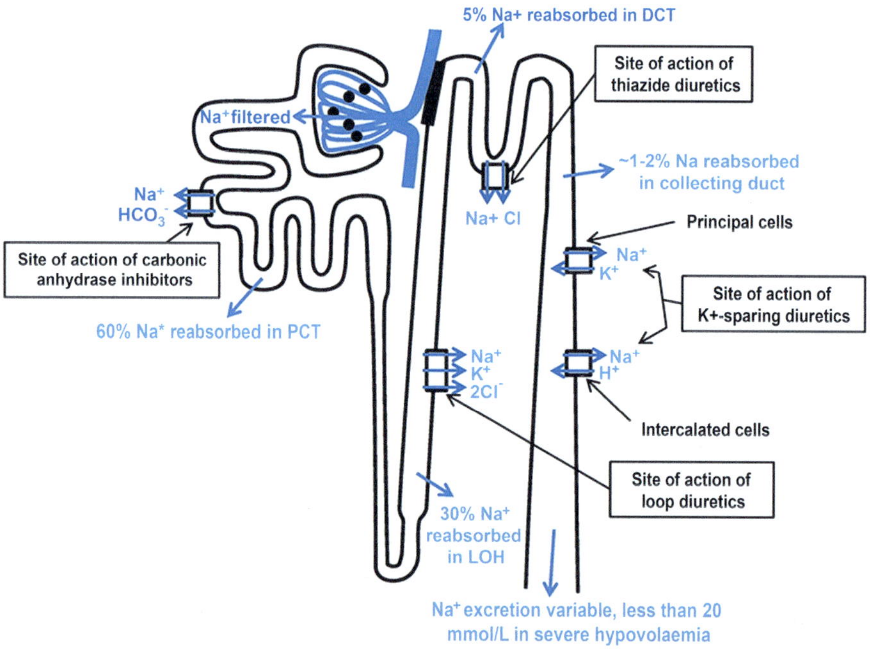

Figure 13.4. Role of the kidneys in electrolyte regulation.

Source: https://static.cambridge.org/binary/version/id/urn:cambridge.org:id:binary:20230303112412116-0846:9781108565011:46399fig69_4.png?pub-status=live.

13.1.1. Mechanisms of Electrolyte Reabsorption

The kidney's function in maintaining electrolyte balance through the complex mechanisms of reabsorption is critical and primarily occurs in the nephron. Electrolytes such as sodium, potassium, and chloride are vital for several physiological processes, such as muscle contraction and conduction of nerve impulses. Reabsorption begins in the proximal convoluted tubule, where approximately

65-70% of the filtered sodium is actively reabsorbed, along with water and other solutes, through both transcellular and paracellular pathways. The process is supplemented by the activity of sodium-potassium ATPase pumps, which maintain a low intracellular sodium concentration, thereby enhancing the driving force for sodium reabsorption. The dynamic nature of this reabsorption is critical, not only for maintaining blood volume and blood pressure, but also for the effective operation of downstream nephron segments to further modulate electrolyte and fluid balance, and consequently influence overall renal function and homeostasis. Nephron segments develop, particularly in the thick ascending limb of the loop of Henle, with changes in mechanisms of sodium reabsorption. Sodium reabsorption in this instance is achieved by the Na^{+}-K+-2Cl-cotransporter, which is sensitively responsive to variation in dietary sodium. This segment of the loop plays a critical role in diluting urine and in the formation of the hyperosmolar medullary interstitium, which is required for urine concentration downstream in the collecting duct. Active sodium reabsorption also plays a crucial role in forming the counter-current multiplier system, which is vital to urine concentration. Any dysregulation of these transport mechanisms at this segment has the potential to cause profound disturbances in sodium homeostasis, which can then manifest as hypertension, especially in cases of high dietary salt intake or underlying renal disease (Dominiczak et al., 2017). The final process of reabsorption of electrolytes occurs in the collecting duct, wherein the subtle adjustment of electrolyte and water balance is effectively governed. Epithelial cells within this segment have tight junctions with specific claudins (Cldn-3, Cldn-4, Cldn-7, Cldn-8) that control paracellular ion and water movement, which is vital to the conservation of transepithelial potential differences (Leiz et al., 2019). Hormonal regulation, specifically by aldosterone, enhances sodium reabsorption while secreting potassium, a vital component for homeostasis. This ability of the segment to adjust to changes in body fluid volume or composition only serves to highlight its essential role in maintaining protection against electrolyte imbalance and acid-base disturbances. Functional impairment of the collecting duct's epithelial barrier, therefore, has extreme pathophysiological ramifications, highlighting the integrative role of renal mechanisms in regulating electrolytes in disease.

13.1.2. Impact of Kidney Function on Electrolyte Levels

The kidneys play a pivotal role in regulating homeostasis through maintaining the balance of electrolytes, which is crucial for various physiological functions. Whenever renal function is compromised, it significantly impacts the kidneys' ability to process blood and eliminate excess electrolytes. For instance, the glomerular filtration rate (GFR) is directly related to electrolyte balance; a reduction in GFR leads to the retention of potassium, sodium, and phosphorus, resulting in hyperkalemia, hypernatremia, and hyperphosphatemia, respectively. These retentions not only disturb fluid balance but also acid-base balance, and are highly hazardous to chronic kidney disease (CKD) and acute kidney injury (AKI) patients. Understanding the relationship between the action of the kidneys and electrolyte levels is vital to the development of proper treatment protocols and management of the potential complications arising from dysregulated mineral metabolism. The collecting duct, a significant segment of the nephron, is primarily responsible for the precise control of electrolyte secretion and reabsorption. This component of the nephron is characterized by its epithelium, which includes claudin-containing tight junctions that regulate paracellular transport of ions and solutes. Disruption of this epithelial barrier can lead to the dysregulation of electrolytes, having a profound impact on fluid balance and blood pressure. For instance, defects in certain claudins lead to diminished sodium reabsorption and altered potassium secretion, exacerbating hyperkalemia in individuals with kidney damage (Leiz et al., 2019). These physiological alterations highlight the function of the collecting duct in maintaining electrolyte balance and how kidney disease can make substantial contributions to pathological electrolyte disturbances. Correction of electrolyte disturbances secondary to kidney damage is crucial in the treatment of patients, especially in acute care facilities.

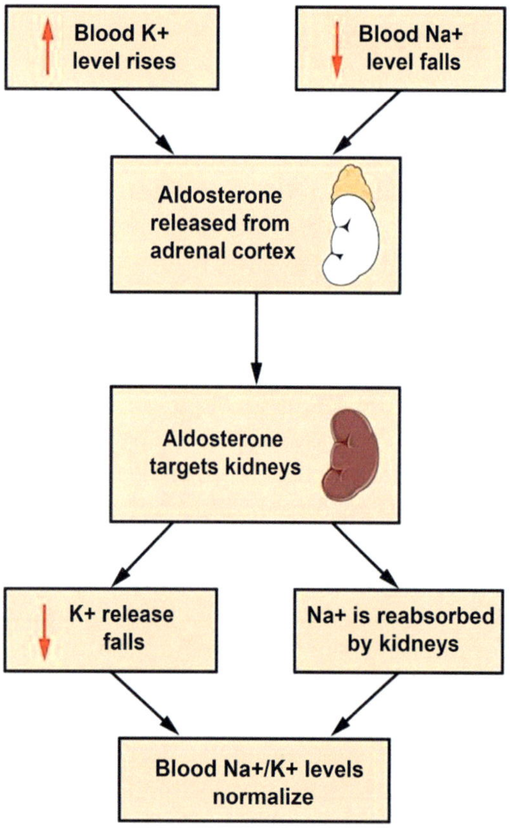

Figure 13.5. Impact of kidney function on electrolyte levels.

Source: https://textimgs.s3.amazonaws.com/osanp/m46414/2711_Aldosterone_Feedback_Loop-01.jpg.

Hyperkalemia, a common electrolyte imbalance in patients with compromised renal function, can lead to lethal cardiac arrhythmias. The traditional therapeutic measures, such as insulin and glucose administration, or β-2 agonist treatment, aim to lower serum potassium; however, these treatments also incur added risks, including dysglycemia and cardiac arrhythmias (Dépret et al., 2019). Therefore, a synergistic strategy integrated with active surveillance of electrolyte compositions, customized treatment strategies, and consequent interventions is necessary in minimizing the harmful effects of unregulated electrolyte metabolism in patients with kidney complications (Figure 13.5).

13.1.3. Consequences of Impaired Electrolyte Regulation

The effect of impaired electrolyte control, particularly in the setting of renal disease, is significant and multifaceted with substantial clinical implications. Disruptions in sodium, potassium, calcium, and magnesium homeostasis can manifest as several disease states. For instance, hyperkalemia, or elevated potassium, can result from renal disease and complicate cardiac arrhythmias that can be potentially lethal if uncontrolled. Similarly, hyponatremia with decreased sodium levels usually occurs due to disorders such as the syndrome of inappropriate antidiuretic hormone secretion. The condition is concerning because it can result in cerebral edema, particularly in acutely ill patients, and thus requires close monitoring and control. Failing to regulate these electrolyte imbalances complicates current kidney disease and even triggers a cascade of systemic consequences that underscore the importance of electrolyte regulation in treating the patient (Crocker et al., 2006). The pathophysiological background of electrolyte imbalances is a multidimensional interaction that renders clinical regulation challenging. Dilutional and depletional hyponatremia illustrate the duality of fluid and electrolyte physiology, which demands understanding of each patient's unique situation. Depletional hyponatremia, for example, may result from gastrointestinal losses or diuretic administration, causing the body to retain water in a futile attempt to compensate. On the other hand, dilutional hyponatremia typically follows excess ingestion of fluid, diluting the levels of sodium, usually present with massive fluid resuscitation. Treatment of such conditions requires clinicians to balance quick correction—reserved for acute cases—with the risk of osmotic demyelination in the case of too aggressive therapies. Understanding how fluid balance leads to the release of vasopressin is critical in treating hyponatremia; thus, the acknowledgment of the significant role electrolyte regulation must play when it comes to kidney disease (HJ A et al., 2008). Outside of direct clinical implications, long-term health effects can result from chronic electrolyte derangement, affecting the overall patient's quality of life. Altered calcium and phosphorus metabolism, for example, is common in chronic renal disease and leads to secondary hyperparathyroidism and to bone disease as renal osteodystrophy. Additionally, persistent hyperkalemia can lead to dietary restrictions, which in turn affect nutritional status and patient compliance. By recognizing the chronic complications of deranged electrolyte control, healthcare professionals can implement preventive measures for surveillance and management. This involves serial electrolyte monitoring and patient-tailored treatment regimens based on the individual's specific deficiencies and excesses that may arise from the multifactorial nature of kidney disease. Lastly, managing the long-term consequences of electrolyte imbalances is crucial for improving patient outcomes and the quality of care in this high-risk group (Crocker et al., 2006).

13.2. Common Electrolyte Disorders in Kidney Disease

The kidneys play a crucial role in maintaining electrolyte balance, and their dysfunction can lead to severe electrolyte disorders. The most common disorder among patients with kidney disease is hyperkalemia, characterized by an elevated blood potassium level. Hyperkalemia develops as a result of reduced renal excretion of potassium, typically in combination with the use of certain medications such as ACE inhibitors and potassium-sparing diuretics. Hyperkalemia can cause serious complications like cardiac arrhythmias and cardiac arrest, particularly in the more advanced stages of renal failure. Treatment of this electrolyte imbalance involves typically dietary modification, administration of diuretics, and dialysis in the most critical cases. Thus, early detection and management are necessary to prevent deleterious cardiovascular effects among patients with chronic kidney disease (Dębska-Ślizień et al., 2023). Another significant electrolyte disturbance with kidney disease is hyponatremia, an abnormally low sodium level in the blood. It may at times be a highly complex condition because it can be due to several causes, including excessive water retention and dilutional effects secondary to renal damage. In chronic kidney disease patients, the inability to properly regulate fluid status can lead to relative water overload over sodium, leading to symptomatic hyponatremia. The clinical manifestations may be as subtle as neurological symptoms or as ominous as seizures or coma. Correction should be made with careful adjustment of the sodium level, which can often only be accomplished through a slow correction to avoid osmotic demyelination. Identifying the etiology of hyponatremia is also essential for effective management, as correction of fluid overload is typically a component of therapy (Cavoli et al., 2011). Lastly, hyperphosphatemia is a common electrolyte disturbance that appears in the setting of chronic kidney disease. As glomerular filtration rate declines, the kidneys' excretory function about phosphate declines, and serum phosphate concentration increases. This accumulation can be detrimental, as it leads to secondary hyperparathyroidism and vascular calcification, which hastens the cardiovascular complications in patients. The treatment of hyperphosphatemia typically includes restricting phosphate intake and administering phosphate binders to prevent gastrointestinal absorption. Dialysis is also effective in removing excess phosphate from the blood. The relationship between phosphate levels and systemic mineral homeostasis highlights the importance of controlling hyperphosphatemia, not only for renal but also for skeletal and cardiovascular health in patients (Dębska-Ślizień et al., 2023) (Figure 13.6).

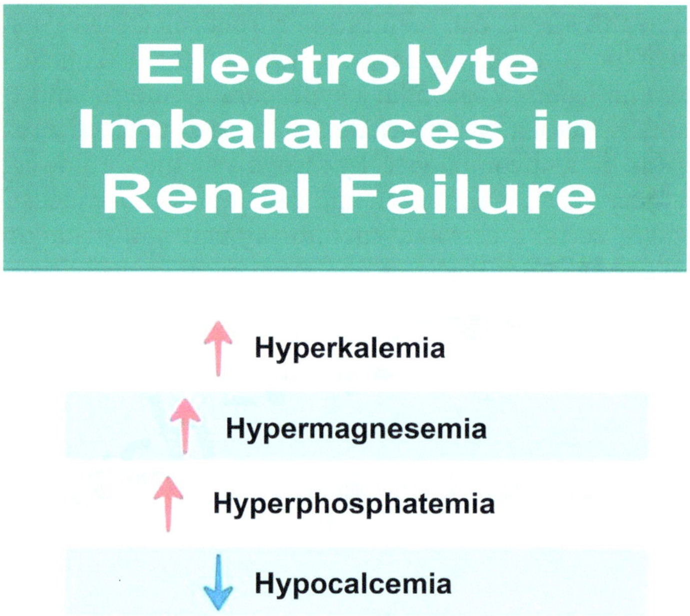

Figure 13.6. Common electrolyte disorders in kidney disease.

Source: https://encrypted-tbn0.gstatic.com/images?q=tbn:ANd9GcRqKQwvQS6ZfAwYflqb44OH_m53w6IKl0eCgQ&s.

13.2.1. Hyperkalemia: Causes and Effects

Hyperkalemia, which refers to an abnormally high concentration of serum potassium, is linked with severe health risks, particularly in patients with kidney disease. The role of the kidneys in regulating potassium homeostasis is critical; hence, any dysfunction leads to an interruption of this process. Underlying conditions that contribute to hyperkalemia include acute kidney injury, chronic kidney disease, and certain medications that inhibit renal potassium excretion. They lead to impaired ability to excrete potassium, culminating in elevated extracellular concentrations. Retention is increased by intake and tissue destruction in patients with impaired renal function, also resulting in hyperkalemia. Life-threatening complications may result from this condition, notably cardiac arrhythmia, highlighting the need to be scrupulously monitored and treated in vulnerable populations, such as renal replacement therapy patients. The interplay of these factors highlights the complexity and clinical relevance of hyperkalemia within the broader context of electrolyte disturbances associated with renal disease. The physiologic impact of hyperkalemia is multifaceted, with specific effects on cardiac and neuromuscular function due to the key role of potassium as a cation in these systems. Serum hyperkalemia can disrupt the resting membrane potential, altering cardiac excitability and conduction. Thus, patients may develop manifestations as mild as palpitations or as extreme as ventricular fibrillation, which can be fatal if not immediately treated. Neuromuscular manifestations, ranging from paralysis to muscle weakness, may also result from hyperkalemia. These manifestations are secondary to alterations in neurotransmission and muscle contraction and add more complexity to the clinical presentation of patients with concomitant renal disease. With these possible outcomes, understanding the causes and effects of hyperkalemia is essential for clinicians to develop appropriate treatment regimens and mitigate the negative impact of the electrolyte disorder. Effective management of hyperkalemia requires an individualized approach tailored to the patient's specific clinical context. Therapeutic management commonly entails pharmacological interventions, such as the administration of insulin and glucose to facilitate the entry of potassium into cells, or beta-2 agonists, which also promote intracellular potassium migration. The interventions, however, carry risks and potential side effects, as described in the literature, necessitating a cautious and patient-specific therapy approach to become critical (Dépret et al., 2019). Besides, renal replacement therapy remains a standard of care for people with severe hyperkalemia, particularly in the acute or chronic failure of the kidneys to eliminate potassium. With continued research into the mechanisms of electrolyte imbalance, renal epithelial barrier function, including tight junctions in the collecting duct, is becoming recognized as a critical area of interest, with implications for potassium regulation and overall kidney function (Leiz et al., 2019). Such deep understanding of the relationship between hyperkalemia and kidney disease is thus critical in successful clinical management and patient outcomes (Figure 13.7).

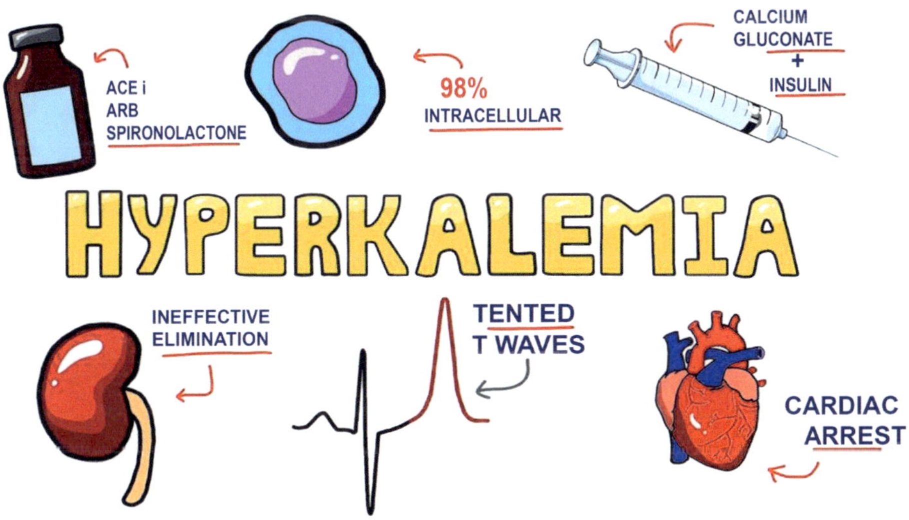

Figure 13.7. Hyperkalemia.

Source: https://i.ytimg.com/vi/2QRcWw97RaM/maxresdefault.jpg.

13.2.2. Hyponatremia: Pathophysiology and Symptoms

Hyponatremia, the condition of abnormally low blood sodium levels, is a tremendous challenge in the context of kidney disease. Pathophysiology of the condition can be broadly categorized into two mechanisms: depletional and dilutional hyponatremia. Depletional hyponatremia is caused by sodium loss due to the employment of diuretics, gastrointestinal losses, or adrenal insufficiency, usually compounded by patients with compromised renal function. On the other hand, dilutional hyponatremia is basically characterized by excessive water retention, which is most frequently met with diseases such as the syndrome of inappropriate antidiuretic hormone secretion (SIADH). Both osmoregulation dysfunctions need accurate diagnostic examinations to characterize the causative disorders because improper treatment can lead to unwanted neurological disorders, including cerebral edema and osmotic demyelination syndromes (Crocker et al., 2006). The clinical picture of hyponatremia can be wide and varied, from mild malaise and headache to profound neurological dysfunction, including confusion, seizures, and coma. These are particularly pertinent in patients with acute-onset hyponatremia, where the brain is most susceptible to osmotic changes. Those with chronic hyponatremia might present more insidiously with features of fatigue and gait instability. Because hyponatremia impacts the central nervous system, the sodium level is kept under close monitoring by medical professionals, especially in critically ill patients. Additionally, recognizing the complications of fluid overload in patients with renal disease, such as pulmonary edema, can be crucial to providing comprehensive patient care (Crocker et al., 2006). Its management optimal, and it depends on its etiology in that it is aimed at treating the cause. The treatment may include fluid restriction, salt supplementation, or administration of a vasopressin receptor antagonist. The management needs to be individualized based on the etiology, as it has the potential to lead to osmotic demyelination if the sodium correction is done too quickly, particularly in chronic hyponatremia. Therefore, interventions should be implemented slowly. Hence, a physiology-oriented approach to hyponatremia management must emphasize tailored patient evaluation, eschewing dependence on single laboratory results to make clinical decisions. This method aims to optimize the treatment of hyponatremia, with a focus on patient safety and resolving electrolyte disturbances associated with renal impairment (HJ A et al., 2008) (Figure 13.8).

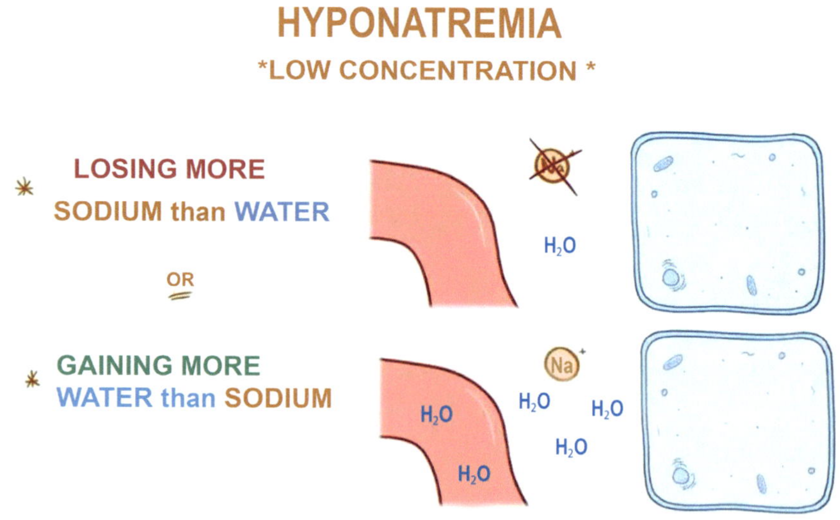

Figure 13.8. Hyponatremia: Pathophysiology and symptoms.

Source: https://www.osmosis.org/_next/image?url=https%3A%2F%2Fd16qt3wv6xm098.cloudfront.net%2FCF62W32RT9Ww-Hhz4tQgfGHjTaKfYDwf%2F_.jpg&w=3840&q=75.

13.2.3. Hypocalcemia: Relationship with Kidney Function

The interaction between hypocalcemia and kidney function is complex and has significant implications for understanding electrolyte and acid-base disturbances in patients with renal insufficiency. Hypocalcemia, as low serum calcium, usually occurs in CKD because of impaired calcium metabolism, which is reflected by reduced renal production of 1,25-dihydroxyvitamin D. This lack of vitamin D inhibits calcium absorption in the intestine and evokes a compensatory increase in parathyroid hormone (PTH) secretion, which also increases bone resorption and leads to secondary hyperparathyroidism.

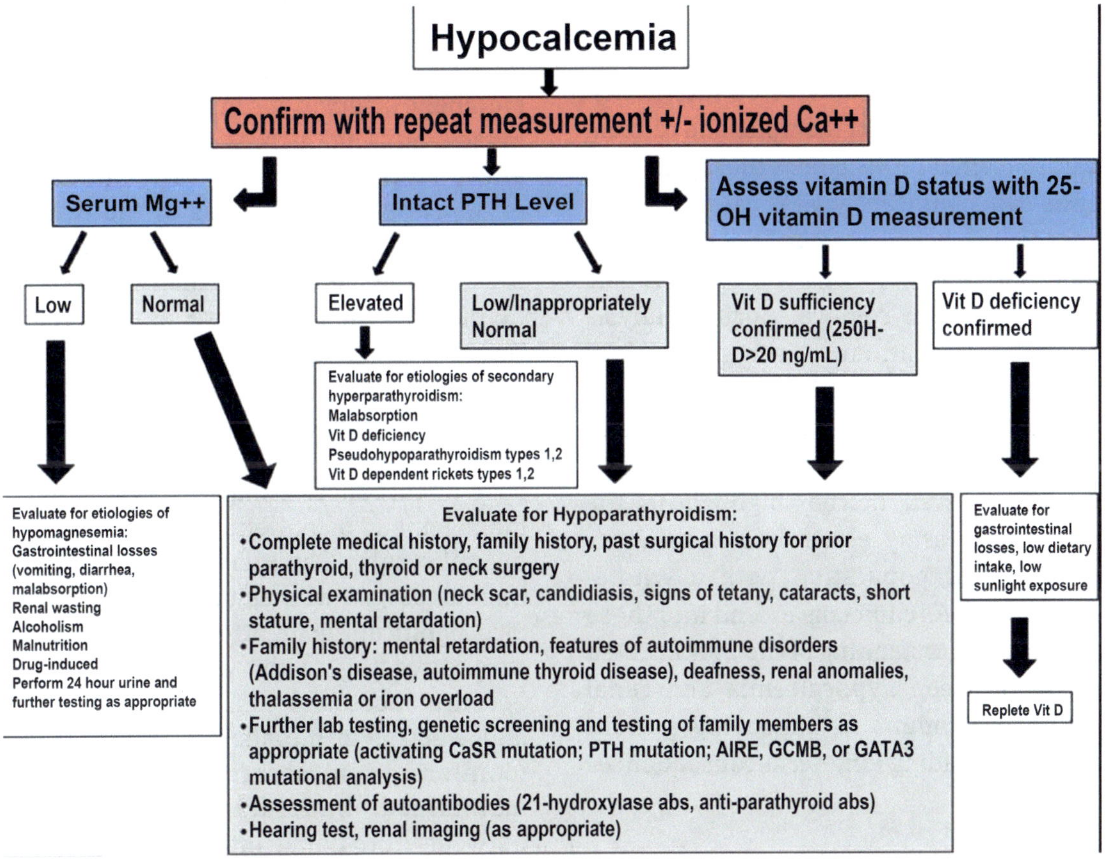

Figure 13.9. Hypocalcemia: Relationship with kidney function.

Source: https://onlinelibrary.wiley.com/cms/asset/0939889b-9e04-4827-8395-393b52ac589c/mfig001.jpg.

Abnormal kidney function promotes these mechanisms, thus creating a vicious cycle that not only leads to hypocalcemia but also to bone fragility and related complications, thereby highlighting the interaction between renal function and calcium status. In addition, the development of hypocalcemia in patients with renal failure can pose a risk for cardiovascular complications because calcium has a vital role in cardiac muscle contraction and electrical conduction. Patients who present with acute kidney injury (AKI) are particularly susceptible to disturbances in serum electrolytes like calcium. AM A et al. (2011) note that such electrolyte disturbances are likely to require close clinical care as they can cause high morbidity and mortality. If the kidneys function improperly, it becomes difficult to maintain calcium homeostasis, which can lead to a higher rate of cardiovascular disease. The interconnection between hypocalcemia and renal function, therefore, not only influences bone health but also carries significant implications for the cardiovascular status of such patients in general. In addition to the direct effects of hypocalcemia on the skeletal and cardiovascular system, there is also a multifaceted interaction between renal replacement therapies and calcium homeostasis. Renal replacement therapies such as dialysis can significantly alter calcium levels and hence induce hypocalcemia if not controlled. The dialysate chemistry of solutions and the dynamics of calcium removal during dialysis can dramatically influence serum calcium concentration. Dépret et al. (2019) identify that individualized therapeutic interventions need to be instituted in a bid to counteract the risks of hyperkalemia as well, thereby highlighting the urgency of addressing electrolyte imbalances among the renal population with a whole-person approach. As clinicians extend into these intricacies, an understanding of the multifaceted interaction between hypocalcemia and renal function is paramount to improving patient outcomes and avoiding long-term consequences (Figure 13.9).

13.3. Acid-Base Balance and Kidney Function

The kidneys play an essential role in the regulation of acid-base balance, a part of the entire process of homeostasis. Acid-base status is regulated within the body primarily by the excretion of hydrogen ions and the reabsorption of bicarbonate by the kidneys. This complex process demonstrates the kidneys' ability to regulate the concentration of several electrolytes, thereby influencing the acid-base status. As soon as kidney function is compromised, as with CKD or AKI, acid-base balance regulation can be seriously compromised. The patients, therefore, develop metabolic acidosis, characterized by a decrease in blood pH and bicarbonate concentration and underscoring the significant role of the kidneys in acid neutralization within the body. The acid-base disturbances of which kidney disease is so frequently a cause, left uncorrected, have severe health implications. Metabolic acidosis, for instance, may exacerbate muscle wasting, increase bone resorption, and affect cardiovascular status. Clinicians need to appreciate the fineness of the disorders of electrolytes and their relationship with acid-base derangement, particularly in the critically ill patient. Targeted care also encompasses the use of pharmacological interventions, including bicarbonate supplementation, in an attempt to correct the underlying acidosis. In addition, understanding the cause of acid-base disturbances enhances the treatment and management of patients, leading to improved overall results. The identification of electrolyte imbalances, as well as acid-base alterations, is also significant in an attempt to provide holistic care according to the patient's requirements. For the successful management of acid-base and electrolyte imbalances in kidney disease, monitoring and assessment must be closely maintained. Understanding the interaction between nutritional intake and renal function may provide indications for optimal nutritional management, especially among patients suffering from acute kidney injury or undergoing renal replacement therapy. Correct nutrition allows the provision of required macronutrients to patients with the prevention of further worsening of renal function. Supplementation of certain vitamins and minerals associated with renal dysfunction is also important; electrolyte imbalances can cause potentially lethal complications if not treated. By the use of a forward-looking approach and adaptation of treatment to the clinical presentation of the patient, clinicians are able to minimize the harmful impact of both electrolyte and acid-base disturbances, enhancing the quality of treatment provided to patients with renal pathologies (Crocker et al., 2006; AM A et al., 2011) (Figure 13.10).

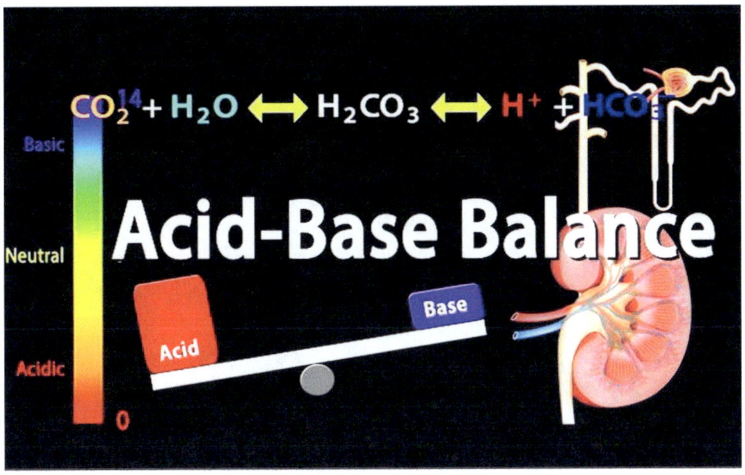

Figure 13.10. Acid-base balance and kidney function.

Source: https://i.ytimg.com/vi/VzEEs00v-JU/sddefault.jpg.

13.3.1. Normal Acid-Base Homeostasis

In maintaining normal acid-base balance, the human body relies on a complex interplay of body mechanisms that regulate the blood levels of hydrogen ions, bicarbonate, and carbon dioxide. This equilibrium is necessary for normal cellular function because deviations by small margins can lead to a range of severe medical conditions. The kidneys, the lungs, and the blood buffer systems all collaborate to maintain pH levels within a particular range of 7.35 to 7.45. The kidneys, through renal excretion and reabsorption, are the primary organs responsible for maintaining bicarbonate and hydrogen ion content. The lungs, on the other hand, control carbon dioxide content through respiratory rate mechanisms. Therefore, these systems play a critical role not just for normal metabolic function but also in the regulation of disturbances that can arise secondary to a wide variety of physiological or disease states concerning overall body homeostasis. An understanding of the significance of acid-base balance is particularly important when managing kidney disease. The kidneys, which are directly responsible for the filtration of blood and maintaining acid-base balance, are most typically injured in patients with kidney disease of any type. Such conditions lead to impaired renal function, resulting in metabolic acidosis characterized by an increase in hydrogen ions and a decrease in bicarbonate levels. It is prevalent in critically ill children who have been found to manifest a high rate of acid-base derangements, thereby necessitating early detection and intervention (Khairunnisa et al., 2025). The occurrence of respiratory alkalosis, as well as metabolic acidosis, in these patients is a common phenomenon, indicating the extent to which renal failure can disrupt normal acid-base homeostasis and lead to adverse clinical consequences. Recent advances in molecular biology have shed light on the renal mechanisms involved in acid-base regulation, particularly in the context of chronic kidney disease. Research with single-nucleus RNA sequencing has revealed special cell populations in the kidney and the role played by various nephrons and their underlying pathways in maintaining acid-base homeostasis (Chen et al., 2019). This is vital in understanding the changes at the molecular level during diseased states, as shifts in gene expression related to these processes can predispose a person to additional disorders. By establishing the cellular and molecular characteristics of the kidney, researchers can determine possible therapeutic targets for reversing normal acid-base balance in these patients and enhancing a crucial aspect of treating electrolyte and acid-base disorders in kidney disease (Figure 13.11).

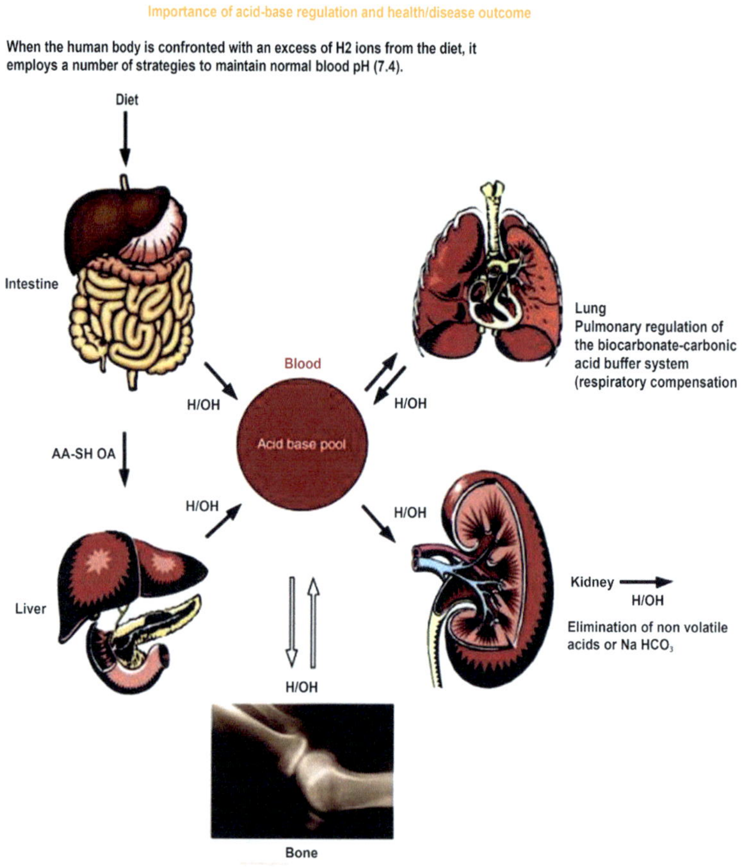

Figure 13.11. Acid-base homeostasis.

Source: https://ars.els-cdn.com/content/image/3-s2.0-B9780123750839000295-f00029-03-9780123750839.jpg.

13.3.2. Role of Kidneys in Maintaining pH Levels

Kidneys regulate the acid-base balance of the body, which is critical to ensure the body performs optimally. Kidneys accomplish this by maintaining the processes of filtration, reabsorption, and secretion of various ions, most notably bicarbonate (HCO_3^-) and hydrogen ions (H^+). By selectively excreting H+ and reclaiming HCO_3^-, the kidneys maintain the blood pH between extremely close limits of 7.35 to 7.45. Once respiratory or metabolic disturbances have developed, the kidneys initiate compensatory processes such as increased secretion of ammonia, which sequesters H+ ions and allows for their excretion. This complex process is crucial in preventing acid-base disorders, which can develop in the event of compromised kidney function and lead to disease states such as metabolic acidosis or alkalosis, significantly impacting overall health (Araujo et al., 2022). In the setting of kidney disease, the ability to attain acid-base homeostasis is severely impaired. Renal tissue injury limits the kidneys' ability to maintain proper pH levels, thereby precipitating electrolyte imbalances and consequent acid-base disorders. For instance, in chronic kidney disease (CKD), renal tubules lose the ability to reabsorb bicarbonate and secrete hydrogen ions efficiently. This dysfunction may lead to metabolic acidosis, an altered state of low blood pH and an accumulation of hydrogen ions. With the kidneys unable to excrete the excess acid, the bicarbonate buffering capacity of the entire system is compromised, highlighting the kidneys' crucial role in maintaining pH homeostasis and illustrating how disturbances can cascade to cause more severe physiological problems (Hayes et al., 2015). Additionally, the kidneys have an impact on extracellular fluid volume and blood pressure, both of which are directly related to maintaining a stable pH balance. The kidneys regulate sodium and potassium levels through selective reabsorption and secretion, thereby playing a fundamental role in maintaining proper acid-base balance. Retention of sodium, for example, can lead to an increase in the volume of extracellular fluid with hemodynamic effects on blood pressure and renal perfusion—thus impacting the kidneys' ability to regulate pH. Furthermore, changes in renal perfusion can also affect the glomerular filtration rate (GFR), thereby further exacerbating acid-base imbalance. Therefore, renal function imbalances may disrupt the complex system of electrolytes that the body is involved in, helping to regulate both pH and overall homeostasis, highlighting the critical role played by the kidneys in acid-base and electrolyte regulation within the body (Araujo et al., 2022).

13.3.3. Consequences of Acid-Base Imbalance

Acid-base imbalance has a significant impact on human physiology, particularly in relation to electrolyte disorders associated with kidney disease. The human body maintains a delicate homeostasis of pH levels to ensure optimal cellular function. In cases where the acid-base balance is disrupted, consequences can manifest in various systems, particularly affecting enzymatic reactions and metabolic processes. For example, acidosis can lead to a decrease in calcium levels, causing disruptions in neuromuscular excitability and potentially resulting in symptoms such as muscle weakness, fatigue, and confusion. Similarly, alkalosis may result in hypokalemia, characterized by low potassium levels, which can disturb cardiac rhythms and lead to dangerous complications like arrhythmias. These physiological repercussions underscore the critical importance of managing acid-base balance, particularly in populations susceptible to kidney dysfunction. Kidney disease exacerbates the risk of acid-base imbalances, with consequences that extend beyond typical metabolic disturbances. The kidneys play a vital role in regulating electrolyte balance and maintaining acid-base homeostasis. Impaired renal function can hinder the excretion of hydrogen ions and the reabsorption of bicarbonate, leading to metabolic acidosis —a common complication in chronic kidney disease. As noted in studies, prolonged metabolic acidosis not only worsens kidney function but can also lead to systemic effects, including bone demineralization and increased risk of cardiovascular events. The interplay between acid-base status and electrolyte levels is complex, as disruptions in one can cascade into additional imbalances. For instance, disturbances in sodium and potassium levels are often intricately linked to the body's overall acid-base status, underscoring the interconnectedness of these physiological processes in patients with kidney disease (Araujo et al., 2022). Furthermore, the consequences of acid-base imbalances are not limited to immediate physiological effects; they can have long-term implications for health, particularly in populations with underlying conditions such as diabetes. According to findings, diabetes is associated with electrolyte disturbances, which may be exacerbated by acid-base imbalances during hyperglycemic crises (Girija et al., 2018). For instance, fluctuations in sodium and potassium levels can lead to complications like diabetic ketoacidosis, which further complicates the management of both diabetes and kidney disease. Chronic acid-base imbalance can contribute to the progression of diabetic nephropathy, reinforcing the need for vigilant monitoring and management of electrolyte levels. As such, a holistic approach to treatment that considers the intricate relationship between acid-base status and overall health is crucial for improving outcomes in individuals affected by this condition (Figure 13.12).

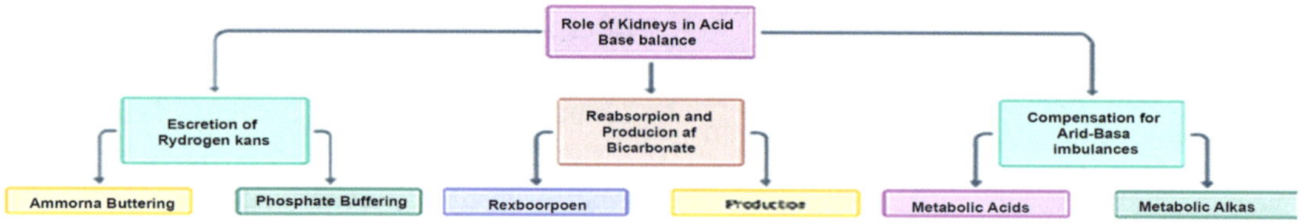

Figure 13.12. Role of kidneys in acid base balance.

Source: https://static.wixstatic.com/media/31186f_22076654d6b940ff8c68b4fbf7c6f855~mv2.png/v1/fill/w_568,h_134,al_c,q_85,usm_0.66_1.00_0.01,enc_avif,quality_auto/31186f_22076654d6b940ff8c68b4fbf7c6f855~mv2.png.

13.4. Types of Acid-Base Disorders in Kidney Disease

The intimate relationship between renal function and acid-base balance underscores the relevance of knowledge of disturbances in acid-base balance in the context of renal disease. The kidney plays a crucial role in homeostasis by excreting hydrogen ions and reabsorbing bicarbonate ions, which are essential for neutralizing acids in the body. In individuals with chronic kidney disease (CKD), the ability of the kidneys to carry out these functions is compromised, such that they become susceptible to metabolic acidosis. Metabolic acidosis is characterized by a decrease in serum bicarbonate, which can result from the loss of bicarbonate reabsorption and hydrogen ion secretion. Also, the accumulation of metabolic acids such as sulfates and phosphates exacerbates the acidosis, indicating that acid-base balance needs to be strictly monitored to be able to manage kidney disease effectively. Renal disease also induces metabolic alkalosis alongside metabolic acidosis, although to a lesser degree. Kidney patients' metabolic alkalosis usually arises from conditions such as vomiting or augmented diuresis, which cause the excretion of hydrogen ions. In primary hyperaldosteronism, for instance, the high concentrations of aldosterone cause the kidneys to excrete excess hydrogen and retain sodium, thereby raising serum bicarbonate levels. This apparently paradoxical situation underlies the complex interactions between hormonal regulation and electrolyte derangements potentially related to renal failure. These mechanisms are crucial for clinicians to understand so that they can employ appropriate therapeutic measures, such as administering potassium-sparing diuretics or replacing potassium, based on the underlying disorder of each patient. Correction of acid-base disturbances in renal disease is often several times more significant than correcting the underlying electrolyte derangements, most notably hyperkalemia. Hyperkalemia can result from diminished renal clearance and further disrupt the acid-base status. In the management of acidosis, one must consider potassium management lest aggressive treatment create dramatically low serum potassium levels by mistake. Conversely, in metabolic alkalosis, maintaining adequate potassium levels is crucial for effectively restoring the body's acid-base balance. More advanced therapeutic strategies, including sodium bicarbonate infusion and phosphate binder administration, can help correct acidosis and manage associated renal mineral imbalances. These comprehensive strategies highlight the multi-aspect nature of electrolyte and acid-base disturbances in patients with kidney disease, which requires patient-specific treatment regimens to optimize patient outcomes (Figure 13.13).

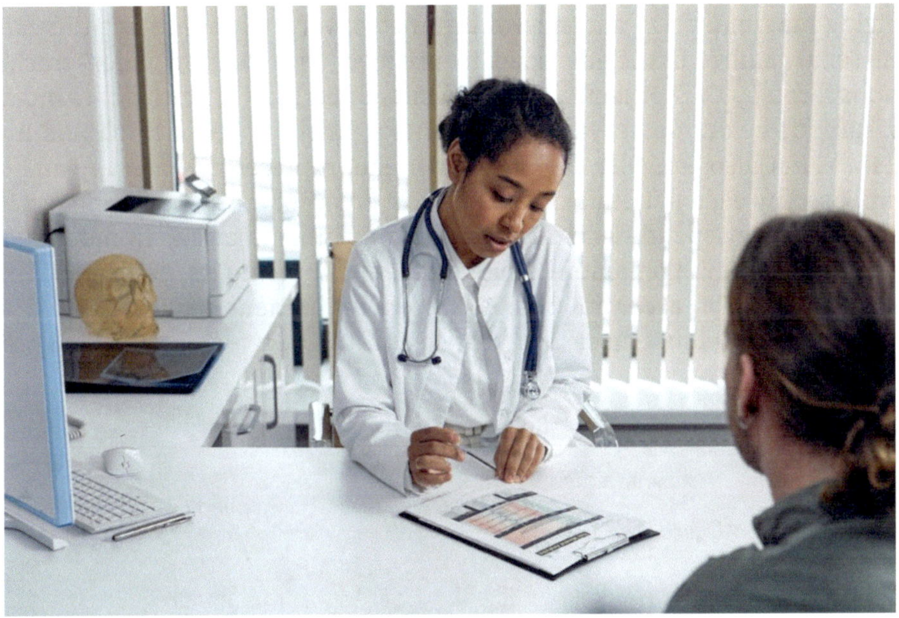

Figure 13.13. Acid-base disorders in kidney disease.

Source: https://texaskidneyinstitute.com/wp-content/uploads/2022/12/doctor-and-patient-going-over-chart.jpg.

13.4.1. Metabolic Acidosis: Causes and Clinical Implications

Metabolic acidosis is a severe electrolyte and acid-base disorder that occurs frequently in patients with kidney disease. Metabolic acidosis develops when the body retains excess hydrogen ions or loses bicarbonate, resulting in a lowered blood pH. In renal patients, a significant cause of metabolic acidosis is diminished acid excretion due to reduced renal function, which is frequent in chronic kidney disease (CKD). Because the kidneys cannot effectively filter and eliminate excess metabolic waste products, organic acids accumulate, thereby exacerbating acidosis. Furthermore, conditions such as diabetes mellitus and sepsis are also known to trigger metabolic acidosis, highlighting the multi-factorial pathogenesis of this condition among patients with kidney diseases, necessitating a mandate for vigorous clinical assessment and management based on the individual patient's needs. The clinical impact of metabolic acidosis is extensive and multifaceted, involving not just acid-base but also overall morbidity and mortality in patients with kidney disease. With progressing metabolic acidosis, cardiac performance is altered, bone metabolism is affected, and protein-energy wasting (PEW) may develop, contributing to the challenges faced by these patients. Of singular significance has been the discovery of a relationship between metabolic acidosis and PEW, with chronic acidosis being observed to increase catabolic function, exacerbating muscle loss and endangering mortality. For patients, symptoms have included weakness, fatigue, and shortness of breath, necessitating strict monitoring of serum bicarbonate levels and acid-base status in a bid to prevent complications. Effective treatment of metabolic acidosis may involve interventions such as the use of buffering agents, such as sodium bicarbonate, or dietary modifications to restore normal acid-base homeostasis. Beyond this, attention to the nutritional concern of metabolic acidosis is of paramount importance in the patient with renal disease. There is a growing consensus on the value of optimizing macronutrient and micronutrient delivery to counteract the catabolic effects of acidosis and renal failure. Clinicians need to proceed with caution when tracking the usual dietary limitations faced by CKD patients, as such limits often lead to inadequate intake of essential nutrients necessary for health preservation. An optimal nutrition regimen should not only rectify inherent imbalances but also consider the impact of renal replacement therapy and the individual requirements imposed by each patient's unique clinical environment. As metabolic acidosis has the potential to increase energy spending and initiate chronic inflammation, an individualized therapy that corrects underlying derangements in metabolism, supplements deficiencies, and provides sufficient caloric intake plays a central role in improving patient results as well as preventing increased complications of kidney disease (AM A et al., 2011; Carrero et al., 2013) (Figure 13.14).

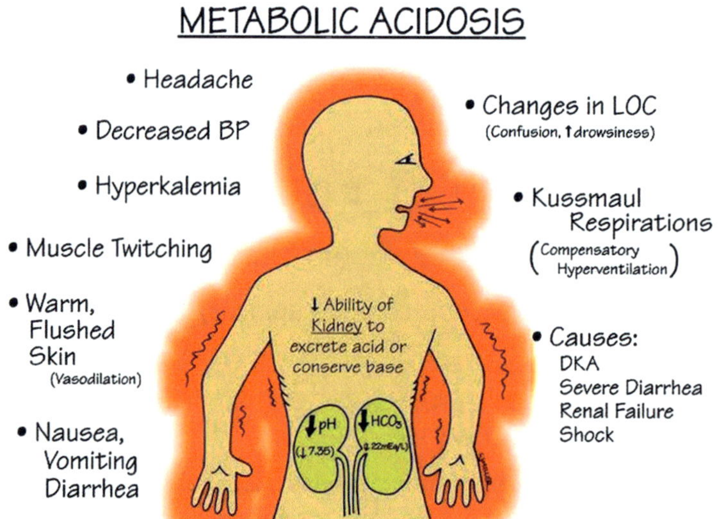

Figure 13.14. Metabolic acidosis.

Source: https://sa1s3optim.patientpop.com/assets/images/provider/photos/2703127.jpeg.

13.4.2. Metabolic Alkalosis: Mechanisms and Effects

Metabolic alkalosis is a condition characterized by elevated blood pH due to elevated bicarbonate ions or the removal of hydrogen ions. In kidney disease, the pathophysiology for metabolic alkalosis is multifaceted. The kidneys regulate acid-base balance, and any disruption in their functioning has a tendency to upset this equilibrium. For instance, diseases such as chronic vomiting can lead to a significant loss of chloride and hydrogen ions, thereby predisposing individuals to alkalosis. Diseases of the renal tubules also compromise the kidney's ability to excrete bicarbonate, further aggravating alkalosis in patients with renal insufficiency. Understanding these mechanisms is critical because it will guide the following therapeutic interventions in patients with renal-related electrolyte and acid-base disturbances.

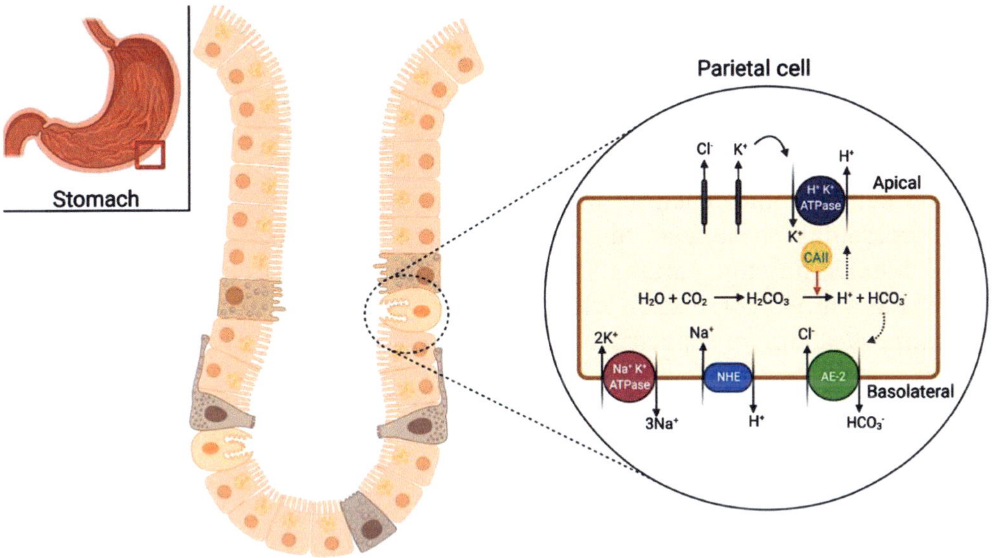

Figure 13.15. Metabolic alkalosis.

Source: https://www.ajkd.org/cms/10.1053/j.ajkd.2021.12.016/asset/73074a31-c3fd-4423-9c00-51cf04b8062a/main.assets/gr3_lrg.jpg.

The impact of metabolic alkalosis can extend far beyond mere biochemical change, influencing a wide range of physiological systems and the general state of health. One of the extremely unsettling consequences is induction of hypokalemia, typically resulting from potassium concentration changes secondary to acid-base disturbances. Patients with metabolic alkalosis can experience excessive potassium loss in their kidneys, leading to further complications such as muscle weakness and cardiac dysfunction. In addition, as proposed by existing evidence, metabolic alkalosis can also arise secondary to underlying psychological illnesses such as anorexia nervosa and bulimia nervosa, with the ability to engender extreme renal involvement as well as disturbance of electrolytes via mechanisms like chronic dehydration and hypokalemia (Cavoli et al., 2011). An appreciation of the intricate dynamics between metabolic alkalosis and kidney disease is therefore crucial for effective clinical management. Furthermore, the complicated interaction of metabolic alkalosis with genetic factors has begun to be given more attention in recent times. Mutations in certain genes encoding ion channels and transporters can lead to conditions characterized by recurrent hypokalemia and metabolic alkalosis. For example, patients with congenital disorders such as Bartter's syndrome or Gitelman's syndrome have these acid-base derangements secondary to renal tubular impairment, which interferes with the management of chloride and bicarbonate (Alazami et al., 2010). These conditions underscore the importance of a thorough search for acquired and congenital causes of hypokalemia and metabolic alkalosis, as awareness of these pathways can aid in refining diagnostic and therapeutic approaches. Comprehensive clinical evaluation is thus of utmost value in distinguishing multiple etiologies and attaining optimal management of patients complicated with electrolyte and acid-base derangements (Figure 13.15).

13.4.3. Respiratory Acidosis: Connection to Renal Function

Knowledge of the relationship between renal function and respiratory acidosis is crucial for managing electrolyte and acid-base disturbances. Respiratory acidosis occurs when there is retention of carbon dioxide (CO_2) due to inadequate ventilation, resulting in an increase in hydrogen ion concentration and a concomitant decrease in blood pH. Kidneys play a crucial role in compensating for this acid-base imbalance by excreting excess hydrogen ions and reabsorbing bicarbonate (HCO_3^-). It is important and essential renal reaction; in its absence, acid-base homeostasis would be severely compromised, worsening the effects of respiratory acidosis. Hypercapnia (elevated CO_2 levels) damages renal tubular function, ultimately affecting acid and base excretion, as renal net acid excretion (NAE) has a direct correlation with plasma bicarbonate and hydrogen ion concentrations, entailing the kidneys' adaptive capacity in acid-base regulation (Hulter et al., 1983).

The relationship between renal response and respiratory function is not only one of compensation but also indicative of underlying metabolic phenomena intrinsic to renal function. When disease conditions, particularly those involving the kidneys, impair their ability to maintain acid-base equilibrium, acute kidney injury (AKI) can predispose to a metabolic environment that is more readily susceptible to respiratory acidosis. The kidneys may fail to maintain acid-base homeostasis due to deranged glomerular filtration and impaired tubular function, making the scenario even more complicated. In acute illness, such as in AKI, clinicians must acknowledge that deranged renal function can worsen respiratory acidosis; thus, a careful assessment of the patient's metabolic status and the need for early intervention to prevent further systemic derangements (AMA et al., 2011). Finally, management of respiratory acidosis due to chronic kidney disease (CKD) requires an understanding of renal physiology and electrolyte management.

The relationship between CO_2 status and renal compensation is crucial in ensuring adequate bicarbonate balance. In CKD, hydrogen ion excretion by the kidneys diminishes, leading to acid retention and worsening acidosis. This reduction in function increases the value of nutritional management and electrolyte balance, with patients having to be monitored for deficiencies that could complicate their conditions. Studies have shown that dietary changes influence plasma acid-base balance, highlighting the interdependence of renal function, intake, and respiratory control (Hulter et al., 1983). Identifying these associations, medical practitioners can create more effective strategies for managing the response to the challenge of respiratory acidosis in kidney disease (Figure 13.16).

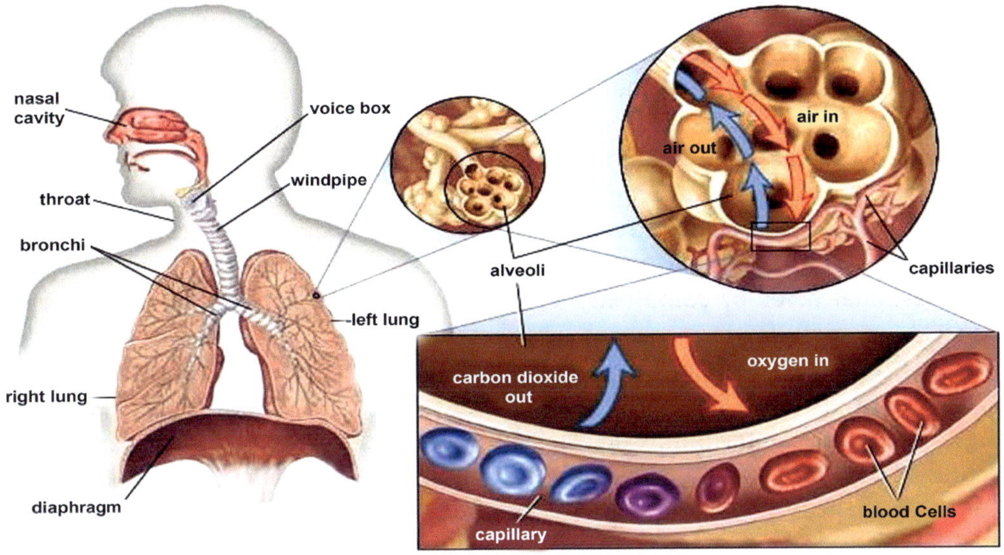

Figure 13.16. Respiratory acidosis.

Source: https://cdn.britannica.com/37/92937-004-1E4EA526/alveoli-capillaries-lungs-oxygen-carbon-dioxide-Imbalances.jpg.

13.5. Diagnosis of Electrolyte and Acid-Base Disorders

Diagnosis of acid-base and electrolyte disorders in the patient with kidney disease is a complex task that requires a nuanced understanding of underlying pathophysiologies. Chronic kidney disease (CKD) significantly alters the balance of electrolytes, particularly calcium and sodium homeostasis. For instance, hypercalcemia can be prevalent in CKD patients, but has traditionally been detected by measuring total calcium concentration (tCa), which cannot provide an accurate indication of physiological imbalances since renal failure can introduce confounding effects on this measurement. It has been demonstrated by studies that tCa is highly specific for establishing ionized hypercalcemia but low in sensitivity, and therefore, the risk of underestimation, especially in instances of low bicarbonate levels. Hence, clinicians must use tCa results in combination with clinical presentation and other biomarkers to accurately diagnose and treat hypercalcemia and potential complications in patients with CKD (Abdi et al., 2017). The clinical management of electrolyte abnormalities in renal disease requires thorough diagnostic processes, particularly in terms of sodium and water balance. Sodium disturbances, which are common among patients with renal diseases, can be due to numerous etiologies leading to conditions like hyponatremia or hypernatremia. In neurologically impaired groups, it is essential to note the prevalence of sodium disturbances since they may serve to worsen existing conditions or cause new complications. Diagnosis of diseases such as the syndrome of inappropriate antidiuretic hormone secretion (SIADH) or cerebral salt wasting requires precise diagnostic techniques, i.e., clinical evaluation and laboratory investigations. Precise diagnosis is crucial and must be carried out early because it will determine the treatment options, which can influence the outcome in patients with these diseases, and thus is vital in this instance of electrolyte imbalance to have a formal method of diagnosis (Crocker et al., 2006). Additionally, the interplay between renal function and acid-base disturbances provides an additional layer of complexity to diagnosis. Acid-base disturbances may range from mild metabolic acidosis to alkalosis, which is usually emergent in patients with renal disease. Diagnosis requires determining arterial blood gas analysis in addition to electrolyte measurements to identify the primary acid-base disturbance and any corresponding compensatory mechanisms. For example, the CKD patient with associated metabolic acidosis may exhibit suggestive bicarbonate changes that would necessitate investigation for the underlying etiology. Thus, a proper evaluation involving biochemical assessment, along with clinical correlation, is necessary for effective diagnosis and management of acid-base disturbances in renal disease, thereby optimizing patient care and outcomes.

13.5.1. Laboratory Tests for Electrolyte Levels

Laboratory testing measurement of electrolyte balance is significant in the management and diagnosis of electrolyte and acid-base imbalance, particularly in patients with kidney disease. Sodium, potassium, chloride, and bicarbonate are some of the critical electrolytes that play numerous roles in the body, including maintaining fluid balance, regulating muscle contraction, and facilitating nerve impulse transmission. Kidney disease significantly disrupts the homeostasis of these electrolytes and may result in serious complications. Regular monitoring through blood work enables clinicians to make an early diagnosis and implement proper interventions. Interpretation must consider the patient's general clinical presentation, other lab results, and symptoms because the ability of the kidneys to excrete or retain electrolytes depends upon the underlying disease. Of particular significance is the investigation of sodium, as derangements can indicate underlying pathological states that are exacerbated by kidney disease. Hyponatremia and hypernatremia are common occurrences that numerous etiologies, including volume depletion, congestive heart failure, or inappropriate release of antidiuretic hormone can cause. A valuable laboratory test of sodium concentration provides insight into a patient's fluid status and potential need for intravenous fluids or diuretic therapy. The sodium balance in renal disease cannot be overstated in its impact on patient management. Clinicians must be aware of signs of sodium imbalance and adjust treatment as necessary, emphasizing the importance of early detection and intervention in maintaining renal function and overall health (Crocker et al., 2006). Moreover, plasma potassium must be tightly controlled in kidney disease patients since the kidneys have the primary function of eliminating potassium. Hyperkalemia, which refers to elevated potassium levels, is highly likely to lead to cardiac arrhythmias and other severe complications. Hypokalemia, while less common, can occur due to excessive diuresis or inadequate intake. Adequate laboratory investigations to accurately detect potassium levels are not only critical for diagnosis but also for making informed decisions regarding treatment, particularly in the modulation of drugs that affect electrolyte dynamics. Aside from sodium, potassium testing is often used to direct more comprehensive electrolyte panels that encompass other significant ions, such as calcium and magnesium, to provide a broader picture of a patient's metabolic status. The tests form the core of developing effective treatment plans for electrolyte disturbances and ultimately patient management in kidney disease (Garshnek et al., 2025) (Figure 13.17).

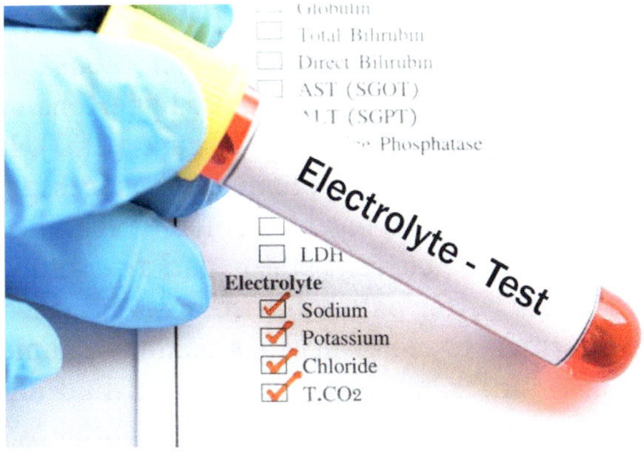

Figure 13.17. Laboratory tests for electrolyte levels.

Source: https://img.mlo-online.com/files/base/ebm/mlo/image/2025/02/67afc72eb5e8b27c9acbe0f7-shutterstock_1079579519.png?auto=format,compress&fit=max&q=45&w=640&width=640.

13.5.2. Arterial Blood Gas Analysis for Acid-Base Status

Arterial blood gas (ABG) analysis is an essential diagnostic test in establishing the acid-base status of patients, particularly those with intrinsic renal disease. In the context of acid-base imbalance, this test provides valuable information about the respiratory and metabolic components of the patients condition. Changes in blood pH, bicarbonate levels, and partial pressures of carbon dioxide and oxygen can provide clues about the body's compensatory mechanisms in response to renal failure. Kidney disease typically leads to the accumulation of acids, leading to metabolic acidosis, which can be diagnosed using the findings of ABG. By rationally correlating with the findings, clinicians can identify the etiology of acid-base disturbances and provide interventions in a more focused manner, especially in the setting of chronic kidney disease, where an early correction is crucial for the prognosis of the patient. In the context of electrolyte and acid-base abnormalities, it is essential to understand where ABG analysis intersects with clinical presentation in patients with kidney disease. For example, an intense study can reveal hyperkalemia or hypocalcemia, conditions that are commonly found in renal failure. Electrolyte imbalances have a significant impact on acid-base status, contributing to the overall clinical picture of the patient. Measurement of bicarbonate and pH, along with electrolytes, allows for a multi-dimensional approach to treatment planning. In particular, careful interpretation of ABG can guide therapeutic decision-making, such as the requirement for bicarbonate correction or dialysis to reverse an acute or chronic imbalance. The interconnectedness of these diagnostic variables highlights the importance of ABG analysis as a vital component of comprehensive patient assessment. In addition, the value of ABG analysis extends beyond simple diagnosis; it becomes imperative in management plans of ongoing patient care for patients with kidney disease. Repeated monitoring of acid-base status through ABG by health care providers enables them to track the efficacy of therapeutic interventions and alter treatment regimens accordingly. For instance, the development of metabolic acidosis necessitates immediate intervention to ensure metabolic homeostasis. The delicate balance of acid-base status and electrolytes is pivotal in maximizing the recovery of renal function or supporting the stabilization of transplant wait-list patients. In response, the utilization of ABG analysis not only facilitates the detection of common conditions but also provides actionable intelligence that can inform long-term care plans, ultimately maximizing patient quality of life and vitality, particularly with the vagaries of chronic kidney disease (Cremer et al., 2018; Amelia et al., 2023).

13.5.3. Clinical Assessment and Patient History

Careful clinical assessment and a comprehensive patient history are key factors in diagnosing renal disease-related electrolyte and acid-base disturbances. The initial evaluation should involve careful scrutiny of the patient's medical, surgical, and family histories that could unveil conditions that predispose the patient to electrolyte disturbances. For example, a history of diabetes or hypertension may warn healthcare practitioners about the risk of developing chronic kidney disease (CKD). In addition, a meticulous drug history, such as nonprescription drugs and supplements, is necessary since some drugs can cause renal dysfunction or exacerbate underlying electrolyte imbalance. Recognition of these background conditions aids in diagnosing the current status and also allows for the creation of tailored treatment plans, paving the way for better patient outcomes. A physical examination, complementing the historical presentation, is critical to the clinical assessment. Edema, hypertension, or altered mental status can provide valuable information regarding the fluid and electrolyte balance of the patient. Monitoring of vital signs and a focused physical examination can help identify complications of acute electrolyte disorders, such as hyperkalemia or metabolic acidosis. These presentations may require immediate interventions to prevent further renal damage or systemic complications. Repeated monitoring of pertinent laboratory values, including serum electrolytes and arterial blood gases, also aids clinical assessment by providing quantitative data to measure the magnitude of electrolyte and acid-base imbalances. These integrated methods will help clinicians adopt effective methods when treating patients with kidney disease. Lastly, the emphasis on structured methods, as evidenced by the call for uniform phenotypes of drug-induced kidney disease, is essential in clinical assessment. Awareness of the heterogeneous presentations of renal insufficiency through some phenotypes allows more subtle recognition of probable drug-induced complications, which are now extremely common etiologies of acute kidney injury. The classification systems presented in recent reviews provide standards that may be compatible with clinical data, patient history, and biochemical results. Adoption of these innovations into routine clinical practice can enhance the accuracy of measurements and enhance multi-disciplinary management of electrolyte disturbances. By such systems, healthcare workers can systematically evaluate and manage the complications of renal disease, thus increasing patient care outcomes in this high-risk population (Awdishu et al., 2015).

13.6. Management and Treatment Strategies

Management of acid-base and electrolyte imbalances in renal disease is inherently complex due to the intricate interplay of underlying pathophysiological mechanisms. Therapeutic options require a comprehensive understanding of the distinctive imbalances observed in the patient. For instance, when treating sodium imbalance, physicians must differentiate between hyponatremia and hypernatremia, each requiring a distinct approach. In acute hyponatremia, urgent correction may be needed to be able to alleviate cerebral edema, but this must be carried out with extreme care not to cause complications such as osmotic demyelination syndrome. Thus, early diagnosis and appropriate treatment are crucial in minimizing the complications associated with such conditions (Crocker et al., 2006). Strategies should also include scrupulous monitoring of sodium levels and supervision of personalized treatments, emphasizing conservative management in minor disturbances to prevent unnecessary intervention. Fluid administration remains one of the pillars of treatment for electrolyte derangements in renal insufficiency. Particularly, depletional and dilutional hyponatremia should be differentiated for successful management. For instance, measuring vasopressin levels can be used to determine whether fluid restriction or fluid resuscitation is required. Clinicians are advised not to overdepend on extraneous laboratory reports but instead focus on thorough investigations that consider each patient's unique clinical context. The introduction of vasopressin receptor antagonists has brought new therapeutic options, with both opportunity and challenge, as they have the potential to improve outcomes in certain hyponatremias but also need to be handled with caution due to potential adverse effects (HJ A et al., 2008). As each new treatment is developed, it is increasingly crucial that nephrologists remain current on best practice as well as therapy. In addition, management strategies must extend beyond the immediate correction of electrolyte imbalances to encompass long-term maintenance and prevention of recurrence. These include follow-up on an outpatient basis to monitor renal function, electrolytes, and acid-base balance, and education of patients on lifestyle modification, dietary modification, and treatment regimen compliance. With an understanding of the ongoing state of kidney disease, healthcare providers must participate in a collaborative endeavor with patients to optimize self-management techniques, allowing patients to maintain a steady electrolyte balance. With nephrology's increasing role in clinical guidelines, the integration of evidence-based practices will prove vital in optimizing patient outcomes. Overall, the effective management of kidney disease electrolyte and acid-base abnormalities involves not only adequate diagnosis and appropriate therapy but also anticipatory and preventive interventions to ensure long-term well-being and good health (Figure 13.18).

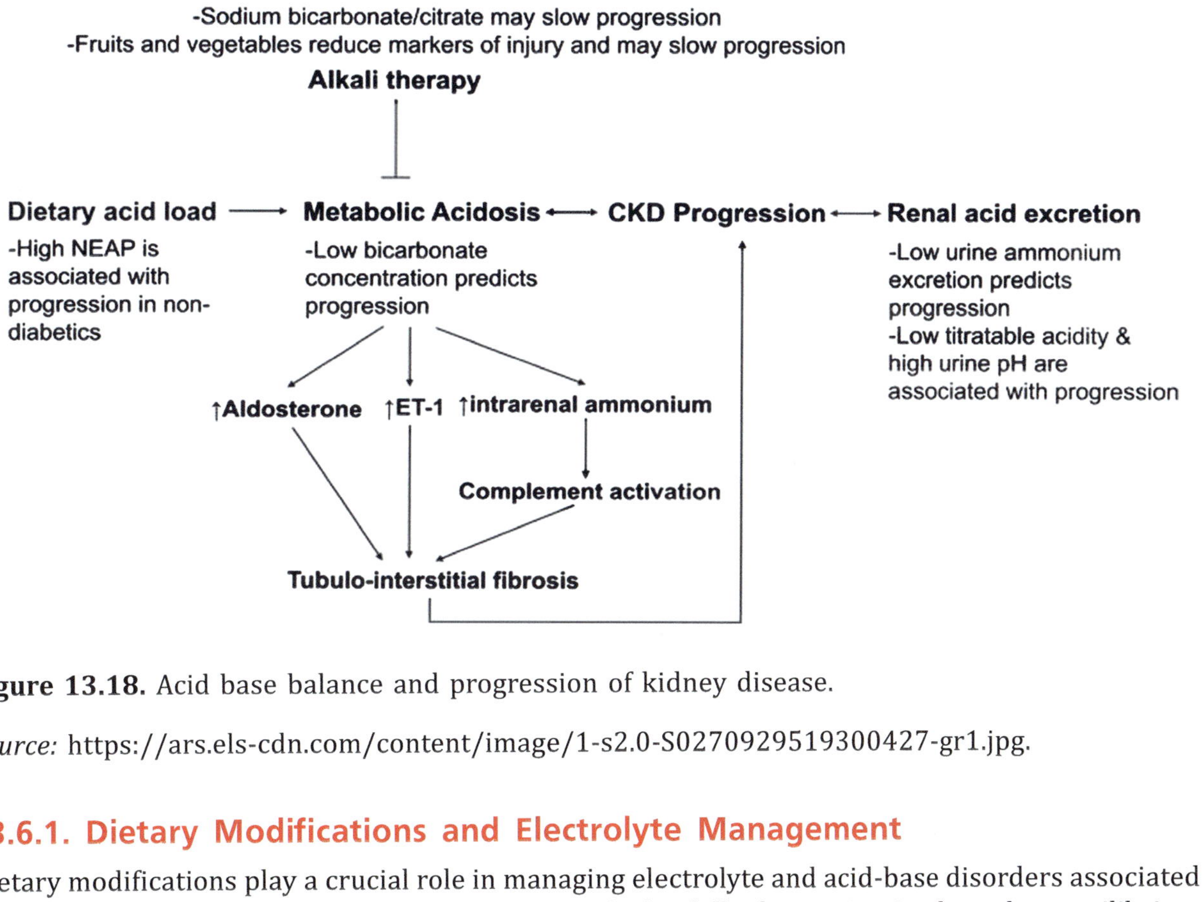

Figure 13.18. Acid base balance and progression of kidney disease.

Source: https://ars.els-cdn.com/content/image/1-s2.0-S0270929519300427-gr1.jpg.

13.6.1. Dietary Modifications and Electrolyte Management

Dietary modifications play a crucial role in managing electrolyte and acid-base disorders associated with renal disease. Patients with poor renal function find it difficult to maintain electrolyte equilibrium due to the dysfunction of the kidneys' excretion and filtration functions. Hence, the application of dietary restrictions to limit the intake of specific electrolytes, such as potassium, sodium, and phosphorus, is highly essential. For example, low-potassium intake can avert hyperkalemia, a common complication caused by reduced renal clearance. Furthermore, interventions involving the restriction of processed foods, which are typically high in sodium and phosphorus content, can significantly contribute to enabling patients to manage their electrolytes efficiently. Thus, clinical professionals must collaborate with nutrition professionals in developing individualized dietary plans that are palatable to patients and tailored to their customized metabolic needs for optimal health benefits. Electrolyte balance in the context of dietary modification is particularly critical in preventing the formation of calcium oxalate (CaOx) uroliths due to an incorrect dietary composition. Recent research has highlighted the increasing prevalence of CaOx stones, prompting a call for targeted dietary interventions. Although some stone prevention diets exist, they are often of limited efficacy, and greater emphasis must be placed on identifying dietary risk factors, such as oxalate intake. The contribution of high dietary oxalate to stone formation must be explored extensively to inform nutritional interventions. Specifically, knowledge of the metabolic processes involved in the body's formation of oxalate will assist dietitians in creating diets that minimize the likelihood of stone formation without compromising other nutritional requirements for the care of kidney disease. Therefore, a detailed diet evaluation and adjustments based on research are crucial for patient care. Furthermore, the integration of dietary modification can significantly aid in managing electrolytes in patients with acid-base disorders secondary to renal disease. In particular, the application of dietary carbohydrates has been examined regarding its impact on endogenous oxalate metabolism, with a promising pathway for intervention. Specifically, reducing carbohydrate intake can enhance global metabolic balance, which in turn affects oxalate status. This association supports the need for an overall strategy to change the diet, taking into account potential biochemical interactions within the organism. Patients must also be educated about the potential impact of different food groups on their overall electrolyte balance and motivated to make informed choices. By facilitating patient participation in their own dietary regimen, healthcare professionals can promote heightened compliance with prescribed dietary therapy, ultimately leading to more effective regulation of both electrolyte status and acid-base homeostasis in patients with kidney disease.

13.6.2. Pharmacological Interventions

The treatment of electrolyte and acid-base imbalances in renal pathology can involve a plethora of pharmacologic interventions to restore balance to the body. Three of these medications are commonly utilized to correct metabolic acidosis, a frequent disorder in CKD. This condition results from decreased renal excretion of hydrogen ions and impaired bicarbonate reabsorption, leading to low blood pH. Sodium bicarbonate infusion can effectively correct serum bicarbonate and, subsequently, system pH. The therapy, however, needs to be determined appropriately since excess bicarbonate leads to alkalosis or fluid retention in patients with underlying cardiac conditions. Hence, patient-specific needs should be individualized in the optimization of outcomes regarding acid-base management in CKD. Apart from sodium bicarbonate, management of electrolyte disturbances using drugs also involves the use of diuretics and electrolytes. Diuretics, such as furosemide and loop diuretics, are typically used to correct fluid overload and hypervolemia, particularly in patients undergoing dialysis. These medications facilitate the excretion of sodium and water and relieve symptoms of kidney disease-induced hypertension and edema. Furthermore, potassium binders are also used in the treatment of hyperkalemia, which is a common and potentially dangerous condition in advanced renal disease. These medications act by exchanging potassium for other cations in the intestinal lumen, thereby facilitating their removal in the feces. However, it is still necessary to monitor the level of electrolytes regularly and adjust these drugs accordingly, as they may inadvertently exacerbate other electrolyte disturbances, particularly with CKD (Kitsiou et al., 2013). Recent studies have highlighted the importance of considering cognitive function when evaluating pharmacological therapy for electrolyte and acid-base imbalances in renal disease. Chronic kidney disease patients are at elevated risk for cognitive impairment, complicating management of electrolytes as well as compliance with treatment. Interventions that decrease the physiological burden of CKD, such as managing anemia and secondary hyperparathyroidism, will have a secondary effect of potentially improving cognitive outcomes through enhanced overall health and function. Both pharmacologic and nonpharmacologic strategies must be integrated. While there are many promising agents, the existing literature indicates a paucity of targeted studies examining the cognitive impact of these interventions. Therefore, ongoing research is crucial to establish an integrated approach that considers both cognitive health and the complex complications characteristic of CKD (et al., 2023).

13.6.3. Dialysis and Its Role in Correcting Disorders

The evolution of kidney disease leads to serious complications, with significant electrolyte and acid-base disturbances being one of them. Dialysis is one of the primary therapies for this complication that acts as a renal replacement therapy to reverse uncorrected disturbances. By the elimination of excess electrolytes like potassium, dialysis helps to correct hyperkalemia—a dangerous condition associated with cardiac disturbances. In addition to eliminating solutes, dialysis also facilitates the restoration of acid-base balance in the body, thereby correcting metabolic acidosis. Dialysis plays a dual role as an important therapeutic measure in kidney disease treatment, where the preservation of electrolyte equilibrium and pH are vital factors for patient survival and overall health outcomes. The highly sophisticated work of dialysis machines allows specific approaches to restore electrolyte imbalance. Techniques such as a four-stream dialysis fluid delivery system enable the strict control of dialysis solution composition, allowing for the treatment of dysnatremias and metabolic acid-base disturbances in combination. The system enables clinicians to adjust sodium and bicarbonate concentrations in the dialysis solution to more closely match the individual patient's needs. With such innovative methods practiced by practitioners, they also gain the ability to adjust treatment regimens dynamically monitored by ongoing assessments of electrolyte and acid-base status. Such developments enhance the efficacy of dialysis and make it a cornerstone for renal therapy of electrolyte and acid-base disturbances. Although dialysis can successfully treat electrolyte and acid-base disturbances, it is essential to remain aware of its associated risks and complications as well. For instance, while dialysis successfully lowers serum potassium levels in the occurrence of hyperkalemia, it may also lead to complications such as cardiac dysrhythmias (as per Dépret et al. (2019). The invasive nature of renal replacement therapy requires a balanced approach, where the benefits of dialysis are weighed against the risks. Knowledge of the pharmacodynamic interactions between other forms of treatment for hyperkalemia is also essential for optimizing patient management. To these complex dynamics, it is apparent that continued advances in dialysis technology, combined with individualized patient therapy, will remain fundamental to treating disorders related to kidney disease effectively.

SUMMARY

It is of utmost importance to understand electrolyte and acid-base disorders in order to treat kidney disease successfully. The kidneys maintain electrolytes and acid-base balance with ideal homeostasis. Dysregulation leads to fatal complications such as arrhythmias, weakness, and metabolic acidosis, complicating the clinical profile of the patients. Successful management regimens must be adapted to the unique presentation of disorders reported by patients based on their primary medical conditions and kidney function. This entails an accurate assessment of electrolyte status and acid-base balance to ensure interventions are based on clinical standards tailored to the individual needs of each patient. Multidisciplinary treatment, involving nephrologists, dietitians, and nursing staff, is also crucial for maximizing care. Given the complex interplay between renal function and nutritional status, clinicians must consider variables such as dietary intake and the use of renal replacement therapy. Through cooperation, there is an enhanced understanding of how to prevent or minimize electrolyte imbalance, resulting in improved outcomes for the patient. The inclusion of personalized dietary alterations has been found promising for regulating kidney disease-associated complications of electrolyte and acid-base disturbances, and thus, nutrition should occupy a prime position in kidney management as a whole. Eventually, the comprehensive treatment of kidney disease-associated electrolyte and acid-base disturbances will be based on an integrated approach that considers both physiological and nutritional aspects. The recent emphasis on this increase in nutrients, particularly micronutrients and electrolytes, emphasizes the importance of a paradigm shift in treatment protocol. Providers have to give priority to correcting deficiencies while simultaneously managing overages, as outlined in the current literature. The insights gained from studies indicate that the urinary excretion of potassium, sodium, and chloride, as well as the metabolic alterations found with acute kidney injury, provide sufficient justification to plan and monitor this replacement meticulously. Clinicians are encouraged to stay abreast of evolving practice to achieve optimal management and improve the quality of life in patients with these complex disorders, as attested by the growing literature on renal health.

Kidney disease and electrolyte disorders interact and are significant in understanding patient treatment outcomes and care. Sodium, potassium, and calcium are vital electrolytes in various physiological events, including nerve transmission and muscle contraction. The kidneys' ability to control electrolyte balance is compromised in an individual with kidney disease, and as a consequence, potential disorders may occur. These patients usually come to the doctor with some condition like hyperkalemia or hyponatremia, which can turn out to be catastrophic if they are not treated effectively. Inadequate diagnosis and treatment at an early point are required to cut down on life-threatening consequences of such imbalances, demonstrating the need for clinicians to remain vigilant to check for electrolyte balance throughout the progression of kidney disease. Acid-base imbalance is equally significant in renal insufficiency, particularly because the kidneys play a crucial role in maintaining a stable blood pH level. Metabolic acidosis is typically observed in patients with chronic renal disease when the body fails to secrete sufficient acid or retain bicarbonate. This further aggravates the already compromised metabolic functions of the body and contributes to complications. Furthermore, acute acid-base disturbances may result in a variety of disparate underlying diagnoses, like that seen in acute kidney injury. Treatment includes not only the management of the underlying renal impairment but also the timing of therapeutic interventions to correct acid-base disturbances, such as bicarbonate supplementation or dietary adjustments. An understanding of these interactions enables the clinician to develop balanced treatment plans tailored specifically to the needs of patients with kidney disease. Finally, a thorough understanding and assessment of acid-base and electrolyte disorders are necessary to optimize the treatment of patients with kidney disease. Some syndromes will emerge, resulting in individualized clinical presentations that can be effectively treated with targeted approaches. For instance, in the neurologic patient, derangements in sodium balance can be created by conditions like the syndrome of inappropriate antidiuretic hormone secretion, which can lead to additional complications of kidney disease. Therefore, there is a need for clinicians to recognize the complexity of these interrelations, as evident in the literature documenting the cyclical nature of such disorders and their impact on patient outcomes. By encouraging an integrative approach to treatment and assessment of patients, medical practitioners can offer better recovery models to patients who are struggling with the challenges of electrolyte and acid-base disorders as manifested in kidney disease (Crocker et al., 2006; Andant et al., 2019).

CLOSER LOOK

HYPEROSMOLAR MEDULLARY INTERSTITIUM

The hyperosmolar medullary interstitium is an essential component of the kidney's ability to concentrate urine and maintain fluid and electrolyte balance. It occurs within the renal medulla, ideally where the loop of Henle and collecting duct lie, where a highly concentrated interstitial fluid is instrumental in advancing water reabsorption. The interstitium in the medullary area has increasing osmolarity from cortex through the inner medulla, to a concentration of 1200 mOsm/kg, primarily due to the accumulation of sodium chloride (NaCl) and urea. This osmotic gradient serves the countercurrent multiplication mechanism, in which the kidneys produce either dilute or concentrated urine depending on the body's level of hydration. The thick ascending limb of the loop of Henle excretes Na^+ and Cl– ions from the tubular fluid into the interstitium in an active process that does not allow water to follow them, thus creating a hyperosmotic environment. Meanwhile, the thin descending limb is permeable to water but not to solutes, allowing water to leave into the hyperosmotic interstitium, concentrating the tubular fluid. Recycling of urea contributes to the inner medullary osmolarity, especially under the influence of antidiuretic hormone (ADH), which enhances urea permeability of the collecting ducts of the inner medulla. The vasa recta, hairpin-arranged peritubular capillaries, are functionally specialized countercurrent exchangers that preserve the medullary osmotic gradient by allowing exchange of solute and water without extraction of the interstitial solutes. This intricate architecture is such that the interstitium remains hyperosmolar even in the presence of continuous blood flow. This hyperosmolarity is essential for the reabsorption of water in the collecting ducts under the influence of ADH, which increases water permeability by translocating aquaporin-2 channels into the apical membrane. Across this membrane, water flows osmotically from the dilute tubular fluid into the concentrated interstitium and subsequently into the blood. Disruption of this osmotic gradient, through processes such as loop diuretic treatment, ischemia, or medullary washout during polyuria, may impair the kidney's capacity to concentrate and lead to water loss and electrolyte imbalance. Further, the balance between solute transport, oxygenation supply, and metabolic demand in the medulla is precarious and vulnerable to hypoxic damage. Maintenance of a hyperosmolar interstitium in the medulla is therefore not only a physiological marvel but also an artful mechanism liable to pathological injuries. Recent insights from imaging, molecular transport studies, and experimental nephrology have added richness to our understanding regarding the role of various ion transporters, urea channels (UT-A1, UT-A3), and water channels (aquaporins) in the upkeep of this osmotic milieu. The relationship between structural specialization and endocrine regulation enables the kidneys to control urine concentration with precision, allowing for homeostatic control of plasma osmolality and blood pressure. Lastly, the hyperosmolar medullary interstitium is a renal structural foundation of physiology that allows efficient preservation of body water, precise control of electrolytes, and adaptation to variability in states of hydration and systemic requirements.

References

1. Van Den Broek, D., Chang, Y., Elliott, J., & Jepson, R. (2017). Chronic kidney disease in cats and the risk of total hypercalcemia. *Journal of Veterinary Internal Medicine*, *31*(2), 465–475. https://doi.org/10.1111/jvim.14643Abdullah, S. M., Arunachalam, S., Ganesan, V., Kathamuthu, S., et al. (2018). Exploring the interrelationship between electrolytes, anemia, and glycosylated hemoglobin (HbA1c) levels in type 2 diabetics. https://core.ac.uk/download/477853758.pdf (accessed on 25th June 2025).
2. Adedoyin, O. T., Anoba, S., Ibrahim, O. R., Katibi, I., et al. (2013). Current trends in the management of acute kidney injury in children. https://core.ac.uk/download/478304394.pdf (accessed on 25th June 2025).
3. Adrogue, H. J., Anderson, R. J., Aw, T. C., Bankir, L., Beukhof, C. M., Bourque, C. W., Burbach, J. P., et al. (2008). Hyponatremia revisited: Translating physiology to practice. https://core.ac.uk/download/18602109.pdf (accessed on 25th June 2025).
4. Alazami, A., Andelfinger, G., Bailey, M., Bates, B., Bettinelli, A., Bockenhauer, D., Borthwick, G., et al. (2010). A practical approach to genetic hypokalemia. https://core.ac.uk/download/pdf/8528690.pdf (accessed on 25th June 2025).
5. Alkhunaizi, A. M., Berger, M. M., Canada, T. W., Druml, W., Feinstein, E. I., Fiaccadori, E., et al. (2011). Nutrition support in acute kidney injury. https://core.ac.uk/download/62428883.pdf (accessed on 25th June 2025).
6. Amelia, F., Gunawan, M., R. C. F., ZulfaIchsanniyati, Resyana, A., et al. (2023). IRIS-stage 4 CKD in a dog: Diagnostic approaches and staging of chronic kidney disease: A case study. https://core.ac.uk/download/560706350.pdf (accessed on 25th June 2025).
7. Andant, A., Anderson, B., Andersson, C., Badawy, D., Balwani, M., Bissell, D. M., et al. (2019). Acute hepatic porphyrias: Review and recent progress. https://core.ac.uk/download/323074395.pdf (accessed on 25th June 2025).
8. Araujo, J. P., Galeska, E., Kowalczyk, A., Wrzecinska, M., et al. (2022). Reproductive consequences of electrolyte disturbances in domestic animals. https://core.ac.uk/download/551875474.pdf (accessed on 25th June 2025).
9. Arici, M., Barbieri, M., Bruchfeld, A., et al. (2023). Cognitive disorders in patients with chronic kidney disease: Approaches to prevention and treatment. https://core.ac.uk/download/610639328.pdf (accessed on 25th June 2025).
10. Awdishu, L., Cerda, J., Chakaravarthi, R., Davenport, A., et al. (2015). Phenotype standardization for drug-induced kidney disease. https://core.ac.uk/download/323065889.pdf (accessed on 25th June 2025).
11. Baal, J., van Dijcker, J. C., Hendriks, W. H., et al. (2011). Influence of nutrition on feline calcium oxalate urolithiasis with emphasis on endogenous oxalate synthesis. https://core.ac.uk/download/pdf/29235447.pdf (accessed on 25th June 2025).
12. Carrero, J. J., Cuppari, L., Franch, H. A., Ikizler, T. A., et al. (2013). Etiology of the protein-energy wasting syndrome in chronic kidney disease: A consensus statement from the International Society of Renal Nutrition and Metabolism (ISRNM). https://core.ac.uk/download/37739312.pdf (accessed on 25th June 2025).

13. Chen, S., Gao, D., Gaut, J., Hoshi, M., et al. (2019). A single-nucleus RNA-sequencing pipeline to decipher the molecular anatomy and pathophysiology of human kidneys. https://core.ac.uk/download/223009535.pdf (accessed on 25th June 2025).
14. Christie, D. A., & Tansey, E. M. (2000). *Intestinal Absorption.* https://core.ac.uk/download/30696173.pdf (accessed on 25th June 2025).
15. Cortellini, S., & Humm, K. R. (2018). Abdominal trauma in dogs 2: Management. https://core.ac.uk/download/158350518.pdf (accessed on 25th June 2025).
16. Crocker, M., Smith, M., Tisdall, M., Watkiss, J., et al. (2006). Disturbances of sodium in critically ill adult neurologic patients: A clinical review. https://core.ac.uk/download/1671042.pdf (accessed on 25th June 2025).
17. De Cremer, L., Michielsen, A., Pardon, B., Proost, J. H., et al. (2018). General anesthesia for surgical treatment of urethral obstruction in nine goats. https://core.ac.uk/download/275703490.pdf (accessed on 25th June 2025).
18. Dębska-Ślizień, M. A., Ferrandiz-Pulido, C., Kurnatowska, I., Lizakowski, S., et al. (2023). Nephron-oncology: Clinical and biochemical aspects of kidney disease and cancer. https://core.ac.uk/download/581114783.pdf (accessed on 25th June 2025).
19. Dépret, F., Legrand, M., Liu, K. D., Peacock, W. F., et al. (2019). Management of hyperkalemia in the acutely ill patient. https://core.ac.uk/download/323062803.pdf (accessed on 25th June 2025).
20. Dickson, K. J., Hess, E., Powers, J. V., Wallace-Robinson, S., et al. (2025). Publications of the space physiology and countermeasures program, regulatory physiology discipline: 1980–1990. https://core.ac.uk/download/pdf/42811395.pdf (accessed on 25th June 2025).
21. Dominiczak, A., Ferreri, N. R., & Graham, L. A. (2017). The role of renal transporters and novel regulatory interactions in the TAL that control blood pressure. https://core.ac.uk/download/82893296.pdf (accessed on 25th June 2025).
22. Garrett, R. E., Glew, R. H., Ing, T. S., Lew, S. Q., et al. (2025). Concurrent control of sodium and bicarbonate serum concentrations using a four-stream hemodialysis fluid delivery system. https://core.ac.uk/download/648214697.pdf (accessed on 25th June 2025).
23. Garshnek, V., Hooke, L. R., Radtke, M., Rowe, J., et al. (2025). *USSR Space Life Sciences Digest, issue 3.* https://core.ac.uk/download/pdf/42842161.pdf (accessed on 25th June 2025).
24. Girija, P., Navya, G., Shirisha, Y., Sirisha, M., et al. (2018). Effect of *Momordica charantia* and *Syzygium cumini* extract on serum electrolytes in alloxan induced diabetic rats. https://core.ac.uk/download/482241166.pdf (accessed on 25th June 2025).
25. Hayes, A., Mann, B., Rose, B., Hao, C. M., Heller, D. A., et al. (2015). Effect of cyclooxygenase (COX)-1 and COX-2 inhibition on furosemide-induced renal responses and isoform immunolocalization in the healthy cat kidney. https://core.ac.uk/download/36778990.pdf (accessed on 25th June 2025).
26. Hulter, H. N., Kurtz, I., Maher, T., Schambelan, M., et al. (1983). Effect of diet on plasma acid-base composition in normal humans. https://core.ac.uk/download/pdf/81977214.pdf (accessed on 25th June 2025).
27. Khairunnisa, A. R., Peryoga, S. U., Widiasta, A., et al. (2025). Acid-base and electrolytes profile in critically ill pediatric patients admitted to Pediatric Intensive Care Unit (PICU). https://

core.ac.uk/download/653319304.pdf (accessed on 25th June 2025).

28. Kitsiou, A. L. P., Caforio, A., Porta-Sanchez, A., Vahanian, A., Iung, B., Carrera, C., Szymanski, C., et al. (2013). *ESC Core Curriculum for The General Cardiologist (2013).* https://core.ac.uk/download/55756305.pdf (accessed on 25th June 2025).

29. Leiz, J., & Schmitt-Ott, K. M. (2019). Claudins in the renal collecting duct. https://core.ac.uk/download/286097290.pdf (accessed on 25th June 2025).

30. Li Cavoli, G., Mulè, G., & Rotolo, U. (2011). Renal involvement in psychological eating disorders. https://core.ac.uk/download/53273765.pdf (accessed on 25th June 2025).

31. Wallace, P. M. (2025). *USSR Space Life Sciences Digest, volume 1, no. 3.* https://core.ac.uk/download/pdf/42858752.pdf (accessed on 25th June 2025).

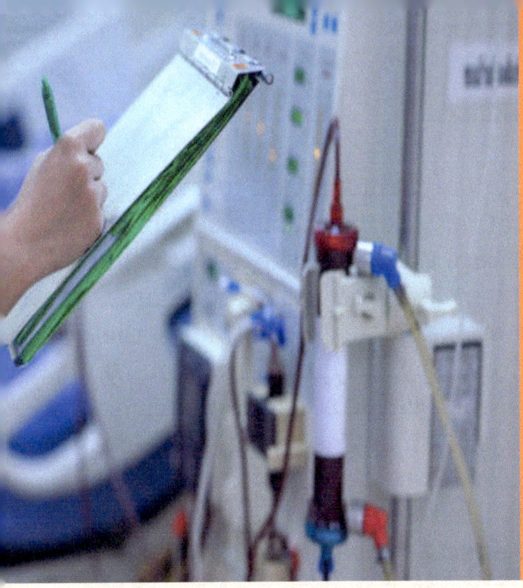

Chapter 14

RENAL REPLACEMENT THERAPY (RRT) AND DIALYSIS

Contents

Introduction

The value of renal function cannot be overstated, as the kidneys play a crucial role in maintaining homeostasis by regulating fluid balance, electrolyte levels, and waste removal. However, when kidneys lose function due to disease, trauma, or other processes, the body can quickly verge on crisis. This condition necessitates medical intervention, mainly in the form of renal replacement therapy (RRT) consisting of various modalities intended to substitute the usual function of the kidney. The most well-documented forms of RRT are hemodialysis, peritoneal dialysis, and kidney transplantation. Each modality has specific merits and demerits, and therefore necessitates an understanding of the underlying principles and factors related to the patient, which influence therapeutic intervention by the clinician. RRT is an indispensable lifeline for patients with end-stage renal disease (ESRD), providing a solution for controlling the symptoms and complications of renal failure. One must appreciate that the initiation of RRT is profoundly impacted by patient-specific factors such as age, comorbid conditions, and quality of life. Moreover, the evolving nature of medicine and technology continually revises best practices in the delivery of dialysis and patient care. Beyond its direct clinical application, the cost aspect of RRT cannot be overlooked, as health care systems struggle with the cost of long-term dialysis therapy and the need for a kidney transplant in appropriate candidates. Hence, awareness of RRT is imperative both for the patient and the clinician in relating to the complexities of the therapy modes. In addition, renal replacement therapy is typified by ongoing controversy regarding the timing and selection of therapy treatment. Whereas some clinicians advocate early dialysis in an attempt to avoid complications, others caution against early initiation that may deplete patient resources with little benefit. Patient-centered care becomes essential to the process, as caregivers must consider the patient's preferences, lifestyle, and treatment goals. This cautious decision-making highlights the importance of patient education, communication, and support in facilitating the patient's adoption of RRT. With the increasing population of patients with chronic kidney disease, the necessity to understand more about renal replacement therapy will be higher, and this necessitates large-scale educational practices that will enable patients and further enhance their involvement in their healthcare process (Figure 14.1).

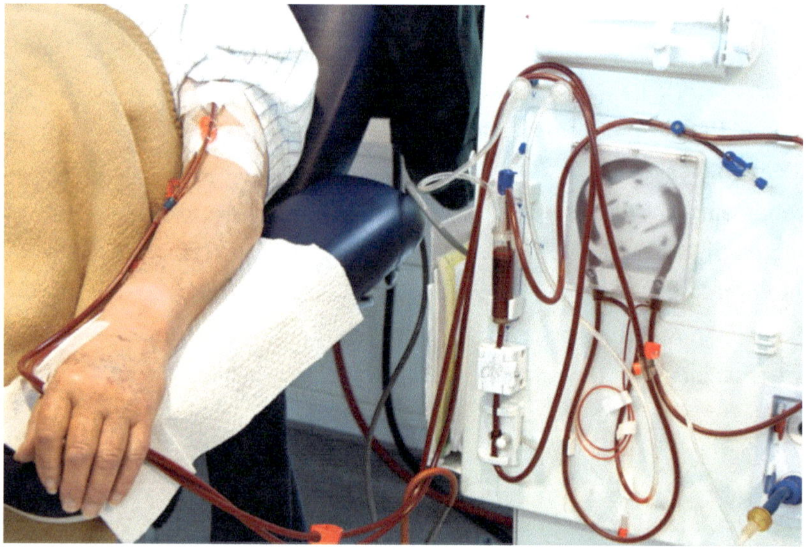

Figure 14.1. Renal replacement therapy.

Source: https://www.thelancet.com/cms/10.1016/S0140-6736(14)60721-2/asset/98dcde66-129f-4c9c-94af-dc6cd953096d/main.assets/fx1.jpg.

Definition of Renal Replacement Therapy (RRT)

RRT encompasses various treatment modalities designed to perform the kidney's functions in patients with renal failure. The therapy is necessary when the kidneys are unable to filter waste products from the blood adequately, maintain electrolyte balance, or regulate fluid volume, which typically occurs in acute kidney injury (AKI) or chronic kidney disease (CKD). RRT primarily comprises dialysis—hemodialysis or peritoneal dialysis—and kidney transplantation. Whereas dialysis effectively removes excess from the blood, renal transplantation is a more permanent solution to the process of normal kidney function. The modality of RRT used depends on the patient's health status, etiology of kidney failure, and patient preference, highlighting the importance of individualization to achieve the maximum therapeutic response. Understanding the definition of RRT is crucial, as it enables healthcare professionals to recognize when such interventions are necessary and manage patient treatment effectively.

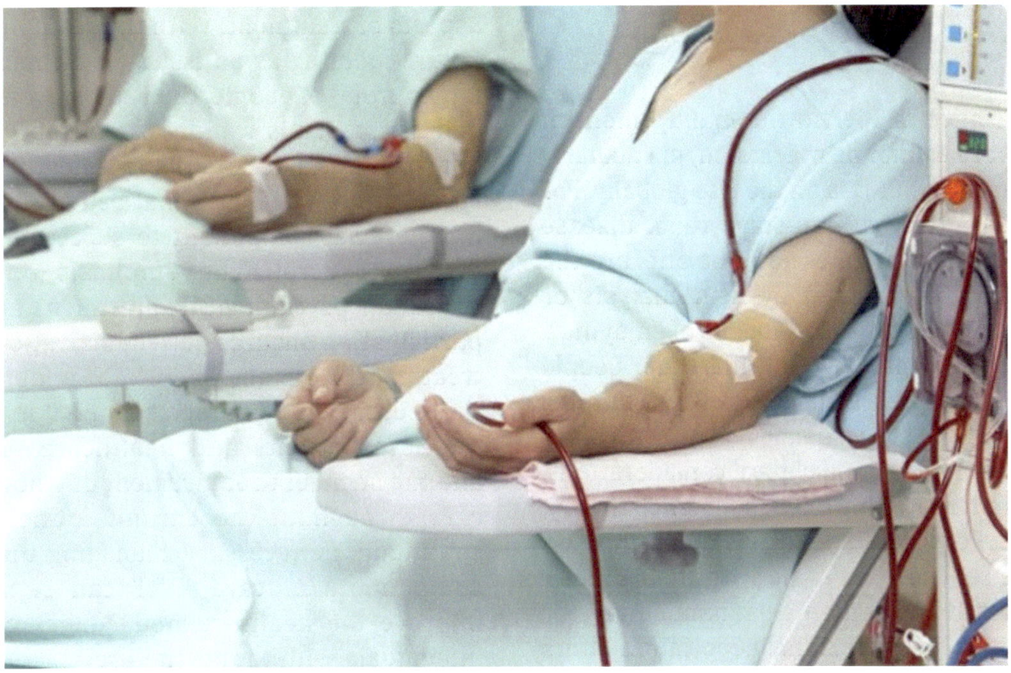

Figure 14.2. Renal replacement therapy (RRT) encompasses the various treatment modalities designed to perform the functions of the kidneys in individuals experiencing renal failure.

Source: https://d2jx2rerrg6sh3.cloudfront.net/image-handler/picture/patient%20monitored%20by%20electronic%20sphygmomanometer%20during%20dialysis%20session-Picsfive_thumb.jpg.

According to guidelines established, RRT is indicated when conservative therapy fails, especially when patients develop complications of AKI or CKD. KDIGO recommendations define the limit for AKI as an acute decline in kidney function within seven days, and for CKD as a condition lasting longer than 90 days (Dewitte et al., 2017). Demand for RRT is typically associated with the consequences of these conditions, including fluid overload, metabolic acidosis, and critical electrolyte disturbances. A clear understanding of these definitions enables clinicians to initiate RRT early, thereby improving patient outcomes by avoiding potentially lethal expressions of renal insufficiency. The evolving situation of RRT has also facilitated research and innovation aimed at improving the efficacy and safety of renal replacement modalities. As highlighted in recent literature, the increasing incidence of AKI, particularly in critically ill patients, necessitates enhanced understanding of RRT use and the development of targeted treatments for promoting recovery (Benoit et al., 2016). Initiatives are underway to more precisely define and establish criteria for the commencement of RRT, particularly in AKD, which is the status that follows AKI but does not involve full recovery of renal function. Continued study into renal replacement therapy shows a commitment to improving clinical practice and suggests that the future will bring advancements allowing for the prevention and management of patient groups of AKI and CKD. Hence, the term RRT is more than a matter of clinical naming; it represents a paradigm shift in treatment ethos and patient care (Figure 14.2).

Importance of RRT in Managing Kidney Failure

The importance of RRT in the management of kidney failure cannot be overstated, particularly given the fact that CKD is on the rise globally. For individuals getting to end-stage renal disease (ESRD), RRT is a lifeline, not just offering the survival that is provided by hemodialysis or peritoneal dialysis but also a means of enjoying a semblance of normalcy in daily life. Older people with more advanced CKD have a very complex decision-making process that typically involves both socio-emotional and clinical considerations. As noted in Negotiating a Safe Existence theory, the majority of older patients feel that they want to achieve safe care, struggle with their illness, and understand what their treatment entails for them. This multi-dimensional negotiation offers a glimpse into how they are able to arrive at RRT decisions, typically highlighting the need for safety in their care environments, ultimately leading to their treatment pathway (Sedgewick et al., 2017). The second essential characteristic of RRT is its impact on a patient's overall wellness, extending beyond physical health. Shifting to RRT necessitates holistic multidisciplinary care, not just medical management, but also social and psychological care. Effective management of CRF patients implies early management to offer the optimal treatment options together with the prevention of associated cardiovascular complications. These measures, as evoked in recent practice, are crucial in facilitating a smooth transition into RRT and improving quality of life. Early referrals also enable healthcare providers to counsel patients on preemptive kidney transplantation and self-dialysis, thereby involving them in the decision-making process. This combined approach facilitates more straightforward adaptation of care plans to suit diverse patients' needs and attain optimal health benefits (Karkar et al., 2011). In conclusion, the RRT's role in kidney failure highlights the importance of a holistic patient care approach that combines the medical and individualized aspects of treatment. With the reality of kidney failure looming as an issue for an increasingly larger group of people, the need for intervention and assistance is rapidly established. RRT not only provides a necessary physiological function by substituting failed renal activity but also a most crucial component to successful chronic disease control. The emphasis on patient education, psychological adjustment, and family participation ensures patient activation in their treatment regimen. Therefore, understanding the multifaceted character of RRT is essential for both patients and healthcare providers, and the stringent requirement of whole-person care throughout the chronic kidney disease continuum is necessary. Managing the various components of care, RRT can significantly improve the health-related quality of life for individuals with kidney failure.

14.1. Types of Renal Replacement Therapy

RRT encompasses a range of treatment modalities utilized to substitute kidney function when kidneys are no longer able to maintain homeostasis in the presence of conditions such as AKI or chronic kidney disease. The major categories of RRT are hemodialysis, peritoneal dialysis, and CRRT. Hemodialysis involves withdrawing blood from the body, cleansing it in a dialyzer, and subsequently returning the purified blood, typically performed in a medical setting several times a week. Peritoneal dialysis utilizes the peritoneal cavity as a living filter, continuously filling and draining a dialysate solution, making it more flexible in scheduling and promoting patient autonomy. All methods possess specific benefits and limitations, designed to serve the changing needs of patients with various medical conditions affecting renal function. CRRT is most suited for critically ill patients requiring continuous removal of fluid and solute, as opposed to the intermittent pattern used in standard hemodialysis. It is mainly used in intensive care units for treating AKI or profound fluid overload to avoid hemodynamic instability. The CRRT process continues uninterrupted for 24 hours, providing a non-violent method of solute removal and fluid management that is critical in sustaining patient stability. Innovations in CRRT technology, as outlined in expert consensus reports, emphasize the need for customized treatment protocols tailored to the individual patient's characteristics and clinical conditions. These strategies have paved the way for the development of new specialized approaches that optimize RRT efficacy in patients with severe illness, with an emphasis on continuous evaluation of treatment techniques (Bagshaw et al., 2016). Furthermore, the indications for RRT are wider compared to conventional dialysis conditions. New technologies, including therapeutic plasma exchange and multi-organ support systems, demonstrate the crossover ability of extracorporeal treatments for emergent illnesses, such as sepsis and multi-organ dysfunction syndrome. The evolving framework of RRT is guided by ongoing investigations, reinforcing the need to standardize definitions and protocols across various therapeutic fields to reduce variability in treatment outcomes. Guidelines established by specialist panels have a critical function in standardizing protocols and optimizing patient care. The implementation of well-delineated treatment protocols ensures that clinicians have a better chance of addressing the complexities of AKI management and renal replacement, ultimately enhancing patient outcomes for such severe health conditions (Kellum et al., 2013) (Figure 14.3).

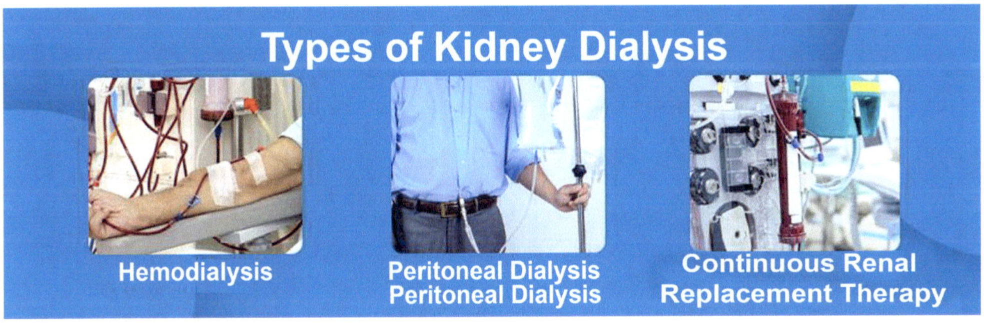

Figure 14.3. Types of renal replacement therapy.

Source: https://www.felixhospital.com/sites/default/files/inline-images/types-of-kidney-dialysis.jpg.

14.1.1. Hemodialysis

Hemodialysis is a component of RRT that serves all ESRD patients. It is a process that removes waste products and excess fluid from the blood, mimicking the filtering function of healthy kidneys. The patient's blood is taken out through a system of tubes and an artificial kidney, or dialyzer, cleaned, and then reintroduced, allowing for the regulation of electrolyte balance and homeostasis. Because of its widespread use, hemodialysis not only demonstrates the progress in technology in nephrology but also points to the need for constant monitoring and assessment of patients' health outcomes. Therefore, it is crucial to appreciate the relationship between hemodialysis and both physical and psychosocial aspects of health, with a focus on long-term patient outcomes and quality-of-life enhancement. The psychosocial effects of hemodialysis cannot be overlooked, as treatment on a regular schedule causes anxiety and depression in patients. Evidence is utilized to demonstrate that such emotional problems directly affect the subjective happiness and health of patients. A study aimed to explore the associations between life satisfaction, humor, and measures of mental health among hemodialysis patients and determined that subjective happiness had a positive relationship with life satisfaction and humor. Conversely, higher levels of depression were negatively correlated with their subjective well-being, indicating that mental health significantly influences patients who are facing the ordeal of hemodialysis therapy (Antunes et al., 2019). This interconnection between psychological health and treatment efficiency points to the necessity for an integrated approach to patient care, which should include both medical treatment and psychological guidance. Interprofessional care models are becoming increasingly important in the management of chronic kidney disease and the administration of hemodialysis therapy. Interprofessional models of care have been applied to promote collaboration among health professionals to enhance the delivery of holistic care that addresses the needs of patients. A retrospective study highlighted the pivotal role of interprofessional care, which is associated with improved quality outcomes and high patient satisfaction scores (Awdishu et al., 2019). Several quality measures, such as blood pressure control and renal care education, were significantly enhanced, indicating a clear association between collaborative care behaviors and patient outcomes. By promoting effective communication and shared decision-making behaviors, interprofessional teams can effectively address the complex needs of hemodialysis patients, ultimately contributing to the enhanced overall effectiveness of renal replacement therapies and improved quality of life for individuals living with this chronic illness (Figure 14.4).

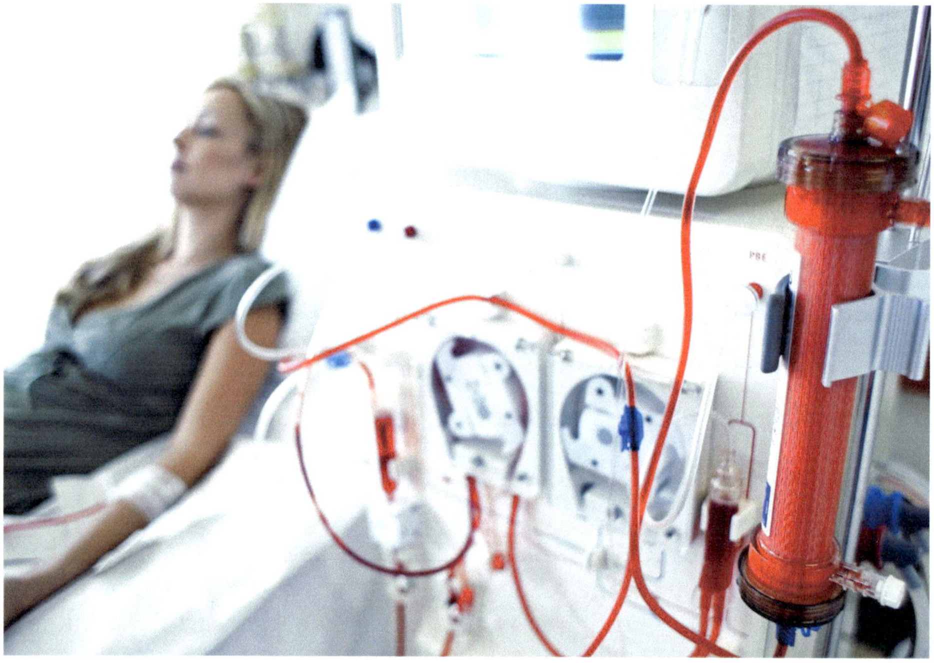

Figure 14.4. Hemodialysis.

Source: https://www.verywellhealth.com/thmb/1H8W0YcrxGs8GDScmoQ4Mpr6CyY=/1500x0/filters:no_upscale():max_bytes(150000):strip_icc()/RENAL_DIALYSIS-56a275235f9b58b7d0cac1e2.jpg.

14.1.2. Peritoneal Dialysis

In the RRT context, peritoneal dialysis (PD) stands as a pioneering option for treating patients with end-stage renal disease. PD takes advantage of the patient's peritoneum as a semipermeable membrane with solute and fluid exchange potential through dialysate instilled within the peritoneal space. It can be performed either continuously with ambulatory peritoneal dialysis (APD) or automatically with automated peritoneal dialysis (APD), allowing for the potential to tailor treatment protocols. When compared to hemodialysis (HD), which involves repeated visits to a dialysis unit, PD may be more patient-independent and therefore more desirable for patients who prefer home care. Nevertheless, the relative effectiveness and results of PD over HD have sparked significant controversy, prompting extensive studies to establish its advantages and limitations in various clinical settings. Evidence regarding long-term outcomes of peritoneal dialysis versus hemodialysis is multifaceted and often contentious. Various observational studies have sought to compare these two modalities, with evidence indicating that PD may offer some survival advantage to specific patient populations, namely in the short term of therapy. A case in point is patients initiating RRT on PD who tend to have better short-term survival on treatment compared with initiating RRT on HD. But with more time elapsed, other research indicates that after the two-year mark, the survival benefits of PD diminish and eventually yield similar outcomes among the modalities. Observational studies, such as those of Perl and others, attempt to address these dilemmas through advanced statistical analysis intended to minimize confounding effects inherent in patient selection for both treatment modalities. Nonetheless, heterogeneity of populations and methods across studies renders results challenging to interpret and requires further study. The situation in different geographic areas, such as Croatia, is also characteristic of the multiplex position of PD within RRT. According to local data, Croatian nephrologists are making particular efforts to promote PD use, which has yielded promising initial results in terms of both technique success and patient survival. Though only 7% of RRT patients in Croatia are treated with PD, five-year survival for those who begin treatment with this modality is considerably higher than for those who start with HD.

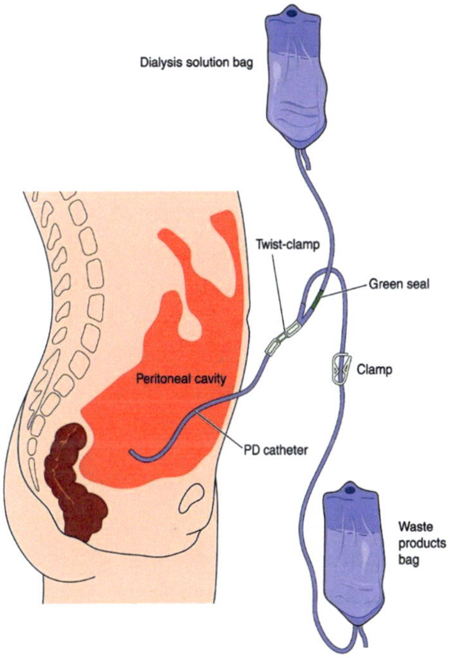

Figure 14.5. Peritoneal dialysis.

Source: https://medschool.cuanschutz.edu/images/librariesprovider74/transplant-surgery/peritoneal-dialysis-catheter-diagram-1-1000x1350.jpg?sfvrsn=aed570b9_4.

The Croatian Registry for Renal Replacement Therapy has provided valuable data indicating that a significant percentage of patients opting for PD continue to do so for more than five years, which demonstrates good long-term outcomes. This evidence emphasizes the potential for growth of PD programs with an emphasis on PDs value as a first-line therapy for RRT. In attempting to maximize patient care, in today's more globalized community of nephrology, ongoing evaluation of PD's role remains vital in determining the most effective means of dialysis (Figure 14.5).

14.1.3. Kidney Transplantation

Of all the various modalities of RRT, renal transplantation is the most effective of the long-term modalities for ESRD patients. Unlike dialysis, which merely substitutes for renal function, transplantation has the potential for improved quality of life and improved survival rates. Furthermore, successful transplantation significantly reduces cardiovascular ESRD complications, which is important because cardiovascular disease remains a leading cause of death in these patients. The improved survival and morbidity outcomes for transplantation can be primarily attributed to the restoration of normal renal function, thereby mitigating the complications provoked by chronic kidney disease.

The kidney transplant is therefore often considered the treatment of choice in planning long-term patient management protocols for renal replacement modalities. Despite its advantages, a kidney transplant is not without challenges and may be complicated by many factors post-operatively. For instance, recipients typically experience complications related to immunosuppression, which are employed to prevent graft rejection. The complications may take the form of infections, malignancies, and cardiovascular disease; therefore, post-transplant care is vital for maintaining graft function as well as patient health. Additionally, patients with end-stage renal disease who are kept on dialysis have greater morbidity and mortality, as evidenced by the outcomes of a Maltese dialysis patients' study indicating high mortality risk tied to age and transplant status. This supports the necessity for early transplantation as a means of enhancing the patient's overall prognosis and managing their chronic ailments, as precipitated by international pressures demanding a transplant compared to prolonged dialysis. Optimization of post-transplant outcomes requires the control of cardiovascular risk factors. As kidney transplant candidates often have pre-existing risk factors such as hypertension, diabetes, and dyslipidemia, these must be controlled by interventions aimed at them to mitigate their detrimental effects. Pharmacologic therapy may include the use of antihypertensive agents and lipid-lowering drugs to avert these problems beforehand. Additionally, dietary changes and regular physical activity should be encouraged among the recipients to further enhance their overall well-being. By personalizing immunosuppression and using integrated cardiovascular risk management, the quality of life and survival of kidney transplant patients can be significantly improved by healthcare providers, thereby maintaining the procedure's status as the best practice for treatment in renal replacement therapies (Jardine et al., 2014; Abdilla et al., 2019) (Figure 14.6).

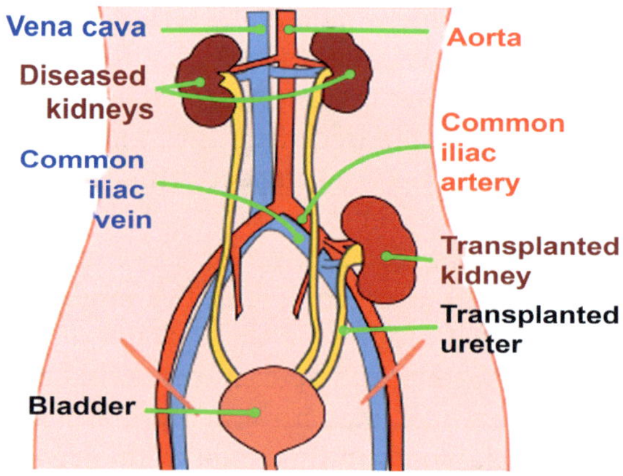

Figure 14.6. Kidney transplantation.

Source: https://upload.wikimedia.org/wikipedia/commons/thumb/4/4e/Kidtransplant.svg/1200px-Kidtransplant.svg.png.

14.2. Indications for RRT

The indications for RRT are numerous and primarily driven by the need to manage significant complications of acute and chronic kidney injury. AKI needs to be treated urgently, particularly in the patient with substantial metabolic derangements such as hyperkalemia, acidosis, or fluid overload. These complications threaten patient stability, and therefore, RRT becomes a valuable addition to the treatment arsenal. AKI is also typically found in patients with cancer, in whom this complication is prevalent due to multiple etiologies, including nephrotoxicity from anticancer agents and increased incidence of underlying CKD (Benoit et al., 2016). The timing of RRT in AKI is typically adjusted to the severity of the renal injury and the associated physiological derangements that require correction. CKD also presents compelling reasons to support the application of renal replacement therapy. The integration of AKI and CKD treatment emphasizes the importance of initiating RRT early before irreversible damage. Proper guidelines have established benchmarks that indicate RRT is increasingly necessary as CKD progresses, particularly when glomerular filtration rates fall below certain thresholds, leading to the accumulation of waste products in the circulatory system. In addition, CKD is associated with comorbidities that render it more challenging to treat the patient, necessitating close monitoring and possible intervention with RRT as the kidney function weakens (Dewitte et al., 2017). By treating CKD using RRT, medical professionals can alleviate symptoms such as uremia, resulting in improved quality of life and clinical outcomes in patients suffering. In the critical care setting, initiation of RRT can also be guided by the development of certain clinical eventssuch as acute tumor lysis syndrome that usually complicates , such as acute tumor lysis syndrome, which often complicates the management of oncologic patients. The syndrome is characterized by increased cell lysis, which can potentially trigger disastrous metabolic derangements, thereby positioning RRT as a life-sustaining intervention (Benoit et al., 2016). The implication of implementing RRT in such high-risk groups cannot be overstated; injudicious delays in treatment may result in serious risks like elevated morbidity and mortality. Indications of RRT for both AKI and CKD guidelines, therefore, need to shift dynamically, integrating new evidence and clinical practice to enhance patient care strategies (Dewitte et al., 2017). By being aware of the subtle cues for RRT, clinicians can more effectively navigate this complex setting, ensuring that appropriate patients receive timely interventions.

14.2.1. Acute Kidney Injury

AKI is a harmful and increasingly significant condition in the past few years, with its very high prevalence and adverse prognostic meaning for the patient. This generally reversible renal insufficiency may arise as a result of various insults to the kidney, including nephrotoxins, ischemia, and infection, which compromise renal function. Defined in the Kidney Disease: Improving Global Outcomes (KDIGO) guidelines, prompt detection and staging of AKI are vital for its effective intervention and treatment (Bagshaw et al., 2016). Proper diagnosis of AKI not only facilitates early treatment but is also crucial in enhancing survival. In acutely ill patients, a clear understanding of AKI facilitates easier integration of RRT into the management stage so that the patient is given the necessary support to uphold homeostasis and limit additional damage to the organs. A multi-strategy approach is needed in treating AKI, particularly with respect to RRT. RRT encompasses several modalities, including hemodialysis and continuous renal replacement therapy. These modalities are applied based on the patients clinical condition and the conditions being treated. The consensus report on RRT methods emphasizes the need for a universal definition and operational framework to enhance the effectiveness of interventions in acutely ill patients (Bagshaw et al., 2016). These modalities not only correct renal function but also address fluid overload, electrolyte imbalances, and metabolic derangements that are often associated with AKI. Successful initiation of RRT is best accomplished by close coordination between healthcare staff to ensure the modality chosen is suitable for the patient's clinical needs and individual preferences. This emphasis underscores the need for meticulous monitoring and adjustment of therapeutic interventions to achieve the optimal patient outcome in the context of acute illness. In critically ill patients, the interplay between AKI and systemic complications is extreme, and hence an evidence-based management approach is required. The KDIGO guidelines emphasize the importance of aggressive risk stratification and management techniques aimed at reducing the incidence of AKI and related complications (Kellum et al., 2013). Additionally, RRT evaluation ensures the relative superiority of the available choices to avoid additional renal injury and promote recovery. As highlighted in the current literature, the efficacy of therapeutic management is measurable based on systematic reviews and clinical trials that underpin the best evidence in the treatment of AKI in the intensive care unit. Familiarity with recent advances in RRT techniques can be advantageous to practitioners in providing quality care while navigating the complexities associated with AKI, thereby promoting patient prognosis and quality of life despite renal adversity (Figure 14.7).

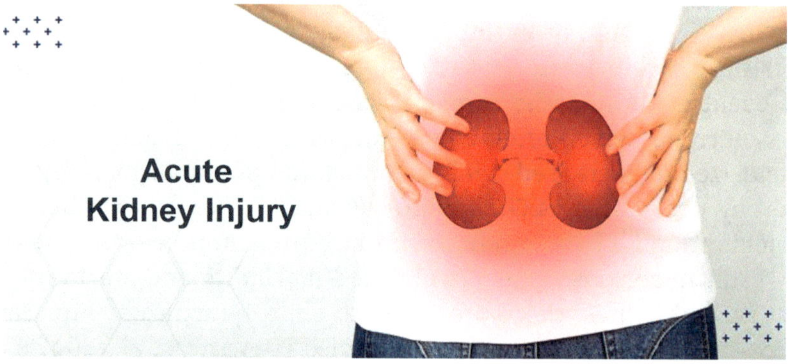

Figure 14.7. Acute kidney (Renal) injury or failure.

Source: https://ainuindia.org/blogs/img/acute-kidney.jpg.

14.2.2. Chronic Kidney Disease

CKD is a growing public health issue with a substantial impact on the need for RRT, particularly in developing countries. CKD progressing to ESRD may require dialysis or transplantation of the patient. CKD is etiologically multifactorial with diabetes, hypertension, and other lifestyle elements, which are ubiquitous in developed as well as developing nations. In sub-Saharan Africa, CKD is compounded by the co-prevalence of communicable and non-communicable disease conditions that impose an extra burden on healthcare systems. The lack of proper preventive practices also worsens the control of CKD, highlighting the importance of timeliness in interventions that can be utilized to target populations at risk and devise means of managing existing conditions before they reach the endpoint of end-stage kidney disease (Tupper et al., 2016). The renal replacement therapy environment varies significantly across different regions of the globe, particularly in low-resource settings. Hemodialysis has emerged as the most prevalent form of RRT in sub-Saharan

Africa, even though it is extremely expensive and not accessible to the majority of the population. Peritoneal dialysis is also promising, as it can be performed in resource-limited environments; however, constraints, including poor infrastructure and the absence of proper training among healthcare workers, prevent its widespread use. In addition, access to kidney transplantation is still narrow, with only a few nations providing such facilities, usually limited to the urban elite. With the increasing burden of CKD, it is essential that healthcare policymakers not only increase the availability of RRT modalities in these areas but also promote local capacity-building initiatives for sustainability (Tupper et al., 2016). To address the rising burden of CKD and increase the accessibility of renal replacement therapy, new funding models like public-private partnerships are gaining attention. A prime example is that of the National Kidney Foundation Singapore (NKFS), which has developed long-term partnerships with the private and NGOs to offer chronic dialysis therapy to a vast majority of its ESRD population. These collaborations have the potential to expand the quality and coverage of CKD management programs. Through sharing resources and combining skills, public-private collaborations have the potential to facilitate the scaling up of RRT in resource-limited settings. In addition, these collaborations can prioritize preventive approaches, facilitating community education and screening programs that aim to reduce the burden of CKD (Figure 14.8).

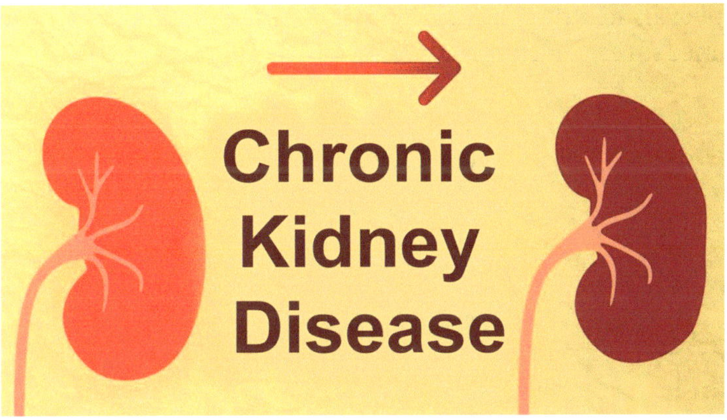

Figure 14.8. Chronic kidney disease.

Source: https://cdn-images.ausmed.com/ausmed-articles/20220502_cover.jpg.

14.2.3. End-Stage Renal Disease

ESRD refers to the final stage of chronic kidney disease, wherein kidney function worsens to the point that the organs are no longer able to sustain life on their own. It needs RRT to survive, and options are either dialysis or a kidney transplant. Diagnosis of ESRD typically occurs after decades of cumulative kidney damage, with common causes being diabetes, hypertension, or glomerular diseases. Since the kidneys do not remove the waste products in the blood, patients usually present with a broad spectrum of symptoms like hypertension, anemia, electrolyte disturbances, and fluid overload. In cardiac patients, the incidence of developing ESRD is remarkably high, demonstrating a reciprocal relationship between renal and cardiovascular function. Therefore, early detection and effective management of underlying comorbidities are crucial in preventing the onset of ESRD. When ESRD ensues, the selection of renal replacement treatment is crucial to improving survival and overall quality of life. The two most prevalent methods of RRT are hemodialysis and peritoneal dialysis, both of which have merits and demerits. Hemodialysis involves the withdrawal and cleansing of blood using external machinery, typically performed in hospitals three times a week. Alternatively, peritoneal dialysis utilizes the patient's peritoneal space for filtration, with the potential for more freedom and autonomy, although with potential complications like peritonitis. A recent study emphasizes that kidney transplantation offers patients the most favorable survival rates after ESRD, noting its superiority to both forms of dialysis. Specifically, when ESRD had been established, renal transplantation meant a median survival of 6.4 years compared to just 2.2 and 0.3 years for dialysis and conservative care, respectively (Brugts et al., 2020). This necessitates referring all patients early for transplantation evaluation. In children, the management of ESRD has unique challenges, particularly in the frequency of transplantation and the impact of obesity. Obesity is strongly correlated with decreased rates of transplantation and elevated mortality in children with end-stage renal disease. As peritoneal dialysis for glucose is the treatment of choice in such children, systemic glucose absorption and weight gain are concerns. Current studies endeavor to establish whether peritoneal dialysis plays a significant role in causing obesity and thus delays kidney transplantation candidacy. Through the measurement of a year's weight fluctuation in children receiving peritoneal dialysis, researchers anticipate more refined renal replacement therapy regimens to achieve improved results (Belliveau et al., 2016). This comprehensive understanding of how the patient's overall health interacts with treatment modality will ultimately lead to the improvement of care measures for children facing ESRD (Figure 14.9).

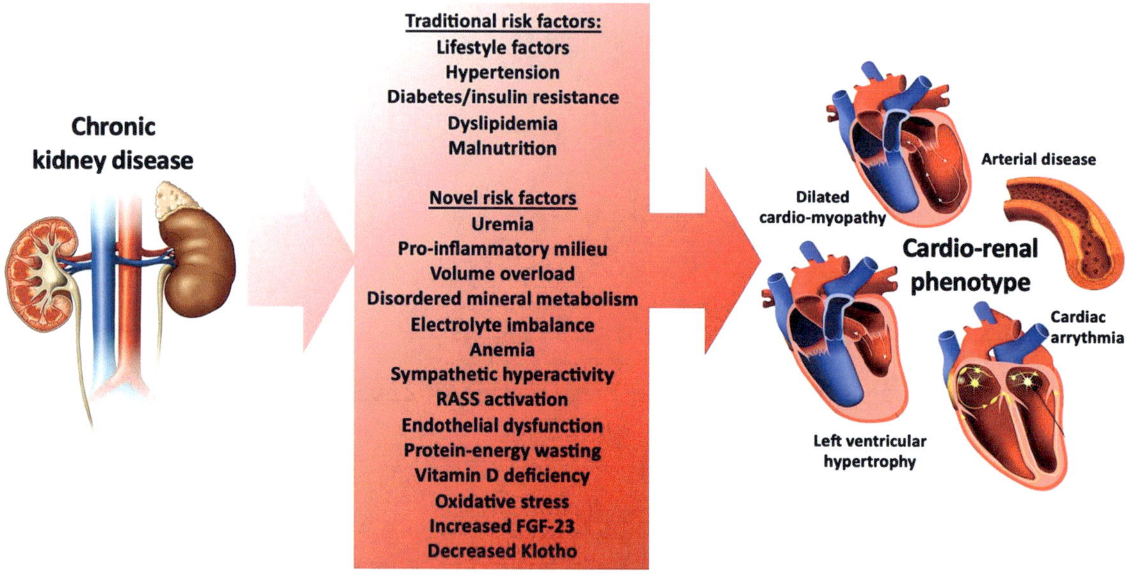

Figure 14.9. End-stage renal disease (ESRD) signifies the final stage of chronic kidney disease, where kidney function declines to the point that the organs are unable to sustain life independently.

Source: https://www.frontiersin.org/files/Articles/572355/fphys-11-572355-HTML/image_m/fphys-11-572355-g001.jpg.

14.3. Mechanisms of Dialysis

Dialysis is a central procedure in RRT with the purpose of clearing waste materials and excess fluid from the blood, thereby very closely mimicking the filtering activity in normal kidneys. There are two predominant modalities—hemodialysis and peritoneal dialysis—operating on different mechanisms to achieve this critical function. Hemodialysis utilizes an artificial kidney, or dialyzer, to filter the blood outside of the body, while peritoneal dialysis uses the patient's peritoneum as a natural filter, introducing a dialysis solution directly into the abdominal cavity. The efficacy of the two procedures strongly relies on the principles of ultrafiltration, osmosis, and diffusion that govern the transport of solutes and fluid through semipermeable membranes for the purpose of removing toxins, water, and electrolytes from the body to sustain individuals with renal insufficiency. The physiological process of dialysis has the potential to result in hemodynamic alterations that can impact a patient's hemodynamic stability.

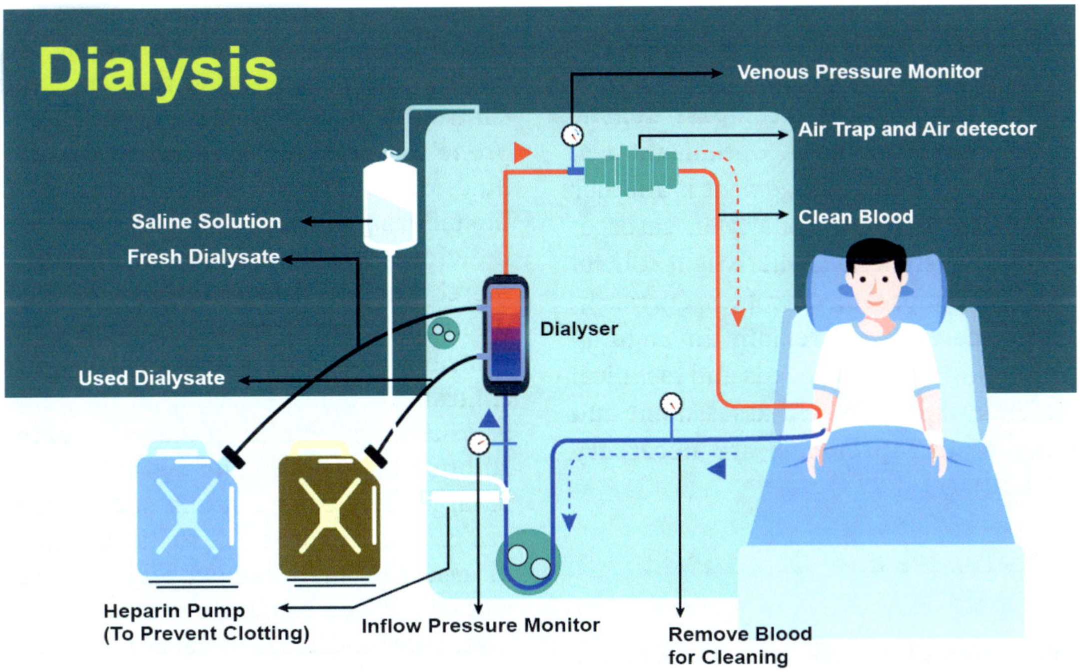

Figure 14.10. Mechanisms of dialysis.

Source: https://media.geeksforgeeks.org/wp-content/uploads/20240212111751/Dialysis.png.

The hemodialysis process itself, for example, tends to result in lowered blood pressure, hemodialysis-induced hypotension, which may cause complications such as myocardial stunning. These physiological responses over the long term may result in complications such as left ventricular hypertrophy and congestive heart failure, highlighting the delicate interaction between dialysis and cardiac function. Furthermore, the bio-incompatibility of dialysis membranes can induce an increase in oxidative stress and inflammation, resulting in a condition referred to as dialysis-induced cardiorenal syndrome (CRS) (Evgeny et al., 2021). These all-encompassing interactions are stereotypical in demonstrating the need for cautious monitoring of both dialysis procedures and patient well-being to prevent unfavorable consequences. The current advancements in RRT demonstrate new approaches for enhancing the efficiency of dialysis with minimal side effects. For instance, a unified effort has been initiated to standardize names and procedures for various dialysis techniques, aiming to clarify communication in medicine and practice (Bagshaw et al., 2016). This is necessary in the context of increasing the use of extracorporeal therapies, such as therapeutic plasma exchange and multiple organ support therapies, to extend the scope of dialysis beyond renal support and encompass holistic care for critically ill patients. Optimization of volume status and fluid management is another crucial consideration, particularly in cases of multiple organ dysfunction, where tight control has a significant impact on outcomes. Currently, the dialysis mechanisms remain an ongoing field, responding to clinical needs and technical advancements; thus, repeated assessment and fine-tuning of RRT protocols are necessary (Figure 14.10).

14.3.1. Diffusion and Osmosis in Hemodialysis

The mechanisms of osmosis and diffusion are integral to the effectiveness of hemodialysis, a main RRT. In hemodialysis, blood is pumped through a dialyzer, an artificial filter that substitutes for kidney function. Through diffusion, waste products such as urea and creatinine can move from the blood into a dialysate solution, whose concentration of these solutes is lower than that of the blood. The role of this process is to re-establish metabolic balance by effectively removing built-up toxins within the clinical setting of renal failure. Convective transport, alongside diffusion, also ensures the transport of excess fluid and small solutes, allowing patients to achieve maximum clearance of metabolic waste through the treatment procedure. The delicate interdependence among these physical processes is essential for the successful recovery of patients undergoing hemodialysis. Osmosis is also vital in hemodialysis because it regulates fluid balance in patients with failing kidneys. During the process, the presence of a hypertonic dialysate creates an osmotic gradient that influences the movement of water. Water moves from an area of reduced solute concentration in the blood towards the dialysate, which is optimized to have an ideal concentration of electrolytes. This water movement not only helps in the elimination of fluid excess but also controls the blood pressure in patients who are prone to exhibiting a variation due to excess fluid. Moreover, knowledge of osmosis enhances the tailoring of dialysis prescriptions for better individualization of patients' requirements, thereby improving the efficacy of the overall treatment. Such precision in hemodialysis can contribute significantly to patient well-being and clinical outcomes, attesting to the importance of osmotic principles in dialysis treatment. In addition to diffusion and osmosis, the removal of larger solutes and toxins, such as cystatin C, has gained attention due to its potential for use in assessing dialysis adequacy. Both diffusion and convection remove cystatin C and provide a sensitive indicator of renal function and the quality of dialysis. Studies have proven that cystatin Cs clearance is positively influenced by blood flow rate and treatment length, with little variation across treatments, and thus constitutes an adequate measure of residual renal function in dialysis patients. This is a manifestation of the intricate processes involved in hemodialysis, where diffusion, osmosis, and solute-specific clearance work in tandem to maximize therapeutic effectiveness in patients with end-stage kidney disease. Technological advancements in dialysis continue to upgrade these treatments and enhance patients' well-being, underscoring the importance of ongoing research in this life-critical area of renal therapy (Shih-Han et al., 2015; Dang et al., 2021) (Figure 14.11).

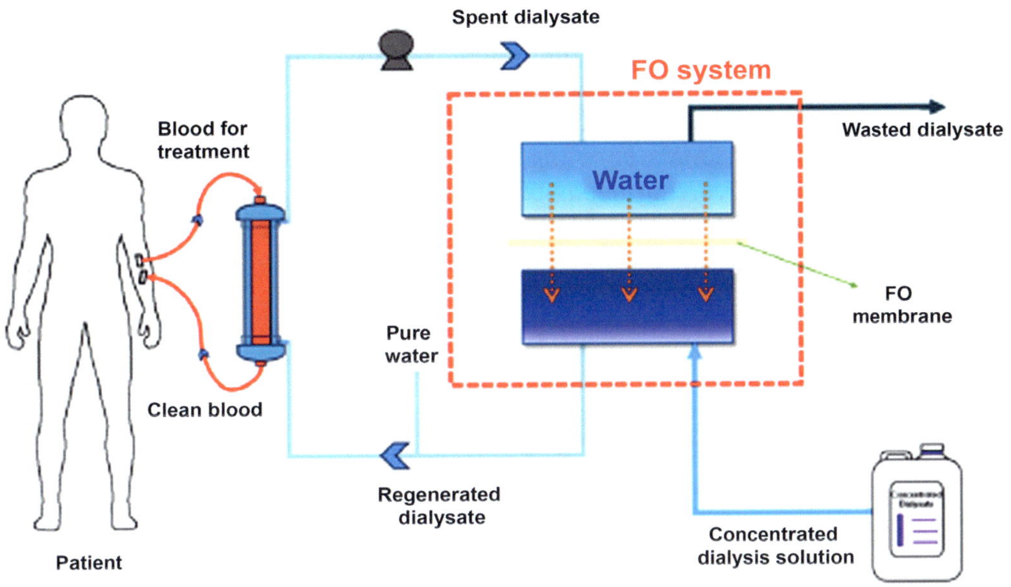

Figure 14.11. Diffusion and osmosis in hemodialysis.

Source: https://pub.mdpi-res.com/membranes/membranes-10-00438/article_deploy/html/images/membranes-10-00438-ag.png?1608285780.

14.3.2. Dialysate Composition and its Role

The concentration of dialysate is a key determinant of the success of RRT and dialysis. The composition is designed to facilitate the movement of waste products, toxins, and excess electrolytes from the blood into the dialysate through the dialysis process. The typical formula of dialysate involves varying concentrations of electrolytes, such as sodium, potassium, calcium, and bicarbonate, tailored to the patient's specific needs. The precise formulation can significantly impact patients' biochemical stability and overall well-being while undergoing dialysis. For instance, in hyperkalemia patients, increasing the level of potassium in the dialysate can be avoided, thereby preventing other complications due to elevated levels of potassium. This degree of dialysate tailoring puts a high value on clinical monitoring vigilance and adjustment based on the patients' continually evolving health status, and thus it is the model of the individualized care required in maximum renal care. Dialysate serves a function beyond toxin removal; it is also crucial in maintaining acid-base balance and supporting metabolic processes. One of the most important applications of bicarbonate as a buffer is in the dialysate, as it neutralizes acidosis, a common condition among patients with renal failure. Bicarbonate regulation can, by itself, determine patient outcome and, besides systemic pH, avert worsening complications related to acid-base imbalance. Moreover, adjustments in the composition of the dialysate may be necessary for different patient groups, such as the elderly and those with certain comorbidities. Aceto et al. (2018) provide that the nutritional and metabolic parameters must be monitored for elderly peritoneal dialysis patients and also that custom-made dialysate compositions directly affect the quality of life as well as the clinical condition of these patients. Additionally, the science of designing and maintaining best-in-class dialysate formulations is a continually evolving field of research and clinical practice guideline development. Research consistently indicates the complexity of achieving optimal dialysate compositions tailored to individual patient categories. For example, the Standards for Dialysis Units, presented in Fox et al. (2019), emphasize the importance of regular assessment of the major constituents in dialysate, thereby facilitating a response to new evidence and clinical practice. Such guidelines provide a framework for healthcare professionals, enabling them to better care for patients through evidence-based practice. The constantly evolving needs of patients demand dialysate solutions that evolve in parallel with advances in clinical research, thereby keeping renal replacement therapy a safe and effective modality for all patient groups (Figure 14.12).

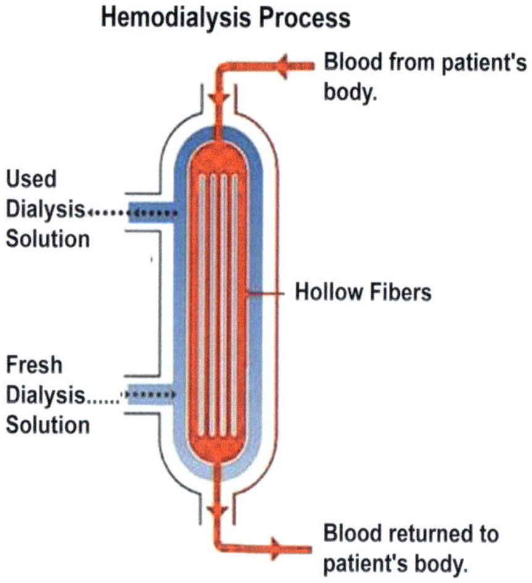

Figure 14.12. Dialysate composition and its role.

Source: https://ars.els-cdn.com/content/image/3-s2.0-B9780323958844600008-ELSST281-intro-gr39.jpg.

14.3.3. Peritoneal Dialysis Process and Exchange

The cycle of peritoneal dialysis utilizes the peritoneal cavity as a natural filter to clear away the wastes, utilizing the semipermeable nature of the peritoneal membrane. It is a process of introducing a sterile dialysis solution into the peritoneal space, where it dwells for a while, permitting waste products and excess water in the blood to diffuse and osmosis into the solution. Following the dwell phase, the used solution is discarded, and new dialysate is introduced, bringing about the exchange process. The mechanism of exchange is crucial not only for efficient removal of solutes but also to manage fluid balance and, therefore, is an integral component of renal replacement therapy. These exchanges can generally be performed at home, providing more autonomy to the patient, but require vigilant attention to aseptic measures to avoid complications, including peritonitis, which can undermine the effectiveness of treatment and the quality of life for the patient. Choosing the method of catheter insertion is central to the success of peritoneal dialysis, as it has a direct influence on potential complications and overall results. Various methods, including laparoscopic, percutaneous, and open surgery, are employed to implant the dialysis catheter, each with its own advantages and complications. Laparoscopic implantation is accompanied by fewer complications than traditional open surgery, which has hazards such as postoperative hemorrhage and peritonitis (Andras et al., 2017). Furthermore, correct catheter placement is crucial for ensuring proper drainage and minimizing catheter failure risks. Through the identification and implementation of the optimal insertion technique, healthcare practitioners can significantly enhance patient safety, thereby improving clinical outcomes for patients initiating peritoneal dialysis. Moreover, understanding the physiological impact of peritoneal dialysis exchanges is equally essential for achieving optimal therapy outcomes.

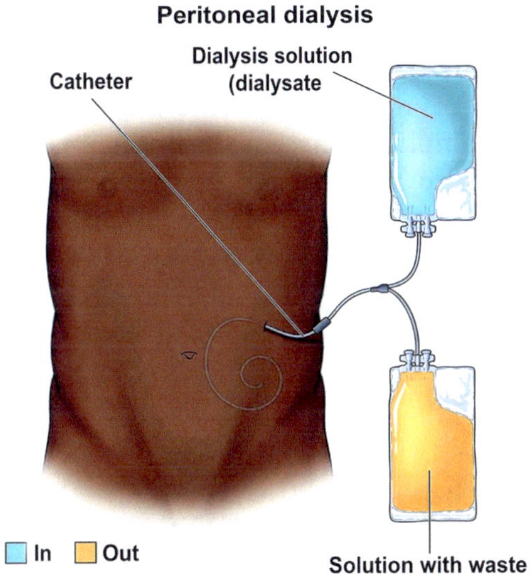

Figure 14.13. Peritoneal dialysis process and exchange.

Source: https://my.clevelandclinic.org/-/scassets/images/org/health/articles/peritoneal-dialysis.

Dwell time, dialysate volume, and composition play a significant role in solute transport and ultrafiltration rate. Elevated glucose concentration in the dialysate enhances osmotic fluid flow but may lead to hyperglycemia and its associated metabolic consequences over the long term. On the other hand, the use of biocompatible solutions can reduce the impact on peritoneal membrane status and potentially enhance patient comfort while preserving residual renal function. Continuous monitoring of kidney function and dialysis parameter optimization based on individualized clinical patient status is critical in maximizing dialysis efficacy. Through tight control of these parameters, clinicians minimize chronic kidney disease complications, thus enabling enhanced quality of life in renal replacement patients (Anders et al., 2017) (Figure 14.13).

14.4. Benefits of RRT

The benefits of RRT extend far beyond mere survival, significantly enhancing the quality of life in patients with acute or chronic renal failure. RRT is a lifesaving treatment for the management of fluid overload, electrolyte disturbance, and accumulation of toxic waste products, all of which are extremely common in patients with renal failure. By applying methods such as dialysis, RRT facilitates the removal of such harmful substances, allowing for better homeostasis of the body. RRT also stabilizes critically ill patients, especially those with underlying disease, thereby reducing the risk of complications of AKI. As the number of AKI patients with more than one condition, like cancer, rises, so does the need for effective RRT (Benoit et al., 2016). In addition to physically aiding, RRT plays a significant psychological and social role in patients' lives as well. Having RRT at hand allows patients some level of autonomy and control over their care. Hemodialysis and peritoneal dialysis can often be performed at home, giving the patient the freedom to adapt the treatment to their own scheduling and desires, which can abate the feelings of powerlessness so common a complaint of chronic disease.

The improvement in health status can also lead to greater emotional well-being, enabling patients to function more effectively in social interactions and activities. This combined optimization is significant, especially in the case of chronic kidney disease that stems from acute complications. By managing not only the somatic but also the psychosocial aspect of kidney disease, RRT serves to enhance patient satisfaction and quality of life (Black et al., 2014). Finally, RRT is an essential driver for reducing long-term healthcare costs by preventing severe complications attributable to unchecked kidney failure. Enlightening. As renal impairment worsens without proper intervention, patients are subjected to heightened hospitalization, more complex disease management, and overall increased healthcare costs. RRT is an anticipatory strategy that prevents these complications, allowing for timely treatment and lessened chances of developing ESRD, which requires expensive long-term dialysis or transplant. Additionally, the early implementation of RRT not only improves prognostic outcomes among critically ill patients but has also been associated with better long-term survival rates. By effectively executing RRT, health systems are positioned to mitigate the economic burden on both providers and patients, thereby emphasizing the economic advantages inherent in early and effective renal replacement therapy (Benoit et al., 2016).

14.4.1. Symptom Relief and Quality of Life Improvement

The benefits of RRT extend far beyond mere survival, significantly enhancing the quality of life in patients with acute or chronic renal failure. RRT is a lifesaving treatment for the management of fluid overload, electrolyte disturbance, and accumulation of toxic waste products, all of which are extremely common in patients with renal failure. By applying methods such as dialysis, RRT facilitates the removal of such harmful substances, allowing for better homeostasis of the body. RRT also stabilizes critically ill patients, especially those with underlying disease, thereby reducing the risk of complications of AKI. As the number of AKI patients with more than one condition, like cancer, rises, so does the need for effective RRT (Benoit et al., 2016). In addition to physically aiding, RRT plays a significant psychological and social role in patients' lives as well. Having RRT at hand allows patients some level of autonomy and control over their care. Hemodialysis and peritoneal dialysis can often be performed at home, giving the patient the freedom to adapt the treatment to their own scheduling and desires, which can abate the feelings of powerlessness so common a complaint of chronic disease.
The improvement in health status can also lead to greater emotional well-being, enabling patients to function more effectively in social interactions and activities. This combined optimization is significant, especially in the case of chronic kidney disease that stems from acute complications. By managing not only the somatic but also the psychosocial aspect of kidney disease, RRT serves to enhance patient satisfaction and quality of life (Black et al., 2014). Finally, RRT is an essential driver for reducing long-term healthcare costs by preventing severe complications attributable to unchecked kidney failure. Enlightening. As renal impairment worsens without proper intervention, patients are subjected to heightened hospitalization, more complex disease management, and overall increased healthcare costs. RRT is an anticipatory strategy that prevents these complications, allowing for timely treatment and lessened chances of developing ESRD, which requires expensive long-term dialysis or transplant. Additionally, the early implementation of RRT not only improves prognostic outcomes among critically ill patients but has also been associated with better long-term survival rates. By effectively executing RRT, health systems are positioned to mitigate the economic burden on both providers and patients, thereby emphasizing

the economic advantages inherent in early and effective renal replacement therapy (Benoit et al., 2016) (Figure 14.14).

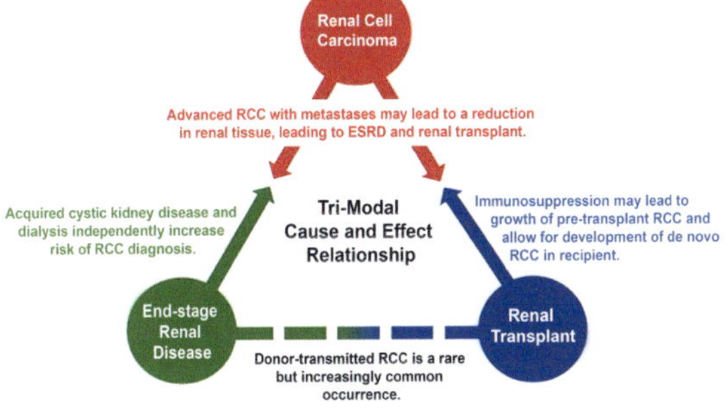

Figure 14.14. The management of end-stage kidney disease (ESKD) through renal replacement therapy (RRT) and dialysis plays a critical role in symptom relief and overall quality of life improvement.

Source: https://www.mdpi.com/cancers/cancers-16-00003/article_deploy/html/images/cancers-16-00003-g001.png.

14.4.2. Life Expectancy and Survival Rates

The correlation of RRT and survival in patients has a significant influence on life expectancy in patients with chronic kidney disease, particularly dialysis patients. Literature indicates a bleak picture in maintenance dialysis patients, with cumulative survival rates reflecting the extent of their illness. In a cohort study of patients starting dialysis in Malta from 2009 to 2012, cumulative adjusted survival at 5 years was approximately 36%, and only 25% survived to the 8-year mark. These figures underscore the morbid state of patients on dialysis and guide healthcare practices and patient management strategies to optimize outcomes and lifespan (Abdilla et al., 2019). Lastly, the imperative for novel treatments and potential improvement in care monitoring must take precedence so that better chances for survival can be attained for this vulnerable group. The influence of age and suitability for transplant on survival also makes the outcome of patients receiving RRT more complex. As patients age, their survival probability tends to decline; in the Maltese cohort, the hazard ratio of death increased by 3% with each additional year of life, demonstrating the significant impact of demographic factors on survival. Transplant status was also an important factor, with non-transplanted patients having 7% greater risk of mortality. As approximately 22% of the study population eventually underwent transplants, it is apparent that renal transplantation access can be a turning point intervention in decreasing mortality rates. Identifying proper candidates and streamlining the referral process for transplantation becomes essential in guaranteeing the survival rate of patients with end-stage renal disease (Abdilla et al., 2019). Recently, attention has also been given to the management of older patients requiring RRT, i.e., renal transplantation, which has been shown to provide better survival rates compared to dialysis in various studies. More guidelines are favoring the inclusion of elderly patients in renal transplant programs, as age is no longer a constraining factor. The evidence suggests that transplantation, especially from expanded criteria donors, significantly enhances survival rates for older patients compared with continued dialysis. Widespread assessments of comorbidities and overall health status can contribute to effective decisions regarding the suitability of elderly patients for transplantation. As transplant waiting lists continue to grow, evolving strategies for the inclusion of older candidates can ultimately lead to improved patient outcomes and survival within this population, rendering renal transplantation a viable and potentially rewarding option.

14.4.3. Flexibility and Lifestyle Considerations

Flexibility in RRT is also crucial for improving the quality of life for ESKD patients. Options like home hemodialysis (HD) and peritoneal dialysis (PD) allow patients to personalize their treatment with their daily routine rather than being bound to tedious in-center therapy. Home HD, for instance, empowers patients by giving them autonomy in terms of keeping their cleaning and treatment habits, ultimately conforming to their personal and work commitments. Research indicates that home HD patients not only experience improved survival rates but also satisfaction with balancing treatment with other aspects of life. But medical professionals must defeat the obstacles to some groups, particularly indigenous and poor patients, promoting equal access to home dialysis therapy as highlighted in current literature (Howard et al., 2017). The quality-of-life implications of choosing between different dialysis modalities are considerable and can potentially impact one's sense of normalcy and overall well-being. Patients receiving peritoneal dialysis report that home therapy is more convenient and less invasive than that offered in the center. This autonomy provides greater freedom for work and social life, and these are significant contributors to world satisfaction with life. Patient interviews on PD have also demonstrated the way in which the integration of treatment into the routine of life improves independence and stability, as such patients are able to proceed with customary family and community activities throughout their treatment period (Airheart et al., 2016). Hence, patient-centered approaches in dialysis modality selection are essential because they play a significant role in facilitating continuity of lifestyle. Lastly, the promotion of flexible dialysis therapy is key to improving health and patient satisfaction with RRT. As the increasing recognition of the role of lifestyle variables in treatment decision-making develops, clinicians are encouraged to facilitate collaborative decision-making models that focus on individual preferences and circumstances. Not only do these approaches empower patients, but they also enhance compliance with treatment. By supporting a culture where patients are empowered to take active roles in their care decisions, the medical community can help alleviate some of the burdens of ESKD management. This patient-centered approach contributes significantly to improved quality of life and empowers individuals in their health, thereby further highlighting the value of universal access to all dialysis modalities that address the heterogeneity of patients' needs (Airheart et al., 2016; Howard et al., 2017).

14.5. Risks and Complications of Dialysis

Dialysis, one form of RRT, is not free from risks and complications. Patients undergoing dialysis are at a high risk for numerous cardiovascular diseases because the procedure itself may subject the heart to too much stress. Hemodynamic alterations that result from dialysis sessions may be responsible for abrupt changes in blood pressure, with resultant potential hypotension. In addition, fluid removal accelerates pre-existing cardiovascular disease, again requiring strict monitoring and management. Lastly, complications from vascular access, such as thrombosis or infection at the site of insertion, further complicate patient care. Providers must be aware of these risks from an early stage and adopt preventive measures to minimize adverse dialysis effects, placing the utmost emphasis on patient safety during treatment. Besides cardiovascular complications, dialysis patients are also prone to infections, particularly when vascular access is obtained using catheters. Catheter-related bloodstream infection (CRBSI) is a significant issue and can lead to severe sepsis, more extended hospital stay, and even increased mortality. The underlying condition of most dialysis patients being immunocompromised raises their risk of other infections, like peritonitis in patients on peritoneal dialysis. Adequate infection control practices, including aseptic procedure at the time of access and ongoing surveillance, are needed to reduce the incidence of infectious complications. Compliance with guidelines by both patients and healthcare workers, through health education, can significantly reduce risks of infection, while prompt detection and treatment are critical in preventive management among this high-risk population. Finally, metabolic imbalances are also a vital dialysis complication. These result from shifts in the electrolyte balance during dialysis treatment. Dialysis treatment can lead to the removal of waste products and excess electrolytes, resulting in imbalances in the quantities of potassium and phosphorus. Hyperkalemia, or the condition of having high levels of potassium, can be fatal and can lead to cardiac arrhythmias if not successfully treated. Hypophosphatemia, on the contrary, is a result of dialysis itself and results in bone disease and has implications on mineral homeostasis as a whole. Laboratory test monitoring and necessary adjustments to the dialysis regimen are important steps in minimizing such metabolic derangements. According to the literature, dialysis patients often develop multifactorial complications and therefore require an integrated and patient-tailored approach to care to enhance quality of life, as well as mitigate the dangers associated with renal failure therapy (Kellum et al., 2013; Stomel et al., 2017) (Figure 14.15).

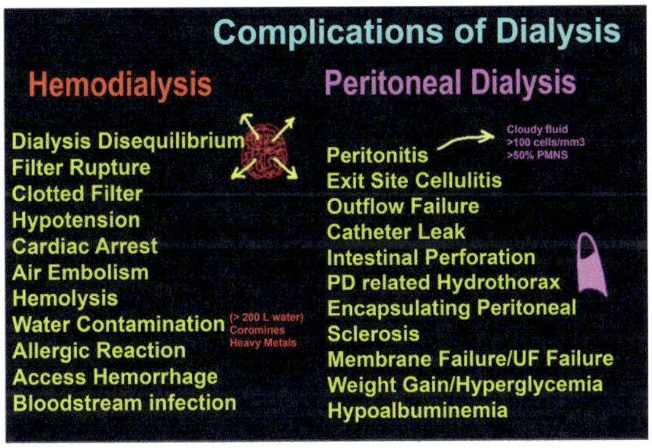

Figure 14.15. Dialysis complications.

Source: https://i.ytimg.com/vi/VwaBwHE5pXA/maxresdefault.jpg.

14.5.1. Infection and Access Site Complications

Increased reliance on vascular access for RRT is a significant reason for alarm from a perspective of infection and access site complications. Central venous catheters (CVCs), the most common means of initiating hemodialysis, are particularly susceptible to infectious processes due to their prolonged dwell time and the invasive nature of their placement. The risk of CRBSIs is apprehensive, considering that the infections not only delay hospitalization, but also can double the cost of healthcare. Proper aseptic practice, strict catheter handling, and appropriate site care are crucial factors to avoid such risks. However, with tight protocols, the occurrence of infection is still an unfortunate reality for the majority of patients; therefore, there must be ongoing debate regarding optimal access techniques and infection prevention methods in RRT. When treating access site complications, it is essential to distinguish between the types of vascular access used in RRT, including central venous catheters, arteriovenous (AV) fistulas, and arteriovenous grafts. While AV fistulas remain the gold standard for long-term vascular access due to reduced rates of infection and longevity, problems continue to occur with their timely maturation and development, particularly with patients starting dialysis emergently. Relying on CVCs for emergent initiation of hemodialysis increases the risk of infection and causes added morbidity. According to existing evidence, most patients with end-stage renal disease initiate RRT in an unplanned manner, presenting an area where pre-dialysis care can be optimized to minimize the use of CVCs and complications (Cabrita et al., 2020). Resolving these issues may lead to improved patient outcomes among individuals undergoing dialysis. New evidence regarding urgent-start peritoneal dialysis presents a promising solution to counter the morbidity caused by CVCs. The use of peritoneal dialysis as an emergency measure has the potential to avoid the infectious complications associated with central venous access. Research suggests that this modality yields outcomes comparable to those of traditional hemodialysis methods, thereby contradicting the conventional use of CVCs in emergencies. Yet, despite the increasing amount of literature promoting urgent-start peritoneal dialysis, most practitioners remain cautious, primarily due to institutional barriers or a lack of training (Cabrita et al., 2020). Awareness of the importance of quick adaptation to peritoneal dialysis can enhance patient management methods, leading to better patient outcomes and lower infection rates associated with vascular access in the context of RRT (Figure 14.16).

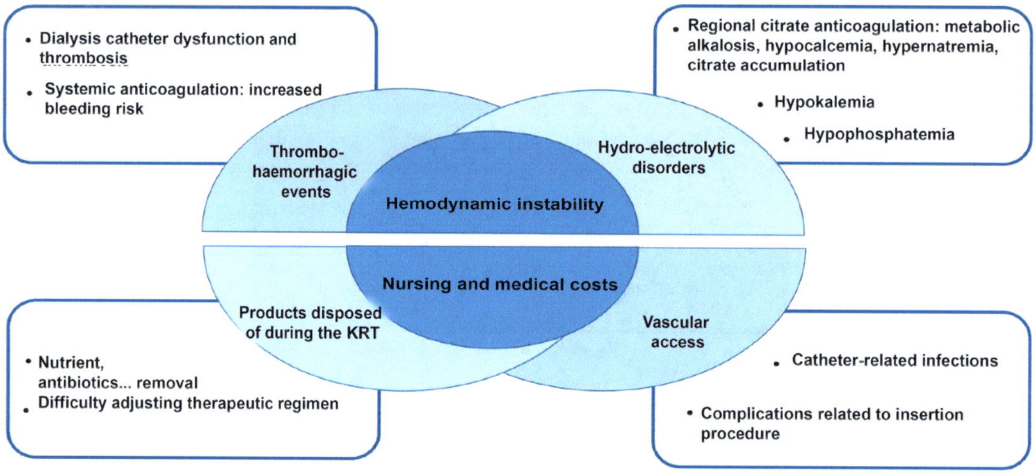

Figure 14.16. The increased reliance on vascular access in renal replacement therapy (RRT) raises significant concerns surrounding infection and access site complications.

Source: https://www.mdpi.com/jcm/jcm-13-00579/article_deploy/html/images/jcm-13-00579-g001.png.

14.5.2. Electrolyte Imbalances and Fluid Overload

Electrolyte imbalance is a common consequence of renal failure and carries severe consequences for patient status and effectiveness of RRT. The kidneys regulate sodium, potassium, calcium, and phosphate levels under normal circumstances, maintaining balance and proper physiological function. Electrolyte imbalance in dialysis patients can exacerbate intrinsic states and initiate complications such as arrhythmias or cardiac arrest, particularly due to profound hyperkalemia. Serum electrolyte monitoring should be constant with RRT, as the treatment process itself can influence the amount of electrolytes; thus, cautious, individualized fine-tuning of the dialysis prescription is necessary. As advised by recent studies, goal-directed approaches are capable of correcting these imbalances without risking patients' safety and improving outcomes (Btaiche et al., 2005). Fluid overload is another significant issue suffered by patients with renal impairment, particularly those undergoing dialysis. In the normal person, the kidneys control fluid balance normally, but in patients with renal failure, fluid retention can lead to hypertension, pulmonary edema, and congestive heart failure. For the RRT patient, management of fluid is essential and generally requires the addition of ultrafiltration techniques to dialysis therapy. Fluid status is dynamic and needs frequent assessment and adjustment of dialysis orders. Effective control of fluid overload is especially crucial for children, whose risks during extracorporeal circulation differ substantially from those of adults (Garzotto et al., 2014). The balance of fluid is an essential part of achieving the optimal dialysis result, which is why proper planning and observation during treatment are of maximal value. The reciprocal relationship among electrolyte imbalances, fluid overload, and renal replacement therapy demonstrates how complex dealing with patients suffering from renal failure can be. Not only does dialysis substitute for failing kidney function, but it also needs constant adjustment to control the fluctuating dynamics of fluid and electrolyte balance. Furthermore, these elements need to be customized individually in accordance with a patient's general health, comorbidities, and individual needs. As RRT continues to progress, advancements in dialysis technology and methodology can facilitate even more accurate balancing of these imbalances, leading to enhanced patient safety and quality of life. Subsequent studies on individualized RRT modalities are likely to further illuminate the optimization of care for patients with such acute needs. The implementation of multimodal approaches is, consequently, imperative to improve the therapeutic setting for patients requiring advanced renal treatments (Btaiche et al., 2005).

14.5.3. Psychological Impacts and Emotional Challenges

The process of undergoing RRT and dialysis has profound psychological effects and emotional burdens on patients dealing with CKD. Diagnosis usually triggers a series of emotions such as anxiety, depression, and fear as the patient realizes that they have a life-threatening illness. According to research, the emotional suffering that patients go through is usually compounded by the radical changes in lifestyle that dialysis and other RRT modalities impose. Patients frequently experience fear of loss not only of their physical well-being but also of control and independence in their lives. Such psychological load may have a significant impact on overall well-being and adherence to the treatment regimen; therefore, it is essential to provide widespread psychological support in conjunction with medical management throughout the treatment duration. Transitions from one dialysis modality to another, e.g., home-based to in-center hemodialysis, pose additional psychological issues. A qualitative patient transition study identified convergent experiences of how patients react emotionally during the process. Some patients indicated a relief of the responsibility that comes with treatment at home, while others felt loss of independence and control and, as a result, experienced helplessness and frustration. This paradox highlights the importance of understanding individual patients' emotional needs when providing care. By responding to these convergent emotional responses, healthcare professionals can create a care setting that allows patients to go through these transitions with ease and uncertainty (Combes et al., 2020). Personalizing the approach to meet the emotional needs of the patients is crucial to enhancing their overall experience of RRT. The socio-economic factors of CKD and treatment that accompany it further intertwine with patients' emotional health as well. Almost all of these patients with renal disease have to deal with a huge economic burden from the expense of continued dialysis, drugs, and potential lifestyle modification. All this can increase depression and anxiety as the patients worry about how they will keep maintaining themselves and meeting the needs of their homes. A qualitative study examining the lived experiences of patients found that the socio-economic impact of hemodialysis extended beyond monetary concerns to influence their psychological and emotional resilience (Gatchalian et al., 2023). Health care professionals should thus employ an integrated strategy involving mental support as well as socio-economic considerations alongside generating a multidimensional care plan to combat the complex dynamics of the emotional battle of RRT patients.

14.6. Advances in RRT Technology

The RRT profession has also experienced a dramatic emergence of adulthood in technological advancement, which has transformed the management of acute and chronic kidney disease. Dialysis equipment now utilizes intelligent technology, resulting in enhanced accuracy in delivering treatment tailored to the patient's individual physiological needs. For example, machine learning models are being increasingly employed to detect patient risk and rationalize treatment modalities, leading to improved outcomes and reduced complications during RRT. Furthermore, the development of portable dialysis machines has increased the flexibility of treatment, allowing patients to receive care in various environments, which aligns with the trend towards patient-centered care in renal therapy. With advances in technology, advancements in renal replacement modalities have expanded therapeutic potential for practitioners. CRRT is now a standard part of the care of critically ill patients with acute kidney injury. Continuous rather than intermittent performance of CRRT facilitates better volume control and toxin removal, which is crucial in intensive care unit practice. This technology is particularly beneficial in hemodynamically unstable patients, where intermittent dialysis can be more risky. As Echeverri et al. (2018) stress, the effective application of CRRT is greatly reliant on specialized teams, training, and protocol implementation, which are vital in delivering optimal clinical outcomes. Furthermore, there have been significant breakthroughs in the treatment of complications associated with conventional dialysis therapies. Technological advancements in biocompatible dialyzer membranes and anticoagulation regimens have diminished inflammatory responses and clotting risks, so patients are more comfortable and protected during the procedure. In addition, studies on the use of bioengineered products for dialysis membranes still hold promise for improved transport characteristics and reduced side effects. These advances not only advance the quality of care but also underscore the impact of evidence-based practice on kidney therapy. Adopting suggestions from systematic guidelines, as outlined by Kellum et al. (2013), demonstrates the importance of harmonizing clinical evidence with technological innovation in accelerating RRT.

14.6.1. Innovations in Dialysis Machines

The evolution of dialysis machines has significantly impacted RRT, particularly in extending the capabilities of treatment for vulnerable populations, including infants and children. Innovations over the past two decades have focused on developing technologies tailored specifically to these groups, resulting in advancements in pediatric dialysis. One notable innovation is the design of new CKRT machines specifically tailored for small infants, which feature a reduced extracorporeal volume. This reduction not only minimizes the volume of blood needed to prime the system but also enhances volume control with smaller catheter diameters without affecting blood flow rates. These developments indicate a shift toward more precise and safer dialysis modalities, ultimately contributing to improved patient outcomes and reducing clinical challenges in pediatric acute kidney injury treatment (Ceschia et al., 2023). Moreover, the technological modernization of dialysis extends beyond building developments to encompass the global user experience as well as clinical efficacy. Evolutions in volumetric monitoring and continuous blood volume monitoring on more sophisticated dialysis machines enable more precise ultrafiltration rate control. These are important in curbing discomfort and possible adverse effects, including hypotension and seizures, during dialysis therapy. In kids, the use of chronic internal jugular venous catheters and anesthetic ointments has also improved the patient experience in terms of pain relief from needle insertion. All of these advancements, combined with non-invasive patient condition monitoring technologies, are reducing healthcare costs while improving quality of care. These developments represent a significant step toward personalized pediatric dialysis as an integrated therapy, rather than symptomatic treatment (Edefonti et al., 2005). Moreover, the advancement of "ultrapure" dialysate and biocompatible synthetic membrane technology is a strong development in dialysis machine technology. Ultrapure dialysate eliminates microbiological contamination and endotoxins, which are critical to maintain patient safety and well-being while undergoing procedures. Enhanced dialyzer and tubing material biocompatibility allows for improved patient tolerance and reduced inflammatory reactions during treatment. With the background of new treatment therapies, such as hemodiafiltration with online capacities, the potential for expanded phosphate control and cardiovascular advantages becomes clear, particularly in high-risk pediatric patients. This ongoing scientific progress in dialysis machine technology not only reiterates the importance of a correct dialysis dose but also reassures clinicians that RRT has a life-saving and life-maintaining capacity in children with issues due to chronic renal failure (Ceschia et al., 2023; Edefonti et al., 2005) (Figure 14.17).

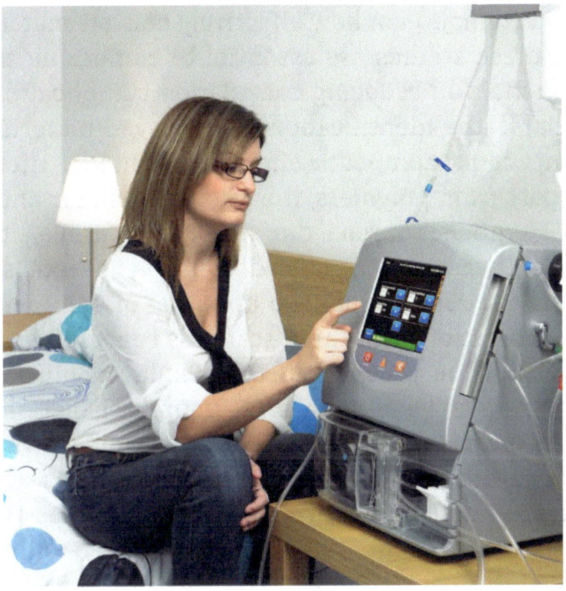

Figure 14.17. Innovations in dialysis machines.

Source: https://www.ingenia.org.uk/media/g4ejrgjn/6464-astwood-11-small.jpg?width=1000&format=webp&rnd=133573159769430000.

14.6.2. Development of Biocompatible Materials

The development of biocompatible materials is essential for enhancing the safety and effectiveness of RRT and dialysis. Biocompatibility ensures that materials used in such medical devices do not induce undesirable responses, an aspect that is especially crucial given the prolonged exposure times patients endure during treatment. Advances in material technology have also led to the creation of advanced polymers and composites with enhanced blood and tissue biocompatibility, resulting in decreased inflammatory response and improved patient outcomes. For instance, dialysis membrane surface modification has been shown to significantly enhance the biocompatibility of the membrane, ensuring improved blood filtration rates without promoting clotting. As long as optimum dialysis materials are still being sought, the addition of new biocompatible compounds will be central in setting new standards of performance and safety in RRT. Technological improvements in the aspect of biocompatible materials have introduced a diverse set of methodologies for evaluating and enhancing material properties in dialysis. Recent micro-CT scanning research has set a benchmark for the quantitative determination of the thrombogenicity of hemodialyzer fibers. With the offer of an objective, non-invasive measurement of fiber patency and blockages, this approach allows for an improved determination of how effectively dialysis material operates within physiologic systems. The findings of these studies are essential to comparing treatment modalities and materials to establish best practices in reducing coagulation complications and fiber blocking. These developments not only enable the identification of improved materials but also gain additional insight into the design's impact on therapeutic effectiveness in RRT, thereby building a brighter future for dialysis technology. Apart from polymers, the study of cellular and biomimetic materials is a cutting-edge approach in the synthesis of renal therapy biocompatible alternatives. Recent advances in biomimetic tissues have opened new avenues for designing synthetic scaffolds that facilitate cell growth and incorporation into the renal niche. The potential of using mesenchymal stem cells derived from other tissues in combination with these scaffolds represents a significant stride towards enhancing renal function. Despite the prospect of using induced pluripotent stem cells bringing promising avenues, more effort must be undertaken to optimize isolation and differentiation protocols further. These advances can ultimately lead to improved regenerative approaches in RRT, where biocompatible materials serve not only as passive supports but as active facilitators towards healing, which can rewrite the horizon of renal replacement therapies (Bosnakovski et al., 2013).

14.6.3. Future Directions in Kidney Transplantation

The future of renal transplantation is marked by the peak of RRT, driven by advances in medical technology and shifts in patient demographics. As the incidence of CKD increases, new strategies are required to meet the expanding demand for kidney transplantation. Enhancing organ preservation techniques has been a focus area, which could improve the viability of donor kidneys and expand the donor pool. This can involve the implementation of machine perfusion methods and other organ preservation solutions to allow for the kidneys to maintain function. Such improvement is significant not only for augmenting the transplant supply but also for optimizing post-transplant outcomes, thereby reducing the hurdles presented by waitlist mortality and organ shortages in the recipient population. Moreover, advancements in genetic engineering and regenerative medicine hold auspicious hopes for the future of kidney transplantation. CRISPR tools and advances in stem cells have the potential to lead to the development of bioengineered kidneys with greater immunological proximity to the recipient, thereby minimizing the risk of rejection. This can, in itself, lead to a turn away from the reliance on traditional donor organs, reducing the disparities faced by patients for transplant. In addition, the study of xenotransplantation, which involves the use of genetically modified pig kidneys, is a different avenue that could provide potential alternatives for patients with ESKD who have limited options in the form of human donor organs. As such regions continue to evolve, the influence for practice and care of kidney transplantation will be immense. At a more systemic level, the transcendence of socio-economic and educational barriers to kidney transplantation will also be pivotal. Enhanced awareness and outreach can facilitate informed decision-making for patients and healthcare providers alike. Emphasis on making the patient more independent with education about transplant possibilities, such as home hemodialysis, presents a mechanism for improving quality of life after transplant. The collaborative approach to enhancing transplant preparedness is not just about integrating clinical considerations but also considering individual patient circumstances and patient choice, which may result in better compliance with medical counsel. Collectively, these novel directions in kidney transplantation represent an intersection of technological progress, ethics, and patient-centered care that can potentially revolutionize the practice of RRT and enhance patient outcomes for those with CKD and ESKD.

SUMMARY

The quest for RRT and dialysis underscores the importance of these interventions in managing acute kidney injury and chronic kidney disease. RRT encompasses a myriad of modalities, including hemodialysis and peritoneal dialysis, each with intrinsic advantages and limitations. The dynamic nature of renal failure necessitates a personalized approach to therapy, whereby clinicians must analyze patient-specific variables as well as the etiology of renal failure. The use of newer technologies, such as intensive hemodialysis, has been productive, particularly in patients with complicated diseases like multiple myeloma. This indicates not only the need for personalized treatment protocols but also the growth of RRT in response to new clinical challenges. On a deeper look, it is seen that the productivity of RRT can be largely determined by early intervention strategies and overall management of comorbid conditions. Early intervention, particularly in cases of acute kidney injury, is associated with improved recovery rates of the kidneys, as evidenced by a comparison of intensive and standard methods of dialysis. Proof shows that early vigorous treatment strategies for the removal of nephrotoxins, like serum-free light chains in multiple myeloma, can lead to favorable clinical outcomes. Specifically, the research highlights the importance of ongoing research and treatment protocol adjustments, which have a direct impact on patient prognosis and overall survivability (Mahajan et al., 2015). RRT implications extend beyond immediate care to include the long-term management of patients and their quality of life. The decision-making process regarding dialysis initiation, modality selection, and transitioning to kidney transplantation requires multidisciplinary care to achieve optimal outcomes. There is strong evidence for individualized, evidence-based processes that take into account patient preferences and socioeconomic status. As the field advances, continuous measurement of RRT protocols from a patient-outcomes angle will be needed to optimize practices and enhance the effectiveness of dialysis therapies. Therefore, as we are at the intersection of innovation and patient care, the future of renal replacement therapy promises much potential to be a vibrant field, destined to make substantial contributions to nephrology (Mahajan et al., 2015).

The complexities of RRT demand a specific understanding of its core principles and clinical applications. Above all, renal replacement therapy involves multiple modalities to replace the kidney's natural process of filtering blood, which is crucial in patients with ESRD or AKI. The most common form of RRT is dialysis, where the patient can live his or her life while addressing the life-threatening complications of renal failure. Differentiation between the two primary types of dialysis, hemodialysis and peritoneal dialysis, needs to be made, with each having certain benefits and drawbacks appropriate to their patients' condition. Their efficacy and patient preference generally dictate the most appropriate management and treatment in the realm of renal health. AK has become a significant public health issue affecting millions across the globe and typically causing serious side effects. AKI, with an acute onset and possible progression to CKD, calls for an integrated strategy for proper management. The Kidney Disease: Improving Global Outcomes (KDIGO) guideline has standardized definitions and clinical practice guidelines for AKI, enabling better identification, staging, and treatment recommendations for high-risk patients. Of particular significance, AKI and CKD have been recognized as related conditions, with the supposition that early effective intervention in AKI could potentially forestall long-term kidney impairment. An understanding of such interactions is essential for renal health professionals who facilitate the management and timely initiation of RRT as needed. The evolving definitions underscore the need for continuous education and research aimed at improving the management of kidney disease (Dewitte et al., 2017). Furthermore, it is essential to highlight the systemic implications of renal replacement therapy within the broader healthcare system. Renal replacement therapy management extends beyond treatment and requires careful risk assessment, preventive measures, and attention to patient-specific factors. The KDIGO guidelines include comprehensive guidance for non-dialytic management of both CKD and AKI, in keeping with the overriding imperative of intervening before patients become candidates for RRT. Growing evidence and professional opinion give top priority to maximizing outcomes, as in the value of individualized patient care plans. Such interventions are not only crucial to the preservation of current renal function but are also critical to optimizing patients overall quality of life, raising awareness about the necessity of research into effective management pathways in renal medicine (Kellum et al., 2013).

CLOSER LOOK

CARDIORENAL SYNDROME

CRS is a bidirectional and multifaceted pathophysiological state in which chronic or acute heart or kidney failure leads to acute or chronic failure of the other organ. It highlights the close interdependence between cardiac and renal function, which is conducted through hemodynamic, neurohormonal, and inflammatory processes. CRS is further classified into five subtypes based on the primary organ involved and whether the dysfunction is of a chronic or acute nature: Type 1 (acute cardiorenal), Type 2 (chronic cardiorenal), Type 3 (acute renocardiac), Type 4 (chronic renocardiac), and Type 5 (secondary cardiorenal secondary to illnesses like sepsis or diabetes). In acute decompensated heart failure (Type 1), reduced cardiac output leads to decreased renal perfusion, stimulation of the renin-angiotensin-aldosterone system (RAAS) and sympathetic nervous system, all of which work to increase sodium and water retention, further stressing the already failing heart. In chronic heart failure (Type 2), chronic hypoperfusion and neurohormonal overdrive gradually compromise renal function, typically resulting in incapacitating CKD. Conversely, in Types 3 and 4, renal impairment leads to cardiac dysfunction. AKI can result in volume overload, electrolyte imbalance (e.g., hyperkalemia), and accumulation of uremic toxins, causing myocardial depression, arrhythmias, and increased preload and afterload. Chronic kidney disease leads to left ventricular hypertrophy, fibrosis, and vascular calcification, and to cardiovascular events. The fifth is systemic diseases, such as sepsis or lupus, in which both organs are simultaneously attacked by generalized inflammation, oxidative stress, or endothelial dysfunction. Key mediators of CRS include angiotensin II, aldosterone, vasopressin, endothelin, and inflammatory cytokines, which contribute to a maladaptive remodeling process and organ injury. The clinical presentation of CRS is based on its etiology, typically involving dyspnea, edema, fatigue, elevated jugular venous pressure, oliguria, and worsening of renal biomarkers, such as serum creatinine and BUN. Management of CRS is also highly challenging in the sense that fluid removal needs to be sustained without compromising renal function, especially with the application of diuretics. Loop diuretics remain at the forefront of volume control but can cause diuretic resistance or further renal damage. In such cases, combination diuretic therapy, vasodilators, inotropes (for low perfusion), or ultrafiltration can be initiated. RAAS inhibitors such as ACE inhibitors and ARBs have cardio-renal protective effects but need to be used cautiously to avoid hyperkalemia and further renal damage. Newer therapies such as SGLT2 inhibitors are helpful in improving cardiac and renal outcomes in diabetics with heart failure. Monitoring strategies include repeated assessments of renal function, volume, and cardiac function using echocardiography, BNP/NT-proBNP, and imaging studies. Management of CRS typically necessitates multidisciplinary involvement with cardiologists, nephrologists, and intensivists. Prevention targets early detection of high-risk patients, optimization of the treatment of hypertension, diabetes, and heart failure, and minimization of exposure to nephrotoxins. Understanding the interdependent pathophysiology of cardiorenal syndrome is needed for individualized therapy and best outcomes in this high-risk population.

References

1. Baldacchino, I., Debattista, S., Debattista, D., Balzan, G., Abdilla, S., Baldacchino, L., Borg, G., Buttigieg, S., Stafrace, N. C., Cutajar, K., Galea, M., Sciberras, W., Xerri, T., Camilleri, L., & Farrugia, E. (2019). National analyses on survival in Maltese adult patients on renal replacement therapy started during 2009–2012. *European Medical Journal*, 117–123. https://doi.org/10.33590/emj/10313216Aceto, P., Amabile, M. I., Bargagli, M., Gnerre Musto, R., et al. (2018). Peritoneal dialysis in older adults: Evaluation of clinical, nutritional, metabolic outcomes, and quality of life. https://core.ac.uk/download/188827791.pdf (accessed on 25th June 2025).
2. Airheart, J. W. (2016). Lived experiences of individuals with end-stage renal disease on peritoneal dialysis. https://core.ac.uk/download/84457992.pdf (accessed on 25th June 2025).
3. Andermatt, R., David, S., Dutkowski, P., Erlebach, M., et al. (2024). Comparative study of acute kidney injury in liver transplantation: Donation after circulatory death versus brain death. https://core.ac.uk/download/613615066.pdf (accessed on 25th June 2025).
4. Anders, H. J., Glassock, R., Jager, K. J., Levin, A., et al. (2017). Chronic kidney disease. https://core.ac.uk/download/351115971.pdf (accessed on 25th June 2025).
5. Andras, A., Briggs, V. R., Campbell, M., Fotheringham, J., et al. (2017). Catheter insertion techniques for improving catheter function and clinical outcomes in peritoneal dialysis patients (Protocol). https://core.ac.uk/download/74235688.pdf (accessed on 25th June 2025).
6. Antunes, A. V., José, H. M. G., Marques-Vieira, C. M. A., Silva, C., et al. (2019). Subjective wellbeing, sense of humor and psychological health in hemodialysis patients. https://core.ac.uk/download/232112842.pdf (accessed on 25th June 2025).
7. Awdishu, L., Moore, T., Morrison, M., Trzebinska, J., et al. (2019). A primer on quality assurance and performance improvement for interprofessional chronic kidney disease care: A path to Joint Commission certification. https://core.ac.uk/download/323064308.pdf (accessed on 25th June 2025).
8. Azancot Rivero, M. A., Bermejo García, S., Bestard, O., Gironella, M., et al. (2023). Role of light chain clearance in the recovery of renal function in multiple myeloma: Another point of view. https://core.ac.uk/download/581115336.pdf (accessed on 25th June 2025).
9. Badowski, M., Batabyal, P., Bayat, A., Benedetti, E., Berger, S., Bhagani, S., et al. (2016). Criteria for and appropriateness of renal transplantation in elderly patients with end-stage renal disease: A literature review and position statement on behalf of the European Renal Association-European Dialysis and Transplant Association Descartes Working Group and European Renal Best Practice. https://core.ac.uk/download/287582224.pdf (accessed on 25th June 2025).
10. Bagshaw, S. M., Balducci, A., Baldwin, I., Barbarigo, F., et al. (2016). Nomenclature for renal replacement therapy and blood purification techniques in critically ill patients: Practical applications. https://core.ac.uk/download/153365476.pdf (accessed on 25th June 2025).
11. Barros, I., Bicho, L., Carrelha, S., Chumbinho, M., et al. (2023). New tool for signal patients at risk. https://core.ac.uk/download/591216219.pdf (accessed on 25th June 2025).

12. Belliveau, L. (2016). Effect of peritoneal dialysis on weight change in pediatric patients. https://core.ac.uk/download/482106249.pdf (accessed on 25th June 2025).
13. Benoit, D., Lameire, N., Van Biesen, W., Vanholder, R., et al. (2016). Acute kidney injury in critically ill cancer patients: An update. https://core.ac.uk/download/55807820.pdf (accessed on 25th June 2025).
14. Black, C., Fluck, N., & Marks, A. (2014). Chronic kidney disease–Where next? Predicting outcomes and planning care pathways. https://core.ac.uk/download/20664050.pdf (accessed on 25th June 2025).
15. Boone, M., Dhondt, A., Dierick, M., Eloot, S., et al. (2018). Micro-computed tomography for the quantification of blocked fibers in hemodialyzers. https://core.ac.uk/download/158344454.pdf (accessed on 25th June 2025).
16. Bosnakovski, D., Curic, D., Efremov, L., Kanjevac, T., et al. (2013). Perspectives on regeneration of alveolar bone defects. https://core.ac.uk/download/35339538.pdf (accessed on 25th June 2025).
17. Brennan, F., Davidson, B., Krause, R., Wearne, N., et al. (2020). Renal palliative and supportive care in South Africa–A consensus statement. https://core.ac.uk/download/386359520.pdf (accessed on 25th June 2025).
18. Brugts, J. J., Caliskan, K. C., Ciszek, M., Constantinescu, A., et al. (2020). Incidence of end-stage renal disease after heart transplantation and effect of its treatment on survival. https://core.ac.uk/download/287757399.pdf (accessed on 25th June 2025).
19. Btaiche, I. F., Good, K. L., & Wooley, J. A. (2005). Metabolic and nutritional aspects of acute renal failure in critically ill patients requiring continuous renal replacement therapy. http://deepblue.lib.umich.edu/bitstream/2027.42/141368/1/ncp0176.pdf (accessed on 25th June 2025).
20. Cabrita, A., Carvalho, M. J., Lima, A., Rodrigues, F., et al. (2020). Urgent-start peritoneal dialysis–A viable option? A case report and literature review. https://core.ac.uk/download/334531839.pdf (accessed on 25th June 2025).
21. Čala, S. (2007). Peritoneal dialysis in Croatia. *Peritoneal Dialysis International, 27*, 238–244. https://www.semanticscholar.org/paper/c07367bbd9fe4545f98a3b7f062880cb6cb5e056 (accessed on 25th June 2025).
22. Castledine, C., & Caskey, F. (2013). Dialysis modality after renal transplant failure. *Peritoneal Dialysis International, 33*, 600–603. https://www.semanticscholar.org/paper/5de7443e37e2762eeacce6d1cdad9ac71fb9ac6f (accessed on 25th June 2025).
23. Ceschia, G., Parolin, M., & Vidal, E. (2023). New perspectives in pediatric dialysis technologies: The case for neonates and infants with acute kidney injury. https://core.ac.uk/download/576928440.pdf (accessed on 25th June 2025).
24. Chang, Y., Chou, J., Ferrey, A., Inrig, J., et al. (2017). There's no place like home: 35-year patient survival on home hemodialysis. https://core.ac.uk/download/231897282.pdf (accessed on 25th June 2025).
25. Combes, G., Davies, S., François, K., Holvoet, M., et al. (2020). Patients' experiences of transitioning between different renal replacement therapy modalities: A qualitative study. https://core.ac.uk/download/299792286.pdf (accessed on 25th June 2025).

26. Dang, B. (2021). A portable artificial kidney system using microfluidics and multi-step filtration. https://unsworks.unsw.edu.au/bitstreams/68df0f6b-d252-4ad6-814b-7d09d82678a6/download (accessed on 25th June 2025).

27. Dewitte, A., Ishani, A., Morden, A., Pai, A. B., Schneider, A. G., Lewington, A. J., et al. (2017). Acute kidney disease and renal recovery: Consensus report of the Acute Disease Quality Initiative (ADQI) 16 Workgroup. https://core.ac.uk/download/84041861.pdf (accessed on 25th June 2025).

28. Durai, T. T., Hsu, S. I. H., & Ramirez, S. P. B. (2003). Paradigms of public-private partnerships in end-stage renal disease care: The National Kidney Foundation Singapore. https://core.ac.uk/download/pdf/82396250.pdf (accessed on 25th June 2025).

29. Echeverri, J., Huerfano, M., & Larrarte, C. (2018). Continuous renal replacement therapy specialized teams: A challenge to improve quality performance. https://core.ac.uk/download/322439229.pdf (accessed on 25th June 2025).

30. Edefonti, A., Watson, A., Bakkaloglu, S. A., Bell, L., Besbas, N., Block, D., Bour, S., et al. (2005). Hemodialysis in children: General practical guidelines. https://core.ac.uk/download/pdf/7514796.pdf (accessed on 25th June 2025).

31. Fox, A., Ashby, D., Borman, N., Burton, J., et al. (2019). Renal Association Clinical Practice Guideline on Haemodialysis. https://core.ac.uk/download/287582168.pdf (accessed on 25th June 2025).

32. Garzotto, F., Ronco, C., & Zanella, M. (2014). The evolution of pediatric continuous renal replacement therapy. https://core.ac.uk/download/604638128.pdf (accessed on 25th June 2025).

33. Gatchalian, P. A., Lacambra, G. M., Manalo, J. C., Osuna, L., et al. (2023). Lived experiences of patients with chronic kidney disease receiving in-center hemodialysis at a tertiary hospital in Laguna, Philippines. https://core.ac.uk/download/591835327.pdf (accessed on 25th June 2025).

34. Howard, K., Morton, R. L., & Walker, R. C. (2017). Home hemodialysis: A comprehensive review of patient-centered and economic considerations. https://core.ac.uk/download/554168969.pdf (accessed on 25th June 2025).

35. Huang, S. S. H. (2015). The kinetics of cystatin C: A marker for dialysis adequacy. https://core.ac.uk/download/61661510.pdf (accessed on 25th June 2025).

36. Jardine, A. G., Mark, P. B., & Stoumpos, S. (2014). Cardiovascular morbidity and mortality after kidney transplantation. https://core.ac.uk/download/42353945.pdf (accessed on 25th June 2025).

37. Karkar, A. (2011). Caring for patients with CRF: Rewards and benefits. https://core.ac.uk/download/pdf/8566581.pdf (accessed on 25th June 2025).

38. Kellum, J. A., & Lameire, N. (2013). Contrast-induced acute kidney injury and renal support for acute kidney injury: A KDIGO summary (part 2). https://core.ac.uk/download/55800526.pdf (accessed on 25th June 2025).

39. Kellum, J. A., & Lameire, N. (2013). Diagnosis, evaluation, and management of acute kidney injury: A KDIGO summary (part 1). https://core.ac.uk/download/55846642.pdf (accessed on 25th June 2025).

40. Kring, D. L. (2008). Using the revised Wilson and Cleary model to explore factors affecting quality of life in persons on hemodialysis. https://core.ac.uk/download/149228825.pdf (accessed on 25th June 2025).

41. Mahajan, A., Avenell, A., Kamper, A. M., Johnston, A. T., Di Iorio, B., van Hout, B. A., Workeneh, B. T., et al. (2015). Does oral sodium bicarbonate therapy improve function and quality of life in older patients with chronic kidney disease and low-grade acidosis (the BiCARB trial)? Study protocol for a randomized controlled trial. https://core.ac.uk/download/30664447.pdf (accessed on 25th June 2025).

42. Martingo, M. L. (2024). Insect chitosan bioinspired approach for hemodialysis treatment. https://core.ac.uk/download/614521557.pdf (accessed on 25th June 2025).

43. Sedgewick, J. M. (2017). Older peoples' views of choice and decision-making in chronic kidney disease: A grounded theory study of access to the social world of renal care. https://core.ac.uk/download/157800807.pdf (accessed on 25th June 2025).

44. Shutov, E., & Filatova, N. (2021). Cardiorenal syndrome in patients on renal replacement therapy. https://core.ac.uk/download/479935620.pdf (accessed on 25th June 2025).

45. Stomel, J. (2017). Perceptions of HIV-positive kidney donations to HIV-positive recipients. https://open.bu.edu/bitstream/2144/26938/5/Stomel_bu_0017N_13181.pdf (accessed on 25th June 2025).

46. Tupper, H. (2016). Confronting the growing burden of kidney disease: The sub-Saharan landscape. https://open.bu.edu/bitstream/2144/19210/1/Tupper_bu_0017N_11986.pdf (accessed on 25th June 2025).

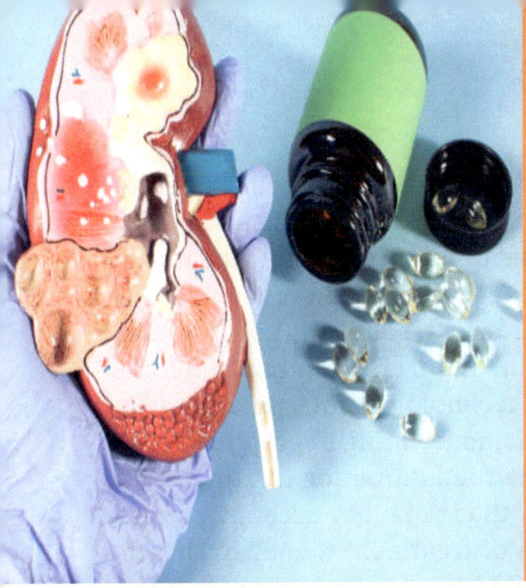

Chapter 15

KIDNEY TRANSPLANTATION AND IMMUNOSUPPRESSIVE THERAPY

Contents

Introduction

Kidney transplant has emerged as an essential treatment modality for patients suffering from end-stage renal disease (ESRD), significantly improving the quality of life and survival. As a surgical intervention, it involves the transfer of a healthy kidney from a donor to a recipient, circumventing the limitations of long-term dialysis. The urgency of transplantation cannot be overstated, as it allows the patient to regain functional renal function and avoids the cumbersome restrictions of other renal replacement modalities. Kidney transplantation, being advantageous, has complex medical and ethical challenges, such as donor access, stringent recipient screening, and management of post-operative complications. Easily the most essential part of kidney transplantation is the immunosuppressive therapy that recipients must endure to prevent organ rejection. The immune system, with its inherent role in defending the body against foreign cells, recognizes the transplanted kidney as a potential threat, and this may lead to acute or chronic rejection if not prevented. To prevent this from happening, patients are treated with a regimen of personalized immunosuppressants that dampen the body's immune response. Though such drugs significantly enhance the success rates of transplant, their side effects, e.g., increased susceptibility to infection and certain types of cancer, indicate the delicate balance required in the post-transplant scenario. Knowledge about different classes of immunosuppressants and to grasp the nuances of successful kidney transplantation, as their mechanisms of action are crucial. Moreover, the field of immunosuppressive management is continually evolving due to advancements in medical science and technology. More potent agents with enhanced efficacy and fewer side effects are being designed, demonstrating ongoing efforts to maximize transplant results. Standard regimens have served as the foundation for treatment, but there is growing recognition of individually optimized treatments that take into account patient-specific factors and possible genetic modifiers. This customization of treatment demonstrates the dynamic nature of transplant medicine and the necessity of interprofessional collaboration between nephrologists, transplant surgeons, and pharmacologists. Hence, with the evolving field of kidney transplantation, the relationship between patient care and immunosuppressive therapy remains a priority area of practice and investigation, aimed at improving the lifespan and quality of life of transplant recipients (Figure 15.1).

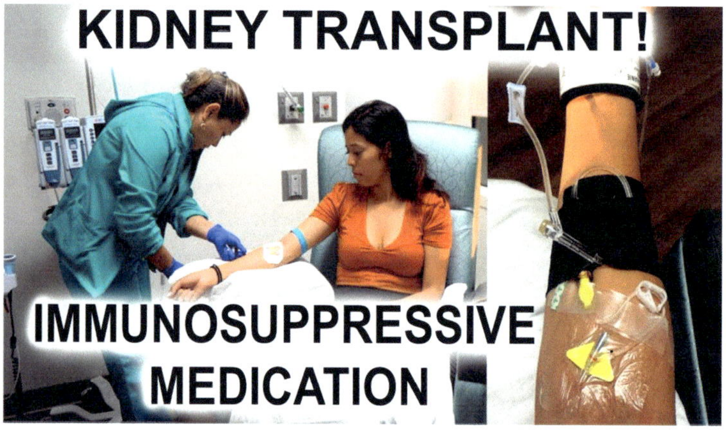

Figure 15.1. Kidney transplant medication.

Source: https://external-content.duckduckgo.com/iu/?u=https%3A%2F%2Fi.ytimg.com%2Fvi%2F08PwOpWyL4s%2Fmaxresdefault.jpg&f=1&nofb=1&ipt=0b42b3616e0d16c5532f282b65d502e3bfb26b9fa24ec431258b43cf0f400688.

Definition of Kidney Transplantation

The concept of kidney transplant is best understood by reading about its definition and mechanism. Essentially, a kidney transplant involves the surgical implantation of a donor's healthy kidney, either from a living or deceased donor, into a recipient whose kidneys are no longer capable of working properly, typically referred to as end-stage renal disease (ESRD). This procedure is not only aimed at achieving kidney function but also improving the well-being of individuals with kidney failure who suffer from crippling symptoms. While the operation itself has become more sophisticated, with refinements in technique and technology, its success relies heavily on effective immunosuppressive therapy to prevent rejection of the donated organ. Understanding kidney transplant consists in grasping the central role of immunology. The human immune system is such that it identifies and degrades alien tissue, including transplanted tissues. Hence, effective immunosuppressive therapy becomes imperative to counter the body's response to the donated kidney. The treatment method utilizes various pharmacologic drugs with the purpose of suppressing the immune system's activity, thus reducing the risk of acute rejection. Research has revealed that advances in immunosuppressive medications have significantly enhanced graft survival, demonstrating the delicate balance between preventing rejection and infection. Furthermore, ongoing research continues to explore novel avenues, emphasizing the importance of personalized medicine in achieving optimal results for transplant recipients. Recent breakthroughs into microchimerism have also revolutionized the dynamics of kidney transplantation. This phenomenon involves the long-term survival of small numbers of donor cells in the recipient's body, which may be involved in immune tolerance. What this means is that successful kidney transplantation is not so much about completely suppressing the immune system as it is about enabling the donor and recipient cells to coexist peacefully and knowing how microchimerism works can lead to new treatments for inducing long-term tolerance with reduced immunosuppression. Experiments have confirmed that such bidirectional interaction between recipient and donor is central to achieving maximum transplant success and minimizing complications, the reason for further investigation here to maximize technique in kidney transplantation as well as immunosuppressive therapy (Delaney et al., 1996; Hsieh et al., 2013) (Figure 15.2).

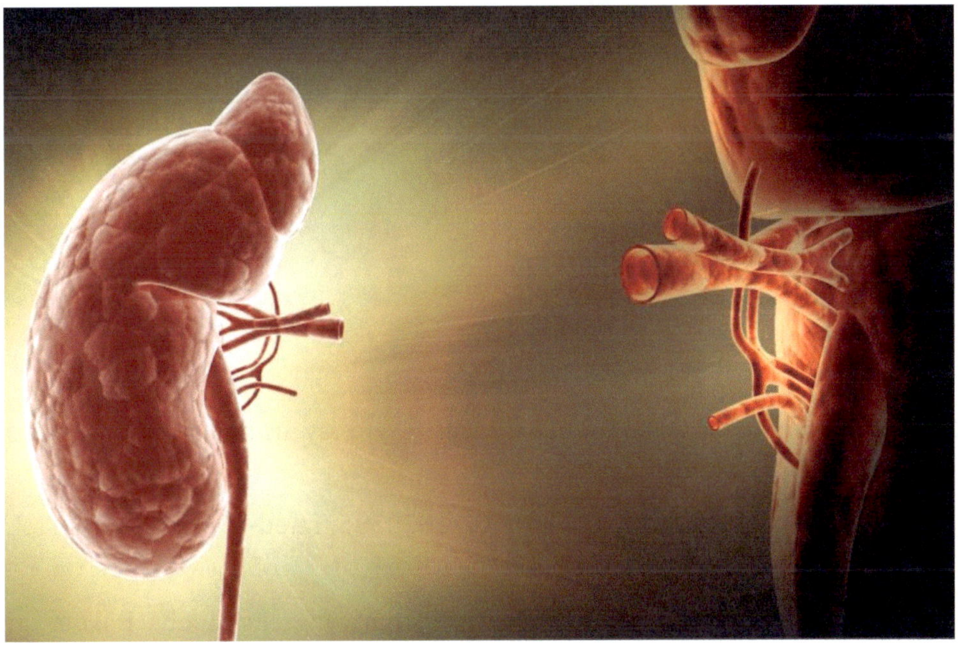

Figure 15.2. Kidney transplantation.

Source: https://external-content.duckduckgo.com/iu/?u=https%3A%2F%2F2.bp.blogspot.com%2F-n7sN1Sv6_CM%2FXElQHWqwiwI%2FAAAAAAAAAAw%2FFY7cQyLLA-o2pkR_V6LJ7KJUQzhWIvP9QCLcBGAs%2Fs1600%2Fkidney%252Btransplant.jpg&f=1&nofb=1&ipt=2a37ccee0ea34d2c07688632e433940cc1f75b92850ed5f140a9896bc75999e0.

Importance of Immunosuppressive Therapy

Immunosuppressive therapy is necessary in kidney transplantation as it lowers the risk of organ rejection by a significant percentage. The recipient's immune system recognizes the new organ as foreign upon transplant and targets it with an immune response to destroy it. To counteract this protective mechanism, immunosuppressants are employed to induce an immunosuppressed state. This enables the transplanted kidney to function normally without being attacked by the host's immune cells. Success with a kidney transplant in the long term relies on the careful balancing of immunosuppressive regimens, which must be tailored to the patient to achieve optimal allograft survival with minimal toxicity. Hence, the importance of this therapy cannot be overstated, as efficient management and compliance are crucial in achieving good outcomes in transplant recipients. The long-term reliance on immunosuppressive drugs presents challenges to kidney transplant patients.

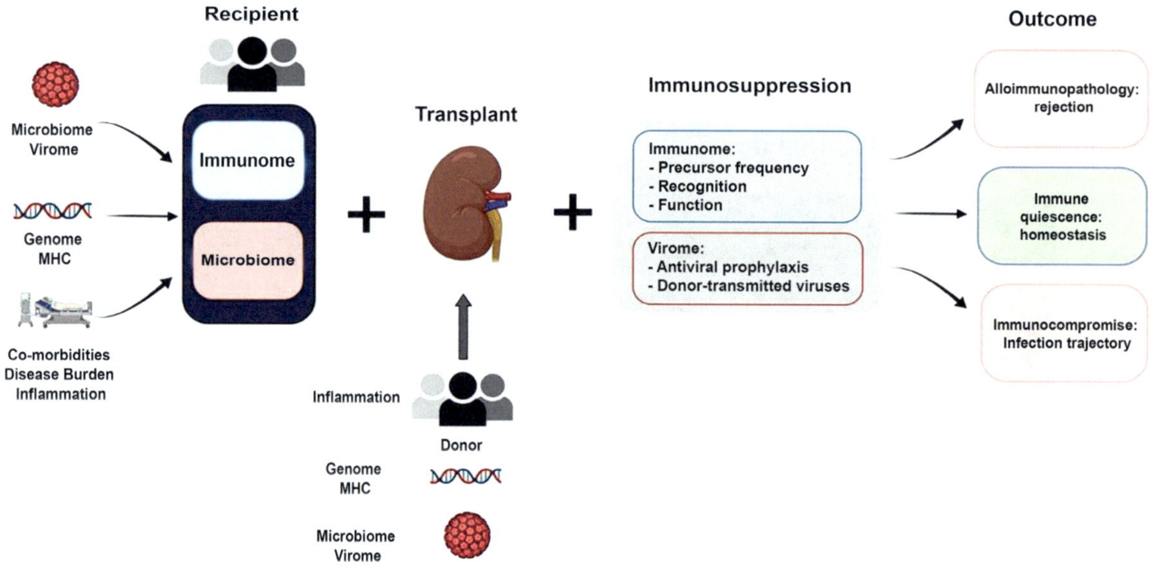

Figure 15.3. Immunosuppressive therapy is critical in kidney transplantation as it significantly reduces the risk of organ rejection.

Source: https://www.frontiersin.org/files/Articles/1070385/fmed-09-1070385-HTML/image_m/fmed-09-1070385-g001.jpg.

Though such drugs are imperative to prevent rejection, ongoing feedback from the recipients identifies lifelong drug burden as one of their significant concerns. It is common for patients to demand a treatment regimen that decreases the amount of drugs consumed daily, making life better. A sound system should meet minimal drug requirements while ensuring proper immunosuppression. Recent research emphasizes the need for optimizing therapeutic regimens to enhance patient compliance, which is crucial for long-term graft survival. The complications of non-adherence are severe, including acute rejection episodes that lead to irreversible graft damage, which underscores the need for effective immunosuppressive therapy during the post-transplant period (Greene et al., 2014). Immunosuppressive therapy is also complex and requires a thorough understanding of pharmacodynamics, as well as patient-related factors. It has been established that the risk is very high for both under-immunosuppression and over-suppression, which can lead to adverse effects such as rejection or increased susceptibility to infections and malignancies. All patients react differently to immunosuppressive drugs; variability in genetics and health could affect drug metabolism and effectiveness. Thus, treatment regimens need to be personalized, and therapeutic drug monitoring is employed routinely to keep drug levels within the therapeutic range. Pharmacogenetics and biomarker-based are in the pipeline, but their use in routine clinical practice is still under development. As the specialty further develops, individualized optimized immunosuppressive therapy will increasingly be tailored to meet the unique needs of each transplant recipient and continue to underpin the necessity for meticulous management in kidney transplantation (Abboudi et al., 2012) (Figure 15.3).

15.1. The Need for Kidney Transplantation

The increasing prevalence of chronic kidney disease (CKD) has necessitated possible solutions, and among those, kidney transplantation as a life-saving intervention. Patients with end-stage renal disease are likely to develop debilitating symptoms that compromise their quality of life severely, including fatigue, fluid overload, and repeated dialysis requirements. Kidney transplantation emerges as a potential solution, offering patients notable improvements in overall well-being and quality of life. Moreover, studies have determined that transplant recipients can experience a better quality of life than dialysis patients, highlighting the necessity and benefits of transplantation (Greene et al., 2014). Thus, while the prevalence of CKD increases globally, an understanding of the necessity for kidney transplant becomes increasingly imperative in alleviating this significant public health problem. The necessity for a kidney transplant persists, while the complexity surrounding immunosuppressive therapy post-transplant provides several levels of decision-making. After a kidney transplant, patients have to adhere to long-term immunosuppressive regimens to prevent organ rejection, which is onerous for the majority. The management of immunosuppressive medications is complex, as numerous medications have the potential to induce side effects and require frequent monitoring (Greene et al., 2014). The regimens should be used to attain optimal suppression of the immune system without causing unwanted effects. The struggle against these drugs can influence patient compliance, and thus healthcare providers seek means of ensuring patients adhere to their medication regimen. Therefore, the interaction between the needs of kidney transplantation and the complexity of therapy that comes with it emphasizes the necessity of comprehensive post-transplant care. The evolving nature of kidney transplantation underscores the need for ongoing research to optimize patient outcomes and ensure adherence to immunosuppressive therapy. Clinical trials, such as those that evaluate the effectiveness of various drug combinations, provide valuable data toward achieving enhanced graft survival rates. For instance, a comparative analysis of different immunosuppressive regimens revealed considerable differences in both patient and graft survival rates based on the treatment approach followed. By having patient-centered care at the forefront, emphasis on tailoring regimens can improve not just outcomes but quality of life in transplant patients. Finally, planning for kidney transplantation involves a whole-person approach that combines effective immunosuppressive therapy with patient education and support systems to overcome obstacles in life after transplant (Figure 15.4).

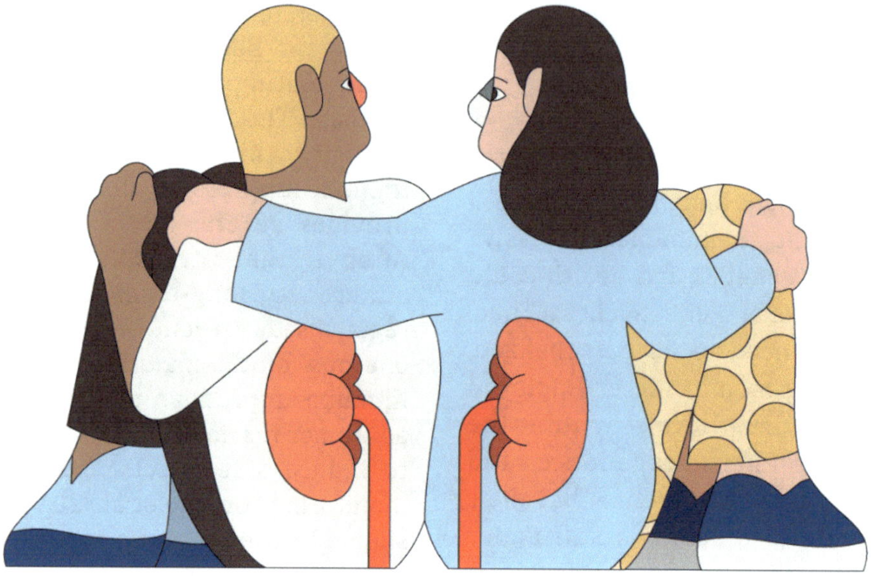

Figure 15.4. The need for kidney transplantation.

Source: https://external-content.duckduckgo.com/iu/?u=https%3A%2F%2Fliveandletlive.montefiore.org%2Fstatic%2Faf9df14807b64b8736d929f5e9dd99fd%2Ff3cf8%2F03%252520-%252520Living%252520Kidney%252520Donor.png&f=1&nofb=1&ipt=e7ee4ab5ed68e6947563afc108512d23c0e0bca8d614de5e6c187aa6c86249fb.

15.1.1. Causes of Kidney Failure

The etiology of renal failure encompasses a wide range of conditions that may contribute to the impairment of renal function. Diabetes mellitus is one of the most prevalent causes and accounts for a substantial proportion of end-stage renal disease (ESRD) in the United States. The long-term hyperglycemia in diabetes results in the destruction of the microvasculature of the kidney and diabetic nephropathy. In addition, hypertension is also a significant etiology that often acts together with diabetes in accelerating renal damage. Untreated hypertension can cause damage to the glomeruli and progressive scarring and impairment. With the decreased efficiency of the kidneys in waste filtration, the need for interventions such as kidney transplantation becomes increasingly possible, highlighting the significant demand for effective immunosuppressive therapy in post-transplantation care (Ellis et al., 1995). Furthermore, glomerulonephritis, or inflammation of the kidney's filtering structures, contributes significantly to kidney failure. It can be caused by autoimmune diseases, infection, or other illnesses in the body that cause varying degrees of damage to renal architecture. Chronic glomerulonephritis can also be insidious and will often have few symptoms until severe damage has already been inflicted. In the majority of instances, the glomerulonephritis patients will ultimately require transplantation and hence the use of immunosuppressive medications to prevent acute organ rejection (Fung et al., 2000). Polycystic kidney disease, where numerous cysts form in the kidneys, and obstructive uropathy, where there is urinary tract obstruction by anatomical abnormalities, leading to renal damage, are also causes of kidney failure. The influence of lifestyle and environmental problems cannot be overestimated when it comes to the causation of kidney failure. Risk factors such as obesity, smoking, and dietary habits significantly contribute to one's vulnerability to contracting kidney-related problems. The intake of high-protein and high-sodium diets exacerbates the already present conditions, such as diabetes and hypertension, and it also hastens the degeneration of kidney function. Moreover, AKI from dehydration, infections, or even nephrotoxic medication can cause CKD if left untreated. Where kidney damage progresses to the point where transplantation is necessary, aggressive immunosuppressive treatment is required to maintain graft function and patient health, thereby allowing the long-term function of the transplanted kidney despite such odds (Ellis et al., 1995) (Figure 15.5).

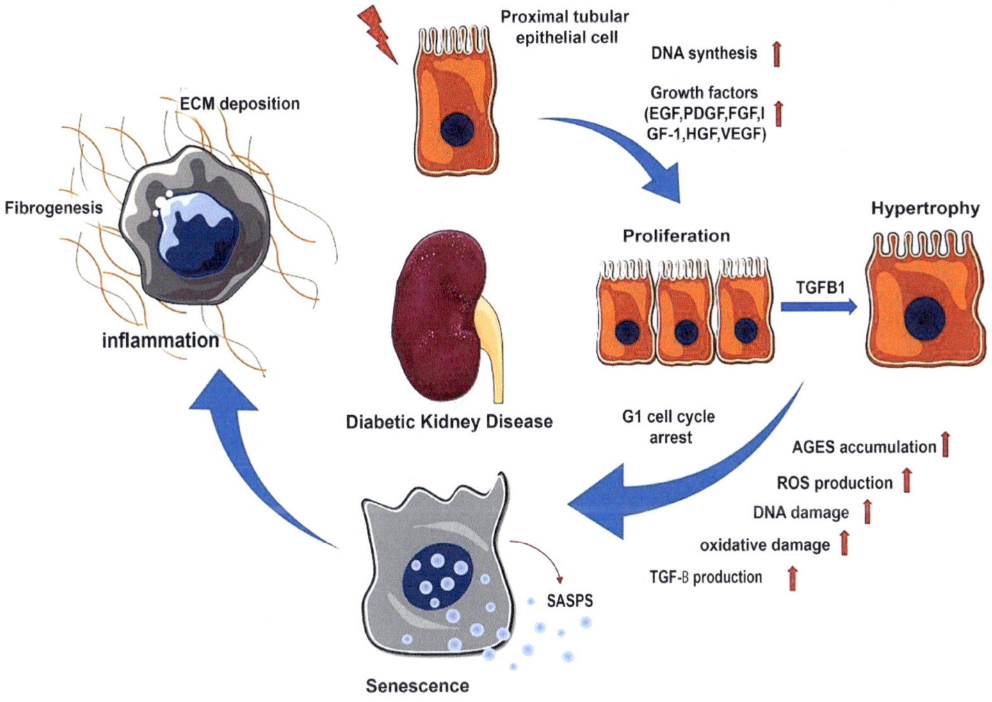

Figure 15.5. The chronic hyperglycemia associated with diabetes damages the microvasculature of the kidney, resulting in diabetic nephropathy.

Source: https://www.frontiersin.org/files/Articles/1238927/fendo-14-1238927-HTML/image_m/fendo-14-1238927-g001.jpg.

15.1.2. Impact of Kidney Failure on Quality of Life

Kidney failure significantly impairs quality of life, providing an assortment of physical, emotional, and social challenges that must be tolerated by patients daily. End-stage renal disease patients mostly endure incapacitating symptoms such as fatigue, insomnia, and pain, resulting from poisons in the body caused by the inefficiency of the kidneys. This physical decline not only limits their ability to perform daily tasks but also may lead to psychological distress, such as depression and anxiety. As patients go through continuous dialysis or wait for transplantation, the burden of their health care becomes heavy, typically leading to a reduced sense of well-being and lower life satisfaction. Thus, understanding the impact of kidney failure on quality of life is crucial for clinicians who aim to provide holistic care that addresses both physical and emotional needs. Furthermore, the psychosocial impact of kidney failure cannot be ignored since the disease affects numerous aspects of a patient's life, such as interpersonal relationships and employment. Most of those with kidney failure need to change their way of life to suit regular doctor visits and treatments, which disrupts their working and social life. This disruption usually leads to feelings of loneliness and frustration and further exacerbates the emotional impact of the disease. Moreover, the cost of continuous treatment and possible loss of a job creates extreme stress. As investigated in more recent studies, these psychosocial factors are of utmost importance to overall health and rehabilitation and demand a holistic approach in the management of kidney failure beyond the mere medical (Burke et al., 2000).

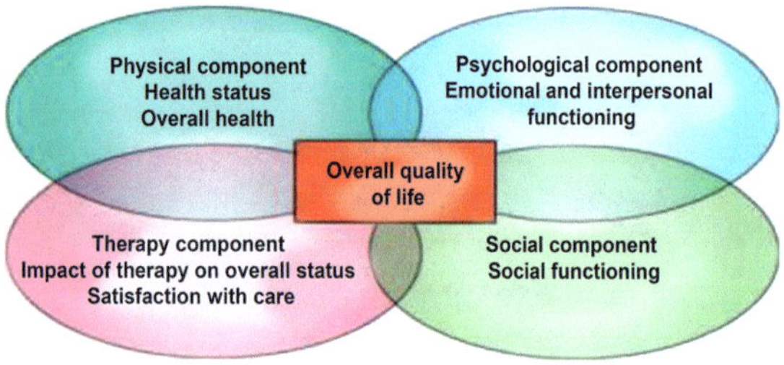

Figure 15.6. Health related quality of life and the CKD patient.

Source: https://ars.els-cdn.com/content/image/1-s2.0-S0085253815541045-gr1.jpg.

The transition to kidney transplantation offers a potential quality of life improvement but is associated with its own challenges. The recipients commonly experience the demanding task of adhering to immunosuppressive therapy to prevent organ rejection, an additional health burden and which complicates the process of recovery. Research indicates that although transplantation can restore function and reduce the need for dialysis, frequent medication requirements can impact patients' lifestyles, including dietary restrictions and increased susceptibility to infection. Nonetheless, studies have shown that successful transplantation is linked with marked improvements in emotional health and overall life satisfaction. Improved metabolic control and freedom from dialysis not only enhance physical health but also allow patients to reassert control over their lives, underscoring the potentially transformative potential of kidney transplantation in conjunction with adequate immunosuppressive regimens (Balamurugan et al., 2002) (Figure 15.6).

15.1.3. Statistics on Kidney Transplantation Success Rates

Kidney transplantation has emerged as the treatment of choice for ESRD patients with clear improvements in survival and quality of life over dialysis. The one-year graft survival rate after a kidney transplant from a deceased donor is approximately 93%, and for live donor transplants, the success rates are even higher at approximately 97% (Stomel et al., 2017). Over five years, these rates remain robust, with about 85% of transplant recipients retaining functional grafts. Additionally, advancements in immunosuppressive therapy have significantly contributed to improving these rates. As protocols have evolved, the application of personalized medicine and tailored immunosuppressive regimens has resulted in improved management of organ rejection and reduced toxicity, significantly influencing patient outcomes and overall transplant success rates. Statistics over decades indicate a dramatic advancement in success rates for renal transplants, the major reason being advancements in surgical technique, donor selection, and post-transplant care. For instance, innovation in induction therapy and the advancement in maintenance immunosuppression strategies have been important in countering the immune hurdles of transplantation. The latest statistics from the Scientific Registry of Transplant Recipients indicate that the ten-year survival rate for the graft exceeds 50%, varying according to factors such as patient age, underlying medical conditions, and donor-recipient matching (Kovacevic et al., 2016). The enhanced success rate is not only a testament to the importance of fastidious medical protocol but also to the evolving understanding of the immunological landscape that governs transplant viability. One of the most significant factors to the success of kidney transplants is the application of immunosuppressive therapy following transplantation. Tailoring immunosuppressive protocols based on the recipient's genetic profile and certain risk factors has been demonstrated to improve graft survival and reduce side effects. With findings highlighting the potential of pharmacogenetic testing, initial findings suggest that tailoring can optimize compliance and avert over- or under-immunosuppression-related complications. Its financial implications also matter, as it has been established that preemptive testing would be cost-effective in the long run, even while genetic analysis takes the initial bite (Kovacevic et al., 2016). The use of innovative methods within immunosuppressive therapy is hence not only driving improved kidney transplant outcomes but also paving the way for more sustainable medicine.

15.2. The Kidney Transplantation Process

The kidney transplantation process is a sequential critical process to ensure the successful grafting of the donor kidney into an end-stage renal disease recipient. A critical assessment of the recipient begins with a review of their medical history, physical examination, and laboratory studies to determine compatibility. Additionally, potential donors are tested for their organ viability, tissue compatibility, and blood type to minimize the risk of rejection. Once a suitable donor is found, the procedure is scheduled. The surgery lasts a few hours, during which the donor kidney is transplanted into the patient's body carefully. Surgical method and early postoperative management are critical to allow for an optimal result because any delay during this time may have a far-reaching consequence on the long-term function of the graft. The success of transplantation does not depend just on surgery but also on adherence to a strict protocol of immunosuppression. Post-transplant management is an essential aspect of the kidney transplant process, where immunosuppressive therapy plays an important part. On completion of the surgery, the recipient must undergo a regimen of drugs to suppress their immune system so that the transplant kidney will not be rejected as a foreign body. These medications, such as glucocorticoids and calcineurin inhibitors, should be closely monitored to achieve immunosuppression against infections and other complications. Notably, adherence to the prescribed immunosuppressive medication is of utmost importance for graft success; a lack of adherence is associated with increased rejection and lower graft survival. Health practitioners thus stress educating patients on the need for constant drug intake and side effects monitoring. This is vital to care and points out the delicate balance necessary in managing the immune system and maintaining the recipient's general health. The long-term success of kidney transplantation, beyond the transplantation procedure and early postoperative care, is largely dependent on continued research into immunosuppressive management. Advances aim to maximize the therapeutic effect of immunosuppressants with minimal adverse effects and improve the patient's quality of life. Other adjunctive therapy research that could further maximize graft acceptance includes thoracic duct drainage, which, in early trials, has been shown to reduce acute rejection in certain patient groups (Iwatsuki et al., 1981). These techniques need to be supplemented, however, with intense maintenance treatments to sustain graft function beyond the first year. The problem remains how to create a universal immunosuppressive protocol that balances the burden of long-term medication against maximizing graft survival and patient health. This continued research suggests that the solution involves a patient-specific approach where personal preference and situation are considered, ultimately to improve patient adherence and satisfaction with the transplant experience (Greene et al., 2014) (Figure 15.7).

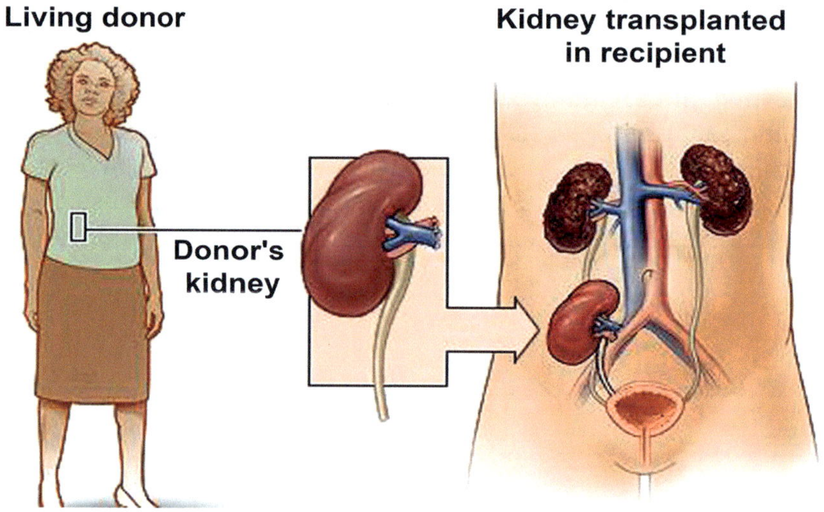

Figure 15.7. The kidney transplantation process.

Source: https://com-dom-neph-a2.sites.medinfo.ufl.edu/files/2011/12/tranplantclinic.jpg.

15.2.1. Pre-transplant Evaluation and Matching

Pre-transplant evaluation is a critical kidney transplant process to determine whether both the donor and recipient are adequately assessed to obtain the best transplant result. A comprehensive evaluation of multiple medical, psychological, and social factors is conducted. Extensive testing by clinicians is performed to assess the recipient's overall health, taking into account kidney function, potential comorbidities, and immune status. Accurate testing can help identify conditions that may complicate surgery or lead to post-transplant complications. Equally important is the evaluation of psychosocial factors, as patient adherence to postoperative immunosuppressive therapy should be ensured to prevent rejection and promote long-term graft survival. Through the systematic management of these factors, healthcare professionals can safely minimize the risks of kidney transplantation, resulting in improved recipient outcomes and overall benefiting the broader healthcare system. Donor-recipient matching by human leukocyte antigen (HLA) typing plays a crucial role in the pre-transplant process, as it directly impacts immunological compatibility and subsequent transplant outcomes. HLA mismatches have the potential to initiate acute rejection episodes, making the post-transplant course problematic. Over the past few years, advances in HLA typing methods have enhanced our capacity to determine compatibility with increased accuracy. These methods allow detection of donor-specific antibodies (DSAs) responsible for antibody-mediated rejection (ABMR). Acute ABMR can develop even in the presence of effective HLA matching; hence, understanding the subtleties of pre-transplant immunological parameters becomes critical. As underscored in recent literature, the correlation between HLA matching and the incidence of graft rejection highlights the importance of stringent matching protocols, ultimately leading to improved patient prognosis and a reduced incidence of unnecessary complications post-transplantation (Matsuda et al., 2016). Equally significant are equity issues related to organ allocation, aimed at offsetting the inequalities that persist in the transplantation system. Research has established that females and certain racial and ethnic groups have longer waiting times and lower rates of transplantation, demonstrating a pressing need for fairer policies in kidney procurement and allocation. These differences are exacerbated by differential cultural beliefs, socioeconomic circumstances, and geographic distribution, presenting a multifaceted challenge that extends beyond the hospital setting. By applying frameworks that examine these disparities and inequalities, health care systems can identify root causes of disparities and inequalities, so it becomes feasible to create effective interventions. Resolution of these disparities not only complies with ethical norms but also results in a more effective and fair allocation of organs, thereby enhancing the success rates of transplantation and overall outcomes for patients (Wells et al., 2012) (Figure 15.8).

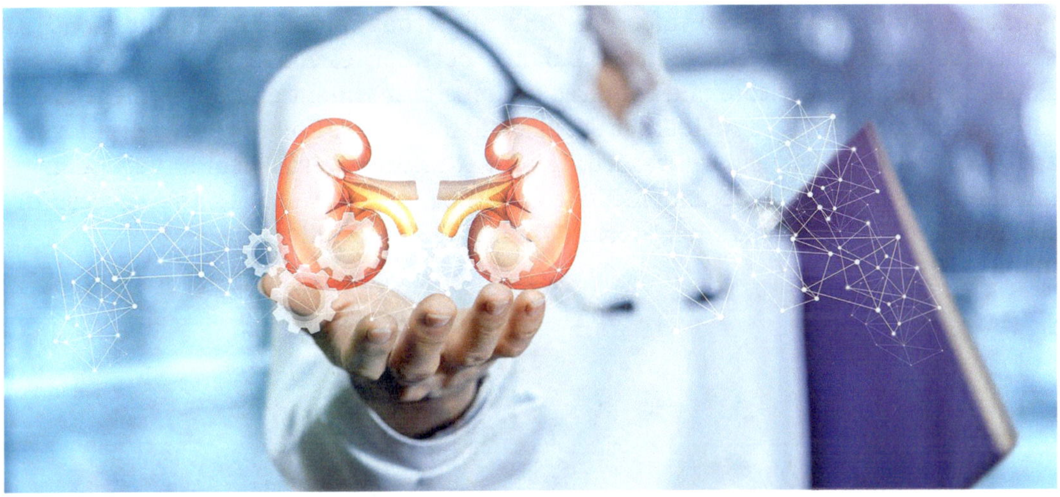

Figure 15.8. The pre-transplant evaluation is a critical step in the kidney transplantation process, ensuring that both the donor and recipient are appropriately assessed to maximize transplant success.

Source: https://thesunshinehospital.co.in/wp-content/uploads/2023/08/Pre-Post-Kidney-Transplantation.jpg.

15.2.2. Surgical Procedure for Kidney Transplantation

The surgical method in kidney transplant is a well-organized procedure that calls for extensive preoperative assessment to obtain maximum outcomes. The donor and recipient are tested before the procedure with meticulous examinations that include blood studies, imaging studies, and immunologic studies. These preliminary measures are designed to find compatible donors to reduce the risk of rejection. The surgery itself lasts three to four hours, in which the recipient's diseased kidney is usually removed and the donor kidney is placed in the lower abdomen. The transplanted kidney is then connected to the recipient's blood vessels and bladder, and continues to function as a ureteral drain. This very sophisticated application of medical expertise not only highlights the surgical complexity but also sets the stage for subsequent immunosuppressive therapy, which is imperative for preventing graft rejection following transplantation. The recipient postoperatively is kept in a state of critical care, wherein meticulous monitoring is essential to prevent complications such as infections and organ rejection. This is also a time of urgency, as postoperative infections have been causally linked with the intensification of immunosuppressive regimens used to prevent graft rejection. Studies have revealed that infectious disorders were prevalent among most recipients of renal homotransplantation and that specific pathogens like staphylococci and Pseudomonas species became prime offenders in postoperative infections (Marchioro et al., 1964). The interplay of immunosuppressive therapy with an increased risk of infection emphasizes the necessity of an individualized pharmacological approach. Each recipient's therapy schedule must be tailored, in consideration of their personal immunological background and the potential hazards of infections and other complications following the transplant procedure. The course of immunosuppressive therapy following kidney transplantation is a crucial part of patient care, to ensure the long-term function of the transplanted organ. Immunosuppressants play a crucial role of suppressing the recipients' immune system from rejecting the foreign kidney. But then there arises a series of risks, including increased vulnerability to infections and numerous metabolic complications. As noted in numerous research studies, the delicate balance between effective immunosuppression and minimizing side effects is intricate and requires ongoing assessment and adjustment of treatment protocols (di Luca et al., 2017). Providers must also ensure that recipients are well-informed about the potential side effects, particularly regarding how it affects overall health. Particularly, proper education about drug compliance and lifestyle modification is crucial to the success of kidney transplantation and the recipient's long-term health (Figure 15.9).

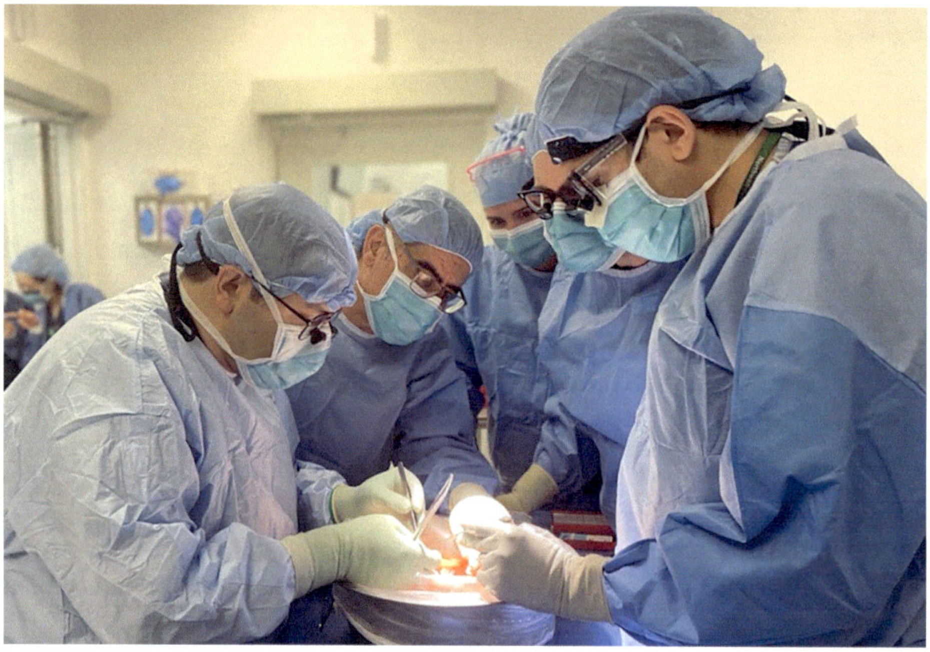

Figure 15.9. Surgical procedure for kidney transplantation.

Source: https://external-content.duckduckgo.com/iu/?u=https%3A%2F%2Fdam.northwell.edu%2Fm%2F4962c3b8fd679e5c%2FDrupal-NEWS_kidney-transplant-surgery-2024.jpg&f=1&nofb=1&ipt=4415ebcaacdecba3fa8a16d80ead6fbc4f3ad4841f57e2f66037944688fe47ab.

15.2.3. Post-Operative Care and Recovery

Post-operative care in a kidney transplant plays a crucial role in ensuring effective recovery and minimizing complications. Patients are transferred to a supervised recovery unit after the operation, where their vital signs and kidney function are closely monitored. Any sign of graft rejection or infection needs to be identified promptly, as they are major complications of overall recovery. Studies have shown that most transplant patients experience at least one significant complication during the post-operative period, and hence, constant monitoring and intervention strategies are a prerequisite (Shaw et al., 1985).

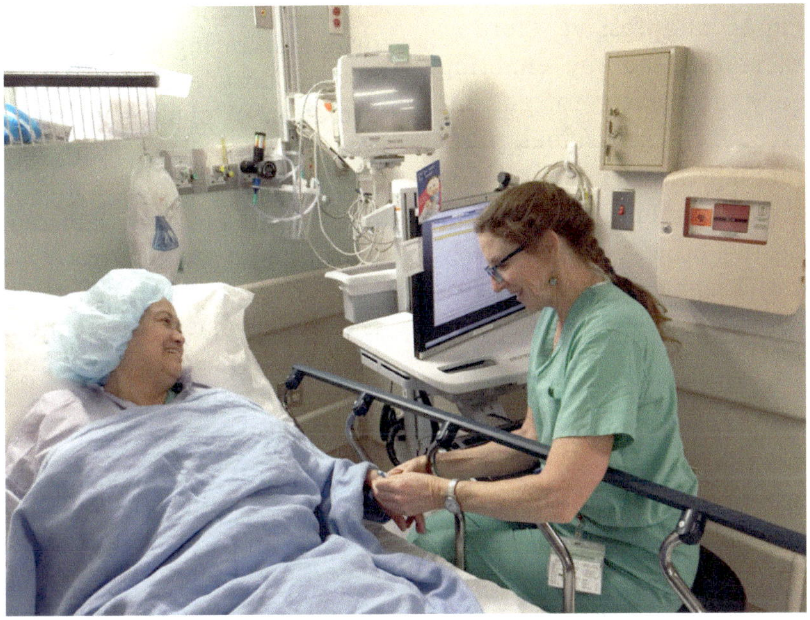

Figure 15.10. Post-operative care and recovery for kidney transplantation.

Source: https://external-content.duckduckgo.com/iu/?u=https%3A%2F%2Fhealth.ucdavis.edu%2Fsurgicalservices%2Fimages%2Fsame%2520day%2520surgery%2FPre-op-2-web.jpg&f=1&nofb=1&ipt=1c8ed7a006961cd7fa9e5c87ae6ae3433b7af2e3c447f384cf405d0e96c849e6.

These anticipatory measures can enhance the patient's outcome by facilitating early diagnosis of incipient complications and enabling rapid treatment, thereby leading to an uneventful postoperative course. Additionally, the role of immunosuppressive therapy in recovery following surgery cannot be overstated. Drugs such as Tacrolimus have been instrumental in preventing organ rejection following kidney transplantation. Their availability has introduced a paradigm shift in the treatment of post-transplant patients, resulting in significantly improved graft survival rates. As healing occurs, the immunosuppressive approach is gradually modified to establish a proper balance between preventing rejection and minimizing the risk of infection (Doyle et al., 1996). Consequently, individualized adjustments in medication levels are made based on each patient's tolerance and response, exhibiting the dynamic nature of post-operative care in ensuring the viability of the transplanted kidney. Patient education and counseling are also integral parts of post-operative recovery.

Informing patients about their care plan, including medication adherence and lifestyle modifications, is instrumental in achieving long-term success. Psychosocial rehabilitation in the post-transplant period can help address the emotional issues of transplantation, particularly concerns about potential complications. Additionally, regular follow-up after discharge facilitates comprehensive assessments of renal function, immunosuppressive therapy, and overall health status, thereby enabling an interdisciplinary approach to patient management. Consequently, meticulous post-operative care planning, involving intensive monitoring, drug management, and patient education, is responsible for excellent recovery outcomes following kidney transplantation (Figure 15.10).

15.3. Immunosuppressive Therapy Overview

Immunosuppressive therapy is a cornerstone of post-kidney transplantation medicine, essential for the avoidance of organ rejection with precise juggling of immune response. The complexities of these therapies are due to their limited therapeutic range, wherein under-treatment and over-treatment can both yield catastrophic outcomes. Inadequate suppression has the potential to induce organ rejection, ultimately handicapping or causing loss of the transplanted kidney. Conversely, excessive immunosuppression significantly increases susceptibility to infections and malignancies, as well as specific complications such as diabetes mellitus and nephrotoxicity. Individualized treatment protocols have become standard, necessitating personalized drug dosing based on a patient's unique clinical profile and risk factors, thereby ensuring that patients achieve optimal therapeutic outcomes without undue risk (Abboudi et al., 2012). The variety of immunosuppressants currently available can facilitate the development of individualized regimens for transplant patients, but incorporating these agents into an overall regimen has its own limitations. Contemporary protocols typically involve the use of calcineurin inhibitors, corticosteroids, and antiproliferative drugs, each with its characteristic pharmacologic properties and toxicities. Notably, the pharmacokinetic-pharmacodynamic interaction can be challenging to predict, and therefore, careful therapeutic drug monitoring is necessary to determine the optimal drug levels for each patient. The recent evolution of pharmacogenetics holds promise for improving personalized medicine in this regard, but the clinical utility of this approach has yet to be fully realized. As researchers continue to design newer biomarker-based methods for monitoring and risk stratification, it is expected that these technologies will improve the long-term success of kidney transplantation, as well as the overall health of the patient (Abboudi et al., 2012). Care after transplantation involves more than just immunosuppressive therapy, as kidney transplant patient care often requires proactive management of other clinical conditions and potential surgical interventions. As patient survival improves, it has become increasingly common for such patients to need further surgery unrelated to their transplant. Such cases necessitate careful preoperative evaluation, with particular attention to the condition of the transplanted organ and the specific immunosuppressive regimen being utilized. The anesthesiologist plays a key role in this process since he/she assesses the individual patient's circumstances, screens for potential drug interactions, and weighs the risks and benefits of invasive management in immunosuppressed patients. It is of paramount importance to preserve optimal graft function while addressing other medical complications, underscoring the necessity of a multidisciplinary management plan for the care of the transplant recipient (Figure 15.11).

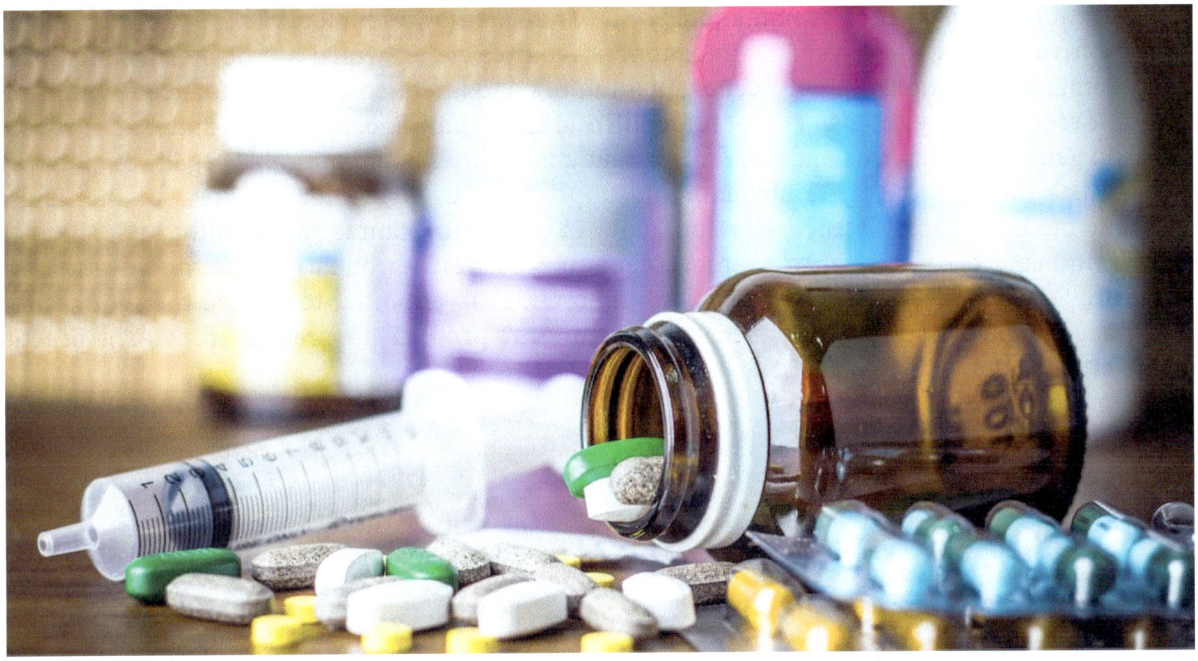

Figure 15.11. Immunosuppressive therapy is a cornerstone of post-kidney transplantation medicine.

Source: https://external-content.duckduckgo.com/iu/?u=https%3A%2F%2Fwww.neoteryx.com%2Fhubfs%2Fshutterstock_544348294%2520(1)%2520(1).jpg&f=1&nofb=1&ipt=10264e98bfe7603f3cd25fb8e7b61bb0f08ffac19f3ac2e87b4f2b19dc12ae21.

15.3.1. Definition and Purpose of Immunosuppressive Therapy

Immunosuppressive therapy is a cornerstone of kidney transplant to prevent the immune system from rejecting the transplanted organ. Immunosuppressants are essentially drugs that suppress or modulate the immune response to reduce the likelihood of the host's immune system recognizing the graft as foreign. This is a necessary therapy, given that the body naturally mounts an immune response to foreign tissue, which is then followed by rejection. Treatment of these agents tends to be long-term, often spanning the life of the transplant recipient, emphasizing their importance in graft survival and patient well-being. A better understanding of immunosuppressive regimens is critical because minor modifications in regimens can impact transplant outcomes profoundly, both short-term and long-term survival of the transplanted kidney. The function of employing immunosuppressive therapy extends beyond merely inhibiting rejection; it also involves the long-term survival of the graft, accompanied by a synergy of potential side effects. The sophistication of these therapies underscores the need for individualized treatment patterns, one that considers patient-specific parameters, such as immunological risk profiles and the corresponding type of transplanted organ. Certain agents can target specific immune pathways, and this can create synergistic interactions, enhancing the protection against rejection with diminished toxicity. Of greater significance is the evidence that optimizing immunosuppressive regimens has the potential to reverse IRI, a common complication of kidney transplantation that has significant adverse effects on early graft function as seen in studies of the protective capacity of agents like bilirubin and biliverdin (Thomas et al., 2011). Moreover, the continuous evolution of immunosuppressive strategies parallels the maturation of the science of immunology and transplantation biology. There are increasingly more selective drugs with newer immunosuppressive properties, which are designed to maintain essential immune functions that protect against tumors and infections. This avoidance is vital since transplant recipients are often at risk of infection due to the immunosuppressed state. Additionally, studies on genetic engineering and novel therapeutic modalities could optimize organ compatibility and minimize the need for aggressive immunosuppression, ushering in a new era for the field of transplant medicine. For instance, developments in xenotransplantation, recently highlighted in research, indicate the potential to overcome immune barriers through genetic modification and thus improve the success of organ transplantation, with the potential to reduce the requirement for prolonged immunosuppressive therapy, a significant problem in present transplant practice (Ayares et al., 2012) (Figure 15.12).

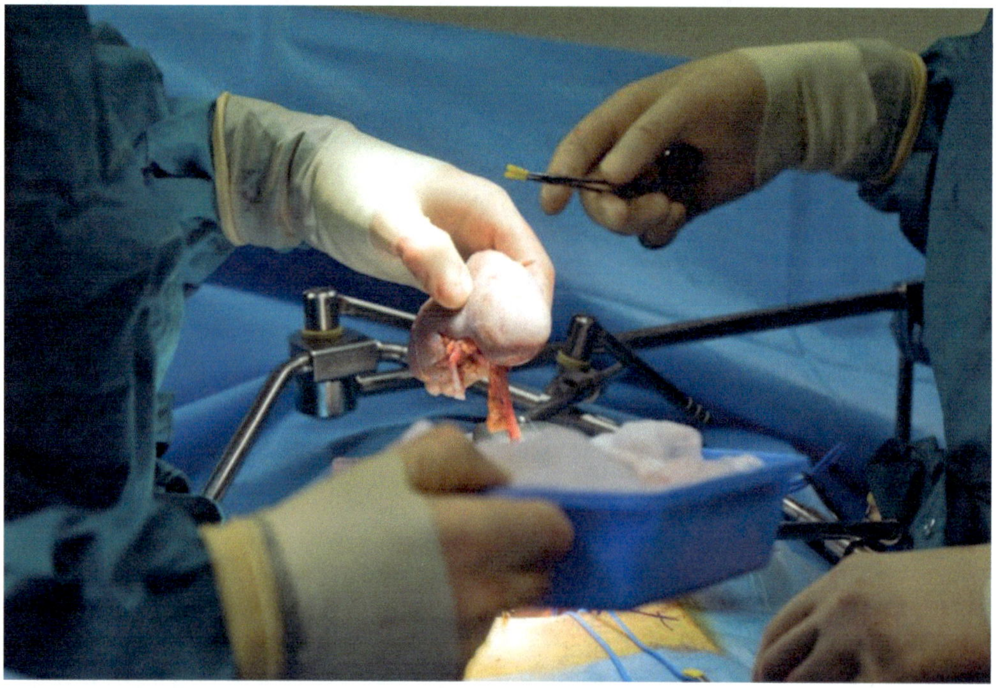

Figure 15.12. Immunosuppressive therapy is a cornerstone of kidney transplantation, designed to prevent the immune system from rejecting the transplanted organ.

Source: https://media.springernature.com/lw703/springer-static/image/art%3A10.1038%2Fnature.2012.10188/MediaObjects/41586_2012_Article_BFnature201210188_Figa_HTML.jpg.

15.3.2. Types of Immunosuppressive Medications

Immunosuppressive medications play a critical role in ensuring that kidney transplantation is successful by preventing the rejection of an organ. Corticosteroids, such as prednisone, are a primary class of immunosuppressive drugs. Corticosteroids act by controlling the body's immune system so that the inflammation and activation of white blood cells that can enter the transplanted kidney are prevented. While effective in the immediate posttransplant period, chronic corticosteroid use can lead to significant adverse effects, e.g., osteoporosis and increased risk of infection. Therefore, clinicians must balance the need for a necessary immunosuppressive effect with minimizing adverse effects. The relative effectiveness of corticosteroids versus other immunosuppressive agents highlights the complexities of selecting the appropriate drug regimen for each patient in the context of kidney transplantation. A second class of primary immunosuppressive agents is the calcineurin inhibitors, including cyclosporine and tacrolimus. They act by inhibiting the activation of T-lymphocytes, which is a key component of the immune response to transplanted organs. Calcineurin inhibitors have revolutionized transplant care since their introduction, significantly improving graft and patient survival rates. They are, however, burdened with their own drawbacks, including nephrotoxicity, which is particularly troublesome in renal transplant recipients. The narrow therapeutic window of the drugs necessitates tight monitoring of drug levels to avoid toxicity while still maintaining adequate immunosuppression. In addition, future interactions with other medications and the role of individual metabolic variations underscore the need for patient-specific approaches to immunosuppressive therapy after transplantation. Antimetabolites represent another class of immunosuppressants used in renal transplantation. Agents such as azathioprine and mycophenolate mofetil are currently popular agents for inhibiting lymphocyte proliferation, further reducing the risk of rejection. These agents are particularly valued for their ability to amplify the effects of glucocorticoids and calcineurin inhibitors, allowing for the use of reduced doses of the latter and minimizing their concomitant side effects. Interestingly, recent data suggest that mycophenolate mofetil, in addition, exhibits an improved side effect profile compared to older antimetabolites and is the drug of choice among clinicians. A balance between efficacy and safety is crucial, as evidenced by recent research on their long-term outcomes and adverse effects, which can inform better clinical practice within the complex arena of kidney transplant and immunosuppression therapy (Wells et al., 2012; Esteban et al., 2016) (Figure 15.13).

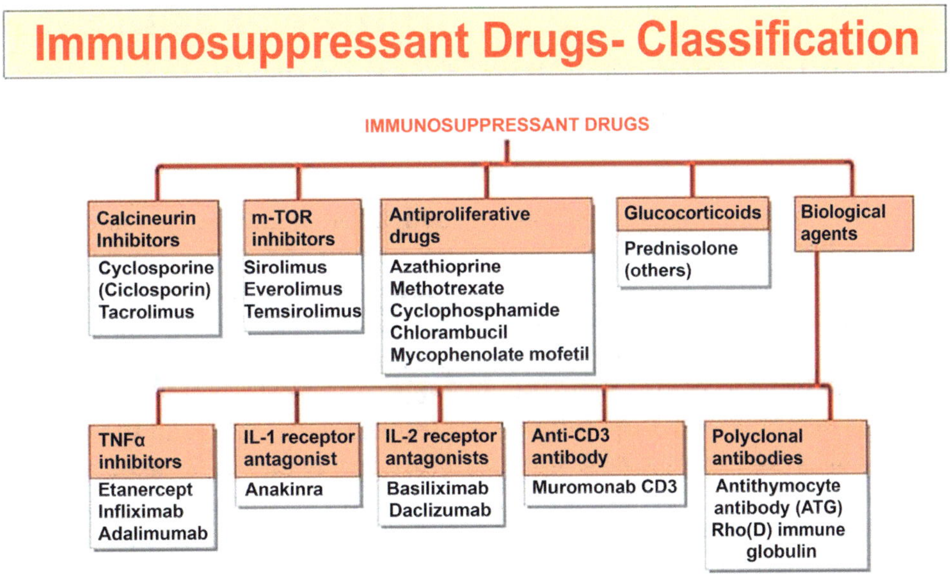

Figure 15.13. Types of immunosuppressive medications.

Source: https://i.ytimg.com/vi/p4KwQFrc_cM/hq720.jpg?sqp=-oaymwEhCK4FEIIDSFryq4qpAxMIARUAAAAAGAElAADIQj0AgKJD&rs=AOn4CLAqLePTO0nhb5QZCn9Yy5zEu9wVNg.

15.3.3. Mechanisms of Action of Immunosuppressants

Understanding the mechanisms of action of immunosuppressants is crucial to the successful management of kidney transplantation. The dominant mode of action of immunosuppressants is the inhibition of the immune response that would reject an organ transplant through more than one pathway. CNIs, such as cyclosporine and tacrolimus, inhibit T-lymphocyte function by blocking calcineurin activation. This phosphatase protein removes phosphate from NFAT. This interference blocks the transcription of interleukin-2, a critical growth factor for T-cells, thereby suppressing the general immune response against the donor organ. The CNIs are thus a foundation of maintenance immunosuppression regimens that require careful dose handling to ensure therapeutic efficacy while minimizing the side effects of their administration, as revealed by various minimization approaches highlighted in clinical practice (Andrade-Sierra et al., 2018). In addition to CNIs, other drugs with alternative mechanisms of action further limit the regulation of kidney transplantation. Mycophenolate mofetil (MMF) inhibits the enzyme inosine monophosphate dehydrogenase (IMPDH), which is crucial in the de novo pathway of purine synthesis, thereby selectively suppressing lymphocytes that rely on this pathway for proliferation. This preferential suppression not only inhibits T-cell and B-cell activation but also reduces the side effects on other actively dividing cells, enhancing patient safety. Initial findings reveal a reduction in side effects, such as gastrointestinal discomfort, when MMF is administered at low doses, thus confirming the importance of personalized immunosuppressive regimens according to patient needs (Andrade-Sierra et al., 2018). These new mechanisms are instrumental in advancing immunosuppressive regimens, resulting in improved long-term graft survival. Nevertheless, effective use of immunosuppressive therapy has implications regarding potential complications, such as the development of new onset diabetes after transplantation (NODAT). NODAT is a significant side effect frequently associated with corticosteroid and CNIs administration in transplant recipients. Interestingly, NODAT may increase death rates as a result of cardiovascular events and predispose individuals to infection, thus harming graft survival. Prevention of these risks involves meticulous patient monitoring and an investigation into the use of alternative immunosuppressants, which may pose a lower risk of metabolic side effects. Through the identification of high-risk patients and the use of preventive interventions, healthcare providers can maximize results and improve long-term prognosis for kidney transplant recipients, showing that modes of immunosuppressant activity are more than mere therapeutic efficacy, involving a more holistic concept of patient management.

15.4. Indications for Immunosuppressive Therapy

The need for immunosuppressive therapy after a kidney transplant is probably because of the body's own immunity, which recognizes the new organ as foreign. The reaction may lead to acute rejection attacks, during which the graft is explicitly targeted by the immune system. To prevent this from happening, recipients typically receive a course of immunosuppressants soon after the transplant, and this serves to improve graft survival. There are several factors that may influence the specific immunosuppressive regimen employed, including the overall health of the patients, the presence of comorbidities, and the histocompatibility of donor and recipient tissues. It has been established through studies that the choice of immunosuppressive drugs may play a significant role in determining long-term outcome, with some of these combinations of medicines offering improved patient and graft survival compared to others, reflecting the application of individualized therapy for optimizing outcomes after transplantation (Fung et al., 2000). Dosage and timing of the immunosuppression also play an essential role in achieving success in kidney transplants. Immunosuppressants are often administered with high initial doses to suppress immune activity rapidly and prevent acute rejection. The dosage may gradually be tapered according to the patient's response and the appearance of any side effects. Ongoing monitoring is crucial in striking a balance between providing sufficient immunosuppression to protect the graft and minimizing side effects, such as infections and malignancies, that can arise from long-term immune suppression. In this respect, newer data show that individualized immunosuppressive protocols improve long-term outcomes with fewer side effects (Abu-Elmagd et al., 2004). The individualized regimens are indicative of the move in transplant medicine towards newer modes of therapy. Also, there are more recent immunosuppressive medications that have potential for increasing the benefits of kidney transplant patients. For instance, medications such as tacrolimus have been shown to be effective in reducing acute rejection and improving graft survival rates. Clinical evidence has established that patients receiving tacrolimus-based regimens experience significantly fewer episodes of rejection compared to patients receiving traditional therapies, thus making it critical to use appropriate immunosuppressive treatment. The long-term outcomes of kidney transplant recipients have indicated increased survival in more recent protocols with the use of both established and novel immunosuppressants. This underscores the importance of ongoing research to optimize existing therapies and develop new modalities targeting specific patient groups, thereby enhancing graft survival and improving the quality of life for recipients (Fung et al., 2000; Abu-Elmagd et al., 2004).

15.4.1. Prevention of Organ Rejection

Organ rejection is a prevalent factor in kidney transplantation, and the outcome of the transplant is heavily reliant upon the host's acceptance of the graft. During the immediate post-transplantation period, the occurrence of acute rejection can be significantly curbed by the administration of immunosuppressive drugs. The purpose of these drugs is to suppress the recipients' immune system against the transplanted kidney, reducing the chances of rejection. However, the use of these drugs is not without its challenges; patients must tread the fine line between proper immunosuppression to prevent rejection and the associated risks of overimmunosuppression, which can lead to infections and other complications. As research continues, other regimens, such as immunomodulatory interventions, are being explored to enhance graft acceptance while reducing the adverse effects previously noted with traditional immunosuppressants (MJ B et al., 2024). The individualized nature of immunosuppressive therapy is essential to ensuring the optimal outcome of kidney transplantation. No two patients have the same immunological picture, and an individualized therapeutic regimen is thus needed. The complexity of this issue is compounded by the narrow therapeutic range for most immunosuppressants: under-treatment can precipitate acute rejection, while over-treatment leads to severe side effects, such as nephrotoxicity and increased susceptibility to infections (Abboudi et al., 2012). Therapeutic drug monitoring plays a significant role in the dosing adjustment to provide the best drug concentrations with decreased toxicity. In addition, emerging pharmacogenetic studies offer potential for further individualization of immunosuppressive therapy. These advances can help clinicians determine the most effective and least toxic drug regimens for a particular group of patients, thereby maximizing patient safety as well as graft survival. While conventional immunosuppressive therapy plays a crucial role in preventing organ rejection, newer modalities need to be adopted to counter the limitations of current methods. Extracorporeal photopheresis (ECP) presents a novel adjunctive therapy for organ rejection prevention, particularly in patients at high risk of transplantation with concomitant comorbid illness or infectious complications. ECP's immunomodulatory activity not only enhances graft tolerance but also reduces the quantities of standard immunosuppressants required, thus circumventing their side effects (MJ B et al., 2024). As research continues to uncover the promise of ECP and other emerging therapies, focus shifts toward integrating these modalities into standard care protocols. Improved insight into biomarker-based risk stratification and pharmacodynamic monitoring will be instrumental in the development of more efficient and safer immunosuppressive regimens, which would ultimately improve patient outcomes after kidney transplantation (Figure 15.14).

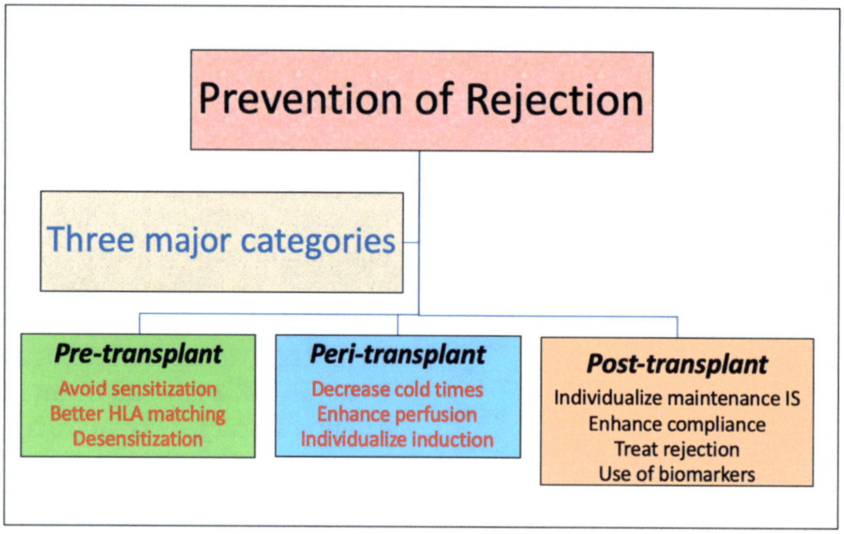

Figure 15.14. The prevention of organ rejection remains a central concern in the field of kidney transplantation, as the efficacy of transplantation heavily relies on the body's acceptance of the graft.

Source: https://www.mdpi.com/jcm/jcm-12-05938/article_deploy/html/images/jcm-12-05938-g001.png.

15.4.2. Management of Autoimmune Responses

Immuneresponse management is a crucial aspect of kidney transplantation and immunosuppressive therapy. Immune reactions can significantly compromise the success of a transplant, and this can lead to acute and chronic graft rejection. Among the various mechanisms, T cell-mediated rejection (TCMR) and antibody-mediated rejection (ABMR) are key players in the pathology of graft rejection. Immunosuppressive therapy must be precisely adjusted to overcome such responses. Adequate immunosuppression can most often control acute TCMR but is ineffective against ABMR, particularly chronic forms that result in permanent graft damage (Matsuda et al., 2016). The complexity of autoimmune responses underscores the importance of ongoing investigation and optimization of immunosuppressive strategies to enhance long-term graft function and survival. Immunotherapy has its drawbacks, including obscuring the management of primary autoimmune diseases. In renal transplant, patients may already have a predisposition to autoimmune diseases so that the post-transplant period is particularly vulnerable. For instance, the history of autoimmune hepatitis presents special difficulties, as the immunosuppressive medications must balance the risk of rejection against the risk of exacerbating ongoing autoimmune processes.

There is recent evidence to indicate that most autoimmune diseases, including autoimmune hepatitis, can be successfully treated with immunosuppression, although relapse is frequent, making long-term management difficult (Miyake et al., 2008). Transplant physicians must exercise a vigilant eye, keeping close watch on patients for the onset of recurrence of autoimmune activity as well as administering adequate immunosuppression. Moreover, the rise of non-HLA antibodies has introduced a new perspective into the management of autoimmune responses after kidney transplantation. Non-HLA antibodies are capable of inducing ABMR regardless of conventional donor-specific HLA antibodies, thus making it extremely important to implement rigorous immunological monitoring before and after transplant. The identification of the source of such non-HLA antibodies and their association with graft rejection underscores the need for an individualized immunosuppressive regimen. Pre-emptive identification of high-risk patients, along with advanced techniques for antibody detection, may enhance the potential for utilizing targeted therapies that can reduce the frequency of rejection episodes (Matsuda et al., 2016). Such multi-modal treatment is essential not only to achieve immediate graft acceptance but also to enhance long-term transplant success and avoid chronic complications.

15.4.3. Long-term Health Considerations for Transplant Recipients

The long-term care problem of transplant recipients involves a multifaceted approach, particularly given the added layer of sophistication provided by immunosuppression. Recipients must be strictly adherent to their drug regimens to prevent the specter of acute rejection and loss of graft. But the medication, significant as it is, carries harmful side effects ranging from increased risk of infection to hypertension to metabolic derangements like diabetes. Notably, the evolution of immunosuppressive therapy has also been accompanied by an increase in the susceptibility of developing cardiovascular disease complications; hence, a close observation and control of cardiovascular status is crucial for the entire life of recipients. With this understanding of the risks, medical staff can advise patients more effectively on lifestyle modifications and intervention in order to promote longevity without jeopardizing the functioning of the donated kidneys. One other key concern in long-term care of transplant recipients is the risk of recurrence of the original disease that led to kidney failure. Diabetic nephropathy is a case in point where continuous monitoring and management of metabolic status needs to be performed to prevent the initial disease from invading the transplanted organ. Although organ transplants are expected to normalize renal function, the underlying disease processes themselves may persist and remain a source of risk to long-term graft survival. Consistently, research has shown that near-optimal control of blood glucose in diabetic recipients is vital to minimizing the risk of complications related to the transplant. Thus, ongoing education and communication among nephrologists and endocrinologists are essential when crafting a comprehensive care plan to maximize health outcomes and quality of life for kidney transplant patients. Lastly, the psychosocial aspects of transplant life necessitate equal emphasis, as emotional and mental well-being significantly influence physical health. Receivers are also plagued by anxiety regarding the ongoing function of their transplant drug side effects and rejection. The addition of psychological support services can assist in coping and encourage compliance with medication. Receivers may also have social concerns, such as work and insurance issues, that could augment feelings of isolation or discomfort. Support group participation and open dialogue with healthcare professionals can reduce some of these accusations and assist in the transplant process, however. As the number of kidney transplant recipients rises, a holistic approach to addressing physical and psychosocial well-being must be considered to maximize long-term health outcomes (Balamurugan et al., 2002; Acan et al., 2018) (Figure 15.15).

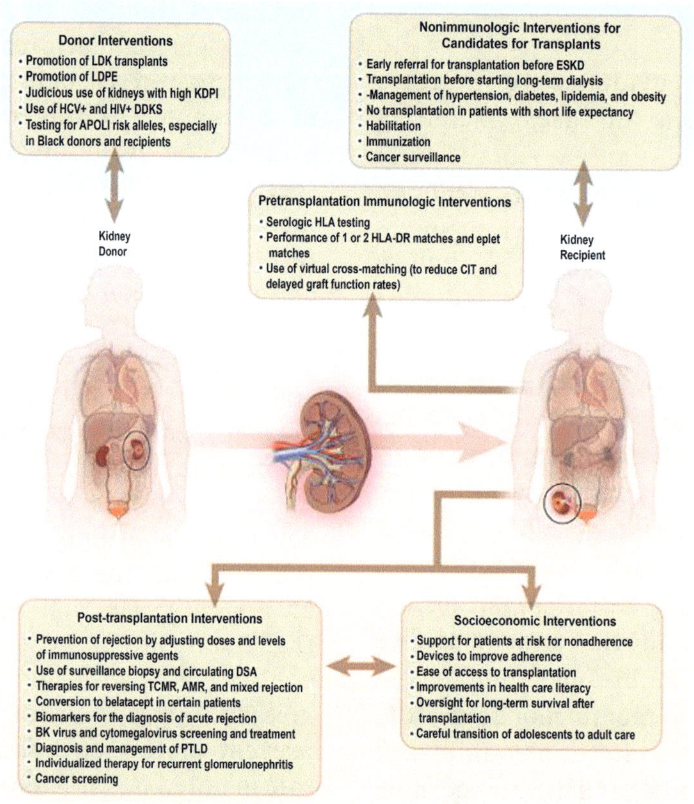

Figure 15.15. Long-term survival after kidney transplantation.

Source: https://www.nejm.org/cms/10.1056/NEJMra2014530/asset/f5945b5b-ea64-46b6-a6b1-d0324e9b7c1d/assets/images/large/nejmra2014530_f1.jpg.

15.5. Side Effects and Risks of Immunosuppressive Therapy

Immunosuppressive therapy has significantly enhanced the success of kidney transplantation, but it is crucial to appreciate the inherent side effects and dangers of the drugs. The mechanism of action of immunosuppressants is based on suppressing the immune reaction to prevent organ rejection;

however, this approach has a narrow therapeutic window, making administration not entirely risk-free. Subtherapeutic dosing leads to rejection episodes, which cause either organ damage or loss. Conversely, over-immunosuppression enhances infection and cancer risk as well as some drug-related complications like diabetes mellitus and nephrotoxicity. Because pharmacokinetics and pharmacodynamics can vary significantly between individuals, tailor-made treatment regimens are crucial to counteract these risks. Therapeutic drug monitoring and precision medicine approaches have thus become a cornerstone of maximizing immunosuppressant therapy following kidney transplantation (Abboudi et al., 2012). Patients typically find it challenging to adopt immunosuppressive regimens due to the side effects and chronicity of the drugs. What transplant recipients tell us is that although the surgery is life-changing, mandatory lifelong drug therapy can compromise quality of life. The best post-transplant scenario would be minimizing the drug burden; however, this remains elusive. While additional research continues to aim to maximize immune management regimens, no regimen to date has allowed patients to stop immunosuppressants entirely. This necessitates a discriminating evaluation of medication compliance factors, including patient satisfaction and psychological health, as non-compliance can threaten long-term allograft survival. This environment highlights the patient-centered approach in determining therapeutic plans (Greene et al., 2014). The therapeutic value of tailored immunosuppressive treatment is notable in light of the implications of response variability to these treatments at the individual level. With the development of pharmacogenetics and novel biomarker-mediated methods, there is also a new avenue for maximizing patient response and minimizing toxicities. These advances would further enhance therapeutic drug monitoring by providing each patient with an individualized metabolic profile and drug response. Moreover, such individually oriented strategies might mitigate the emotional as well as physical cost involved in managing intense side effects. Yet, even with these encouraging results, current treatment protocols require ongoing patient education and support to achieve compliance. Therefore, the investigation of tailored treatment modalities is of critical importance, not only for minimizing risks but also for fostering a concordant relationship between patients and healthcare providers in the context of kidney transplantation (Abboudi et al., 2012).

15.5.1. Common Side Effects of Immunosuppressants

Immunosuppressants are at the forefront of kidney transplantation success because they prevent the body from rejecting the transplanted organ. The drugs, however, are very commonly associated with a chain of harmless side effects that significantly impact patient health and treatment compliance. Unusual side effects include increased susceptibility to infection, as the immunosuppression reduces the body's natural defense barriers. Additionally, patients may also experience gastrointestinal disturbances such as indigestion, diarrhea, and nausea. These side effects reduce the quality of life, prompting people to question the long-term continuation of these treatments. The psychological burden of such side effects can then impact patients' adherence to regimens, emphasizing the need for communication and management between health professionals and patients to overcome such adversity (Greene et al., 2014). Metabolic disorders are also a frequent side effect of immunosuppressants that occur via weight gain, hypertension, and dyslipidemia. These metabolic changes can arise due to the drugs' negative impact on glucose homeostasis and lipid profiles, predisposing to cardiovascular disorders. Hence, kidney transplant patients typically require concomitant management of these metabolic disturbances and immunosuppressive treatment. This multidimensional approach mandates stringent monitoring of blood pressure, cholesterol, and blood sugar, further complicating post-transplant management. Furthermore, the increased risk of developing diabetes, particularly among corticosteroid-treated patients, serves to underscore the importance of a tailored nutritional and exercise program in post-transplant treatment plans. These metabolic side effects in turn serve to emphasize the importance of ongoing patient education and proactive intervention strategies to promote optimal well-being following transplantation (Balamurugan et al., 2002). Long-term adherence to immunosuppressive therapy is necessary for the success of kidney transplantation, yet pervasive side effects can pose significant obstacles to adherence. Patients routinely report emotional and psychological effects, including depression and anxiety, that are likely induced by the chronic nature of drug regimens and their associated side effects. Educating the patient on the importance of compliance and potential side effects can empower them to take an active role in their own care. Immunosuppressant therapy and patients' experience with it should also be monitored regularly by healthcare professionals, adjusting treatment regimens as needed to reduce toxicity without sacrificing allograft function. Active debate about the benefits and challenges of immunosuppressive therapy can lead to better compliance and quality of life for kidney transplant recipients. Lastly, the recognition and management of reversible side effects of immunosuppressants should be prioritized for optimal patient experience and outcomes in kidney transplantation (Greene et al., 2014) (Figure 15.16).

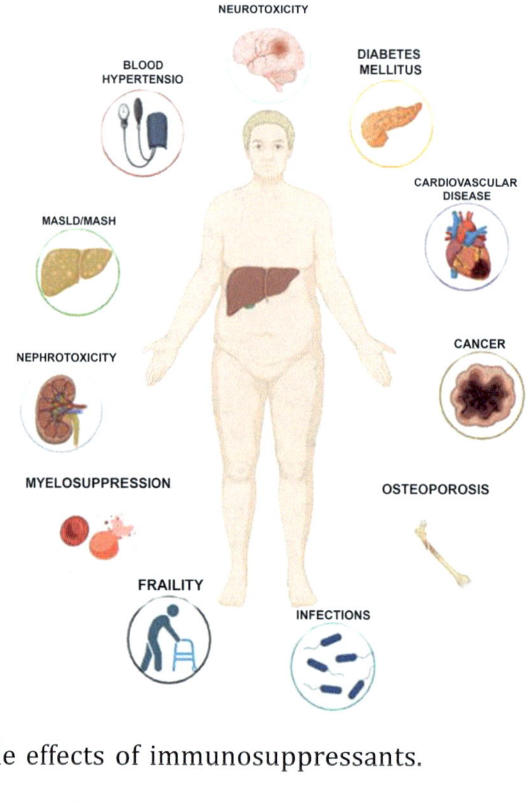

Figure 15.16. Common side effects of immunosuppressants.

Source: https://www.mdpi.com/pharmaceuticals/pharmaceuticals-18-00342/article_deploy/html/images/pharmaceuticals-18-00342-g002.png.

15.5.2. Increased Risk of Infections

The immunosuppressive therapy needed by transplant recipients of kidney transplants significantly increases the risk of infection, and hence, proper monitoring and management need to be ensured. Immune-modulating drugs are administered to the patients, post-transplant, to prevent graft rejection at the cost of their natural and adaptive immune functions, something that they unfortunately pay with their lives. The dual consequences of immunosuppression include an enhanced susceptibility to opportunistic infections and the risk of delayed infection diagnosis due to suppressed inflammatory responses. Thus, such patients become more vulnerable to a range of infectious pathogens, including bacteria, viruses, and fungi, which can potentially lead to life-threatening complications. Moreover, the onset and character of infections that do develop may also vary, typically reflecting the degree of immunosuppression, warranting the employment of particular treatment strategies to combat such threats effectively.

Among the infections that kidney transplant patients are faced with, viral infections, and specifically those by Polyomavirus BK (BKV), deserve special mention. BKV is prevalent among the general population; yet, it presents a particular threat to immunocompromised individuals and particularly kidney transplant recipients. BKV is capable of post-transplantation being the cause of bridging asymptomatic viremia and viruria, which can lead to nephropathy when closely observed. The pathophysiologic mechanisms of susceptibility to BKV in renal transplant patients are yet to be determined. The evidence suggests that patients undergoing kidney transplantation, compared with non-renal solid organ transplant recipients, have an increased rate of BKV infection, perhaps because of the unique immunologic status accomplished after transplant (Mitterhofer et al., 2016). Generally, vigilant surveillance for BKV and other viral infections in these patients is necessary to maximize graft survival. Bacterial and fungal infections are also challenging entities to kidney transplant recipients. Traditional bacterial pathogens may present, along with community-acquired and nosocomial infection, secondary to the patient's immunocompromised status. The impaired immune system often does not respond in the way it should, leading to severe and life-threatening complications. Fungal infections, such as those caused by Candida or Aspergillus species, also pose severe threats, particularly among individuals undergoing intensive immunosuppression therapy (Doyle et al., 1996). The management of such infections often requires aggressive regimens, including prolonged antimicrobial treatment and possible intervention to prevent severe complications. With the possibility of numerous infection threats to kidney transplantation, superior patient care must be complemented by a comprehensive strategy involving active screening, education, and prevention to maximize patient care and long-term health benefits (Figure 15.17).

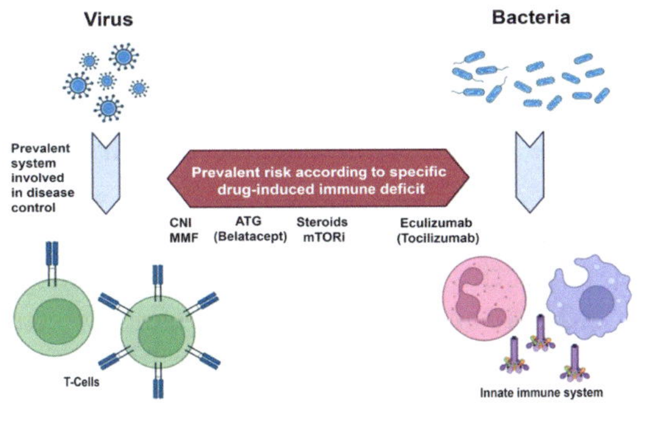

Figure 15.17. Bacterial and viral infection and sepsis in kidney transplanted patients.

Source: https://www.mdpi.com/biomedicines/biomedicines-10-00701/article_deploy/html/images/biomedicines-10-00701-g001.png.

15.5.3. Long-term Health Complications

After they undergo kidney transplantation, patients are faced with a variety of long-term complications in their health that must be managed and followed up closely. Chief among these is the requirement of lifelong immunosuppressive therapy, which, while critical in preventing organ rejection, subjects recipients to a series of side effects. Long-term use of such drugs, including Tacrolimus, has been found to predispose individuals to cardiovascular diseases, infection, and malignancies. Studies have proven that infections following transplant are far more common since the immune system is suppressed, and the patient must tread a delicate balance between preventing rejection and avoiding further disease. Clinicians must therefore embrace a holistic and tailored approach to patient management that seeks to mitigate these risks and deliver the optimal long-term outcome in transplant recipients. In addition to the enhanced risk of infections and cardiovascular morbidity, recipients of a kidney transplant are also afflicted by metabolic complications. Typically accompanied by prolonged immunosuppressive therapy, these include hypertension, dyslipidemia, and diabetes, which further complicate the post-transplant course. For instance, corticosteroid therapy is well-documented to impair glucose metabolism. It can be an etiological factor for the development of new-onset diabetes, thus impacting overall health and quality of life. Additionally, immunosuppressive drug synergism has been associated with reported instances of renal impairment, and such may necessitate further interventions or even a repeat transplant. Such metabolic complications further underscore the importance of continuous monitoring and treatment plan adjustment to manage emerging complications, so that kidney transplant recipients may be able to maintain their health in the postoperative years. Lastly, the psychosocial impact of long-term medical complications cannot be overstated. Those with the sequelae of kidney transplant and immunosuppressive therapy are often beset by psychiatric issues, including depression and anxiety, in accordance with chronic illness concerns and the burdens of treatment compliance. Readjustment to life posttransplant can be challenging, with patients having to deal with the complexity of merely tolerating medications but also with the threat of long-term complications. Furthermore, the financial expense of ongoing medical care can bring yet another stressor. Support systems, including peer support and counseling, are essential for helping patients to cope with these psychosocial concerns, affirming the need for a holistic model of post-transplant care that covers physical and emotional needs.

15.6. Advances in Immunosuppressive Therapy

The art of immunosuppressive therapy has advanced significantly, particularly in kidney transplantation. The traditional regimens have primarily consisted of a combination of calcineurin inhibitors, such as cyclosporine and tacrolimus, with corticosteroids and antimetabolites. However, emerging innovations hold out the hope of increasingly individualized treatment regimens that cover both biological and patient-specific needs. More recent agents, such as mTOR inhibitors and antibodies against unique immune mechanisms, mark a move towards reducing late side effects while maintaining graft function. These individualized regimens demonstrate an emerging perception of the immunology of transplantation with a desire to eliminate broad-spectrum immunosuppressants that result in significant long-term complications. Furthermore, the progressive development of lower toxicity immunosuppressive regimens is underlined by patients' reports that often refer to non-compliance with medication as an utmost challenge following transplantation. Further research focuses on the importance of considering patient satisfaction and quality of life when selecting therapeutic programs. Through the investigation of non-pharmacological options, including lifestyle modification and compliance interventions, healthcare professionals can achieve better outcomes. Greene et al. (2014) suggest that even though the complete elimination of drugs remains a long way off, limiting the number and the complexity of medication regimens prescribed can improve prospects for compliance and thereby guarantee allograft survival while optimizing the overall health of patients. Precision medicine practice is also gaining popularity as an essential component of kidney transplantation immunosuppressive therapy. Using genetic profiling and biomarker discovery, physicians can now determine which patients would benefit most from one immunosuppressive intervention rather than another. Findings from graft viability studies suggest that focusing on protection against rejection, rather than solely on histocompatibility, may prove more successful (Starzl et al., 1971). The more closely researchers understand the intricacies of immune response, the more specific techniques may revolutionize post-transplant care. With the ongoing refinement of immunosuppressive therapy, the potential for achieving a balance between safety and efficacy is increasingly real, ultimately benefiting both patients and clinicians.

15.6.1. Newer Immunosuppressive Agents

The ever-changing landscape of immunosuppressive therapy has witnessed the introduction of newer agents meant to improve patient outcomes following kidney transplantation. Among them, the role of calcineurin inhibitors, such as tacrolimus, has emerged into the limelight, as they are efficient in preventing acute rejection and improving graft survival. Tacrolimus, first used in the late 1980s, has been able to decrease rejection rates by a remarkable extent compared to traditional therapies. With cumulative experience demonstrating that almost 70% of long-term patients achieve stable graft function on this monotherapy, it is easy to understand why tacrolimus remains a cornerstone in immunosuppressive therapy (Abu-Elmagd et al., 1999). But with its benefits, the agent is saddled with several long-term toxicities, primarily renal toxicity and cardiovascular disease, which demand careful management and ongoing research to ensure its optimum use in the clinical arena. Aside from the calcineurin inhibitors, other newer drugs, such as mTOR inhibitors (such as sirolimus and everolimus), offer alternative mechanisms of immunosuppression via halting cell growth and remodeling the immune system. Such molecules have been of interest due to their better side effect profiles, particularly with respect to renal function, compared to calcineurin inhibitors. Evidence shows that mTOR inhibitors not only maintain graft survival but can reduce the incidence of certain malignancies, a significant problem in long-term transplant patients. The application of mTOR inhibitors in immunosuppressive treatment makes regimens more adjustable, as substantiated by the expanding body of literature regarding their synergistic action when applied together with other drugs (Greene et al., 2014). The potential for the individualization of immunosuppressive therapy represents a foremost advancement in perfecting the equilibrium between the prevention of transplant rejection by the body and the minimization of adverse effects. Compliance and patient satisfaction are essential determinants of the success of kidney transplantation. The newer agents of immunosuppression have created much controversy regarding the quality of life of recipients. The majority of patients are anxious about the complexity and burden of lifelong therapy, and they emphasize the need for regimens with low medication load but adequate graft protection (Greene et al., 2014). As clinicians optimize immunosuppressive regimens, patient preference, satisfaction, and global health outcomes must be of the highest priority. It is not only difficult to develop successful therapeutic regimens but also to make the patients adhere to the regimens because non-adherence is one of the main contributing factors to transplant failure. Therefore, patient education assessment, simplification of the regimen, and open communication between patients and healthcare workers are critical to ensuring maximum long-term success in kidney transplantation.

15.6.2. Personalized Medicine Approaches

The integration of individualized medicine approaches into kidney transplantation represents a profound shift towards care tailored to the individual patient, particularly in the administration of immunosuppression. Personalized medicine aims to tailor therapy to the specific characteristics of each patient, including genetic, environmental, and lifestyle factors. In kidney transplantation, this approach cannot be avoided because patients exhibit differential drug metabolism and immunosuppressive response. Such diversity is capable of leading to inadequate immune suppression or over-immunosuppression, both of which can undermine graft survival and patient health. Individualized strategies involving pharmacogenetic analysis can optimize immunosuppressive regimens to achieve maximum effectiveness, allowing for more precise dosing and minimizing side effects, resulting in overall optimal outcomes in kidney transplant patients. In addition, advances in the identification and study of biomarkers are crucial to the individualized design of immunosuppressive treatment for kidney transplant recipients. The identification of personal biomarkers for allograft damage or tolerance necessitates a novel approach to monitoring immunosuppression. It is now possible for investigators to correlate genomic, transcriptomic, and proteomic data from the donor and recipient tissues with clinical results using high-throughput platforms. This interaction will enhance the risk stratification processes and adaptive treatment strategies, which are more than capable of responding meaningfully to dynamic physiological status. Sustained non-invasive blood-based biomarker development will be invaluable in providing clinicians with real-time feedback on graft status, and this will ultimately lead to improved long-term graft function, as well as reduced immunosuppressive-related morbidity (Khatri et al., 2011). The clinical application of personalized medicine strategies depends on the translation of findings into routine practice.

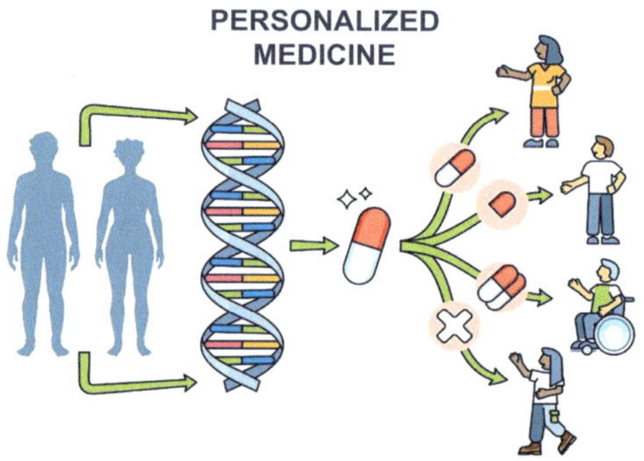

Figure 15.18. Personalized medicine aims to tailor treatment based on the unique characteristics of each patient, including genetic, environmental, and lifestyle factors.

Source: https://www.medznat.ru/uploads/images/post_content/7182/image_3/1690458980image_3.webp.

Therapeutic drug monitoring is standard for several immunosuppressive medications; however, the priority of incorporating pharmacogenetic data and new biomarkers into clinical practice remains. As evidence demonstrates the potential of these strategies, clinicians must weigh their practical usefulness and availability within different clinical settings. The ongoing study of multi-gene expression panels and other novel biomarkers is an attractive avenue for future advances, as it has the capability to predict graft accommodation and establish the baseline risk for allograft injury prior to transplant (Abboudi et al., 2012). Together, these personalized medicine strategies offer the potential to optimize immunosuppressive therapy, enhancing the quality and success rates in kidney transplant recipients (Figure 15.18).

15.6.3. Research on Minimizing Side Effects

Decreasing the unwanted side effects of immunosuppressive therapy in kidney transplantation is a highly critical research area, primarily due to the delicate equilibrium physicians must maintain between preventing graft rejection and managing side effects. The drugs, though essential for organ acceptance, have high risks like increased susceptibility to infections and cancers, and drug-specific side effects such as diabetes and nephrotoxicity. The narrow therapeutic index of immunosuppressants heightens this conundrum, wherein inappropriateness of dosing would either cause rejection or result in toxicities. It is for this reason that present therapeutic practices are centered on tailored treatment regimens following a thorough clinical assessment. This approach deviates from standard practice to a more individualized method, whereby parameters unique to each patient are considered to optimize the drug's efficacy while minimizing the risk of complications (Abboudi et al., 2012). Research has more and more focused on therapeutic drug monitoring as a critical element in the optimalization of immunosuppressive treatment. Through constant monitoring of the drug level in the blood, physicians can more accurately quantify the effectiveness of therapy and minimize side effects. Pharmacokinetics and pharmacodynamics, however, often show significant patient-to-patient variability so that ongoing dosing changes might be needed. Moreover, advances in pharmacogenetics provide the promise of still more tailored immunosuppressive therapy, even though clinical benefits are yet to be fully established. Novel biomarker-based approaches also hold promise with enhanced risk stratification and pharmacodynamic monitoring on the cards, which would maximize dosage in real-time, thus improving patient outcome overall and maximizing graft survival (Abboudi et al., 2012). Apart from monitoring regimens, several new approaches have been invented to limit the side effects of immunosuppressive drugs. Among these, decreasing the dose of calcineurin inhibitors (CNI) while maintaining efficacy has been a promising approach. Present research indicates that tapering doses does not necessarily accompany the rise in acute rejection rates when compared with other immunosuppressives. Other methods include early withdrawal of steroids following transplantation and mycophenolate mofetil dose titration, which has been shown to diminish side effects without compromising graft function. These new immunosuppressive approaches novel therapies, such as alemtuzumab and belatacept, aiming to induce operational tolerance through the use of these therapies. Although initial outcomes of such are encouraging, further experimental testing must be performed to establish their long-term safety and efficacy in reducing the side effects of kidney transplantation.

SUMMARY

The procedure of kidney transplant, as well as the complexity of immunosuppression therapy, underscores the need for personalized medical approaches. The delicate balance between preventing organ rejection and avoiding complications related to over-immunosuppression suggests a vital area of research. Under-treatment could cause rejection attacks, resulting in organ loss, while over-immunosuppression opens the patient to infections and other untoward results. As emphasized in recent investigations, therapeutic drug monitoring remains a cornerstone of immunosuppressive regimen management; however, developments in pharmacogenetics and biomarker-guided strategies hold promise to further streamline this endeavor towards achieving maximized patient outcomes and successful long-term allograft survival (Abboudi et al., 2012). An attitude of patient-centeredness towards immunosuppressive treatment following kidney transplant should be acknowledged. While the clinical efficacy of these medications is firmly established, patient self-report suggests that the lifelong requirement to remain on such regimens is troublesome. While ongoing investigations attempt to minimize medication burden, failure to implement a generic regimen necessitates consideration of the individual needs of each patient. The importance of regimen choice—quality of life and medication adherence—cannot be overstated, since these are critical to long-term organ transplanted function. Discussion of these issues remains essential to improve treatment strategies continually (Greene et al., 2014). Finally, the dynamic nature of kidney transplantation and immunosuppression necessitates an integrated decision-making approach that involves patients actively. Compliance is essential to allograft survival, and interventions taking into consideration lifestyle and preference issues for the patient are now seen as an integral part of the treatment plan. Future therapeutic developments need not only to refine pharmacologic interventions but also to prioritize patient experience, establishing settings that promote compliance maximally through support and education. Lastly, the present research on individualized immunosuppressive regimens promises greater patient satisfaction and improved outcomes, underscoring a steadfast commitment to kidney transplant best practices in the healthcare sector (Greene et al., 2014).

In kidney transplantation, the most critical part for the success of the procedure is the immunosuppressive treatment. Immunosuppressants are used to prevent organ rejection, which occurs when the recipient's immune system identifies the transplanted kidney as foreign. Efficiency in these treatments has significantly increased due to the development of sophisticated drug technology, allowing for fine-tuning of control over rejection processes. Interestingly, studies show that donor hematolymphoid cells can be present long-term in recipients, and through this, they may contribute to the state of microchimerism, in which these cells create a more symbiotic relationship between the graft and the host. This explains that immunosuppressive therapy not only suppresses rejection reactions but also produces a condition that can promote tolerance of the graft, contrary to the early perspective that passenger leucocytes are simple effectors of rejection (Delaney et al., 1996). With improvements in transplant medicine, the quest for other sources of organ transplantation, such as xenotransplantation, comes into the spotlight. The primary barrier is the immune response to xenografts, particularly those from genetically modified pigs. Top-level genetic alterations have made progress in reducing immune activation against porcine cells in primate models. Current experimental work focuses on overcoming coagulation dysregulation, which is challenging to sustain graft survival. The elimination of antibody and cell-mediated responses combined brings hope that advances in xenotransplantation will soon reduce the persistent shortage of human organs. Despite the challenges, successful clinical trials may offer patients with limited renal replacement therapy alternatives options (Ayares et al., 2012). Overall, advances in immunosuppressive treatments and new sources of transplantation demonstrate the dynamic character of kidney transplantation approaches. Incorporating these specializations not only enhances the understanding of the immunological environment post-transplantation but also provides avenues for new therapeutic approaches. Patient outcomes can be significantly improved by customized immunosuppressive therapy tailored to individual response and long-term tolerability. Additionally, advancements in xenotransplantation, if successful, could revolutionize the treatment landscape for individuals with end-stage renal disease. The constant incorporation of research into practice will remain crucial to the advancement of kidney transplantation and governance of immunological issues around it (Delaney et al., 1996; Ayares et al., 2012).

CLOSER LOOK

EXTRACORPOREAL PHOTOPHERESIS

ECP is a treatment that involves harvesting, therapy, and reinfusing a patient's white blood cells after they have been exposed to a photoactivatable drug and ultraviolet A (UVA) light. Initially utilized in the 1980s to treat cutaneous T-cell lymphoma (CTCL), ECP is now recognized to be of clinical benefit in a range of immune-mediated conditions, including graft-versus-host disease (GVHD), solid organ transplant rejection, autoimmune diseases, and certain forms of atopic dermatitis. The treatment begins with leukapheresis, where mononuclear cells are collected from the patient's circulation. The cells are then exposed ex vivo to 8-methoxypsoralen (8-MOP), a psoralen compound that intercalates into DNA. Upon exposure to UVA light, 8-MOP causes cross-linking with DNA and renders the cells apoptotic. After irradiation, the cells are infused back into the patient's circulation. Unlike traditional immunosuppressive treatments, ECP does not cause global immunosuppression. Instead, it triggers explicitly apoptosis in pathogenic T cells and induces tolerance through the regulation of dendritic cells and the promotion of regulatory T cell (Treg) growth. This mechanism is the basis for its wide margin of safety and minimal systemic toxicity. In chronic GVHD, for example, ECP has been shown to reduce involvement of the skin, liver, and lungs, especially in steroid-refractory individuals. Similarly, in CTCL, ECP leads to clinical improvement the elimination of malignant T lymphocytes without compromising host defense mechanisms. ECP is tolerated well, and side effects are limited to catheter-related complications, mild hypotension, or flu-like symptoms. Treatment is administered on an outpatient basis in repeated cycles, with the frequency determined by disease severity and response. One of the unique attributes of ECP is that it can restore immune reactions in balance without jeopardizing the patient with infections or cancer. Thus it is of additional value for long-term therapy of immune disturbances. Patient selection and procedure timing are equally crucial for the efficacy of ECP. Biomarkers, including levels of Tregs, dendritic cell function, and cytokine patterns, are being studied to predict responsiveness and inform treatment protocols. Technical advances in apheresis equipment and procedural automation have improved the efficiency and accessibility of ECP. Despite having its effectiveness proven, however, the underlying cellular and molecular mechanisms by which ECP exerts its effects are not yet clearly understood. Studies show that apoptotic cells generated during the process of ECP stimulate tolerogenic dendritic cells, which induce Tregs and divert the immune system away from an inflammatory phenotype. Furthermore, ECP may influence cytokine environments by reducing pro-inflammatory mediators, such as IL-2 and IFN-γ, while inducing the anti-inflammatory cytokine IL-10. This reduction is in the direction of immune tolerance rather than extensive suppression. As more is known about immunomodulation, ECP can be expected to have an increasingly wider role in the management of chronic immune-mediated diseases. Existing clinical practice guidelines favor its application as second-line or adjuvant therapy, especially when standard treatment has failed or becomes intolerable. Ultimately, ECP is an illustration of a cell-based, targeted form of immunotherapy that holds promise for individuals with multifaceted immunologic disorders who need long-term, safe, and efficacious therapies.

References

1. MacPhee, I., & Abboudi, N. (2012). Individualized immunosuppression in transplant patients: potential role of pharmacogenetics. *Pharmacogenomics and Personalized Medicine*, 63. https://doi.org/10.2147/pgpm.s21743Abu-Elmagd, K., Basu, A., Bond, G., Khan, F., et al. (2004). Pancreatic transplantation at the University of Pittsburgh. https://core.ac.uk/download/12205623.pdf (accessed on 25th June 2025).
2. Abu-Elmagd, K., Fung, J., Jain, A., Kashyap, A., et al. (1999). What have we learned about primary liver transplantation under tacrolimus immunosuppression? –Long-term follow-up of the first 1000 patients. https://core.ac.uk/download/12205513.pdf (accessed on 25th June 2025).
3. Acan, I., & Brusich, K. T. (2018). Anesthetic considerations in transplant recipients for nontransplant surgery. https://core.ac.uk/download/322435451.pdf (accessed on 25th June 2025).
4. Andrade-Sierra, J., Cerrillos-Gutiérrez, J. I., Chávez-Iñiguez, J. S., González-Espinoza, L., et al. (2018). Immunosuppressive minimization strategies in kidney transplantation. https://core.ac.uk/download/322437636.pdf (accessed on 25th June 2025).
5. Ayares, D., & Cooper, D. K. C. (2012). Potential benefits and risks of clinical xenotransplantation. https://core.ac.uk/download/12213803.pdf (accessed on 25th June 2025).
6. Balamurugan, A. N., Alexander, M., Allen, M., Amos, W., Barber, M., Barrou, B., Bartlett, S., et al. (2002). Pancreas and islet cell transplantation. https://core.ac.uk/download/12205582.pdf (accessed on 25th June 2025).
7. Barten, M. J., Fisher, A. J., & Hertig, A. (2024). The use of extracorporeal photopheresis in solid organ transplantation—Current status and future directions. https://core.ac.uk/download/603541967.pdf (accessed on 25th June 2025).
8. Bobbio, E. (2024). Management of heart failure with focus on inflammatory myocardial diseases: A comparison between cardiac sarcoidosis and giant cell myocarditis. https://core.ac.uk/download/620674476.pdf (accessed on 25th June 2025).
9. Burke, C. A. V., Vivas, C., Corry, D., Fioretto, M., Foger, H., et al. (2000). Results of pancreas transplantation after steroid withdrawal under tacrolimus immunosuppression. https://core.ac.uk/download/12205523.pdf (accessed on 25th June 2025).
10. Delaney, C. P., Demetris, A. J., Murase, N., Starzl, T. E., et al. (1996). Prevention of transplant rejection: Can tolerance be achieved with immunosuppressive treatment? https://core.ac.uk/download/12205304.pdf (accessed on 25th June 2025).
11. Demetris, A. J., Fung, J. J., Hakala, T. R., Irish, W., et al. (1995). A prospective randomized trial of FK506-based immunosuppression after renal transplantation. https://core.ac.uk/download/12205089.pdf (accessed on 25th June 2025).
12. di Luca, N. M., Marinelli, E., Montanari Vergallo, G., Zaami, S., et al. (2017). Ethical and medico-legal remarks on uterus transplantation: May it solve uterine factor infertility? https://core.ac.uk/download/153370886.pdf (accessed on 25th June 2025).

13. Doyle, H. R., Fung, J. J., Gayowski, T., Marino, I. R., et al. (1996). Orthotopic liver transplantation in U.S. veterans under primary tacrolimus immunosuppression. https://core.ac.uk/download/12205413.pdf (accessed on 25th June 2025).
14. Esteban, C., Staeck, O., Tresp, V., Yang, J., et al. (2016). Predicting clinical events by combining static and dynamic information using recurrent neural networks. http://arxiv.org/abs/1602.02685 (accessed on 25th June 2025).
15. Friedman, S. B. (2023). Immunosuppression after cardiac transplantation: What is the best approach? https://core.ac.uk/download/616444359.pdf (accessed on 25th June 2025).
16. Fung, J., Green, M., Gronsky, C., Jain, A., et al. (2000). Comparative long-term evaluation of tacrolimus and cyclosporine in pediatric liver transplantation. https://core.ac.uk/download/12205541.pdf (accessed on 25th June 2025).
17. Greene, H., Kyegombe, M., MacPhee, I. A., Popoola, J., et al. (2014). Patient involvement in selection of immunosuppressive regimen following transplantation. https://core.ac.uk/download/29469510.pdf (accessed on 25th June 2025).
18. Hsieh, S. C., Khush, K., Li, L., Luikart, H., et al. (2013). Identification of common blood gene signatures for the diagnosis of renal and cardiac acute allograft rejection. https://core.ac.uk/download/323072492.pdf (accessed on 25th June 2025).
19. Iwatsuki, S., Klintmalm, G. B. G., Schroter, G., Starzl, T. E., et al. (1981). Late follow-up after thoracic duct drainage in cadaveric renal transplantation. https://core.ac.uk/download/12203878.pdf (accessed on 25th June 2025).
20. Khatri, P., Roedder, S., Sarwal, M. M., Vitalone, M. J., et al. (2011). Biomarkers in solid organ transplantation: Establishing personalized transplantation medicine. https://core.ac.uk/download/323074810.pdf (accessed on 25th June 2025).
21. Kovacevic, A., Djordjevic, N., Rancic, N., Vavic, N., Dragojevic-Simic, V., & Segrt, Z. (2016). Economic evaluation of pharmacogenetic tests in patients subjected to renal transplantation: A review of literature. https://core.ac.uk/download/pdf/82847868.pdf (accessed on 25th June 2025).
22. Kukulski, L., Przybyłowski, P., Strojek, K., Wróbel, M., et al. (2020). New onset diabetes after transplantation (NODAT): Scientific data review. https://core.ac.uk/download/395681916.pdf (accessed on 25th June 2025).
23. Marchioro, T. L., Rifkind, D., Starzl, T. E., Waddell, W. R., et al. (1964). Infectious diseases associated with renal homotransplantation: I. Incidence, types, and predisposing factors. https://core.ac.uk/download/12203488.pdf (accessed on 25th June 2025).
24. Matsuda, Y., & Sarwal, M. M. (2016). Unraveling the role of allo-antibodies and transplant injury. https://core.ac.uk/download/323073772.pdf (accessed on 25th June 2025).
25. Mitterhofer, A. P., Muiesan, P., Tinti, F., Umbro, I., et al. (2016). Different behavior of BK-virus infection in liver transplant recipients. https://core.ac.uk/download/54529293.pdf (accessed on 25th June 2025).
26. Miyake, Y., & Yamamoto, K. (2008). Current status of autoimmune hepatitis in Japan. https://core.ac.uk/download/12525881.pdf (accessed on 25th June 2025).
27. Shaw, B. W., Starzl, T. E., & Wood, R. P. (1985). Extrahepatic complications of liver transplantation. https://core.ac.uk/download/12204047.pdf (accessed on 25th June 2025).

28. Starzl, T. E. (1971). The current status of liver transplantation. https://core.ac.uk/download/12203658.pdf (accessed on 25th June 2025).

29. Stomel, J. (2017). Perceptions of HIV-positive kidney donations to HIV-positive recipients. https://open.bu.edu/bitstream/2144/26938/5/Stomel_bu_0017N_13181.pdf (accessed on 25th June 2025).

30. Thomas, M. (2011). The effects of bilirubin and bilirubin-di-taurate on ischemia reperfusion injury in a rat model of kidney transplantation. https://core.ac.uk/download/11033129.pdf (accessed on 25th June 2025).

31. Wells, S. A. (2012). Health disparities in kidney transplantation: An equity analysis. https://digitalscholarship.unlv.edu/cgi/viewcontent.cgi?article=1054&context=jhdrp (accessed on 25th June 2025).

INDEX

Symbols

A

B

C

D

I

K

L

M

N

O

P

Q

R